The AHA Clinical Cardiac Consult

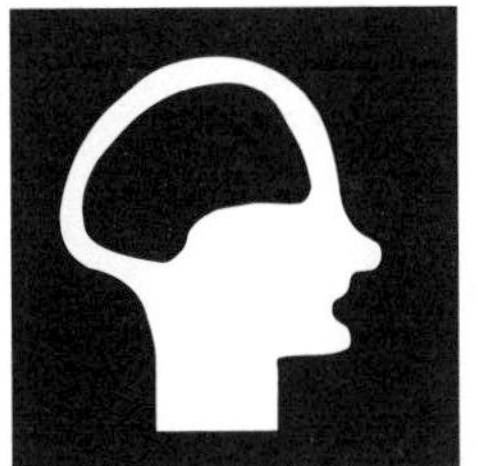
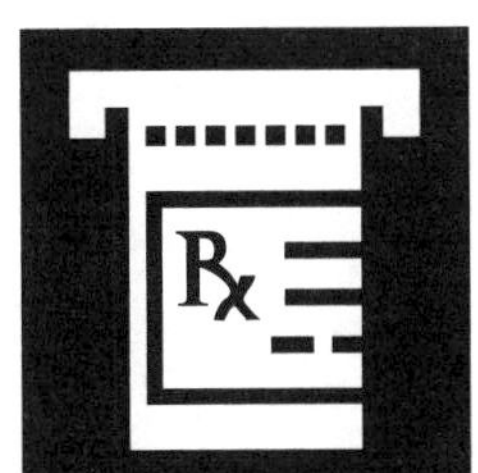

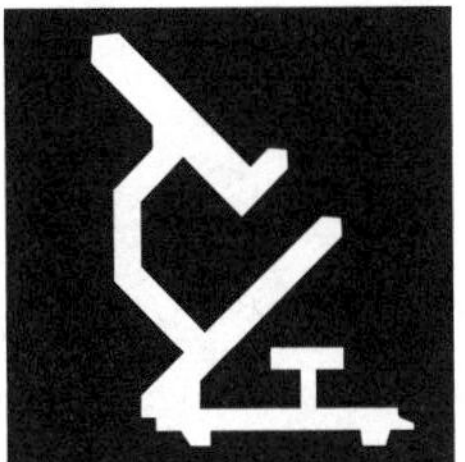
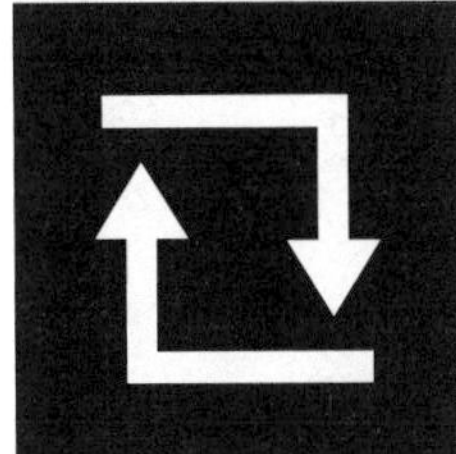
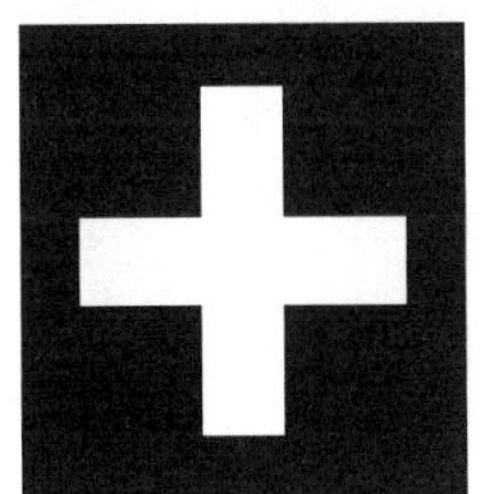
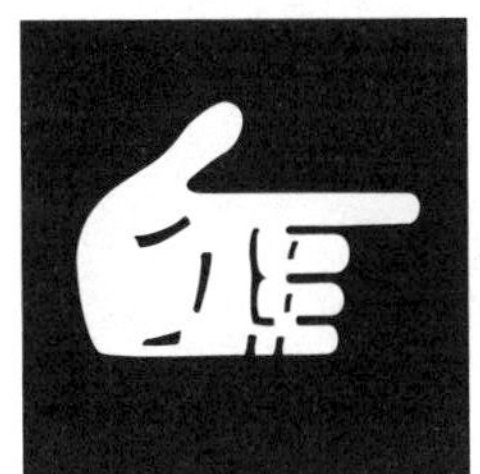

The AHA Clinical Cardiac Consult

EDITOR

JOSEPH S. ALPERT, M.D.

ROBERT S. AND IRENE P. FLINN PROFESSOR OF MEDICINE

HEAD

DEPARTMENT OF MEDICINE

THE UNIVERSITY OF ARIZONA COLLEGE OF MEDICINE

AND HEALTH SCIENCES CENTER

TUCSON, ARIZONA

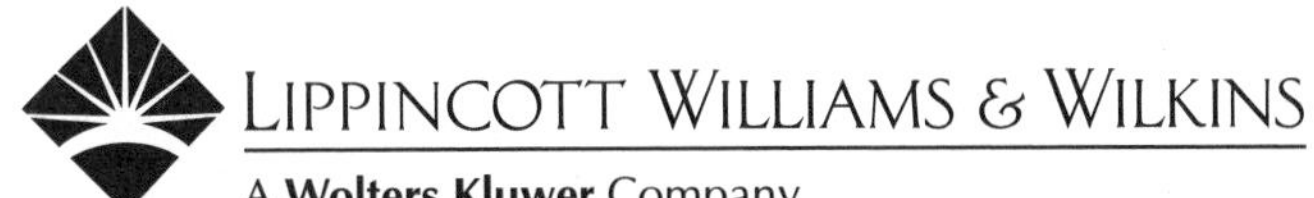
LIPPINCOTT WILLIAMS & WILKINS
A **Wolters Kluwer** Company
Philadelphia • Baltimore • New York • London
Buenos Aires • Hong Kong • Sydney • Tokyo

Acquisitions Editor: Ruth W. Weinberg
Developmental Editor: Ellen DiFrancesco
Supervising Editor: Steven Martin
Manufacturing Manager: Tim Reynolds
Production Service: Colophon
Compositor: The PRD Group, Inc.
Printer: R.R. Donnelley Willard

Library of Congress Cataloging-in-Publication Data

The AHA clinical cardiac consult / editor, Joseph S. Alpert; associate editors, Gerard P. Aurigemma ... [et al.].
p. ; cm.
Includes bibliographical references and index.
ISBN 0-7817-2420-1 (alk. paper)
1. Cardiology—Handbooks, manuals, etc. 2. Heart—Diseases—Handbooks, manuals, etc. 3. Cardiological manifestations of general diseases—Handbooks, manuals, etc. I. Title: Clinical cardiac consult. II. Alpert, Joseph S. III. Aurigemma, Gerard P.
[DNLM: 1. Cardiovascular Diseases—diagnosis. 2. Cardiovascular Diseases—therapy. 3. Diagnosis, Differential. WG 120 A285 2001]

RC669.15 .A36 2001
616.1′2–dc21

00-065518

10 9 8 7 6 5 4 3 2 1

Preface

The publication of this book culminates several years of intense discussion and work within the American Heart Association's Council on Clinical Cardiology. The Executive Committee of the Council began drafting the idea for this book at one of its meetings. Dr. Kathryn Taubert of the AHA senior scientific staff asked me to create a list of topics to be covered and to structure the organization of the text. I, in turn, recruited current and former members of the Council to cover the many topics deemed necessary for a comprehensive but concise overview of cardiovascular disease. In each area, the associate editors have worked closely with their colleagues to produce a high-quality product.

The success of the condensed format employed in this book has been proven over the years in a number of primary care and specialty areas. I anticipate that this text will be equally successful. By spending five minutes with the text, a physician or other healthcare worker can obtain a reasonable understanding of a specific disease entity from a number of view points. In addition, tables and definitions appended to the text are added benefits to the time-conscious seeker of knowledge in cardiovascular disease.

I am extremely grateful to my associate editors who rapidly assigned, obtained, and edited the many topics. Ruth Weinberg and Ellen DiFrancesco from Lippincott Williams & Wilkins were, as always, tremendously efficient and helpful in preparing the text for publication. Kathryn Taubert, Ph.D. at the American Heart Association, with whom I have worked for over 20 years, will always be one of my favorite people at the AHA. Her energy, dedication, and intelligence have been of great assistance in preparing this book. Finally, I would like to thank my administrative assistant, Barbara Raney, without whom many of my academic projects could not be accomplished.

Joseph S. Alpert

Contributing Authors

CHRISTOPHER ABADI, M.D.
Department of Cardiology
Lahey Cardiology at The Medical Center
Nashua, New Hampshire

LINDA J. ADDONIZIO, M.D.
Associate Professor of Pediatrics
Columbia University
College of Physicians and Surgeons
New York Presbyterian Hospital
New York, New York

KATHLEEN M. ALLEN, M.D.
Assistant Professor of Medicine
Division of Cardiology
Director
Cardiac Catheter Laboratory
University of New Mexico School of Medicine
Albuquerque, New Mexico

KAREN ALTMANN, M.D.
Assistant Professor of Clinical Pediatrics
Columbia University
College of Physicians and Surgeons
New York Presbyterian Hospital
New York, New York

HOWARD D. APFEL, M.D.
Assistant Professor of Clinical Pediatrics
Columbia University
College of Physicians and Surgeons
New York Presbyterian Hospital
New York, New York

PHOEBE A. ASHLEY, M.D.
Cardiology Fellow
University of New Mexico School of Medicine
Albuquerque, New Mexico

GERARD P. AURIGEMMA, M.D.
Department of Medicine
Division of Cardiovascular Medicine
University of Massachusetts Memorial Medical Center
University Campus
Worcester, Massachusetts

DAVID S. BADER, M.D.
Department of Cardiology
Boston University Medical Center
Boston, Massachusetts

MARIA CECILIA BAHIT, M.D.
Research Fellow
Duke Clinical Research Institute
Duke University Medical Center
Durham, North Carolina

ROBYN J. BARST, M.D.
Associate Professor of Pediatrics
Columbia University
College of Physicians and Surgeons
New York Presbyterian Hospital
New York, New York

DEEPAK L. BHATT, M.D.
Department of Cardiology
The Cleveland Clinic Foundation
Cleveland, Ohio

TIMOTHY C. BISHOP, M.D.
Cardiology Fellow
University of New Mexico School of Medicine
Albuquerque, New Mexico

DAVID BRICK, M.D.
Instructor in Clinical Pediatrics
Columbia University
College of Physicians and Surgeons
New York Presbyterian Hospital
New York, New York

CRAIG M. BRODSKY, M.D.
Department of Medicine
Division of Cardiology
Emory University School of Medicine
Atlanta, Georgia

BERNARD R. CHAITMAN, M.D.
Professor of Medicine
Director
Cardiovascular Research Department of Internal Medicine
Division of Cardiology
St. Louis University School of Medicine
St. Louis, Missouri

GERALD A. CHARLTON, M.D.
Director
Critical Care Unit
Cardiology Section
Albuquerque Veterans Affairs Medical Center
Albuquerque, New Mexico

RICHARD CHEN, M.D.
Cardiology Fellow
Department of Medicine
Division of Cardiology
Emory University School of Medicine
Atlanta, Georgia

ANDREW B. CHUNG, M.D., PH.D.
Cardiology Fellow
Department of Medicine
Division of Cardiology
Emory University School of Medicine
Atlanta, Georgia

RUBIN S. COOPER, M.D.
Professor of Clinical Pediatrics
Cornell University
New York Presbyterian Hospital
New York, New York

MICHAEL H. CRAWFORD, M.D.
Professor of Cardiology
Department of Medicine
Chief
Division of Cardiology
University of New Mexico School of Medicine
Albuquerque, New Mexico

L. VAN-THOMAS CRISCO, M.D.
Interventional Cardiology Fellow
Department of Medicine
Division of Cardiology
Emory University School of Medicine
Atlanta, Georgia

DAVID CROWE, M.D.
Clinical Instructor in Pediatrics
Cornell University
New York Presbyterian Hospital
New York, New York

HAROLD L. DAUERMAN, M.D.
Department of Medicine
Division of Cardiovascular Medicine
University of Massachusetts Memorial Medical Center
University Campus
Worcester, Massachusetts

STEPHEN J. DEMPSEY, M.D.
Department of Medicine
Division of Cardiology
Emory University School of Medicine
Atlanta, Georgia

CHANDAN DEVIREDDY, M.D.
Resident in Internal Medicine
Department of Medicine
Duke University Medical Center
Durham, North Carolina

CHRISTOPHER K. DYKE, M.D.
Fellow
Division of Cardiology
Duke Clinical Research Institute
Duke University Medical Center
Durham, North Carolina

DEBORAH L. EKERY, M.D.
Fellow
Department of Cardiology
Boston University Medical Center
Boston, Massachusetts

AMR EL-SHAFEI, M.D.
Fellow
Division of Cardiology
St. Louis University School of Medicine
St. Louis, Missouri

ANDREW E. EPSTEIN, M.D.
Professor of Medicine
Department of Medicine
Division of Cardiovascular Disease
The University of Alabama at Birmingham
Birmingham, Alabama

ERIC D. FETHKE, M.D.
Assistant Professor of Clinical Pediatrics
Columbia University
College of Physicians and Surgeons
New York Presbyterian Hospital
New York, New York

GARY S. FRANCIS, M.D.
Professor of Medicine
Director
Coronary Intensive Care Unit
Department of Cardiology
The Cleveland Clinic Foundation
Cleveland, Ohio

SAMER GARAS, M.D.
Cardiovascular Fellow
Department of Medicine
Division of Cardiology
Emory University School of Medicine
Atlanta, Georgia

DEBORAH R. GERSONY, M.D.
Advanced Research Fellow
Columbia University
College of Physicians and Surgeons
New York Presbyterian Hospital
New York, New York

WELTON M. GERSONY, M.D.
Alexander S. Nadas Professor of Pediatrics
Director
Pediatric Cardiology
Division of Pediatric Cardiology
Columbia University
College of Physicians and Surgeons
New York Presbyterian Hospital
New York, New York

HELENE GLASSBERG, M.D.
Department of Cardiology
Boston University Medical Center
Boston, Massachusetts

THOMAS M. GUEST, M.D.
Department of Medicine
Division of Cardiology
Emory University School of Medicine
Atlanta, Georgia

MADHUKAR GUPTA, M.D.
Fellow
Division of Cardiology
St. Louis University School of Medicine
St. Louis, Missouri

CONSTANCE J. HAYES, M.D.
Professor of Clinical Pediatrics
Columbia University
College of Physicians and Surgeons
New York Presbyterian Hospital
New York, New York

WILLIAM E. HELLENBRAND, M.D.
Professor of Clinical Pediatrics
Columbia University
College of Physicians and Surgeons
New York Presbyterian Hospital
New York, New York

STEVEN HERRMANN, M.D.
Fellow
Division of Cardiology
St. Louis University School of Medicine
St. Louis, Missouri

ROBERT HOGAN, M.D.
Interventional Cardiology Fellow
Division of Cardiology
University of Massachusetts Medical School
Worcester, Massachusetts

ALLAN HORDOF, M.D.
Professor of Clinical Pediatrics
Columbia University
College of Physicians and Surgeons
New York Presbyterian Hospital
New York, New York

BRENDA J. HOTT, M.D.
Fellow
Department of Medicine
Division of Cardiology
Emory University School of Medicine
Atlanta, Georgia

DAPHNE T. HSU, M.D.
Associate Professor of Clinical Pediatrics
Columbia University
College of Physicians and Surgeons
New York Presbyterian Hospital
New York, New York

MICHAEL P. HUDSON, M.D.
Senior Staff Cardiologist
Associate Director
Cardiac Intensive Care Unit
Henry Ford Hospital
Detroit, Michigan

VINEET KAUSHIK, M.D.
Fellow
Department of Medicine
Division of Cardiology
Emory University School of Medicine
Atlanta, Georgia

JEFFREY H. KERN, M.D.
Assistant Clinical Professor of Pediatrics
Columbia University
New York Presbyterian Hospital
New York, New York

JAMES A. KONG, M.D.
Resident in Internal Medicine
Department of Medicine
Duke University Medical Center
Durham, North Carolina

PETER KRINGSTEIN, M.D.
Cardiology Fellow
Division of Cardiology
University of Massachusetts Medical School
Worcester, Massachusetts

JARVIS W. LAMBERT, M.D.
Department of Cardiology
Boston University Medical Center
Boston, Massachusetts

JACQUELINE M. LAMOUR, M.D.
Assistant Professor of Pediatrics
Columbia University
College of Physicians and Surgeons
New York Presbyterian Hospital
New York, New York

JONATHAN LANGBERG, M.D.
Department of Medicine
Division of Cardiology
Emory University School of Medicine
Atlanta, Georgia

DONALD LEICHTER, M.D.
Associate Clinical Professor of Pediatrics
Columbia University
College of Physicians and Surgeons
New York Presbyterian Hospital
New York, New York

JERRE LUTZ, M.D.
Associate Professor of Medicine
Department of Medicine
Division of Cardiology
Emory University School of Medicine
Atlanta, Georgia

ZVI S. MARANS, M.D.
Associate Clinical Professor of Pediatrics
Columbia University
College of Physicians and Surgeons
New York Presbyterian Hospital
New York, New York

RICHARD MASCOLO, M.D.
Resident
Department of Medicine
Division of Cardiovascular Medicine
University of Massachusetts Medical Center
Worcester, Massachusetts

ROSEMARY MEHL, M.D.
Staff Physician (Ambulatory Care)
Brockton/West Roxbury Veterans Affairs Medical Center
Instructor in Medicine
Harvard Medical School
Brockton, Massachusetts

THEOFANIE MELA, M.D.
Department of Cardiology
Massachusetts General Hospital
Harvard Medical School
Boston, Massachusetts

JOSEPH I. MILLER III, M.D.
Department of Medicine
Division of Cardiology
Emory University School of Medicine
Atlanta, Georgia

SEEMA MITAL, M.D.
Assistant Professor of Pediatrics
Columbia University
College of Physicians and Surgeons
New York Presbyterian Hospital
New York, New York

CHRISTINE L. NELL, NP-C, MPH, MSN
Preventive Cardiology Nurse Practitioner
Department of Medicine
Division of Cardiology
Emory University School of Medicine
Atlanta, Georgia

LARRY A. OSBORN, M.D.
Associate Professor of Medicine
Internal Medicine Department
Division of Cardiology
University of New Mexico School of Medicine
Albuquerque, New Mexico

ROBERT H. PASS, M.D.
Assistant Professor of Pediatrics
Columbia University
College of Physicians and Surgeons
New York Presbyterian Hospital
New York, New York

STEFANO PERLINI, M.D., Ph.D.
Clinica Medica 1
Department of Internal Medicine
IRCCS San Matteo
University of Pavia
Pavia, Italy

DANIEL T. PRICE, M.D.
Assistant Professor of Medicine
Section of Cardiology
Boston University School of Medicine
Boston Medical Center
Boston, Massachusetts

BETH FELLER PRINTZ, M.D., Ph.D.
Irving Assistant Professor of Pediatrics
Columbia University
College of Physicians and Surgeons
New York Presbyterian Hospital
New York, New York

BRYAN J. REYNOLDS, M.D.
Assistant Professor of Cardiology
Department of Medicine
Division of Cardiology
University of New Mexico School of Medicine
Albuquerque, New Mexico

CARLOS A. ROLDAN, M.D., FACC
Associate Professor of Medicine
University of New Mexico School of Medicine
Director
Echocardiography Laboratory
Veterans Affairs Medical Center
University of New Mexico
Albuquerque, New Mexico

ERIKA BERMAN ROSENZWEIG, M.D.
Assistant Professor of Pediatrics
Columbia University
College of Physicians and Surgeons
New York Presbyterian Hospital
New York, New York

CHERYL RUSSO, M.D.
Resident in Internal Medicine
Department of Medicine
Duke University Medical Center
Durham, North Carolina

SALEM N. SAYAR, M.D.
Department of Medicine
Division of Cardiology
Emory University School of Medicine
Atlanta, Georgia

HELGE U. SIMON, M.D.
Department of Cardiovascular Medicine
University of Massachusetts Medical Center
Memorial Campus
Worcester, Massachusetts

DAVID SOLOWIEJCZWK, M.D.
Associate Clinical Professor of Pediatrics
Columbia University
College of Physicians and Surgeons
New York Presbyterian Hospital
New York, New York

LAURENCE S. SPERLING, M.D.
Department of Medicine
Division of Cardiology
Emory University School of Medicine
Atlanta, Georgia

THOMAS J. STARC, M.D.
Professor of Clinical Pediatrics
Columbia University
College of Physicians and Surgeons
New York Presbyterian Hospital
New York, New York

MARK STEINER, M.D.
Fellow
Department of Medicine
Division of Cardiology
Emory University School of Medicine
Atlanta, Georgia

JOHN S. STROBEL, M.D.
Department of Cardiology
Internal Medicine Associates
Bloomington Hospital
Bloomington, Indiana

ROBERT A. TAYLOR, M.D.
Assistant Professor
Department of Medicine
Division of Cardiology
University of New Mexico School of Medicine
Albuquerque, New Mexico

DONNA M. TIMCHAK, M.D.
Assistant Clinical Professor of Pediatrics
Columbia University
College of Physicians and Surgeons
New York Presbyterian Hospital
New York, New York

KIRSTEN TOLSTRUP, M.D.
Cardiology Fellow
Department of Internal Medicine
Division of Cardiology
University of New Mexico Health Sciences Hospital
Albuquerque, New Mexico

PRADYUMNA E. TUMMALA, M.D.
Fellow
Department of Medicine
Division of Cardiology
Emory University School of Medicine
Atlanta, Georgia

SARAH M. VERNON, M.D.
Assistant Professor of Medicine
University of New Mexico
Director
Cardiac Catheterization Laboratory
Albuquerque Veterans Affairs Medical Center
Albuquerque, New Mexico

NANETTE K. WENGER, M.D.
Professor of Medicine (Cardiology)
Emory University School of Medicine
Chief of Cardiology
Grady Memorial Hospital
Consultant
Emory Heart and Vascular Center
Atlanta, Georgia

BENOY J. ZACHARIAH, M.D.
Fellow in Cardiology
Department of Cardiology
Boston University Medical Center
Boston, Massachusetts

HOWARD ALAN ZUCKER, M.D.
Associate Professor of Clinical Pediatrics
and Clinical Anesthesiology
Columbia University
College of Physicians and Surgeons
New York Presbyterian Hospital
New York, New York

Contents

APPENDIX

APPENDIX TABLES

The AHA Clinical Cardiac Consult

Acromegaly and the Heart

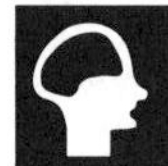

Basics

DESCRIPTION

Excess production of growth hormone, usually from a pituitary adenoma or rarely an ectopic site, results in enlargement of the heart and possible heart failure.

- Due in part to associated hypertension and coronary artery disease
- There may be a causal relationship with high growth hormone levels.

EPIDEMIOLOGY

Up to one-third of patients with acromegaly have ventricular hypertrophy and congestive heart failure.

ETIOLOGY

Excess growth hormone can have a direct effect on cardiac hypertrophy.

- Concomitant hypertension, present in about one-third of patients, leads to ventricular enlargement and failure.
- Difficult to distinguish the mechanism of heart failure in patients with acromegaly, because severe hypertension and obesity frequently coexist.

RISK FACTORS

Hypertension is a risk factor for development of heart failure in the acromegalic patient.

PREGNANCY

- Not advisable in someone with symptomatic congestive heart failure

ASSOCIATED CONDITIONS

- Hypertension
- Diabetes mellitus
- Coronary artery disease
- Hyperthyroidism, especially if arrhythmias are present
- Obesity

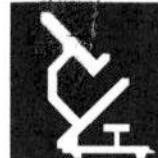

Diagnosis

DIFFERENTIAL DIAGNOSIS

- Other causes of cardiomegaly
- Other possible coexisting causes of hypertension are pheochromocytoma and aldosteronoma.
- Hyperthyroidism should be sought if atrial fibrillation is present.

SIGNS AND SYMPTOMS

- Dyspnea on exertion and at rest
- Orthopnea
- Paroxysmal nocturnal dyspnea
- Arrhythmia
- Cardiomegaly
- Left ventricular hypertrophy
- Left ventricular lift
- S3
- S4
- Hypertension
- Large hands
- Prominent forehead
- Obesity

LABORATORY PROCEDURES

- Elevated serum growth hormone levels at baseline and nonsuppressibility after glucose loading
- Measurement of insulin-like growth factor 1 levels: ECG commonly shows left ventricular hypertrophy (LVH), ST depression, T-wave inversion, bundle branch block, and atrial or ventricular ectopy.

IMAGING STUDIES

- Chest x-ray
  —Shows cardiomegaly by the fifth decade of life
- Echocardiography
  —Shows LVH, right ventricular hypertrophy (RVH), and asymmetric hypertrophy of the septum
  —Diminished ejection fraction and LV dilatation also may be seen.
  —Doppler shows diastolic dysfunction.

SPECIAL TESTS

- Cardiac catheterization often shows premature coronary artery disease. Small vessel disease also may be present.
- Myocardial biopsy can show massive myocardial hypertrophy. Lymphocyte infiltration and interstitial fibrosis also may be seen, although these findings are not specific.

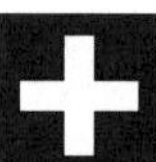

Treatment

GENERAL MEASURES

Low-sodium diet is particularly effective in treating heart failure in these patients.

SURGICAL MEASURES

- Surgery and irradiation of the pituitary gland are the principal types of management for acromegaly and may result in a dramatic improvement in cardiac function.
- Treatment of hypertension is important.
- Heart transplantation has been performed for acromegalic cardiomyopathy.

ADMISSION/DISCHARGE CRITERIA

- Standard for heart failure of any etiology

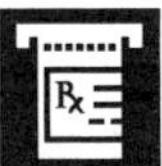

Medications

DRUG(S) OF CHOICE

- Management of the underlying condition, previously with bromocriptine but now with somatostatin, can lead to rapid reversal of even severe ventricular dysfunction.
- Standard therapy for congestive heart failure (CHF)
- Diuretics are particularly effective.
- Antihypertensive therapy

Follow-up

PATIENT MONITORING

- These patients are usually obese.
- At risk for development of diabetes

EXPECTED COURSE AND PROGNOSIS

- Risk of sudden death
- Risk of premature coronary artery disease

PATIENT EDUCATION

- Standard for heart failure of any etiology
- Risks of hypertension, diabetes, coronary artery disease, colon cancer

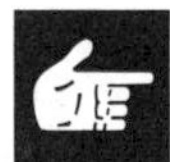

Miscellaneous

ICD-9-CM

428.0 Failure, heart, congestive
425.4 Cardiomyopathy

BIBLIOGRAPHY

Barsness GW, Feinglos MN. Endocrine systems and the heart. In: Topol EJ, ed. *Comprehensive cardiovascular medicine.* Philadelphia: Lippincott-Raven, 1998:961–962.

Williams GH, Lilly LS, Seely EW. The heart in endocrine and nutritional disorders. In: Braunwald E, ed. *Heart disease: a textbook of cardiovascular medicine,* 5th ed. Philadelphia: WB Saunders, 1997:1887–1890.

Martins JB, Kerber RE, Sherman BM, et al. Cardiac size and function in acromegaly. *Circulation* 1977;56:863–869.

McGuffin WL, Sherman BM, Roth J, et al. Acromegaly and cardiovascular disorders—a prospective study. *Ann Intern Med* 1974;81:11–18.

Chanson P, Timsit J, Masquet C, et al. Cardiovascular effects of the somatostatin analog octreotide in acromegaly. *Ann Intern Med* 1990;113:921–925.

Albat B, Leclercq F, Serre I, et al. Heart transplantation for terminal congestive heart failure in an acromegalic patient. *Eur Heart J* 1993; 14:1572–1575.

Authors: Deepak L. Bhatt and Gary S. Francis

AIDS and the Heart

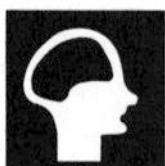

Basics

DESCRIPTION

Clinical syndrome caused by infection with human immunodeficiency virus (HIV)

- An enormous spectrum of clinical presentations secondary to primary effects of HIV, opportunistic infection, neoplastic transformation, and of therapeutic agents themselves
- Cardiac involvement also has been demonstrated with similar diversity in presentation.

EPIDEMIOLOGY

- Prevalence of cardiac involvement uncertain: 5% to 70%
- Estimated incidence of dilated cardiomyopathy in HIV-positive patients: 1.59%/yr

Incidence/Prevalence

In the United States:

- 2 million estimated have been diagnosed with AIDS
- 1 million estimated HIV positive

Globally:

- Estimated 60 to 70 million adults infected with HIV
- 13.9 million deaths since 1981

ETIOLOGY

- HIV retrovirus possessing reverse transcriptase infecting CD4 T-helper lymphocytes; profound immunodeficiency resulting primarily from a progressive quantitative and qualitative deficiency of the subset of T-lymphocytes referred to as helper or inducer T cells
- Etiology of cardiac disease is as broad as range of opportunistic infections in AIDS.
- HIV cardiomyopathy has been identified with causation secondary to HIV myocyte infection or autoimmune process.
- Multiple opportunistic agents also can involve the myocardium, pericardium, or endocardium. Heart failure can result secondary to other comorbidities caused by AIDS.

Method of Spread

- Sexual contact, blood and blood products, maternal-fetal/infant contact

RISK FACTORS

- Homosexual sex
- Intravenous drug abuse
- High-risk sexual practice (unprotected sex, money for sex)
- Use of blood products (hemophiliacs), immigration from area of high prevalence (sub-Saharan Africa, South Asia)

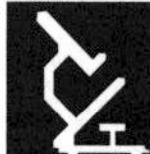

Diagnosis

DIFFERENTIAL DIAGNOSIS

Myocardial Involvement

- HIV-related infections
- Bacterial
  - —*Mycobacterium tuberculosis*
  - —*Mycobacterium avium-intracellulare*
- Fungal
  - —*Cryptococcus neoformans*
  - —*Aspergillus fumigatus*
  - —*Candida albicans*
  - —*Histoplasma capsulatum*
  - —*Coccidiodes immitis*
- Protozoan
  - —*Toxoplasma gondii*
- Viral
  - —Cytomegalovirus
  - —HIV
  - —Herpes simplex
  - —Coxsackievirus

Noninflammatory Myocardial Disease

- Microvascular spasm
- Catecholamine excess
- Coronary artery disease
- Infection
- Toxic drug reaction (antiretroviral therapy)
- Malnutrition (particularly selenium deficiency)

Inflammatory Myocardial Disease

- Autoimmune process induced by HIV or other viruses, systemic lupus erythematosus

Right Ventricular Hypertrophy or Dilation

- Pulmonary infections, pulmonary emboli

Neoplastic

- Kaposi's sarcoma, lymphoma

Pericardial Involvement

- Infectious
  - —Bacterial: *M. tuberculosis, M. avium-intracellulare, Nocardia*
  - —Viral: Herpes simplex
  - —Fungal: *Histoplasma capsulatum, Cryptococcus neoformans*
  - —Neoplastic: Kaposi's sarcoma, lymphoma

Endocardial Involvement

- Marantic endocarditis (nonbacterial thrombotic endocarditis)
- Infective endocarditis (bacterial, fungal)

SIGNS AND SYMPTOMS

- Congestive heart failure
  - —Dyspnea, orthopnea, paroxysmal nocturnal dyspnea, lower extremity edema, tachycardia, pulmonary rales on auscultation, third heart sound (S3), jugular venous distention, ascites
- Pericardial involvement
  - —Inspiratory chest pain, pain relieved by sitting up/leaning forward, pericardial friction rub on auscultation, distant heart sounds and absent PMI (point of maximal impulse) if prominent effusion, tamponade (elevated neck veins, pulsus paradoxus, shock)
- Myocarditis
  - —Chest pain/pressure, shortness of breath, fever, may be asymptomatic

LABORATORY PROCEDURES

- $CD4^+$ T-cell count: useful for prognosis (<200 increased opportunistic events)
- HIV-positive plasma viral RNA level: useful for determining timing of and response to treatment
- Complete blood count (CBC)

IMAGING STUDIES

- Chest x-ray: Nonspecific, but look for cardiomegaly, pulmonary edema, or other source of pulmonary pathology.
- Echocardiography: Evaluate for impaired left ventricular shortening, left ventricular dilation, pericardial effusion, vegetation/thrombus, overall right and left ventricular function

SPECIAL TESTS

- ECG: Nonspecific, but acute myocarditis may mimic ischemia/infarction
- Myocardial biopsy: Current evidence does not support utility.

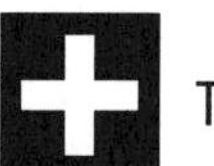

Treatment

GENERAL MEASURES

Currently, a cure for HIV is nonexistent.

- Aggressive antiretroviral therapy to limit the onset of opportunistic pathogens and neoplasms
- Only supportive treatment exists for HIV-specific cardiomyopathy, similar to that of typical congestive heart failure.
- Maintain wide differential, including cardiac etiologies, for any presenting symptoms given the broad spectrum of offending pathology in HIV/AIDS.
- If other causative etiology is found, tailor therapy accordingly (e.g., removal of cardiotoxic agent, antiinfective therapy, dialysis, etc.)

SURGICAL MEASURES

- None. Significant concern exists regarding transmission to health care workers.
- Risk of transmission after documented parenteral exposure in health care setting is 0.29% per exposure.
- Physician may not ethically refuse to treat patient solely because he or she is HIV positive.

ADMISSION/DISCHARGE CRITERIA

- Specific to individual patient presentation

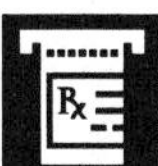

Medications

DRUG(S) OF CHOICE

- Antiretroviral therapy (typically two nucleoside analogues and protease inhibitor, although multiple alternative regimens exist and are in development)
- Antiinfectives should be targeted to etiologic agent if treatment is possible.
- Supportive therapy for congestive heart failure

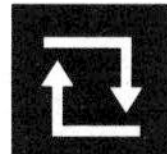

Follow-up

PATIENT MONITORING

- Plasma $CD4^+$ and HIV-positive plasma RNA every 3 to 6 months
- Close monitoring for development of clinical manifestations of opportunistic processes

EXPECTED COURSE AND PROGNOSIS

- Median time from primary HIV infection to the development of AIDS is approximately 10 years.
- Onset of congestive heart failure commonly marks onset of terminal stages of disease.
- Dilated cardiomyopathy on echocardiography is an independent adverse prognostic factor, with 50% mortality within 6 months.
- Patients with congestive heart failure may demonstrate initial symptomatic response to standard agents.

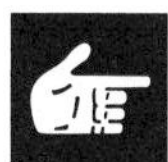

Miscellaneous

ICD-9-CM

421.9 Acute endocarditis, unspecified
422.90 Acute myocarditis, unspecified
422.91 Idiopathic myocarditis
425.4 Idiopathic cardiomyopathy
423.9 Pericardial disease, unspecified

INTERNET RESOURCES

Centers for Disease Control website: http://www.cdc.gov/nchstp/hiv_aids/dhap.htm

BIBLIOGRAPHY

Alexander RW, et al., eds. *Hurst's the heart,* 9th ed. New York: McGraw-Hill, 1998.

Fauci AS, et al., eds. *Harrison's principles of internal medicine,* 14th ed. New York: McGraw-Hill, 1998.

Kaul S, et al. Cardiac manifestations of acquired immune deficiency syndrome: a 1991 update. *Am Heart J* 1991;122:535–544.

Lipshultz SE. Dilated cardiomyopathy in HIV-infected patients. *N Engl J Med* 1998;339: 1153–1155.

Author: Chandan Devireddy

Alcohol and the Heart

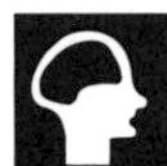

Basics

DESCRIPTION

Excess consumption of alcohol leads to a dilated cardiomyopathy.

- The definition of *excess,* however, is not clear.
- Varying levels of alcohol intake can lead to cardiomyopathy in a particular individual, including amounts considered "social drinking."
- Binge drinking also can lead to cardiomyopathy.
- Individuals with left ventricular dysfunction of any etiology should likely avoid consumption of even small quantities of alcohol, because it can further depress left ventricular function.
- Alcohol can even depress cardiac function in people with normal hearts.
- Although alcohol in small quantities may have a beneficial effect on the lipid profile, the clinical significance of this is controversial.

EPIDEMIOLOGY

- Potentially one-third of cases of nonischemic cardiomyopathy is due to alcohol.
- Found most often in men 30 to 55 years of age with a long history of heavy alcohol consumption, usually for at least a decade
- However, the prevalence of cardiomyopathy is similar among male and female alcoholics.

ETIOLOGY

- Alcohol can damage the heart due to a direct toxic effect on the myocardium.
- Acetaldehyde and acetate, metabolites of ethanol, are known to inhibit myocardial protein synthesis.
- In certain circumstances, iron or cobalt added to alcohol may predispose to cardiomyopathy.
- Certain individuals may have a genetic predisposition to develop alcoholic cardiomyopathy.
- Women may develop this disorder with a lower cumulative intake of alcohol compared with men.
- Nutritional deficiencies also may play a role.
- Thiamine deficiency, known to occur in alcoholics, can cause beriberi.

RISK FACTORS

- Heavy alcohol use
- Malnutrition

PREGNANCY

- Contraindicated in someone who drinks heavily

ASSOCIATED CONDITIONS

- Atrial fibrillation, either due to the cardiomyopathy or to alcohol ingestion, is common.
- Supraventricular arrhythmia
- Cirrhosis of the liver
- Pancreatitis
- Gastritis
- Myopathy
- Hypertension
- Subarachnoid hemorrhage
- Thiamine and folate deficiency

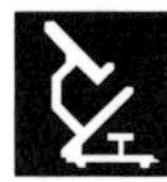

Diagnosis

DIFFERENTIAL DIAGNOSIS

- Other causes of dilated cardiomyopathy

SIGNS AND SYMPTOMS

- Fatigue
- Weakness, especially muscle weakness
- Exertional dyspnea
- Orthopnea
- Paroxysmal nocturnal dyspnea
- JVD (jugular venous distension)
- Edema
- Hypertension
- Narrow pulse pressure
- S3
- S4
- MR (mitral regurgitation), TR murmurs (tricuspid regurgitation)
- Hepatomegaly (either from right-sided failure or alcoholism)
- Telangiectasia
- Spider angiomata

LABORATORY PROCEDURES

- ECG may show atrial arrhythmia, ectopy, or bundle branch block.
- QT interval may be prolonged.
- Poor R-wave progression and hypertrophy also may be seen.

IMAGING STUDIES

- Chest x-ray may show cardiomegaly and pulmonary congestion.
- Echo shows biatrial and biventricular dilatation.
- Both systolic and diastolic dysfunction are present.
- Mitral and tricuspid regurgitation may be present.

SPECIAL TESTS

Myopathy is often present on skeletal muscle biopsy.

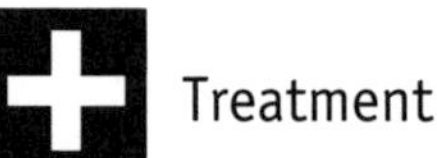

Treatment

GENERAL MEASURES

- Alcohol cessation is mandatory.
- Concomitant tobacco abuse, often present, also should be discouraged.
- Hypophosphatemia, hypokalemia, and hypomagnesemia also may be present and should be corrected.

SURGICAL MEASURES

Heart transplantation would not be considered unless a period of abstinence could be shown.

ADMISSION/DISCHARGE CRITERIA

- As for heart failure of any etiology
- Hospitalization (and observed alcohol cessation) is particularly useful.

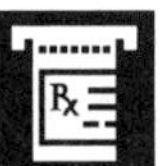

Medications

DRUG(S) OF CHOICE

Intravenous thiamine administration is standard.

Follow-up

PATIENT MONITORING

- Standard for heart failure of any cause
- Observe for any clues that the patient has started drinking again.

EXPECTED COURSE AND PROGNOSIS

- With complete abstinence from alcohol, the cardiomyopathy may partially, or even completely, resolve.
- The majority of improvement occurs in the first several months of abstinence.
- Continued, sometimes covert, drinking makes it difficult to gauge the true effect of abstinence.
- Continued alcohol abuse will lead to myocardial failure and death.
- An increased risk of sudden death, even in the absence of overt cardiac dysfunction

PATIENT EDUCATION

The need for complete abstinence must be stressed.

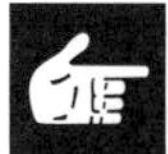

Miscellaneous

ICD-9-CM

428.0 Failure, heart, congestive
425.5 Alcoholic cardiomyopathy

BIBLIOGRAPHY

Kloner RA, Rezkalla S. Substance abuse and the heart. In: Topol EJ, ed. *Comprehensive cardiovascular medicine.* Philadelphia: Lippincott-Raven, 1998:1071–1073.

Rodkey SM, Ratliff NB, Young JB. Cardiomyopathy and myocardial failure. In: Topol EJ, ed. *Comprehensive cardiovascular medicine.* Philadelphia: Lippincott-Raven, 1998:2610–2611.

Wynne J, Braunwald E. The cardiomyopathies and the myocarditides. In: Braunwald E, ed. *Heart disease: a textbook of cardiovascular medicine,* 5th ed. Philadelphia: WB Saunders, 1997:1412–1413.

Fernandez-Sola J, Estruch R, Nicolas JM, et al. Comparison of alcoholic cardiomyopathy in women versus men. *Am J Cardiol* 1997; 80:481–485.

McKenna CJ, Codd MB, McCann HA, et al. Alcohol consumption and idiopathic dilated cardiomyopathy: a case control study. *Am Heart J* 1998;135:833–837.

Jacob AJ, McLaren KM, Boon NA. Effects of abstinence on alcoholic heart muscle disease. *Am J Cardiol* 1991;68:805–807.

Regan TJ. Alcohol and the cardiovascular system. *JAMA* 1990;264:377–381.

Reeves WC, Nanda NC, Gramiak R. Echocardiography in chronic alcoholics following prolonged periods of abstinence. *Am Heart J* 1978;95: 578–583.

Authors: Deepak L. Bhatt and Gary S. Francis

Amyloid Heart Disease

Basics

DESCRIPTION

Deposition of amyloid proteins into the myocardium leads to a restrictive cardiomyopathy.

EPIDEMIOLOGY

- Familial amyloidosis is transmitted via an autosomal-dominant mode of inheritance and can lead to cardiomyopathy in 25% of patients.
- A certain type of amyloidosis, called transthyretin isoleucine 122, is more prevalent among African Americans.

ETIOLOGY

- Primary amyloidosis is due to excess production of immunoglobulin light chain (called AL), whereas secondary amyloidosis is due to production of a protein (called AA).
- Cardiac involvement is much more common in the primary form compared with the secondary form.
- Familial and senile amyloidosis are both due to deposition of a protein called transthyretin (also called prealbumin) and also frequently involve the heart.

RISK FACTORS

- Multiple myeloma

PREGNANCY

- Poorly tolerated, as with other restrictive cardiomyopathies

ASSOCIATED CONDITIONS

- Primary amyloidosis is often associated with multiple myeloma. Renal involvement is common.
- Peripheral and autonomic neuropathy
- Systemic and pulmonary emboli
- Malabsorption

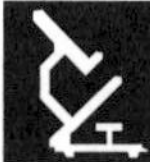

Diagnosis

DIFFERENTIAL DIAGNOSIS

- Other causes of restrictive cardiomyopathy

SIGNS AND SYMPTOMS

- Orthostatic hypotension
- Right-sided heart failure
- Jugular vein distension
- Hepatomegaly
- Splenomegaly
- Edema
- S3
- Mitral and tricuspid valve regurgitation
- Narrow pulse pressure
- Macroglossia
- Angina
- Neuropathy

LABORATORY PROCEDURES

- The ECG classically shows low voltage, despite echocardiographic hypertrophy; this is an important differentiating feature from other causes of left ventricular hypertrophy and is present in about half of cases of cardiac amyloid.
- Q waves may be present.
- Atrial fibrillation is common.
- PVCs (premature ventricular contraction) and ventricular arrhythmias may be seen.
- Sick sinus syndrome and conduction block may be observed.
- Serum and urine protein electrophoresis often can be used to detect a monoclonal protein in primary amyloidosis.

IMAGING STUDIES

- Chest x-ray
  - —May show cardiomegaly, pleural effusions, and pulmonary congestion
- Echocardiography
  - —Massive hypertrophy, with small left and right ventricular cavities
  - —The hypertrophied walls have a sparkling pattern to them due to increased echogenicity.
  - —Both atria are usually dilated, with thickening of the atrioventricular valves.
  - —Valvular regurgitation, and less commonly stenosis, can occur.
  - —A small pericardial effusion is often present.
  - —Abnormal diastolic function, with variable degrees of systolic dysfunction, is present.
  - —Thrombus may be seen in either the atria or ventricles.
- Doppler measurements are able to predict cardiac death more reliably than two-dimensional echocardiography.

SPECIAL TESTS

- Abdominal fat pad biopsy is the easiest way to make the diagnosis.
- Endomyocardial biopsy also can be used to make the diagnosis and is particularly useful when amyloid deposition is localized.
- Using polarized light microscopy and Congo red staining, amyloid fibrils have an apple-green birefringence.
- Square root sign
  - —Diastolic dip and plateau on ventricular pressure waveform
  - —During hemodynamic measurements obtained at cardiac catheterization
- Electrophysiologic study
  - —Can show a prolonged HV interval in AL amyloidosis, which serves as a marker of sudden death

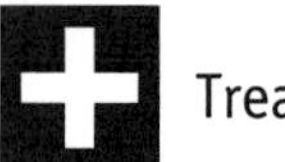

Treatment

GENERAL MEASURES

- Treatment of any underlying disease process, such as multiple myeloma, may help the heart.
- Salt restriction

SURGICAL MEASURES

- Amyloid is generally considered a contraindication to heart transplantation.
- Cardiac transplantation has been used, but results have not been good, due to recurrence of amyloid.
- In the familial form, combined heart and liver transplantation has been performed, because liver transplantation cures the disorder.
- Pacemakers are indicated for advanced heart block.

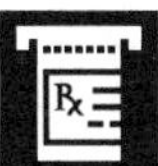

Medications

DRUG(S) OF CHOICE

- Digitalis toxicity can occur at much lower doses than one would expect; if used, caution must be exercised.
- Diuretics can be useful for symptom control, but can precipitate hypotension.
- Calcium channel blockers, by binding to amyloid fibrils, can lead to impaired cardiac contractility and hypotension.
- ACE (angiotensin converting enzyme) can be useful, but would not be prudent if there is preexisting orthostatic hypotension.
- Coumadin is used for treatment of thrombi; bleeding due to vessel fragility can be problematic.
- Intravenous melphalan has been used to treat primary amyloidosis as well as the associated cardiomyopathy.

ADMISSION/DISCHARGE CRITERIA

- As for other etiologies of heart failure

Follow-up

PATIENT MONITORING

- As for other etiologies of heart failure

EXPECTED COURSE AND PROGNOSIS

- Progressive heart failure occurs.
- Heart failure, especially in primary amyloidosis, is associated with a poor short-term prognosis.
- Sudden death can occur as a result of arrhythmias or from infiltration of the conduction system.

PATIENT EDUCATION

- As for other etiologies of heart failure

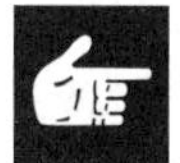

Miscellaneous

ICD-9-CM

428.0 Failure, heart, congestive
277.3 [425.7] Amyloidosis, heart

BIBLIOGRAPHY

Rodkey SM, Ratliff NB, Young JB. Cardiomyopathy and myocardial failure. In: Topol EJ, ed. *Comprehensive cardiovascular medicine.* Philadelphia: Lippincott-Raven, 1998:2606–2609.

Wynne J, Braunwald E. The cardiomyopathies and the myocarditides. In: Braunwald E, ed. *Heart disease: a textbook of cardiovascular medicine,* 5th ed. Philadelphia: WB Saunders, 1997:1427–1429.

Reisinger J, Dubrey SW, Lavalley M, et al. Electrophysiologic abnormalities in AL (primary) amyloidosis with cardiac involvement. *J Am Coll Cardiol* 1997;30:1046–1051.

Kashyap K, Hosenpud J. Cardiac amyloidosis. *Curr Treatment Options Cardiovasc Med* 1999;1:209–217.

McCarthy RE, Kasper EK. A review of the amyloidoses that infiltrate the heart. *Clin Cardiol* 1998;21:547–552.

Klein AL, Hatle LK, Taliercio CP, et al. Prognostic significance of Doppler measures of diastolic function in cardiac amyloidosis: a Doppler echocardiography study. *Circulation* 1991;83: 808–816.

Authors: Deepak L. Bhatt and Gary S. Francis

Anemia and the Heart

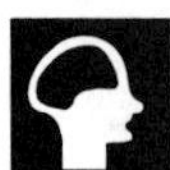

Basics

DESCRIPTION

- Chronically low hemoglobin (<4 g/dL) can lead to high-output heart failure.
- A postulated mechanism is that hemoglobin normally degrades nitric oxide.
- Anemia leads to elevated levels of nitric oxide with resultant vasodilatation.
- Lower viscosity is another potential mechanism leading to elevated cardiac output.
- Neurohormonal activation can be triggered by the low blood pressure and lead to sodium and water retention.
- Acute blood loss does not lead to heart failure.

EPIDEMIOLOGY

- Anemia is common among hospitalized patients.
- Anemia as an isolated cause of heart failure is rare in the United States.
- In the developing world, it is more common due to conditions such as hookworm infection.

ETIOLOGY

- Any cause of profound, chronic anemia
- Hookworm infection (and subsequent chronic blood loss)
- Sickle cell disorder
- Thalassemia

RISK FACTORS

- Poor nutrition (iron, folate, or vitamin B_{12} deficiency)

PREGNANCY

Severe degrees of anemia would need to be corrected before pregnancy to prevent risks to both mother and fetus.

ASSOCIATED CONDITIONS

- Pericarditis is common in thalassemia.
- Pulmonary infarction, stroke in sickle cell anemia

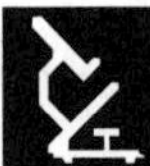

Diagnosis

DIFFERENTIAL DIAGNOSIS

- Other causes of high-output heart failure

SIGNS AND SYMPTOMS

- Pale conjunctivae
- Fatigue
- Exertional chest pain, dyspnea
- S3, S4
- Systolic and diastolic flow murmurs
- Duroziez's sign
- Quincke's pulse
- Edema

LABORATORY PROCEDURES

- Iron, folate, or vitamin B_{12} levels may be low.
- The ECG may show ischemic changes with profound anemia.
- Left ventricular hypertrophy also may be present. In sickle cell anemia right ventricular hypertrophy may occur.

IMAGING STUDIES

- Chest x-ray shows cardiomegaly.
- Echocardiography shows a dilated ventricle with thickened walls.

SPECIAL TESTS

Right heart catheterization reveals increased cardiac output and decreased systemic vascular resistance.

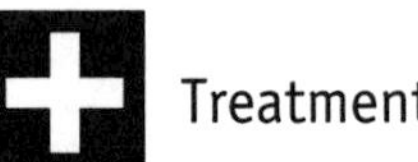

Treatment

GENERAL MEASURES

- Transfusion may be necessary.
  —If performed, red blood cells should be transfused slowly and given with diuretic agents.
- Chelation therapy in cases of iron overload

SURGICAL MEASURES

Splenectomy is useful in patients with thalassemia.

ADMISSION/DISCHARGE CRITERIA

- As for heart failure of any etiology

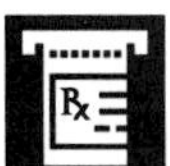

Medications

DRUG(S) OF CHOICE

- Iron, folate, or vitamin B_{12}, as appropriate

Follow-up

PATIENT MONITORING

Follow blood counts.

EXPECTED COURSE AND PROGNOSIS

- Usually, left ventricular function returns to normal once the chronic anemia has been corrected.

PATIENT EDUCATION

Watch for signs of blood loss.

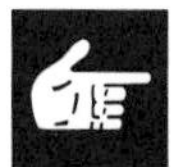

Miscellaneous

ICD-9-CM

428.0 Failure, heart, congestive

BIBLIOGRAPHY

Shulman LN, Braunwald E, Rosenthal DS. Hematological-oncological disorders and heart disease. In: Braunwald E, ed. *Heart disease: a textbook of cardiovascular medicine,* 5th ed. Philadelphia: WB Saunders, 1997:1786–1792.

Amsterdam PB. Hematologic and oncologic disorders and the heart. In: Topol EJ, ed. *Comprehensive cardiovascular medicine,* Philadelphia: Lippincott-Raven, 1998:970–974.

Anand IS, Chandrashekhar Y, Ferrari R, et al. Pathogenesis of edema in chronic severe anemia: studies of body water and sodium, renal function, hemodynamic variables, and plasma hormones. *Br Heart J* 1993;70:357–362.

Authors: Deepak L. Bhatt and Gary S. Francis

Angina, Prinzmetal's, Variant Angina

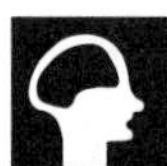

Basics

DESCRIPTION

Variant angina, described in 1959 by Prinzmetal, is characterized by angina at rest associated with transient ST segment elevation on ECG.

- Exercise tolerance is preserved.
- ST segments rapidly return to baseline with relief of chest discomfort.
- Attacks are cyclical.
- Symptoms often occur in the early morning hours.

Systems Affected

- Cardiovascular

Incidence/Prevalence

- Exact incidence and prevalence unknown
- Overall more uncommon than exertional angina

Age-Related Factors

- More often occurs in younger patients than does exertional angina
- Average age 48
- Affects more women than men

Causes

- Transient coronary artery spasm, usually focal, with normal coronary anatomy or at site of atherosclerotic plaque
- IVUS (intravascular ultrasound) often demonstrates plaque at site of spasm even in angiographically normal coronary arteries

Genetics

Increased prevalence in certain geographical locations, including Canada, Italy, and Japan. Recent evidence suggests that specific mutations in the eNOS gene are found with significantly greater incidence in patients with variant angina versus controls.

RISK FACTORS

- Smoking most important risk factor
- Cocaine may precipitate spasm.
- Patients with pure vasospasm younger than patients with exertional angina (average age 48), more likely to be female
- Traditional coronary disease risk factors may be lacking.

PREGNANCY

N/A

ASSOCIATED CONDITIONS

- Migraine headaches
- Raynaud's phenomenon
- Ocular spasm
- Aspirin-induced asthma
- Hypomagnesemia
- Hyperinsulinemia

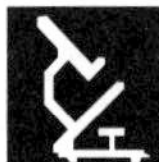

Diagnosis

DIFFERENTIAL DIAGNOSIS

- Angina pectoris
- Pericarditis
- Aortic dissection
- GI disorders
- Neurologic disorders
- Pulmonary processes
- Musculoskeletal disorders
- Psychiatric disorders

SIGNS AND SYMPTOMS

Retrosternal discomfort that may radiate to arms, neck, or jaw usually occurs at rest, often in early morning hours.

- Exercise capacity preserved
- Physical examination usually normal

LABORATORY PROCEDURES

N/A

IMAGING STUDIES

- Coronary angiography recommended
- Consider ergonovine, which produces focal spasm in approximately 90% of patients with variant angina.
- Negative ergonovine test result makes diagnosis unlikely.

SPECIAL TESTS

- ECG during pain and after relief of pain
- Ambulatory ECG monitoring helpful in establishing diagnosis
- Exercise testing may provoke angina, ST elevation.

PATHOLOGIC FINDINGS

Histologic examination of coronary artery plaques revealed neointimal hyperplasia significantly more often in variant angina than in chronic stable exertional angina (68% vs. 8%).

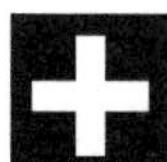

Treatment

GENERAL MEASURES

Symptoms should be treated immediately.

- Chest pain and ECG changes resolve with nitroglycerin.
- Patient is at highest risk for sudden death or myocardial infarction during acute, active phase of disease.
- Treatment goal is prevention of coronary spasm.
- Smoking cessation is of utmost importance.

SURGICAL MEASURES

Consider PTCA (percutaneous transluminal coronary angioplasty)/stenting for patients with significant fixed coronary lesions.

- PTCA with stenting also used successfully in patients refractory to medical treatment
- Recurrence rate of symptoms and angiographic disease after PTCA/stenting higher in patients with variant angina
- Reports of spasm recurring proximal to the stent
- Reports of continued symptoms in occasional patients without demonstrable spasm
- Consider coronary artery bypass grafting in patients with significant multivessel disease.

ADMISSION/DISCHARGE CRITERIA

Hospitalization warranted if symptoms unstable.

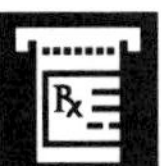

Medications

DRUG(S) OF CHOICE

- Calcium channel blockers
  —Greater than 50% of patients become asymptomatic with calcium channel blocker therapy.
  —High doses may be required.
  —If symptoms not completely relieved with one drug, may be beneficial to add second calcium channel blocker.
  —Calcium channel blocker may decrease risk of myocardial infarction.
- Long-acting nitrates effective, but patients may develop tolerance.
- Sublingual nitrates indicated for acute attacks
- Low-dose aspirin

Contraindications

Beta-blockers may increase duration of attacks.

- Attacks may be provoked by 5-fluorouracil, cyclophosphamide.
- High-dose aspirin may exacerbate attacks by inhibiting coronary vasodilator prostacyclin.

Precautions

Calcium channel blocker withdrawal may cause rebound.

ALTERNATIVE DRUGS

May be effective in refractory cases, but not approved for this use in the United States.

- Amiodarone
- Guanethidine
- Clonidine
- Prazosin

Follow-up

PATIENT MONITORING

- Monitor for relief of symptoms.
- Holter monitoring helpful as some patients have silent attacks

EXPECTED COURSE AND PROGNOSIS

Possible complications include sudden death, myocardial infarction, ventricular arrhythmias, AV block, syncope.

- Greatest risk of adverse outcome during acute, active phase of disease
- Sudden death, myocardial infarction occur most often during acute active phase.
- Acute active phase usually lasts 3 to 6 months, then symptoms often remit.
- Arrhythmias or syncope during attacks increase risk of sudden death.
- ST elevations in inferior and anterior leads on ECG increase risk of sudden death.
- Predictors of poor outcome include extensive and severe coronary artery disease, abnormal left ventricular function, absence of treatment with calcium channel blockers, continued tobacco abuse, ventricular arrhythmias during attacks.
- Once patient is past acute active phase, chance of long-term survival is excellent (89%–97%).

PATIENT EDUCATION

Prevention/Avoidance

- Smoking cessation of utmost importance
- Compliance with medications

Activity

- As tolerated after consulting physician

Diet

- Low-fat, low-cholesterol diet because approximately two-thirds of coronary spasm occurs at site of angiographic atherosclerotic coronary lesion.
- Intracoronary ultrasonography identified atherosclerotic lesions in addition to those identified angiographically.
- Coronary spasm may be contributing factor in development, progression of atherosclerosis.

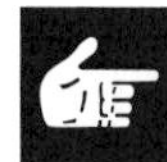

Miscellaneous

SYNONYMS

- Prinzmetal's angina

ICD-9-CM

413.1

ORGANIZATIONS

American Heart Association, National Center, 7272 Greenville Avenue, Dallas, Texas 75231-4596, phone 1-800-242-8721. American Heart Association website: www.americanheart.org

BIBLIOGRAPHY

Theroux P, Waters D. Diagnosis and management of patients with unstable angina. In: Alexander RW, Schlant RC, Fuster V, eds. *Hurst's the heart,* 9th ed. McGraw Hill, 1998:1332–1336.

Gersh BJ, Braunwald E, Rutherford JD. Chronic coronary artery disease. In: Braunwald E, ed. *Heart disease a textbook of cardiovascular medicine,* 5th ed. Philadelphia: WB Saunders, 1997:1340–1343.

Nakayama M, et al. $T^{786} \rightarrow C$ mutation in the 5″-flanking region of the endothelial nitric oxide synthase gene is associated with coronary spasm. *Circulation* 1999;99:2864–2870.

Suzuki H, et al. Histological evaluation of coronary plaque in patients with variant angina: relationship between vasospasm and neointimal hyperplasia in primary coronary lesions. *J Am Coll Cardiol* 1999;33:198–205.

Authors: Brenda J. Hott and Nanette K. Wenger

Angina, Stable

Basics

DESCRIPTION

Stable angina is a symptom complex resulting from insufficient oxygen and nutrient delivery to the heart, with no change in pattern in previous 60 days.

Typical Angina

- Brief (seconds to minutes) chest, jaw, neck, shoulder, back, epigastric, or arm discomfort, aggravated by physical exertion or emotional stress and relieved by rest or nitroglycerin
- Occasional precipitants include smoking, meals, cold air, thyrotoxicosis, anemia, infection, tachyarrhythmia, and uncontrolled hypertension.

Atypical Angina

- Dyspnea, fatigue, or generalized weakness aggravated by exertion or emotional stress and relieved by rest or nitroglycerin

Noncardiac Chest Pain

- Chest discomfort syndromes without the above-listed characteristics

Unstable Angina

See chapter Angina, Unstable.

Angina, Prinzmetal's, Variant

See chapter Angina, Prinzmetal's Variant.

CAUSES

- Coronary atherosclerotic heart disease (CAD) with fixed atherosclerotic plaque, thrombus or plaque with associated thrombus
- Coronary spasm; endothelial dysfunction
- Severe valvular aortic stenosis; insufficiency
- Hypertrophic cardiomyopathy
- Primary pulmonary hypertension
- Severe hypertension or systemic hypotension
- Severe anemia
- Nonatherosclerotic coronary artery disease
  - —Coronary artery anomalies
  - —Primary coronary artery dissection
  - —Coronary embolism
  - —Radiation vasculopathy
  - —Carbon monoxide poisoning
- Arteritis
  - —Kawasaki disease
  - —Takayasu's disease
  - —Polyarteritis nodosa
  - —Systemic lupus erythematosus
  - —Giant cell arteritis
  - —Burger's disease
  - —Syphilis

EPIDEMIOLOGY

Incidence/Prevalence

The initial manifestation of CAD in approximately one half of patients; affects 3 million Americans; costs over $150 billion/yr.

Predominant Age

- Middle-aged and older men and postmenopausal women

Predominant Sex

- More male than female

ETIOLOGY

Genetics

- Genetic susceptibility for CAD; family history very important

RISK FACTORS

- Family history of premature CAD (first-degree relative, ≤55 years of age)
- Primary or secondary dyslipidemia: hypercholesterolemia, elevated LDL, isolated low HDL
- Hypertension
- Tobacco abuse
- Diabetes mellitus
- Male gender
- Advanced age
- Sedentary life-style

PREGNANCY

- Differential diagnosis of anginal symptoms must be considered (coronary artery dissection, pulmonary embolism, etc.).
- Comanagement cardiologist, obstetrician
- Symptoms may increase with hemodynamic changes.
- Treatment options may be limited by pregnancy concerns.

ASSOCIATED DISEASES

- See Risk Factors (above)
- Cerebrovascular or peripheral vascular disease
- Obesity

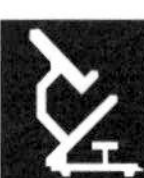

Diagnosis

DIFFERENTIAL DIAGNOSIS

- Acute MI
- Anemia
- Aortic dissection
- Symptomatic cholelithiasis
- Chest wall pain, costochondritis
- Esophageal spasm, esophagitis
- Fibromyalgia
- Gastritis, peptic ulcer disease
- Gastroesophageal reflux disease
- Pancreatitis
- Panic disorder
- Pericarditis
- Pneumothorax
- Pulmonary embolism or hypertension
- Radiculopathy, shoulder arthropathy

SIGNS AND SYMPTOMS

- See above for types of angina.
- Discomfort often radiates to the neck, shoulders, arms, or back.
- Dyspnea on exertion; fatigue
- Discomfort often described as clenching fist over the sternum (Levine's sign)

LABORATORY PROCEDURES

- Hemoglobin (Hgb)
- Fasting glucose, Hgb A1C
- Fasting lipid panel, including total cholesterol, HDL cholesterol, triglycerides, and calculated LDL cholesterol
- If concern for unstable angina pectoris
  - —ECG
  - —Cardiac enzymes (CK + MB, troponin I, myoglobin)

IMAGING STUDIES

Primary utility is diagnostic, risk stratification

- Exercise radionuclide scintigraphy or echocardiography
  - —Useful with complete left bundle branch block; pacemakers; preexcitation (Wolff-Parkinson-White) syndrome; ECG conduction abnormalities; hypertrophy or taking digitalis
  - —Pharmacologic stress imaging tests for patients unable to exercise
- Coronary angiography
  - —Primary utility is risk stratification and evaluation of revascularization need.
  - —Useful for patients who have survived sudden cardiac death; uncertain diagnosis after noninvasive testing; unable to undergo noninvasive testing due to disability, illness, or morbid obesity; occupational requirement for a definitive diagnosis (i.e., pilots); suspected nonatherosclerotic causes of myocardial ischemia; coronary artery spasm is suspected; high pretest probability of left main or three-vessel CAD
- Electron beam CT
  - —Current role in diagnosis and management uncertain

OTHER TESTS

- ECG
  - —Normal in ≤50% of patients with chronic stable angina, does not exclude severe CAD
  - —Prior Q-wave MI on the ECG, ST-T wave changes consistent with myocardial ischemia, or ECG changes of left ventricular hypertrophy favor the diagnosis of angina pectoris
- Chest x-ray with signs or symptoms of heart failure (HF), valvular disease, pericardial disease, or aortic dissection/aneurysm
- Exercise ECG
  - —Primary utility diagnostic; risk stratification
  - —Appropriate if diagnosis remains uncertain after history, physical examination, ECG, and chest x-ray
  - —Greatest utility with intermediate pretest probability of CAD (~50%) based on age, gender, and symptoms
- Echocardiography
  - —Systolic murmur suggestive of aortic stenosis or hypertrophic cardiomyopathy
  - —Evaluate ischemia severity during pain

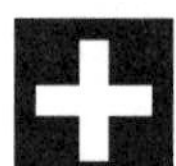

Treatment

GENERAL MEASURES

- Control precipitating; exacerbating conditions

• Risk stratification by history, physical examination, ECG, chest x-ray, exercise ECG, or diagnostic imaging
• Patients with high likelihood (>1 chance in 2) of severe disease: consider angiography
• Treatment of stable angina to:
 —Prevent MI, death, need for revascularization
 —Reduce symptoms of angina, occurrence of ischemia
• A handy mnemonic for appropriate initial health care is A, B, C, D, E:
 —A. Aspirin and antianginal therapy
 —B. Beta-blocker and blood pressure
 —C. Cigarette smoking and cholesterol
 —D. Diet and diabetes
 —E. Education and exercise
• Risk factor modification
 —Blood pressure control JNC VI guidelines
 —Cholesterol lowering to NCEP guidelines
 —Smoking cessation
 —Glycemic control
 —Weight loss
 —Regular aerobic exercise
 —Dietary modification: low fat, low cholesterol, caloric restriction as needed, low-sodium diet for salt-sensitive hypertensive patients
• Stress reduction

SURGICAL MEASURES

• Medical therapy is as effective as PTCA for death, MI outcome.
• PTCA does not improve survival.
• Neither PTCA nor CABG decreases reinfarction.
• Quality of life is better with surgery or angioplasty than with medical therapy.
• Stable angina refractory to medical therapy may benefit from revascularization.
 —Revascularization by PTCA or surgery offered for left main coronary artery stenosis, three-vessel CAD, or two-vessel CAD with proximal left anterior descending coronary artery stenosis
 —Choice of therapy should include patient preference, tolerability of medical therapy

ADMISSION/DISCHARGE CRITERIA

• Unstable symptoms require hospitalization and telemetry monitoring.
• Lack of response to medical therapy or significant; specific angiographic stenosis may indicate need revascularization by PTCA or CABG.

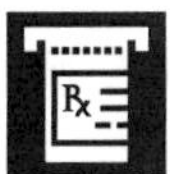

Medications

DRUG(S) OF CHOICE

Pharmacotherapy Shown to Prevent MI and Death and Reduce Symptoms

• Aspirin 325 mg daily, unless contraindications
• Clopidogrel 75 mg daily, when aspirin contraindicated
• Statin-based lipid-lowering therapy target LDL of <100 mg/dL
 —Statins significantly reduce risk of death, MI, stroke, and the need for revascularization in randomized trials
  • Pravastatin 10–80 mg daily
  • Simvastatin 10–80 mg daily
  • Lovastatin 10–80 mg daily
 —Statins likely providing equal benefit (death, MI, stroke, revascularization)
  • Atorvastatin 10–80 mg daily
  • Fluvastatin 10–80 mg daily
  • Cerivastatin 0.1–0.3 mg daily

Pharmacotherapy Shown to Reduce Ischemia and Relieve Symptoms

• Beta-blockers to target heart rate of 50-60 beats/min, improve survival, reduce reinfarction
 —Atenolol 25–100 mg daily
 —Metoprolol 25–100 mg b.i.d.
 —Propranolol 30–100 mg b.i.d.–t.i.d.
• Long-acting calcium antagonists
 —Verapamil 160–480 mg daily
 —Diltiazem 90–360 mg daily
  • Avoid verapamil, diltiazem with decreased left ventricular function, atrioventricular block
 —Amlodipine 5–20 mg daily
 —Nifedipine 30–120 mg daily
  • Short-acting dihydropyridine calcium antagonists should be avoided.
• Long-acting nitrates, sublingual nitroglycerin, or nitroglycerin spray for immediate relief of angina
 —All patients should receive a sublingual nitroglycerin prescription and usage education.
 —Nitrate-free interval of 10–14 hours required with long-acting nitrates
 —Should be prescribed with beta-blocker or calcium antagonist

ALTERNATIVE DRUGS

Possible benefits:
• Low-intensity anticoagulation with warfarin in addition to aspirin
• Promising new drugs under investigation
 —Oral glycoprotein IIb/IIIa platelet inhibitors

Follow-up

PATIENT MONITORING

• Every 4–12 months with ECG
• Testing with changes in clinical status:
 —Chest x-ray and echocardiogram for CHF or MI by history or ECG
 —Echocardiogram for new or worsening valvular heart disease
 —Treadmill exercise ECG if no prior revascularization
 —Pharmacologic stress imaging if no prior revascularization and unable to exercise or with significant ECG abnormalities
 —Stress imaging with prior revascularization
 —Angina within 8 months of PCTA suggests restenosis
• Coronary angiography marked limitation of ordinary activity (CCS class III) despite maximal medical therapy

EXPECTED COURSE AND PROGNOSIS

• Overall annual mortality rate 3%–4%
• Prognosis related to age of onset; disease etiology; disease severity; comorbid conditions; left ventricular function; response to therapy

Possible Complications

• Ischemia, MI, arrhythmia, CHF, sudden death, mitral regurgitation, depression

Age-Related Factors

• Pediatric patients: suspect familial dyslipidemia
• Elderly: special attention to medication side effects, drug interactions

PATIENT EDUCATION

Activity

• Symptom limited, after physician counseling
• Cardiac rehabilitation improves quality of life, functional status, symptom severity.

Diet

Patient specific

• Low-cholesterol, low-fat diet (general population)
• Diabetic diet (diabetics)
• 2-g sodium diet (hypertensives)

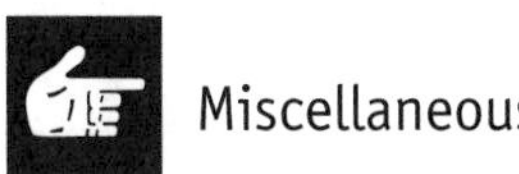

Miscellaneous

ICD-9-CM

411.1 Angina, stable
413 Angina Pectoris
413.1 Prinzmetal's Angina
413.9 Angina, Unspecified

BIBLIOGRAPHY

ACC/AHA/ACP-ASIM Guidelines for the Management of Patients With Chronic Stable Angina. *Circulation* 1999;99:2829–2848.

Heidenreich PA, et al. Meta-analysis of trials comparing beta-blockers, calcium antagonists, and nitrates for stable angina. *JAMA* 1999; 281:1927–1936.

Schlant RC, Alexander RW, et al. *Hurst's the heart,* 9th ed. New York, McGraw-Hill, 1998: 1131–1132, 1266, and 1276–1286.

Authors: L. Van-Thomas Crisco and Nanette K. Wenger

Angina, Unstable

Basics

DESCRIPTION

Symptom complex usually caused by abrupt reduction in coronary flow resulting in mismatch of myocardial oxygen supply and demand

- An acute, dynamic coronary syndrome intermediate on the spectrum between chronic stable angina and acute myocardial infarction (MI)
- May present as new-onset angina (within 2 months), crescendo angina (more severe, prolonged, frequent), angina at rest, postinfarction angina

EPIDEMIOLOGY

- 750,000 hospitalizations per year in United States

Incidence/Prevalence

- More men are affected than women.
- Most frequent in middle-aged or older men
- Incidence in women increases after menopause.
- Diabetes mellitus eliminates benefit of female gender.

ETIOLOGY

- Most commonly coronary atherosclerotic plaque rupture with associated thrombosis; frequently associated with vasoconstriction
- Coronary vasoconstriction (see Prinzmetal's Angina); may occur in normal coronary artery or associated with atherosclerotic plaque
- Progressive luminal narrowing, due to restenosis following PTCA (percutaneous transluminal coronary angioplasty), or progressive atherosclerosis.
- Secondary causes that alter myocardial oxygen supply/demand balance; tachycardia, fever, thyrotoxicosis, cocaine or amphetamine use, hypertension, aortic stenosis are examples of increased demand; anemia, hypoxemia, hyperviscosity states, hypotension are examples of decreased supply

CAUSES

- See Stable Angina

RISK FACTORS

- Advanced age
- Male gender
- Family history of premature coronary artery disease
- Hypercholesterolemia
- Low HDL-C
- Tobacco use
- Hypertension
- Diabetes mellitus
- Sedentary life-style

PREGNANCY

Unstable angina is rare in pregnancy. Consider coronary artery dissection or spasm, hypercoagulable states with coronary thrombosis, and other causes of chest pain such as pulmonary embolism.

AGE-RELATED FACTORS

- Pediatric: Consider familial hypercholesterolemia, homocystinemia, coronary artery anomaly (e.g., coronary arising from pulmonary artery).
- Geriatric: At increased risk for coronary artery disease, but increased benefit with favorable treatment. Consider overall health, concomitant illnesses in treatment decisions. Avoid adverse reactions to medication and drug interactions.

ASSOCIATED CONDITIONS

- Congestive heart failure (CHF)
- Peripheral vascular disease (stroke, transient ischemic attack, renal artery stenosis, aortic aneurysm, claudication)
- Chronic obstructive pulmonary disease (COPD)
- See others above.

Diagnosis

DIFFERENTIAL DIAGNOSIS

- Acute MI
- Esophageal spasm, esophagitis, gastroesophageal reflux
- Pulmonary embolus
- Aortic dissection
- Musculoskeletal disorders: costochondritis, shoulder arthritis
- Pericarditis
- Pneumonitis/pleuritis
- Peptic ulcer disease/gastritis
- Biliary colic
- Pancreatitis
- Pneumothorax
- Herpes zoster
- Panic disorder

SIGNS AND SYMPTOMS

- Chest discomfort similar to classic exertional angina: precordial or retrosternal chest pain or pressure, often radiating to neck, left arm, shoulder.
- Associated with nausea, vomiting, diaphoresis, palpitations, dyspnea, but less often than with acute MI
- Symptoms occur at rest or low levels of exertion; increase in frequency, duration, intensity of symptoms; previously successful medical therapies no longer control symptoms.

LABORATORY PROCEDURES

- Cardiac enzymes: Serial measurements over 24 hours to rule out myocardial infarction; CK and CK-MB (creatine kinase-MB fraction) normal; troponin I and T may be minimally elevated but typically normal; more than minimal elevation of enzymes suggests myocardial infarction.
- CBC: Assess for anemia, thrombocytopenia.
- Lipid profile: LDL, triglycerides often elevated, HDL often low
- Blood glucose or hemoglobin A1C elevation suggests diabetes mellitus.
- Disorders that may alter laboratory results: renal insufficiency; skeletal muscle injury; hypothyroidism may increase CK, CK-MB, troponin T; lipid levels transiently depressed during hospitalization in acute coronary syndromes

IMAGING STUDIES

- Chest x-ray: often normal; look for CHF, aortic dissection, lung disease, pneumothorax, etc.
- Echocardiography: may show transient regional wall motion abnormality during ischemia
- Radionuclide scintigraphy: may demonstrate areas of hypoperfusion
- Possible role of EBCT (electron beam computed tomography) is controversial.
- Coronary angiography: gold standard for diagnosis of coronary artery disease; useful in guiding revascularization

SPECIAL TESTS

ECG

- Often normal; evidence of ischemia includes T-wave flattening or inversion, ST segment depression; transient ST elevation may occur, especially with Prinzmetal's angina; prior MI may be evident; important to compare with prior ECG

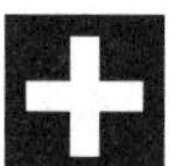

Treatment

GENERAL MEASURES

- Admit to cardiac care unit or telemetry unit depending on severity and acuity of clinical presentation.
- Medical therapy as described below
- Bed rest during initial period of stabilization
- Oxygen if hypoxic
- Low-fat, low-cholesterol diet; low sodium for hypertension, CHF
- Continuous ECG monitoring
- Identify, treat conditions that exacerbate angina: hypoxia, fever, tachycardia, hypertension, anxiety, anemia.
- Consider cardiac catheterization followed by percutaneous or surgical revascularization as needed.
- Identify, treat modifiable risk factors for atherosclerosis.

SURGICAL MEASURES

- Cardiac catheterization, revascularization: generally indicated with angina refractory to medical therapy, left ventricular (LV) dysfunction, postinfarction angina, significant ST deviation during pain; timing, use in lower risk patients controversial
- Intraaortic balloon counterpulsation: effective as bridge to revascularization with medically refractory angina

• Left main coronary artery disease or multivessel coronary artery disease and LV dysfunction: should consider coronary artery bypass surgery; angioplasty usually preferred in one-vessel disease

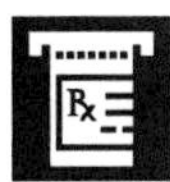

Medications

DRUG(S) OF CHOICE

Antithrombotic Therapy

• Aspirin: 325 mg orally daily
 —First-line antiplatelet agent if no contraindication
• Ticlopidine 250 mg orally b.i.d.; antiplatelet agent useful with aspirin allergy
 —Delayed onset of action
 —Leukopenia, thrombocytopenia, TTP (thrombotic thrombocytopenia purpura) rare side effects; GI upset common
• Clopidogrel: 75 mg orally daily; antiplatelet agent similar to ticlopidine with fewer side effects
 —Leukopenia, thrombocytopenia, TTP far less frequent; not yet studied in unstable angina
• Glycoprotein IIb/IIIa inhibitors: potent platelet antagonists
 —Consider use in high-risk patients (i.e., elevated troponin, marked ST segment abnormalities on ECG, post-MI, or refractory to standard therapy)
 —Contraindications: thrombocytopenia, active bleeding, prior hemorrhagic stroke
• Tirofiban: 10 μg/kg i.v. over 3 minutes then 0.1 μg/kg/min i.v.
 —Eptifibitide 180 μg/kg i.v. bolus then 2 μg/kg/min i.v.; thrombocytopenia infrequent side effect
• Heparin: 80 U/kg i.v. bolus then 18 U/kg i.v. infusion; titrate dose to achieve aPTT (activated partial thromboplastin time) twice the normal level
 —Alternative is low-molecular-weight heparin (enoxaparin, 1 mg/kg s.c. b.i.d.); low-molecular-weight heparin does not require dose titration or PTT monitoring.

Antiischemic Therapy

• Nitrates: 0.2–0.6 mg sublingually (every 5 minutes up to three doses) for acute anginal episodes
 —Topical formulations, long-acting oral nitrates to prevent recurrent angina. Nitrate-free interval of 10–14 h/day necessary to prevent tachyphylaxis
 —Intravenous nitroglycerin (5–10 μg/min titrated up for relief of symptoms) in high-risk patients or with recurrent ischemia
• Beta-blockers: examples are atenolol 25–100 mg orally daily, metoprolol 25–100 mg orally b.i.d.-t.i.d.
 —Titrated as tolerated to achieve heart rate of 50–70 beats/min
 —Use with caution with LV systolic dysfunction, COPD
• Calcium channel blockers do not prevent MI or reduce mortality.
 —Effective in relieving anginal symptoms
 —Use when beta-blockers are contraindicated.
 —Long-acting verapamil 160–480 mg orally daily, diltiazem 90–360 mg orally daily, amlodipine 5–10 mg orally daily preferred
 —Nifedepine and short-acting formulations relatively contraindicated; may increase morbidity, mortality
 —Use diltiazem, verapamil with caution with LV dysfunction
• HMG CoA reductase inhibitors (e.g., simvastatin, lovastatin, atorvastatin) for elevated LDL
• Thrombolytic therapy not indicated in unstable angina

Contraindications

Refer to manufacturer's literature.

Precautions

Refer to manufacturer's literature.

ADMISSION/DISCHARGE CRITERIA

Admission

Most patients with unstable angina should be hospitalized for evaluation.
• Increased risk of death and MI with severe angina at rest or minimal exertion; ECG evidence of ischemia, CHF, or LV dysfunction; and/or abnormal cardiac enzymes warrant admission.
• Selected patients (e.g., new onset of mild exertional angina without indicators of increased risk) may be evaluated with close follow-up as outpatients.

Discharge

• Symptoms well controlled on oral medications
• No CHF, arrhythmia
• Noninvasive testing (exercise or pharmacologic stress test) indicating low risk, or cardiac catheterization performed with definitive therapy as indicated

Follow-up

PATIENT MONITORING

Risk factor modification including:

• Smoking cessation
• Low-fat, low-cholesterol diet
• Regular aerobic exercise
• Lipid-lowering therapy with target LDL of <100 with established coronary artery disease
• Control of hypertension (JNC VI [Joint National Committee on Prevention, Detection, Evaluation, and Treatment of High Blood Pressure, Sixth Report] guidelines)
• Control of diabetes mellitus
• Stress reduction

EXPECTED COURSE AND PROGNOSIS

Prognosis variable

Complications

• Cardiac arrest/sudden death
• Myocardial infarction
• CHF
• Death
• Indicators of high risk include hemodynamic compromise, LV dysfunction, ST segment displacement, elevated cardiac enzymes.

Overall

• Death or MI in 7%–10% within 30 days
• Majority undergo coronary revascularization within 1 year.

PATIENT EDUCATION

Organizations

• American Heart Association, 7320 Greenville Avenue, Dallas, TX 75231. 1-800-AHA-USA1. http://www.amhrt.org.

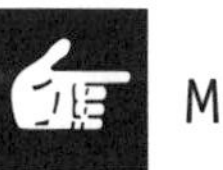

Miscellaneous

ICD-9-CM

411.1 Angina, unstable
413 Angina pectoris
413.1 Prinzmetal's angina
413.9 Angina, unspecified

INTERNET RESOURCE

• Medscape Cardiology, http://cardiology.medscape.com

BIBLIOGRAPHY

Ryan TJ, Antman EM, Brooks NH, et al. 1999 Update: ACC/AHA guidelines for the management of patients with acute myocardial infarction: a report of the American College of Cardiology/American Heart Association Task Force on Practice Guidelines (Committee on Management of Acute Myocardial Infarction). *J Am Coll Cardiol* 1999;34:890–911. Available online at http://www.acc.org/clinical/guidelines.

Theroux P, Fuster V. Acute coronary syndromes: Unstable angina and non Q wave MI. *Circulation* 1998;97:1195–1206.

Theroux P, Waters D. Diagnosis and management of patients with unstable angina. In: Alexander RW, Schlant RC, Fuster V, eds. *The heart,* 9th ed. New York: McGraw-Hill, 1998:1307–1345.

TIMI IIIB Investigators. Effects of tissue plasminogen activator and a comparison of early invasive and conservative strategies in unstable angina and non-Q-wave myocardial infarction: results of the TIMI IIIB trial. *Circulation* 1994;89:1545–1556.

Authors: Stephen J. Dempsey and Nanette K. Wenger

Ankylosing Spondylitis

Basics

DESCRIPTION

Ankylosing spondylitis is a seronegative rheumatic disorder that effects the spine, peripheral joints, and cardiovascular system.

- The aorta in patients with ankylosing spondylitis may become dilated and lead to aortic insufficiency.
- Occasionally, mitral regurgitation results from left ventricular dilation and involvement of the anterior leaflet of the mitral valve.
- Conduction system defects are common and include Wolff-Parkinson-White syndrome and all degrees of atrioventricular (AV) block.
- Left ventricular dysfunction, pericarditis, pericardial effusion, cor pulmonale, aortic arch syndrome, and angina are also described in patients with ankylosing spondylitis.

ETIOLOGY

Genetics

Familial clusterings show a 10- to 20-fold higher incidence of ankylosing spondylitis than the general population. Males are affected 10 times more often than women.

Prevalence

Overall prevalence of ankylosing spondylitis in North American men is 0.2%, with less than 5% of these patients having significant cardiac involvement.

- Up to one-third of the patients with ankylosing spondylitis may have abnormalities noted in the left ventricle by echocardiography, although most are asymptomatic; 10% of patients with ankylosing spondylitis have valvular involvement.
- One-third of patients have abnormalities of the conduction system. Severe left ventricular dysfunction is noted in less than 1% of patients.

Age

Most symptoms occur between the ages of 20 and 40 years.

RISK FACTORS

About 20% of patients with the HLA-B27 develop ankylosing spondylitis.

PREGNANCY

- No contraindication to pregnancy

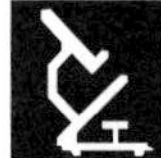

Diagnosis

DIFFERENTIAL DIAGNOSIS

- Rheumatoid arthritis
- Reiter's syndrome
- Systemic lupus erythematosus
- Other causes of aortic insufficiency

SIGNS AND SYMPTOMS

- The most frequent symptom in ankylosing spondylitis is back pain.
- Cardiovascular symptoms include heart failure, shortness of breath, pleuritic chest pain, angina, and syncope.

LABORATORY PROCEDURES

- Erythrocyte sedimentation rate is elevated.
- IgM for rheumatoid factor and antinuclear antibodies are negative.

IMAGING STUDIES

Classic "bamboo spine" on plain film x-ray diagnostic of ankylosing spondylitis.

SPECIAL TESTS

- HLA-B27 phenotype is found in 95% of patients with ankylosing spondylitis.
- There appears to be a correlation to the presence of HLA-B27 antigen and conduction system/valvular disease.

PATHOLOGY

Aorta in ankylosing spondylitis is similar to that seen in syphilis, with adventitial and medial scarring, intimal proliferation, and infiltration of the vaso vasorum with plasma cells and lymphocytes.

- A fibrous commissural bump is often prominent at the aortic valve cusp. The valve cusps shorten and thicken, resulting in regurgitation.
- Fibrosis is common in the conduction system, resulting in the AV conduction abnormalities.

DIAGNOSTICS

- Aortic valve disease generally is diagnosed by finding a diastolic murmur on routine clinical examination.
- Usually, 10–20 years of active ankylosing spondylitis is necessary before aortic valve disease becomes recognized.
- Echocardiography has been used to screen for aortic valve involvement before it becomes clinically important.

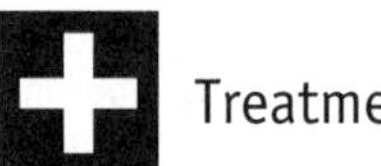

Treatment

GENERAL MEASURES

Aortic insufficiency is treated with afterload reduction.

SURGICAL MEASURES

- Aortic valve replacement may be necessary if aortic insufficiency is symptomatic.
- High-degree heart block may require insertion of a pacemaker.

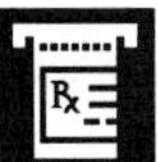

Medications

DRUG(S) OF CHOICE

- Nonsteroidal medications for back and spine pain
- Nifedipine or hydralazine for significant aortic insufficiency

ALTERNATIVE DRUGS

Acetylcholinesterase inhibitors are an acceptable alternative for afterload reduction associated with aortic insufficiency.

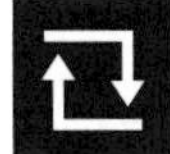

Follow-up

PATIENT MONITORING

Echocardiography is recommended on a yearly basis for aortic insufficiency or when symptoms dictate.

Prevention

Endocarditis prophylaxis is recommended with aortic or mitral valve involvement.

Complications

Endocarditis has been described on the aortic valve as a consequence of ankylosing spondylitis.

EXPECTED COURSE AND PROGNOSIS

Ankylosing spondylitis is generally mild disease with occasional flares. Mortality of patients with ankylosing spondylitis is 80% higher in men at 13 years than age-based controls.

PATIENT EDUCATION

Activity

Activity limited by back and spine discomfort as well as limitation in heart failure symptoms as they develop.

Diet

- Low sodium as symptoms of heart failure develop

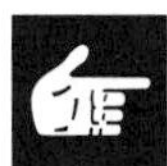

Miscellaneous

SYNONYMS

- Marie-Strumpell Disease

ICD-9-CM

720.0

See also: Aortic Insufficiency, Rheumatoid Arthritis, Heart Block.

BIBLIOGRAPHY

Alexander RW, ed. *Hurst's the heart.* New York: McGraw-Hill, 1998.

Berkrow R, ed. *The Merck manual,* 16th ed. Rahway, NJ: Merck Research Laboratories, 1992.

Braunwald E, ed. *Heart disease: a textbook of cardiovascular medicine,* 5th ed. Philadelphia: WB Saunders, 1997.

Topol EJ, ed. *Textbook of cardiovascular medicine.* Philadelphia: Lippincott-Raven, 1998.

Authors: Steven Herrmann, Amr El-Shafei, Madhukar Gupta, and Bernard R. Chaitman

Anomalous Coronary Arteries

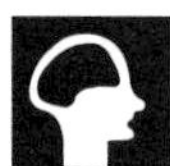

Basics

DEFINITION

Anomalous coronary arteries include abnormal anatomy, origin, course, and/or termination of coronary arteries.

Normal Coronary Anatomy

- Left and right main coronary arteries arise from corresponding aortic sinuses.
- Left main coronary artery (LMCA) divides into left anterior descending and left circumflex, which supply the left ventricular free wall.
- Right coronary artery (RCA) is dominant in 90% of humans. It gives rise to the posterior descending coronary artery, which supplies the posterior interventricular septum, inferior left ventricle, and atrioventricular (AV) node.

ETIOLOGY

Predominantly congenital in origin, they can occur in isolation or in association with other intracardiac malformations.

EPIDEMIOLOGY

Incidence

Anomalies of Coronary Arterial Origin

- Pulmonary arterial origin
  —Anomalous LMCA from pulmonary artery (ALCAPA): 1 in 300,000 live births and 0.5% of all congenital heart disease
  —Origin of RCA or left anterior descending or left circumflex arteries from pulmonary artery
- Origin from inappropriate sinus
  —LMCA from right sinus of Valsalva: 1%–3% of all major coronary anomalies
  —RCA from left sinus of Valsalva: 30% of all major coronary anomalies
  —Left circumflex coronary from RCA: one-third of all major coronary arterial anomalies
  —Single coronary artery arising from a single ostium: 5%–20% of all coronary anomalies

Anomalies of Coronary Artery Termination

- 0.2%–0.4% of all congenital cardiac anomalies and 50% of congenital coronary anomalies
- These include coronary-cameral fistulas (connection between a coronary artery and a cardiac chamber) and coronary arteriovenous fistulas (between coronary artery and coronary sinus, superior vena cava or pulmonary artery).

Anomalies Intrinsic to the Coronary Artery

- Coronary artery aneurysm: congenital or acquired (atherosclerosis, associated with coronary-cameral fistulas, Kawasaki disease, infectious, or traumatic)
- Congenital LCA stenosis or atresia
- Congenital coronary artery hypoplasia
- Myocardial bridges (muscle bridge overlying an epicardial artery) and coronary arterial loops (extreme coiling of the coronary arteries)

Coronary Artery Anomalies Associated with Congenital Heart Disease

- Most commonly seen with tetralogy of Fallot, D- and L-transposition of great arteries, truncus arteriosus, pulmonary atresia, and univentricular hearts

CLINICAL MANIFESTATIONS

Many coronary anomalies are not clinically significant. Serious abnormalities may present with one of the following profiles.

- Anomalous left coronary artery from pulmonary artery: As pulmonary resistance decreases in postnatal life, perfusion pressure decreases, collaterals develop between RCA and LCA, and there may be a pulmonary-coronary steal.
  —Almost 90% of patients with this anomaly present in infancy with episodes of myocardial ischemia, mitral insufficiency with symptoms of congestive heart failure (CHF) (irritability, feeding difficulties, poor weight gain, diaphoresis, respiratory distress). Untreated, 65%–85% die of intractable CHF in the first year of life (infantile type).
  —Some present in later childhood or as young adults with angina of effort or CHF due to mitral incompetence (adult type).
  —15% remain asymptomatic, possibly because of extensive collaterals and a restrictive opening at the origin of the LCA.
  —Anomalous RCA from pulmonary artery: rare, only one-tenth as common as ALCAPA, mostly asymptomatic; occasional cases of syncope, angina, CHF or sudden death may occur, usually during adolescence or young adulthood
  —Anomalous LCA from right sinus of Valsalva: a rare lesion but significantly associated with sudden cardiac death in children and adolescents
  —Common presenting symptoms are syncope, presyncope or chest pain with exercise.
  —Patients in whom the anomalous artery courses between the aorta and pulmonary artery (53%) are at greatest risk for exercise-induced sudden death due to myocardial ischemia secondary to the slitlike ostium or compression of the coronary artery between the aortic and pulmonary roots as they distend during exercise.
- RCA from left sinus of Valsalva: may present with myocardial ischemia, infarction, or sudden death
- Single coronary artery: mostly asymptomatic, except with atherosclerotic occlusion of the artery
- Congenital coronary artery aneurysm, congenital LCA stenosis, or atresia: usually present with symptoms of myocardial ischemia with exercise
- Coronary arteriovenous fistulas: Physiology and presentation depend on the size and location of the shunt. Most patients under 20 years of age are asymptomatic; the majority over 20 years become symptomatic with dyspnea on exertion, fatigue, angina, and palpitations. Most have only small left to right shunts.
  —Fistulas most often occur (in order of frequency) in the right ventricle, right atrium, and pulmonary artery. They also may drain into the left ventricle, left atrium, coronary sinus, or superior vena cava.
  —Complications: CHF, fistula rupture, infective endocarditis, myocardial infarction, aneurysm formation, death

Physical Findings

- Signs of CHF including hepatomegaly, rales, respiratory distress, left ventricular gallop and holosystolic murmur of mitral insufficiency.
- Continuous murmur in patients with coronary arteriovenous fistula or adult type ALCAPA with collaterals
- Mitral regurgitation secondary to papillary muscle infarction in ALCAPA
- Findings of associated congenital heart defects

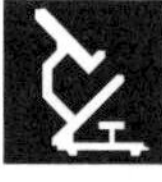

Diagnosis

DIFFERENTIAL DIAGNOSIS

- ALCAPA is most often misdiagnosed as cardiomyopathy or myocarditis because of failure to identify the anomalous coronary artery.
- Every attempt must be made to define coronary artery anatomy in any young patient presenting with apparent cardiomyopathy or unexplained heart failure.

IMAGING STUDIES

ECG

- Resting ECG may be abnormal in symptomatic patients with evidence of myocardial ischemia (ST-T changes), ventricular hypertrophy, and arrhythmias depending on type and location of coronary artery abnormalities.
- Anterolateral infarct in an infant (i.e., abnormal Q waves in leads I, aVL, and precordial leads V4-6 and abnormal R waves or R-wave progression in the left precordial leads) is highly suggestive of ALCAPA in an infant.

Exercise Stress Test

• May uncover ischemia due to underlying coronary anomaly, but is not always conclusive

Echocardiography

Echocardiogram can diagnose most cases. Coronary anatomy is best visualized in the parasternal long, short, and high short-axis views. Echocardiographic features include the following:

• Abnormal attachment of the origin of the coronary artery (in more than one view to avoid problems due to lateral dropout)
• Doppler color-flow mapping showing flow away from the coronary artery into the pulmonary artery indicates ALCAPA.
• A dilated coronary artery on two-dimensional echo should prompt a search for anomalous coronaries, e.g., ALCAPA (dilated RCA) or coronary arteriovenous fistula (dilated proximal portion of the coronary artery that feeds the fistula).
• Intrinsic coronary artery abnormalities like aneurysm, stenosis, atresia, hypoplasia, fistulas
• Chamber dilation secondary to shunting across large coronary fistula
• Abnormalities of left ventricular size and function (i.e., enlarged left atrium and ventricle, diminished left ventricular function, global or regional wall motion abnormalities, endocardial fibroelastosis, and mitral regurgitation), especially in patients with ALCAPA
• Associated congenital intracardiac anomalies and other causes of heart failure (e.g., cardiomyopathy)

Cardiac Catheterization and Angiocardiography

• Remains the gold standard for diagnosis of most coronary anomalies. Injection of contrast into the aortic root and, in cases of anomalous origin, into the pulmonary artery can identify coronary abnormalities.

Other Imaging Modalities

• Ultrafast CT with 3-D reconstruction and MRI may occasionally be useful in defining coronary anomalies.
• Chest x-ray may show cardiomegaly, pulmonary edema in patients with CHF, and abnormal cardiac silhouette in cases of large aneurysm.

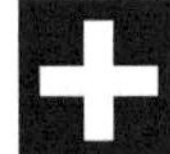

Treatment

GENERAL MEASURES

• Medical treatment is usually supportive.
• Treatment of CHF and arrhythmias to stabilize the patient with left ventricular dysfunction prior to surgery
• Oral anticoagulation (aspirin, warfarin) in patients with aneurysms
• Infective endocarditis prophylaxis

SURGICAL MEASURES

Corrective surgery is the treatment of choice for most coronary anomalies.

Indications for Surgery

• ALCAPA should be repaired urgently once diagnosis is made.
• Anomalies that are associated with significant morbidity and mortality if left untreated should be repaired once diagnosis is made regardless of symptoms (e.g., anomalous LCA from right coronary sinus, large coronary aneurysms, coronary arteriovenous fistulas).
• As part of surgical repair of associated congenital heart defects. Failure to recognize an anomalous coronary artery may result in the artery being injured at surgery or inadequate myocardial protection when cardioplegia is given directly into the major coronary arteries.

Surgical Options

• Anomalous LCA or RCA
  —Direct aortic reimplantation of the anomalous coronary artery (with a button of pulmonary artery around origin) provides the most physiologic repair and is the procedure of choice. The surgical mortality rate is less than 15%. Short-term use of left ventricular assist device in the immediate postoperative period may assist recovery.
  —Alternatives include creation of an intrapulmonary baffle or tunnel (Takeuchi procedure).
  —Most often there is excellent recovery of normal or near-normal left ventricular function and regression of mitral insufficiency, usually within 6 to 24 months of corrective surgery.
• Ligation of aneurysm, aneurysmorrhaphy, aneurysmectomy with interposition of graft
• Coronary artery bypass grafting for coronary stenosis or atresia
• Surgical ligation or transcatheter closure of coronary AV fistulas.

Follow-up

PATIENT MONITORING

• Asymptomatic patients with mild abnormalities should be regularly followed for development of symptoms or electrocardiographic or echocardiographic evidence of progression of lesion (e.g., enlarging aneurysm, chamber enlargement secondary to fistula, thromboembolism).
• According to AHA guidelines, patients with large coronary aneurysms secondary to Kawasaki disease should be followed with serial echoes and exercise stress testing every 6 months to a year.
• Angiography may be required.

PATIENT EDUCATION

• Infective endocarditis prophylaxis for dental and invasive procedures
• Avoid competitive sports for patients with residual coronary artery dysfunction.

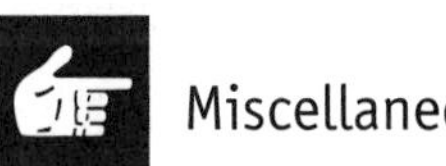

Miscellaneous

ABBREVIATIONS

LMCA, left main coronary artery
RCA, right coronary artery
ALCAPA, anomalous left main coronary artery from pulmonary artery
CHF, congestive heart failure

BIBLIOGRAPHY

Emmanouilides GC, Riemenschneider TA, Allen HD, et al. *Heart disease in infants, children and adolescents,* 5th ed. Baltimore: Williams & Wilkins, 1995.

Garson A, Bricker JT, Fisher DJ, et al. *The science and practice of pediatric cardiology,* 2nd ed. Baltimore: Williams & Wilkins, 1998.

Snider RA, Serwer GA, Ritter SB. *Echocardiography in pediatric heart disease,* 2nd ed. St. Louis: CV Mosby, 1997.

Authors: Seema Mital and Welton M. Gersony

Anomalous Pulmonary Venous Connections, Total

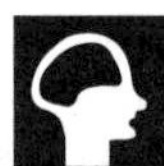

Basics

DESCRIPTION

Total anomalous pulmonary venous connection is a condition in which the pulmonary veins drain to a common pulmonary vein (CPV) that does not connect to the left atrium.

- The CPV drains into one or more alternate channels (embryonic cardinal veins), which eventually reach the right atrium.
- Systemic blood flow is maintained by right-to-left blood flow across a foramen ovale or atrial septal defect to the left atrium.
- If the channels returning blood from the CPV to the systemic venous system are obstructed, a neonate presents with the picture of severe left heart obstruction (e.g., mitral stenosis).
- If obstruction is mild, then the infant will present later with high pulmonary blood flow, pulmonary hypertension, and congestive heart failure.
- With no obstruction, a patient may present later in childhood with the clinical profile of a large atrial septal defect.
- Total anomalous pulmonary venous connections (TAPVCs) are classified as:
  —Supracardiac (55%): retrograde blood flow from CPV to left superior vena cava (vertical vein) to innominate vein to the superior vena cava (SVC) to the right atrium (RA); or less commonly, CPV direct to right SVC
  —Intracardiac (30%): CPV to left SVC to coronary sinus
  —Infradiaphragmatic (13%): CPV to inferior cardinal vein to portal system to liver to inferior vena cava (IVC) to RA
  —Mixed (connections at two or more levels) (2%)

EPIDEMIOLOGY

Incidence

In autopsy series the incidence of TAPVCs varies from 1% to 5% of congenital heart disease.

ETIOLOGY

Genetics

There are limited data.

- The possibility of small chromosome translocations, or a single autosomal gene mutation has been raised.
- There may be a multifactorial inheritance pattern.

RISK FACTORS

N/A

PREGNANCY

Pregnancy should be well tolerated, following successful repair in childhood.

ASSOCIATED CONDITIONS

- Two-thirds of TAPVCs exist as isolated lesions with an atrial communication.
- One-third are associated with other congenital heart lesions
  —Single ventricle
  —Patent ductus arteriosus
  —Truncus arteriosus
  —Atrioventricular canal
  —Hypoplastic left heart syndrome (HLHS)
  —Transposition of the great vessels
  —Pulmonary stenosis and/or atresia
  —Heterotaxy syndrome with anomalies of the atriovisceral situs: asplenia, right isomerism
  —Absent morphologic left atrium and thus virtually always associated with TAPVCs via confluence to the right atrium, or right or left superior vena cava
  —Associated noncardiac malformations include abdominal visceral heterotaxy, malrotation of the gastrointestinal tract, and bilateral right lungs

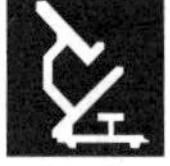

Diagnosis

DIFFERENTIAL DIAGNOSIS

- Newborn
  —Hypoplastic left heart syndrome
  —Interrupted aortic arch or severe coarctation of the aorta
  —Hypoplastic right heart syndromes (tricuspid and pulmonary atresia)
  —Transposition of the great arteries
  —Pulmonary vein stenosis or pulmonary vein atresia
  —Cor triatriatum
  —Persistent pulmonary hypertension of the newborn (PPHN)
  —Respiratory distress syndrome or hyaline membrane disease
- In older infants and children
  —Large atrial septal defect
  —Common atrium
  —Partial anomalous pulmonary venous return

SIGNS AND SYMPTOMS

- Infants with severe obstruction of TAPVC
  —Present with cyanosis and/or respiratory distress shortly after birth or within the first few days of life.
  —Obstruction usually occurs at the connection of the pulmonary venous channel to the systemic venous system (e.g., portal vein, innominate vein, SVC, etc.), rarely at the atrial septum.
  —In the infradiaphragmatic type, severe obstruction is usual, but also may occur with supracardiac connections, especially when the common pulmonary vein connects directly to the right superior vena cava.
- With mild to moderate obstruction, the patient presents later in the first month or two of life with symptoms of heart failure:
  —Dyspnea
  —Difficulty feeding
  —Failure to thrive
  —Cyanosis with saturation of 80%–85%
- Non-obstructed TAPVC patients may escape detection in infancy and present later in childhood, similar to atrial septal defect. Such patients may be asymptomatic.

PHYSICAL EXAMINATION

- Loud murmurs are infrequent, Grade 1 or 2 short systolic pulmonic flow murmurs can occur
- S2 may be loud
- Pulses normal
- Blood pressure generally is normal. In the presence of severe pulmonary venous obstruction or a restrictive atrial communication in a neonate, there is decreased systemic output and low blood pressure.
- Hepatomegaly

LABORATORY PROCEDURES

Oximetry: Arterial oxygen saturation is often reduced to 85%–90%; lower with obstruction. The umbilical venous saturation may be as high (90%–100%), with infradiaphragmatic TAPVC to the portal system.

IMAGING TESTS

Radiography

- Chest x-ray with pulmonary venous obstruction
  —Evidence of a ground-glass appearance with a diffuse linear reticular pattern or pulmonary edema associated with Kerley B lines
  —Heart size is normal or small.
- Chest x-ray without severe pulmonary venous obstruction
  —Heart is enlarged.
  —Pulmonary vascular markings are increased.
  —Supracardiac type may have a "snowman" appearance with TAPVCs to the SVC via a vertical vein to the left innominate vein. This configuation may be obscured by thymus.

Echocardiography

Should be diagnostic for all types of TAPVCs with demonstration of the pulmonary venous confluence draining to the:

- Vertical vein (left SVC) to the left inominate vein, which drains to the right SVC and RA.
- Right SVC
- Coronary sinus or RA
- Portal system or to hepatic sinusoids below the diaphragm

MRI

Multiplane gated MRI in older patients can be useful if transthoracic or transesophageal echocardiography is not diagnostic.

Cardiac Catheterization

- Generally not needed in the newborn period. 2-D echo, Doppler, and Doppler color studies are most often definitive.
- In the presence of pulmonary venous obstruction below the diaphragm, cardiac catheterization may delay surgical treatment and increase morbidity.
- May be necessary to evaluate associated cardiac or pulmonary disease
- Urgent balloon septostomy may be useful in rare cases when the atrial communication is restrictive, and surgery must be delayed.

SPECIAL TESTS

- ECG
  —Right ventricular hypertophy: QR in V3R or V1 or pure R waves in V3R are often present. Upright T waves in V1 and V3R are consistent with systemic pressure in the right ventricle.
  —Left ventricular forces may be decreased.

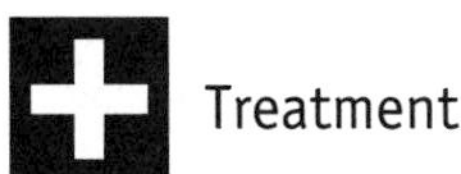

Treatment

GENERAL MEASURES

- Infants with cyanosis or respiratory distress may require ventilator support.
  —Prostaglandin E_1 0.03–0.1 μg/kg/min i.v. may be required to maintain patency of the ductus arteriosus and thus maintain cardiac output.
  —All types of TAPVCs are generally surgically corrected in the newborn period soon after diagnosis.

SURGICAL MEASURES

- Establish connection of confluence of pulmonary veins (CPV) to the left atrium utilizing a generous left atrial anastomosis, usually with pericardial augmentation, as well as ligation of the common vertical vein.
- With prompt surgical intervention, mortality is low, especially with supracardiac and cardiac types.

ADMISSION/DISCHARGE CRITERIA

Any patient diagnosed with a condition with or without obstruction should undergo surgical repair.

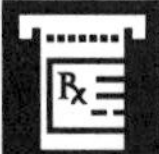

Medications

DRUG(S) OF CHOICE

- Prostaglandin E_1 to maintain patency of ductus arteriosus
- Diuretics and inotropics in the presence of pulmonary venous congestion and obstruction
- Possible use of nitric oxide in the presence of severe pulmonary artery hypertension

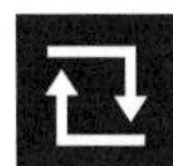

Follow-up

EXPECTED COURSE AND PROGNOSIS

- Long-term postoperative survival of isolated TAPVCs usually is excellent. Early or late postoperative problems could include:
  —Obstruction at the anastomotic site or proximal within the pulmonary veins
  —Obstruction of intrapulmonary venules, causing pulmonary hypertension
- Clinically important atrial arrhythmias may develop in some patients, including sinus bradycardia, supraventricular tachycardia, atrial flutter, and sinus node dysfunction. Ventricular arrhythmias are rare.

PATIENT MONITORING

Postoperatively patients should be monitored for:

- Early and late signs of pulmonary venous congestion and/or obstruction
- Rhythm disturbances
- Pulmonary hypertension

PATIENT EDUCATION

- Full activities and a regular diet appropriate for age
- Patients should be followed by clinicians in a pediatric cardiology or adult congenital heart program.

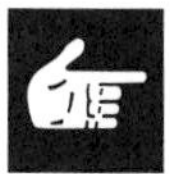

Miscellaneous

ICD-9-CM

747.41

BIBLIOGRAPHY

Freedom RM, Benson LN, Smallhorn JF. *Neonatal heart disease.* New York: Springer-Verlag, 1992.

Freedom RM, Mawson JB, Yoo S, et al. *Congenital heart disease—textbook of angiocardiology.* New York: Futura, 1997.

Garson A Jr, Bricker JT, Fisher DJ, et al. *The science and practice of pediatric cardiology,* 2nd ed. Baltimore: Williams & Wilkins, 1998.

Moss AJ, Adams FH, Emmanouilides GC. *Heart disease in infants, children and adolescents,* 2nd ed. Baltimore: Williams & Wilkins, 1977.

Stark J, deLeval M. *Surgery for congenital heart defects.* New York: Grune & Stratton, 1983.

Authors: Rubin S. Cooper and Welton M. Gersony

Anorexia Nervosa and the Heart

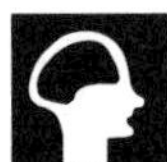

Basics

DESCRIPTION

Refusal to maintain body weight (85% of expected weight), or significant weight loss; intense fear of gaining weight or becoming fat; disturbance in the way in which one's body shape is experienced; in postmenarcheal females, amenorrhea (not due to physical disease)

Several Systems Affected

- Endocrine, GI, metabolic, hematologic, immunologic, dermatologic, cardiovascular, psychiatric

Cardiac Complications

- Arrhythmias, bradycardia, ECG abnormalities, hypotension, left ventricular dysfunction, mitral valve motion irregularities, reduced work capacity, refeeding cardiomyopathy

EPIDEMIOLOGY

Anorexia nervosa occurs in 0.2%–1.3% of the general population, approximately 1% of women. Predominantly affects females during adolescence and young adulthood.

ETIOLOGY

Etiology of anorexia nervosa is unknown, but likely multifactorial (sociocultural, psychological, familial, and genetic factors).

- Some cardiac abnormalities are common adaptations to starvation (bradycardia, low blood pressure).
- Myofibrillar destruction is associated with protein caloric malnutrition.
- Refeeding syndrome is multifactorial in origin and may be the result of restoring of circulatory volume while left ventricular (LV) mass is still reduced.
- Leads to fluid retention; if this is severe, patient may develop CHF.

RISK FACTORS

Perfectionistic personality, compulsivity, low self-esteem, high self-expectations, ambivalence about dependence/independence, stress caused by multiple responsibilities, weight dissatisfaction. Starvation-induced hypophosphatemia, hypokalemia, and hypomagnesemia are risk factors for the refeeding syndrome.

PREGNANCY

- Rare due to amenorrhea

ASSOCIATED CONDITIONS

- Major depression or dysthymia in 50%–70% of patients; obsessive-compulsive disorder in 10% of patients

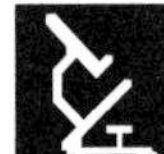

Diagnosis

DIFFERENTIAL DIAGNOSIS

- Depression with loss of appetite
- Inanition due to physical disorder
- Schizophrenia
- Conversion disorder
- Endocrine disorder (hypo- or hyperthyroidism, Addison's disease, diabetes mellitus, panhypopituitarism)
- GI disorders (celiac disease, Crohn's disease, parasitosis)
- Infectious disease (AIDS, tuberculosis, chronic infection)
- Cardiovascular disease (other causes of cardiomyopathy, such as idiopathic, viral, hypertensive, Chagas' disease, rheumatic fever, etc.)
- Malignancy

SIGNS AND SYMPTOMS

- General
  - —Patient is emaciated.
  - —Skin is dry with excessive growth of downy hair.
  - —Skin also may be yellowish due to carotenodermia.
  - —Brittle nails
  - —Thinning scalp hair
  - —Hypothermia
- Cardiovascular
  - —Bradycardia and hypotension are common.
  - —Peripheral edema may be present.

LABORATORY PROCEDURES

- No specific test for anorexia
- Findings related to starvation
  - —Leukopenia, thrombocytopenia, anemia, reduced erythrocyte sedimentation rate, reduced complement levels, low CD4/CD8
  - —Metabolic alkalosis, hypocalcemia, hypokalemia, hypomagnesemia, hypophosphatemia, hypercholesterolemia
  - —Endocrine abnormalities: decreased follicle-stimulating hormone, luteinizing hormone, T4, T3, and estrogens; increased cortisol, growth hormone
  - —Diminished blood urea nitrogen, creatinine clearance
  - —Flat glucose tolerance curve

IMAGING STUDIES

- Transthoracic echocardiogram: mitral valve prolapse, reduced cardiac indices, reduced LV mass, impairment of LV filling

SPECIAL TESTS

- ECG: low voltage, T-wave inversions, nonspecific ST-segment depression, prolonged QT intervals (rare)

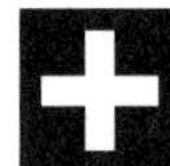

Treatment

GENERAL MEASURES

- A multidisciplinary approach (psychological, medical, and nutritional support) is needed.
- A goal weight should be set and the patient should be initially monitored at least once a week.
- Weight gain should be gradual (1–3 lb/wk) to avoid precipitating congestive heart failure.
- Strategies to avoid refeeding syndrome
  - —Identify patients at risk (chronically malnourished or has not eaten for 7 days).
  - —Measure serum electrolyte level and correct abnormalities before refeeding.
  - —Obtain serum chemistry values every other day for the first 7–10 days, then weekly during remainder of refeeding.
  - —Slowly increase daily caloric intake every 3–4 days.
  - —Monitor patient carefully for development of tachycardia and edema.

SURGICAL MEASURES

N/A

ADMISSION/DISCHARGE CRITERIA

Hospitalization is recommended in the following situations:

- Severe dehydration or electrolyte imbalance.
- ECG abnormalities (prolonged QT interval, arrhythmias)
- Significant hemodynamic instability (hypotension, orthostatic changes)

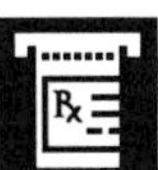

Medications

DRUG(S) OF CHOICE

- Pharmacologic treatment has no role in anorexia nervosa unless major depression or another psychiatric disorder is present.
- Congestive heart failure due to volume overload is treated conventionally (diuretics and vasodilators).

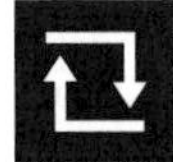

Follow-up

PATIENT MONITORING

- Electrolyte levels, especially during refeeding
- Routine ECG monitoring, especially in patients with prolonged QT interval

EXPECTED COURSES AND PROGNOSIS

- Short-term prognosis is good if a strict program is followed but long-term prognosis is less favorable.
- Approximately 20% make a full recovery, 20% remain chronically ill, and 60% have recurrent episodes.
- Mortality rate 5%
  - —Causes of death: suicide, electrolyte abnormalities, sudden death, starvation

PATIENT EDUCATION

For patient education materials, contact Anorexia Nervosa & Related Eating Disorders, P.O. Box 5102, Eugene, OR 97405, (503)344-1144; National Association of Anorexia Nervosa and Associated Disorders (ANAD), P.O. Box 7, Highland Park, IL 60035, (708)831-3438.

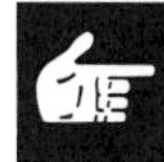

Miscellaneous

ICD-9-CM

307.1 Anorexia nervosa

BIBLIOGRAPHY

de Simone G, et al. Cardiac abnormalities in young women with anorexia nervosa. *Br Heart J* 1994;7:287.

Goroll AH, May LA, Mulley AG, eds. *Primary care medicine,* 3rd edition. Philadelphia: Lippincott-Raven, 1995.

Mehler P. Eating disorders: anorexia nervosa. *Hosp Pract* 1996;31:109–113.

Schocken D, et al. Weight loss and the heart: effects of anorexia nervosa and starvation. *Arch Intern Med* 1989;149:877–881.

Author: Maria Cecilia Bahit

Antiphospholipid Antibody Syndrome

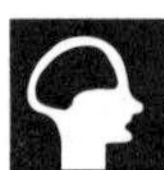

Basics

DESCRIPTION

Clinical constellation of venous and arterial thrombosis, recurrent fetal loss, or both in association with persistent antiphospholipid (aPL) antibodies, either lupus anticoagulant or anticardiolipin antibodies

- Primary aPL syndrome
  - —No evidence of underlying disease.
- Secondary aPL syndrome
  - —In rheumatic and connective tissue disorders [systemic lupus erythematosus (SLE), less commonly rheumatoid arthritis, systemic sclerosis]
  - —In infections (HIV-1, varicella, hepatitis C), in lymphoproliferative diseases, and in drug exposure
- Cardiac manifestations
  - —Valvular disease
  - —Nonbacterial vegetations, valvular thickening, mitral (mainly affected) and aortic insufficiency, and fibrocalcific changes
  - —Pericardial effusion
  - —Myocardial dysfunction
  - —Coronary artery disease: myocardial infarction (MI) in young patients, graft failure after coronary artery bypass grafting
  - —Intracardiac thrombosis
  - —Pulmonary hypertension

EPIDEMIOLOGY

- Young patients (under 45 years)
- aPL antibodies are found in approximately 10% of patients with thromboembolic events.
- Different estimates of aPL antibodies are related to the sensitivity of diverse assays.

ETIOLOGY

- The precise cause of thrombosis is unknown.
- Proposed mechanisms: Inhibition of the protein C pathway, inactivation of factors Va–VIIa, inhibition of antithrombin III activation, impaired fibrinolysis, enhanced platelet activation, Factor Xa generation
- Coronary artery disease due to thrombotic occlusion, early atherosclerosis associated with long-term steroid administration and, less frequently, coronary arteritis
- Cardiomyopathy is associated with thrombotic occlusion of myocardial microcirculation.

Genetics

aPL-positive families exist (association with HLA DR7, DR4, and DQw7 plus DRW53).

RISK FACTORS

- Smoking, atherosclerosis disease, hypertension, long-term steroid administration

PREGNANCY

- Associated with obstetric complications: recurrent fetal loss, intrauterine growth retardation, and preeclampsia

ASSOCIATED CONDITIONS

- Primary aPL syndrome
  - —No evidence of underlying disease
- Secondary aPL syndrome
  - —In rheumatic and connective tissue disorders (SLE, less commonly rheumatoid arthritis, systemic sclerosis)
  - —In infections (HIV-1, varicella, hepatitis C)
  - —In lymphoproliferative diseases
  - —In drug exposure (phenothiazine, chlorpromazine, procainamide, quinine, and quinidine)
  - —Acute alcoholic intoxication

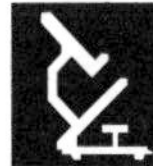

Diagnosis

DIFFERENTIAL DIAGNOSIS

- Patients with thrombosis also should be evaluated for hypercoagulable conditions: deficiencies of protein C, protein S, antithrombin III, and plasminogen resistance.
- Coronary artery disease, atherosclerotic MI
- Atrial myxoma
- Infective endocarditis
- Valvular disease

SIGNS AND SYMPTOMS

- Asymptomatic
- Chest pain and/or shortness of breath
- Aortic or mitral murmurs (due to valve involvement)
- If pulmonary hypertension: right ventricle lift, increased pulmonic second sound
- Acute MI
- Venous or arterial thrombosis
- Stroke, transient ischemic attacks, multiple cerebral infarcts (more frequent in patients with valve abnormalities)
- Peripheral arterial disease
- Pulmonary thromboembolism

LABORATORY PROCEDURES

- Thrombocytopenia (50% of patients)
- Other cytopenias may be associated: autoimmune hemolytic anemia and leukopenia.
- Platelet dysfunction
- Prothrombin time normal or prolonged
- aPTT prolonged
- Plasma clot time prolonged
- Anticardiolipin antibody (IgM and/or IgG) ELISA
- Lupus anticoagulant: sensitive aPTT, the Russell viper venom time, and the kaolin clotting time
- If prolongation of one of these is observed, confirmation requires demonstration of an inhibitor and demonstration of phospholipid dependence
- Anticardiolipin antibody (IgM and/or IgG) ELISA
- False-positive VDRL test result

IMAGING STUDIES

Echocardiography (2-D and Doppler)

- Valve thickening
- Vegetations (Libman-Sacks): particularly in the ventricular surface of the mitral valve, typically sessile, wartlike, and small, firmly attached to the valve surface and showing no independent motion
- Atrial thrombi
- Ventricular enlargement, myocardial dysfunction
- Mitral regurgitation, aortic regurgitation (less frequently)
- Pulmonary artery pressure
- Pericardial effusion

SPECIAL TESTS

- ECG: Myocardial infarction or ischemia

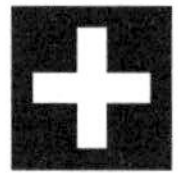

Treatment

GENERAL MEASURES

- Avoid or treat any other risk factor, such as hypertension, hypercholesterolemia, and avoidance of smoking and sedentarism.
- Patients with significant thrombotic events are appropriate candidates for long-term treatment with warfarin (INR >3).
- Treatment of asymptomatic patients with aPLS (antiphospholipid antibody syndrome) has not been defined, because only 10%–15% will develop life-threatening events.

SURGICAL MEASURES

Consider valve replacement according to severity and symptoms.

ADMISSION/DISCHARGE CRITERIA

Consider hospitalization in life-threatening thromboembolic events.

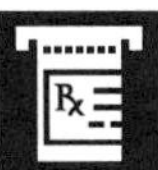

Medications

DRUG(S) OF CHOICE

- Anticoagulants
  —Unfractionated heparin
  —Low-molecular-weight heparins, such as enoxaparin (1 mg/kg s.c. every 12 hours), obviate the need for laboratory monitoring.
  —Oral anticoagulants (warfarin) on a long-term basis, if INR >3.
- Aspirin
  —Uncertain, but recommended as prophylaxis in asymptomatic patients
- Corticosteroid
  —Uncertain; reserved for treatment of underlying comorbid conditions such as active lupus
- Immunosuppressive agents: uncertain

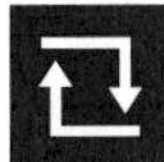

Follow-up

PATIENT MONITORING

Monitor INR in patients on warfarin regularly (INR goal >3).

EXPECTED COURSE AND PROGNOSIS

- Only 10%–15% of asymptomatic patients with aPL antibodies will develop life-threatening thromboembolic events.
- Patients receiving oral anticoagulants have had no recurrence over 8 years; patients in whom this drug has been discontinued have had a 50% probability of recurrent thromboembolic episodes after 2 years.
- Catastrophic aPL syndrome has been reported in a small number of cases, including renal dysfunction, cerebrovascular disease, myocardial infarction, and hypertension. This syndrome is fatal.

PATIENT EDUCATION

N/A

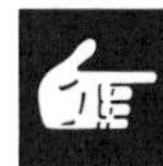

Miscellaneous

ICD-9-CM

286.5 Hemorrhagic disorder due to circulating anticoagulant

BIBLIOGRAPHY

Asherson R, Cervera R. Cardiac manifestations of the antiphospholipid syndrome. *Coronary Artery Dis* 1993;4:1137–1143.

Greaves M. Antiphospholipid antibodies and thrombosis. *Lancet* 1999;353:1348–1358.

Hughes G. The antiphospholipid syndrome: Ten years on. *Lancet* 1993;342:341–344.

Kaplan S, et al. Cardiac manifestations of the antiphospholipid syndrome. *Am Heart J* 1992;124:1331–1338.

Koopman WJ, ed. *Arthritis and allied conditions: a textbook of rheumatology,* 13th ed. Philadelphia: Lippincott Williams & Wilkins, 1997.

Wendell W, Azzudin G, et al. International consensus statement on preliminary classification criteria for definite antiphospholipid syndrome: report of an international workshop. *Arthritis Rheumatism* 1999;42:1309–1311.

Author: Maria Cecilia Bahit

Aortic Aneurysm

Basics

DESCRIPTION

Localized dilatation of the aorta with a diameter at least 1.5 times that of the normal diameter of that segment

- Morphologically, fusiform (symmetrical dilatation) or saccular (localized outpouching)
- The majority are located in the abdominal aorta.
- Thoracic aortic aneursyms (TAAs) are classified according to location:
  - —Aortic root/ascending aorta (most frequent)
  - —Transverse aortic arch
  - —Traumatic, usually distal to left subclavian artery
  - —Descending thoracic aorta
  - —Thoracoabdominal aorta

EPIDEMIOLOGY

Abdominal aortic aneurysms (AAAs) are much more common than are TAAs.

Prevalence

- At least 3% of persons over the age of 50 in the United States

Sex

- Male:female 9:1

Incidence

- Increases rapidly after 55 years of age in men and 70 years in women
- Has increased threefold from 8.7/100,000 person-years in 1951–1960 to 36.5/100,000 person-years in 1971–1980

ETIOLOGY

Genetics

- AAAs
  - —Atherosclerosis
  - —Genetic predisposition: 28% of patients with AAAs have a first-degree relative similarly affected.
- TAAs
  - —Atherosclerosis (arch, descending aorta)
  - —Connective tissue disorder or cystic medial necrosis: most commonly Marfan's syndrome (ascending aorta), also Ehlers-Danlos syndrome
  - —Inflammatory disease: granulomatous, giant cell arteritis, Takayasu's arteritis
  - —Syphilis (now rare)
  - —Aortic dissection
  - —Aortic trauma
  - —Infectious: often secondary to direct spread from aortic bacterial endocarditis

RISK FACTORS

- Increased age
- Atherosclerotic disease
- Hypertension
- Hypercholesterolemia
- Smoking
- Aortic dissection
- Connective tissue disorders

PREGNANCY

When aneurysms are present during pregnancy, they typically do so with rupture and shock; mortality rate is 65%.

ASSOCIATED CONDITIONS

- Aortic dissection
- Aortic rupture
- Annuloaortic ectasia
  - —Condition seen in a subset of patients with TAA in whom idiopathic dilatation of the proximal aorta and aortic annulus leads to pure aortic regurgitation

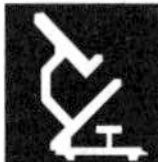

Diagnosis

DIFFERENTIAL DIAGNOSIS

- In AAAs, renal colic, musculoskeletal pain, GI disorder
- In TAAs, congestive heart failure from other causes, musculoskeletal back pain, primary lung process, bronchogenic carcinoma, mediastinal tumor

SIGNS AND SYMPTOMS

Abdominal Aortic Aneurysms

- Majority asymptomatic, often incidentally discovered.
- Most common symptoms:
  - —Hypogastric pain
  - —Low back pain
- Most common signs:
  - —Palpable, pulsatile abdominal mass (occasionally tender)
  - —Abdominal bruit
  - —Diminished femoral/distal pulses

Thoracic Aortic Aneurysms

- 40% are asymptomatic (including traumatic thoracic aneurysms, in which patients often remain asymptomatic for 10–20 years)
- Most common symptoms:
  - —Chest pain/back pain due to compression of intrathoracic structures or bony erosion
  - —Wheezing, cough, dyspnea (may be positional) due to tracheal compression
  - —Hemoptysis, recurrent pneumonitis
  - —Hoarseness due to compression of the recurrent laryngeal nerve
  - —Dyspnea, orthopnea, paroxysmal nocturnal dyspnea, edema due to congestive heart failure from aortic regurgitation and left ventricular failure
  - —Angina/myocardial infarction due to local compression of coronary arteries
  - —Thromboembolism causing stroke, lower extremity ischemia, renal infarction, mesenteric ischemia
  - —Local mass effect precipitating superior vena cava syndrome
  - —Dysphagia due to esophageal compression

Signs

- Include tracheal deviation, aortic regurgitation murmur with or without peripheral manifestations, wide pulse pressure, and, rarely, a left paravertebral bruit with a descending aortic aneurysm

LABORATORY PROCEDURES

N/A

IMAGING STUDIES

- Chest x-ray
  - —Frequently a TAA is initially identified as an incidental finding on chest x-ray; appears as widening of the mediastinal silhouette, dilatation of the ascending aorta, enlargement of the aortic knob, or tracheal deviation.
- Abdominal ultrasonography
  - —Most practical screening method
  - —Nearly 100% sensitive
  - —Can accurately define size to within ±0.3 cm
  - —Unable to define associated mesenteric and renal arterial anatomy or cephalad or pelvic extent of disease
- CT
  - —Extremely accurate for diagnosis and sizing to within ±0.2 cm
  - —Better defines aneurysm and local anatomy than ultrasonography
  - —More expensive, less available than ultrasonography, requires i.v. contrast
  - —Can differentiate TAA from other lung parenchymal/mediastinal masses
- Aortography
  - —Has long been the standard preoperative imaging technique; however, currently debated as to the need for routine use in evaluation of AAA
  - —Cardiac catheterization with aortic root angiogram remains preferred modality for evaluation of TAA with aortic root involvement
  - —Excellent definition of extent of the aneurysm
  - —May underestimate the size of the aneurysm due to the presence of mural thrombus
- Magnetic resonance angiography
  - —Alternative to aortography for preoperative evaluation
  - —Exact role continues to be investigated; may be useful in defining aortic branch vessel anatomy, extent of disease
- Transthoracic echocardiography: not very accurate for diagnosis (limited examination of the thoracic aorta)
- Transesophageal echocardiography: much more accurate than transthoracic echocardiogra-

phy in assessing thoracic aorta; commonly used for detection of aortic dissection

SPECIAL TESTS

N/A

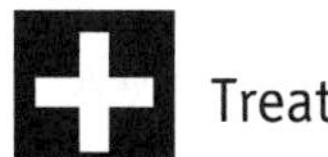

Treatment

GENERAL MEASURES

- Risk factor modification, including cholesterol lowering, smoking cessation, and treatment of hypertension
- Routine ultrasonography or CT scan yearly to detect either rapid expansion or increase in size to 5.0 cm or larger, either of which is an indication for surgery; consider follow-up scan every 3–6 months for higher-risk patients (e.g., those with saccular aneurysms, Marfan's syndrome)
- Traumatic aneurysms that have been present and are asymptomatic >10 years after injury may be periodically observed versus elective excision.

SURGICAL MANAGEMENT

- Size of AAA is the primary indicator for repair of asymptomatic aneurysms
  - —The Society for Vascular Surgery and the International Society for Cardiovascular Surgery recommend elective repair for aneurysms 4 cm or larger; many surgeons consider ≥5.0 cm the indication for surgery.
  - —Approximately half of all perioperative deaths from aneurysm repair are due to myocardial infarction; therefore, preoperative cardiac screening to identify the presence and severity of coronary artery disease is advocated. Cardiac catheterization and revascularization in patients with clinical cardiac disease prior to AAA repair should be considered.
- In general, unless the aneurysm is quite small, prompt excision should be considered for TAAs; most recommend elective surgery for TAAs 5.0–6.0 cm and 7.0 cm or larger in patients at high operative risk.
- In patients with Marfan's syndrome, surgery should be considered at 4.5–5.0 cm given the higher risk of dissection and rupture.
- Surgical repair of AAAs consists of resection of the aneurysm and insertion of a synthetic prosthetic graft.
- Early human trials suggest a successful outcome with the use of percutaneously implanted expanding endovascular stents for AAAs; the use of a transluminally placed endovascular stent graft may be an alternative approach to the surgical management of descending TAAs.
- TAAs are generally resected and replaced with an appropriately sized prosthetic sleeve; when significant aortic regurgitation is present in ascending TAAs, either a separate graft valve or composite graft with a prosthetic valve sewn into one end is used.

ADMISSION/DISCHARGE CRITERIA

Healthier patients may be admitted on the day of surgery; higher-risk patients should be admitted earlier for volume expansion and cardiac optimization.

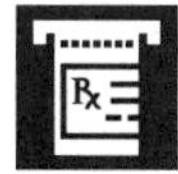

Medications

DRUG(S) OF CHOICE

- Beta-blockers reduce the risk of aneurysm expansion and rupture.
- The long-term outcome of medical management of TAAs has not been examined, however, beta-blocker treatment in patients with Marfan's syndrome significantly slows the rate of aortic dilatation, reduces clinical end points (death, aortic dissection, aortic regurgitation, aortic root >6 cm), and lowers mortality

Follow-up

PATIENT MONITORING

- Preoperatively, as described above in General Measures

EXPECTED COURSE AND PROGNOSIS

- Abdominal aortic aneurysms <4 cm have a 0–9% risk of rupture; >5 cm have a 22% risk of rupture in 2 years, with an overall mortality rate from rupture of 80%.
- Survival following AAA repair has been reported as 1-, 5-, and 10-year survival rates of 93%, 63%, and 40%, respectively.
- Those with concomitant coronary artery disease have a 10% lower rate of survival than those without coronary artery disease.
- The 1-, 3-, and 5-year survival rates for patients with TAAs not undergoing surgery are 65%, 36%, and 20%, respectively.
- Rupture occurs in 32%–68% of patients with TAAs not treated with surgery; mortality rate is 76% at 24 hours after rupture.
- Elective surgical repair of ascending and descending TAAs has a 90%–95% early survival rate.
- The incidence of neurologic injury after aortic arch repair is 0–15%; incidence of paraplegia with descending TAA repair ranges from 0 to 17%, and 5% to 6% at most centers.
- Most common causes of early postoperative death are myocardial infarction, congestive heart failure, stroke, renal failure, hemorrhage, respiratory failure, and sepsis.

PATIENT EDUCATION

Screening with ultrasonography is indicated for relatives of patients with AAAs, because the estimated relative risk for first-degree relatives of affected individuals is 11.6 times greater than for non-first-degree relatives.

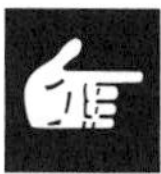

Miscellaneous

ICD-9-CM

441.9 Aortic aneurysm (unspecified)
441.4 Abdominal aortic aneurysm (unspecified)
441.2 Thoracic aortic aneurysm (unspecified)

BIBLIOGRAPHY

Galloway AC, Miller JS, Spencer FC, et al. Thoracic aneurysms. In: Schwartz SI, ed. *Principles of surgery,* 7th ed. New York: McGraw-Hill, 1999:909–929.

Isselbacher EM, Eagle KA, Desanctis RW. Diseases of the aorta. In: Braunwald E, ed. *Heart disease,* 5th ed. Philadelphia: WB Saunders, 1997:1546–1581.

Ouriel K, Green RM. Arterial disease. In: Schwartz SI, ed. *Principles of surgery,* 7th ed. New York: McGraw-Hill, 1999:931–1003.

Author: Helene Glassberg

Aortic Counterpulsation

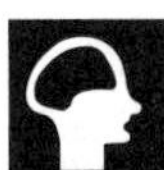

Basics

DEFINITION

Refers to a means of assisting the failing heart by automatically removing arterial blood just before and during ventricular ejection and returning it to the circulation during diastole

- Used as temporary circulatory support in patients with medically refractory cardiogenic shock until more definitive therapy can be undertaken [e.g., coronary artery bypass grafting (CABG) or percutaneous transluminal coronary angioplasty]. More recent indications include medically refractory unstable angina and malignant ventricular rhythms, and prophylactic use in high-risk angioplasty.
- Intraaortic balloon pump (IABP) is indicated for mechanical complications after myocardial infarction (MI) (ventriculoseptal defect, papillary muscle rupture) until cardiac catheterization and CABG can be performed.
- Counterpulsation improves the myocardial oxygen supply/demand balance (85% of coronary perfusion occurs in diastole, the remaining 15% is supplied only to the epicardial area), with modest increase in systemic perfusion.
- Extracorporeal counterpulsation was first introduced in 1961.
- Intraortic balloon pump (IABP) insertion via sheath/dilator was described in 1980.
- IABP is now a standard in circulatory assistance (100,000 placed in the United States in 1993).
- Ventricular assist devices are generally reserved for longer-term support while awaiting cardiac transplantation.
- Recently, enhanced external counterpulsation (sequential inflation of three cuffs from ankle to thigh on each leg during diastole) has been associated with fewer anginal episodes and with longer exercise duration without ECG evidence of ischemia.

Selection Criteria

Cardiogenic shock on maximal inotropic support defined by:

- Cardiac index <1.8 L/min/m^2
- Systolic blood pressure <90 mm Hg
- Left or right atrial pressure >20 mm Hg
- Urine output <20 mL/h
- Systemic vascular resistance >2,100 dynes-sec/cm^5

Exclude if:

- Blood urea nitrogen >100 mg/dL
- Creatinine >5 mg/dL
- Severe chronic lung disease
- Severe chronic liver disease
- Metastatic cancer
- Sepsis
- Significant neurologic deficit
- Incomplete revascularization (if postcardiotomy cardiogenic shock)
- Age >60 years (if used as bridge to transplantation)

Absolute Contraindications

- Significant aortic insufficiency
- Aortic dissection
- Contraindication to femoral placement:
  - —Abdominal aortic aneurysm
  - —Severe calcific aortoiliac or femoral arterial disease
  - —Recent groin incision at proposed site
  - —Surgeons may place via intrathoracic route if femoral route not possible

IABP Insertion

- Balloon catheter is introduced over wire via common femoral artery.
- Balloon diameter should be no more than 80%–90% of aortic diameter; the 40-cc balloon is adequate for most adults (30–34 cc if small, 50 cc if very large patient).
- Tip of catheter is placed in descending aorta, just distal to left subclavian artery.
- Balloon is inflated at dicrotic notch and deflated during isovolumic contraction (pressure monitored via central lumen in IABP catheter).
- If ECG is used to control balloon, inflation occurs on T wave, deflation on R wave. Note: If patient is in atrial fibrillation, deflation on the R wave is the preferred timing method to prevent ventricular contraction against an inflated balloon during a short R-R cycle.
- IABP timing should be adjusted while assisting every other beat (1:2) so that assisted beat waveforms can be compared with normal beats.
- IABP catheter is attached to bedside control/monitoring console.
- Helium gas (30–50 cc) is used to inflate balloon due to its low viscosity (rapid shuttling needed in tachyarrhythmias).

RISK FACTORS

- Diabetes mellitus
- Hypertension
- Female gender
- Peripheral vascular disease
- Extended use (e.g., >5 days)

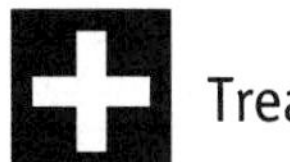

Treatment

GENERAL MEASURES

- Heparin anticoagulation with partial thromboplastin time 50–70 seconds
- Evaluation of the involved limb for ischemia at least every 8 hours
- Daily evaluation for evidence of sepsis, thrombocytopenia, blood loss, hemolysis, vascular obstruction, thrombus, embolus, or dissection
- Thrombocytopenia is expected due to traumatic platelet destruction, but counts rarely fall below 50,000 to 100,000/mL unless some other problem exists (e.g., disseminated intravascular coagulation, heparin-induced thrombocytopenia).
- Monitoring for normal pressure waveform (normally rectangular appearance with brief overshoot and undershoot artifacts)
- If rounding of the waveform occurs, consider a kink in the balloon or connection tubing, an incompletely inflated balloon, or an oversized balloon.
- Patients are kept on bed rest, with restricted hip flexion and head of bed elevated no more than 30 degrees.
- Prophylactic antibiotics (e.g., cefazolin) are not given routinely, but should be given at time of insertion if there is any compromise in sterile technique.

RESULTS

- 75% of patients who develop cardiogenic shock refractory to medication post-MI will respond to IABP therapy (ultimate outcome determined by coronary pathology; patients with operable disease achieve early survival as high as 93%).
- For ventricular septal rupture post-MI, IABP reduces left-to-right shunt; combined with urgent surgery allows 73%–80% survival.
- For papillary muscle rupture post-MI, IABP increases coronary perfusion and reduces ischemic load, mitral regurgitation, and pulmonary capillary wedge pressure; mortality is related to extent of cardiac dysfunction and approaches 55%.
- For postcardiotomy cardiogenic shock, IAPB allows survival in 52% to 66%.
- One-year survival in patients who require IABP pre-transplantation is 72% to 77%.

COMPLICATIONS

- Complication rates range from 6% to 46%.
- Balloon rupture is rare.
- Major complications in 4%–17% (leg ischemia requiring thrombectomy or amputation, aortic dissection, aortoiliac laceration or perforation and deep wound infection requiring debridement)
- Minor complications in 7%–42% (bleeding at insertion site, superficial wound infection, asymptomatic loss of peripheral pulse, and lymphocele)
- Vascular complications are most common (6%–24%). Most are due to insertion procedure.
- If leg ischemia develops, IABP should be removed; if ischemia persists, surgical exploration is indicated.

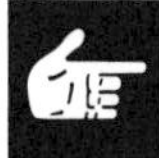

Miscellaneous

BIBLIOGRAPHY

Arora RR, et al. The Multicenter Study of Enhanced External Counterpulsation (MUST-EECP): effect of EECP on exercise-induced myocardial ischemia and anginal episodes. *J Am Coll Cardiol* 1999;33:1833–1840.

Baim D, Grossman W. *Cardiac catheterization, angiography, and intervention,* 5th ed. Baltimore: Williams & Wilkins, 1996.

Braunwald E. *Heart disease: a textbook of cardiovascular medicine,* 5th ed. Philadelphia: WB Saunders, 1997.

Opie L. *The heart.* Orlando: Grune & Stratton, 1984.

Stedman's medical dictionary, 25th edition. Baltimore: Williams & Wilkins, 1990.

Authors: Robert Hogan and Gerard P. Aurigemma

Aortic Regurgitation, Adult

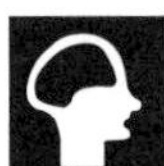

Basics

DESCRIPTION

Back leak of blood from the aorta through the aortic valve during diastole

Prevalence

- Surgical series have reported that aortic regurgitation (AR) accounts for 20%–23% of cases.
- Echocardiographic series reported AR in about 11% of subjects over 50 years of age and 29% of patients over 70.

CAUSES

Common Causes

- Idiopathic dilatation
- Congenital abnormalities of the aortic valve (most notably bicuspid valves)
- Calcific degeneration
- Rheumatic disease
- Infective endocarditis
- Systemic hypertension
- Myxomatous proliferation
- Dissection of the ascending aorta
- Marfan's syndrome

Less Common Causes

- Traumatic injuries to the aortic valve
- Ankylosing spondylitis
- Syphilitic aortitis
- Rheumatoid arthritis
- Osteogenesis imperfecta
- Giant cell aortitis
- Ehlers-Danlos syndrome
- Reiter's syndrome
- Discrete subaortic stenosis
- Ventricular septal defects with prolapse of an aortic cusp

RISK FACTORS

N/A

PREGNANCY

Patients with AR tolerate pregnancy well, but it might precipitate congestive heart failure (CHF) in case of severe AR with left ventricular (LV) systolic dysfunction.

Diagnosis

DIFFERENTIAL DIAGNOSIS

- AR has to be differentiated form other causes of increased pulse pressure.
- Must be differentiated from causes of early diastolic murmur (e.g., pulmonary regurgitation)
- Differential diagnosis of the etiology: refer to Causes.

SIGNS AND SYMPTOMS

- The patient remains asymptomatic, often until the fourth or fifth decade of life, when cardiac reserve is reduced.
- Exertional dyspnea, orthopnea, and paroxysmal nocturnal dyspnea are the main complaints.
- Nocturnal angina–associated diaphoresis that occurs with slowing of the heart rate and reduction of the diastolic blood pressure (BP)
- Abdominal discomfort secondary to splanchnic ischemia
- Palpitations especially on lying down, mostly secondary to increased force of contraction

Examination

Widened pulse pressure is due to increased forward systolic flow and retrograde diastolic flow in the ascending aorta. Peripheral signs (observed only in severe disease):

- De Musset's sign: synchronous movement of the head with heartbeats.
- Corrigan's pulse: water hammer pulse
- Bisferiens pulse: two palpable systolic impulses
- Traube's sign: booming systolic and diastolic sounds heard over the femoral artery
- Muller's sign: systolic pulsation of the uvula
- Duroziez's sign: systolic murmur over the femoral artery when it is compressed proximally and diastolic murmur when it is compressed distally
- Quincke's sign: capillary pulsations, best assessed by transmitting light through the patient's fingertips
- Hill's sign: popliteal systolic pressure exceeds brachia systolic pressure by more than 60 mm Hg.

Cardiac Examination

Apical impulse is hyperdynamic and displaced laterally and inferiorly.

- Auscultation
  —First heart sound is often normal but it might be muffled if the P-R interval is prolonged.
  —Aortic component (A2) of the second heart sound (S2) may be decreased (with valvular disease) or increased (with aortic root disease) depending on the cause of AR.
- Additional sounds
  —Ejection clicks are rare in adult patients.
  —S3 with dilatation of left ventricle
- Murmur of AR
  —Best heard with the diaphragm of the stethoscope in the third and fourth intercostal space to the left of the sternal border in valvular disease and to the right of the border in aortic root disease
  —Starts immediately after A2, and its duration depends on the severity of AR. It is a high-pitched blowing murmur.
  —Best appreciated with the patient leaning forward at end-expiration
- Additional murmurs
  —Austin Flint
    - Low-pitched mid- and late-diastolic apical rumbling murmur
    - Occurs in severe AR and might be secondary to antegrade flow across the mitral valve, which is narrowed by the rapidly increasing left ventricular diastolic pressure or vibration of the leaflet or the LV free wall by the AR jet
  —Ejection systolic murmur secondary to increased forward flow across the aortic valve

LABORATORY PROCEDURES

N/A

IMAGING STUDIES

ECG

- Left ventricular volume overload pattern: increase in Q waves in leads aVL, V5-V6, and I, with relatively small R wave in V1.
- Voltage criteria for left ventricular hypertrophy, which improves with regression of hypertrophy after valve replacement. Those are associated with repolarization abnormalities (strain pattern)

Chest X-ray

- Cardiomegally, dilatation of the ascending aorta, calcification of the wall of the ascending aorta in syphilitic aortitis, calcification of the valve in patients with combined AR and aortic stenosis (AS)

Echocardiography

- Provides reliable evaluation of aortic valve and root anatomy
- Allows identification of the cause of AI in most cases.
- Doppler and 2-D echocardiography allows semiquantitative and quantitative evaluation of the severity of AI.
- Provides reproducible measurement of LV dimensions, volumes, and systolic fuction, which form the cornerstone for decision making and follow-up evaluation.

SPECIAL TESTS

Exercise Testing

- It may be indicated to assess functional capacity and symptomatic responses in patients with equivocal changes in symptomatic status.
- Serial exercise imaging studies to assess LV functional reserve are not indicated in asymptomatic patients or those in whom symptoms develop.

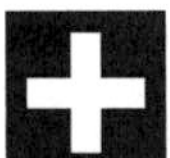

Treatment

GENERAL MEASURES

Prophylaxis against infective endocarditis and recurrent rheumatic fever, if applicable, is indicated.

SURGICAL MEASURES

Indications for aortic valve replacement (AVR) include:

- Severe AI with NYHA class III–IV symptoms and normal ejection fraction (EF)
- Severe AI with Canadian Heart Association class II or greater angina with or without coronary artery disease
- Severe AI with EF of 25%–49%
- Severe AI with NYHA class II symptoms and normal EF but with progressive LV dilatation on serial testing

Medications

DRUG(S) OF CHOICE

Vasodilators

- Therapy is designed to improve forward stroke volume and reduce regurgitant volume.
- These effects should translate into reductions in LV end-diastolic volume, wall stress, and afterload, resulting in preservation of LV systolic function and reduction in LV mass.
- Vasodilators are not indicated in asymptomatic patients with normal systolic function and BP as well as mild AI with preserved LV function.

Nifedipine

- Asymptomatic patients with severe AI and preserved LV function should be treated with long-acting nifedipine when they have elevated BP aiming for the highest dose that completely or partially controls BP.
- Normal BP is rarely achieved secondary to the increased stroke volume.

Precautions

Anorectic drugs also have been reported to cause AR.

ALTERNATIVE DRUG(S)

N/A

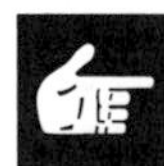

Follow-up

PATIENT MONITORING

- The aim of serial evaluation of asymptomatic patients with chronic AR is to detect the onset of symptoms and objectively assess changes in LV size and function that can occur in the absence of symptoms.
- It should include a detailed history, physical examination, and echocardiography. Serial chest x-rays and ECGs have less value but are helpful in selected patients.
- Asymptomatic patients with mild AR, little or no LV dilatation, and normal LV systolic function can be examined on a yearly basis. Echocardiography can be performed every 2–3 years.
- Asymptomatic patients with normal systolic function but severe AR and significant LV dilatation (end-diastolic dimension >60 mm) should have a history and physical examination performed every 6 months and echocardiography every 6–12 months. In patients with more advanced LV dilatation (end-diastolic dimension >70 mm or end-systolic dimension >50 mm), serial echocardiograms should be obtained every 4–6 months.

Prevention

Prophylaxis against infective endocarditis and recurrent rheumatic fever, if applicable, is indicated.

Complications

- Infective endocarditis
- Congestive heart failure
- Recurrent rheumatic carditis (if the cause was rheumatic heart disease)
- Prosthetic valve-related complications after AVR

EXPECTED COURSE AND PROGNOSIS

The time course between the development of LV dysfunction at rest and the onset of symptoms is relatively short: two-thirds of asymptomatic patients with LV dysfunction develop symptoms requiring operation within 2–3 years.

PATIENT EDUCATION

Patients should be educated about this disease and to report the onset of any new symptoms.

Activity

There are no data to suggest that strenuous exercise accelerates the progression of aortic insufficiency (AI). Asymptomatic patients with normal LV function can participate in all kinds of activity. However, isometric exercise should be avoided.

Diet

- Low-salt diet with the onset of CHF

Miscellaneous

ICD-9-CM

424.1

BIBLIOGRAPHY

Bonow RO. Chronic aortic regurgitation: role of medical therapy optimal timing of surgery. *Cardiol Clin* 1998;16:449–462.

Bonow RO, Carabello B, de Leon AC Jr, et al. ACC/AHA guidelines for the management of patients with valvular heart disease: a report of the American College of Cardiology/American Heart Association Task Force on Practice Guidelines (Committee on Management of Patients with Valvular Heart Disease). *J Am Coll Cardiol* 1998;32:1486–1588.

Otto C. *Valvular heart disease*, 1st ed. Philadelphia: WB Saunders, 1999.

Rahimtoola SH, et al. *Hurst's the heart*, 9th ed. New York: McGraw-Hill, 1998.

Authors: Amr El-Shafei, Steven Herrmann, Madhukar Gupta, and Bernard R. Chaitman

Aortic Regurgitation, Pediatric

Basics

DESCRIPTION

Incompetence of the aortic valve causes leakage of blood into the left ventricle during diastole.

- A regurgitant jet of 20% of the orifice area can double left ventricular output and work.
- In severe cases the diastolic leak can be as much as 60% of the left ventricular stroke volume.
- The increase in left ventricular end-diastolic volume and compensatory reflex peripheral vasodilation results in an increase in total stroke volume.
- With the exhaustion of compensatory mechanisms along with myocardial ischemia, left ventricular failure will ensue.

Systems Affected

- Cardiovascular

ETIOLOGY

Genetics

Isolated congenital aortic regurgitation is a rare congenital malformation.

Incidence/Prevalence

Aortic regurgitation may occur in approximately 5% of whites and up to 50% of Asians with subaortic venricular septal defect. Aortic incompetence is also associated with various forms of left ventricular outflow abnormalities and numerous other entities.

Sex

Predominant sex is related to the specific etiology.

Natural History

Natural history data are available for adult patients only.

- In patients who are asymptomatic and have normal left ventricular function, the rate of development of symptoms or left ventricular dysfunction averages 4.3%/yr.
- Average mortality rate is <0.2%/yr. Conversely, 25% of the patients who die or develop systolic dysfunction do so before the onset of warning symptoms.
- Variables identified as being associated with higher risk for the development of future symptoms, systolic dysfunction, or death include age, left ventricular end-diastolic dimension, and end-systolic dimension.
- On serial longitudinal studies, rate of increase in left ventricular end-systolic dimension and decrease in ejection fraction are reported as independent predictors of outcome.

CAUSES

- Bicuspid aortic valve (congenital)
- Other forms of congenitally abnormal aortic valve
- Aneurysm of the sinus of Valsalva
- VSD with prolapsing aortic cusp
- Marfan's syndrome
- Ehlers-Danlos syndrome
- Osteogenesis imperfecta
- Aortic regurgitation may also occur in association with discrete subaortic stenosis.
- Aortic regurgitation may also occur following intervention for aortic valve stenosis (catheter or surgical) or other cardiac interventions.

Diagnosis

DIFFERENTIAL DIAGNOSIS

Other causes of aortic runoff with similar physical findings include:

- Patent ductus arteriosus
- Ruptured sinus of Valsalva
- Coronary arteriovenous fistula
- Aorta to left ventricle tunnel and aorticopulmonary window
- The diastolic murmur of pulmonary regurgitation in the presence of pulmonary hypertension (Graham Steell's murmur) is also high pitched, similar to that of aortic regurgitation.

SIGNS AND SYMPTOMS

History

- Chronic aortic regurgitation is better tolerated than acute and less likely to have symptoms associated with a given amount of regurgitation. Cardiac awareness may result because of the large stroke volume.
- Excessive sweating and heat intolerance due to vasodilation may be an early symptom.
- Chest pain may occur with exertion.
- Symptoms associated with left ventricular failure include dyspnea, shortness of breath, fatigue.

Physical Examination

- Characteristic peripheral signs are produced by a combination of large pulse volume and vasodilation.
  —With more severe disease the systolic pressure increases and the diastolic pressure decreases.
  —A sharp increase in the pulse gives it a "water hammer quality."
- Apical impulse may be displaced inferiorly and laterally with an apical diastolic thrust.
- Systolic thrill may be palpable over the base.
- Heart sounds are usually normal.
- The typical murmur of aortic regurgitation is heard in early diastole, characterized as a high-pitched decrescendo beginning with the second heart sound and maximally along the left and mid-sternal borders with radiation to the apex.
  —An ejection murmur is often at the base due to increased flow across the aortic valve.
  —With moderate or severe regurgitation a mid-diastolic rumble (Austin-Flint murmur) may be audible over the mitral area.
  —This is due to the regurgitant jet impeding opening of the mitral valve anterior leaflet.

LABORATORY PROCEDURES

N/A

SPECIAL TESTS

ECG

- Normal in mild aortic regurgitation and at times in severe disease
- Severe cases display increased qRS voltage in the left precordial leads with tall and upright T waves
- ST and T wave strain pattern
- Left bundle branch block

Exercise Test and Radionuclide Angiography

In selected patients, exercise and radionuclide studies may be useful.

IMAGING STUDIES

Chest X-ray

- Left ventricle enlargement in an inferior and leftward direction
- Aortic root is dilated.
- Pulmonary venous congestion may be seen in association with left ventricular failure.

DIAGNOSTIC PROCEDURES

Echocardiography

Two-Dimensional Imaging

Useful in assessing potential etiology of aortic regurgitation, including:

- Acquired A1
- VSD with aortic cusp prolapse
- Bicuspid aortic valve
- Subaortic stenosis
- Dilatation of the aortic root and mitral valve prolapse in Marfan's syndrome.

Doppler Imaging

- Assesses the presence and severity of aortic regurgitation
- Holodiastolic reversal of flow can be seen in the descending aorta in patients with moderate severe regurgitation.
- Color Doppler flow mapping of the jet using jet width and area is useful.

M-Mode Imaging

- Useful in the evaluation of secondary changes of the left ventricle resulting from aortic regurgitation, such as dilatation, hypertrophy, and diminished function
- Serial evaluation of left ventricle cavity size and function is important for management decisions.

Cardiac Catheterization

- No longer indicated for the diagnosis of aortic regurgitation
- Occasionally indicated in the management, when questions remain unanswered regarding severity, hemodynamics, or left ventricular function

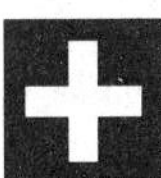

Treatment

GENERAL MEASURES

- Endocarditis prophylaxis
- Management depends on the cause, duration, secondary cardiac changes (ventricular dilatation and function), and associated symptoms.
- Significant symptoms of preoperative left ventricular systolic dysfunction are major indicators of decreased likelihood for optimal postoperative outcome.
- Ideal timing of surgery for aortic regurgitation balances the risk of surgery with the possible prevention of left ventricular dysfunction.

SURGICAL MEASURES

- Pulmonary autograft procedure
  —The patient's pulmonary valve replaces the aortic valve in the left ventricular outflow tract.
  —A homograft is used on the right side of the heart.
  —Intermediate follow-up shows excellent durability of the pulmonary valve in the aortic position in most patients.
  —Growth of the pulmonary valve has been demonstrated in children. There is no need for anticoagulation postoperatively.
- Aortic valve replacement with a mechanical prosthesis
  —Bileaflet mechanical valves such as St. Jude or Carbomedics are durable with excellent function but will need replacement when used in pediatric patients.
  —Anticoagulation is necessary to minimize the risk of thrombosis.
- Aortic valve repair
  —In select patients this is preferable.
- Aortic valve replacement with bioprosthesis
  —A significant risk of valve degeneration and calcification over time requiring replacement
  —These complications are more common in children and adolescents.
- Asymptomatic patients with normal ventricular function
  —Precise timing of surgery in this group of patients is controversial.
  —Patients with left ventricular dysfunction require valve replacement with or without symptoms.
  —Surgery may be recommended in asymptomatic patients with left ventricular end-diastolic dimension >75 mm or left ventricular systolic dimension >55 mm; specific data are not available for infants and children.
  —Patients with ventricular dimensions approaching these values should be followed closely with serial studies.
  —Because of inherent variability in testing, no decision should be made on a single measurement.
- Aortic regurgitation with ventricular septal defect
  —Surgery for aortic regurgitation in association with ventricular septal defect and prolapsing aortic cusp is performed earlier than in most other situations.
  —Although controversy exists as to the precise timing, all would agree that regurgitation which progresses to moderately severe as assessed by both Doppler echocardiography and physical examination warrants surgical repair.
- Aortic regurgitation with Marfan's syndrome or bicuspid aortic valve
  —Timing of surgery is more likely to be determined by the finding of aortic root dilatation.
  —Surgery is generally recommended when the aortic root measures >50 to 55 mm in diameter by echocardiography, at which point the risk of sudden death is thought to outweigh the risk of surgery.
- Aortic regurgitation with discrete subaortic stenosis
  —Timing of surgery for subaortic stenosis is controversial.
  —Aggressive approach is to resect a subaortic membrane when Doppler echocardiographic evidence of aortic regurgitation is present.
  —Many patients exist in whom there are no signs of progression of aortic regurgitation or left ventricular outflow tract obstruction with conservative management.

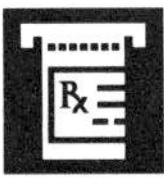

Medications

DRUG(S) OF CHOICE

- Digoxin and diuretic therapy for patients in congestive heart failure
- Vasodilator therapy
  —Nipride, hydralazine, nifedipine, and angiotensin-converting enzyme inhibitors have been shown to reduce systemic vascular resistance, augment forward stroke volume, and reduce regurgitant volume in adults. Standards for children are not available.
  —Criteria for the use of chronic vasodilator therapy in the pediatric patients with mild to moderate aortic insufficiency have not been established. No specific data exist showing long-term benefit in children.

Follow-up

PATIENT MONITORING

- Serial echocardiograms after surgery to assess surgical results and serve as a baseline for late follow-up
- Approximately 80% of the overall reduction in volume occurs within the first 10–14 days postoperatively.
- The magnitude in reduction correlates with the improvement in function and late postoperative period:
  —Patients with persistent left ventricular dilatation should be treated similar to other patients with ventricular dysfunction, including therapy with ACE inhibitors.
  —Repeat clinical evaluation along with echocardiography, if there is significant residual aortic regurgitation, will determine necessity for repeat surgical intervention.

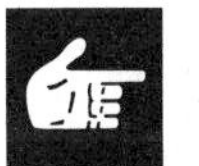

Miscellaneous

BIBLIOGRAPHY

Bonow, et al. ACC/AHA Task Force Report. *J Am Coll Cardiol* 1998;32:1486–1588.

Emmanouilides GC, et al., eds. *Moss and Adams' heart disease in infants, children and adolescents: including the fetus and young adult,* 5th ed. Baltimore: Williams & Wilkins, 1995.

Garson A, et al., eds. *The science and practice of pediatric cardiology,* 2nd ed. Baltimore: Williams & Wilkins, 1998.

Solowiejczwk D, et al. Serial echocardiographic measurements of the pulmonary autograft in the aortic valve position following the Ross operation in a pediatric population using normal pulmonary artery dimensions as the reference standard. *Am J Cardiol* (in press).

Authors: David Solowiejczwk and Welton M. Gersony

Aortic Stenosis, Adult

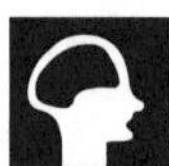

Basics

DESCRIPTION

Obstruction of the outflow of blood from the left ventricle to the aorta

ETIOLOGY

Prevalence

In adults undergoing surgery for aortic stenosis (AS) in the United States, calcific AS accounts for 51% of cases, bicuspid AS 36%, and thematic disease 9%. The prevalence of bicuspid aortic valve in the general population may be as high as 1%–2% of the general population.

Age

- Calcific aortic valve disease presents clinically at 50–60 years in patients with a bicuspid valve versus age 70–80 years in those with trileaflet valve. However, rheumatic AS presents at an earlier age and is usually associated with aortic regurgitation.
- Aortic valve replacement (AVR) is the only option for treatment of symptomatic AS with no age limitations. However, elderly patients have confounding factors, which make aortic valve surgery more risky than in a younger population. These factors include coronary artery disease, left ventricular (LV) dysfunction, and comorbidities. Thus, the decision to proceed with the surgery should take the above-mentioned factors as well as the patient's wishes and expectations into consideration.

PREGNANCY

N/A

RISK FACTORS

N/A

Diagnosis

DIFFERENTIAL DIAGNOSIS

- Supravalvular AS
- Hypertrophic cardiomyopathy
- Subaortic membrane

SIGNS AND SYMPTOMS

Signs

- Pulse: The timing and amplitude of the carotid pulse contour reflects central aortic pressure. With severe AS, the peak occurs later in systole (pulsus tardus) and pulse amplitude is decreased (pulsus parvus).
- Murmur: The second characteristic sign is the ejection systolic murmur over the right second intercostal space. The murmur has a crescendo–decrescendo pattern. Its intensity generally correlates with the severity of obstruction. The presence of a thrill is specific for severe AS. The murmur radiates to the carotids and to the apex (the latter is referred to as the Gallavardin phenomenon).
- The second heart sound is diminished to absent in severe AS and may have reversed splitting because of prolonged ejection time.
- The fourth heart sound (S4) is common and reflects increased atrial contribution to ventricular filling.

Symptoms

- Asymptomatic
  - —Patients remain symptomatic for a long time. The condition is first diagnosed based on detection of a systolic murmur on auscultation that can be explained by the gradual progress of obstruction.
- Dyspnea
  - —The most common initial symptom is exertional dyspnea, which may progress to frank CHF.
- Exertional angina is also a common initial symptom.
- The third classic symptom is exertional presyncope or syncope.

CAUSES

- Calcific (degenerative): the most common cause of valve lesion that requires replacement
- Congenital
- Rheumatic
- Obstructive infective vegetations
- Homozygous type II hyperlipoproteinemia
- Paget's disease of bone
- Systemic lupus erythematosus
- Ochronosis
- Rheumatoid disease
- Irradiation

LABORATORY PROCEDURES

N/A

IMAGING STUDIES

ECG

The classic finding is LV hypertrophy. Other nonspecific changes are left atrial enlargement, left axis deviation, and left bundle–branch block. ECG changes can occur only during exercise despite a normal resting ECG.

Chest Radiography

May be entirely normal. However, poststenotic dilatation of the ascending aorta may be evident. Calcification of the aortic valve is rarely seen on radiography but may be seen on fluoroscopy.

Echocardiography

- Echocardiography is helpful in assessing the severity of AS, the degree of coexisting aortic regurgitation, LV size and function; in estimating pulmonary systolic pressure; and in identifying other cardiac abnormalities.
- Aortic valve area can be estimated, as can the maximum jet velocity, which are the most useful clinical measurements of severity.

Cardiac Catheterization

- Indicated for hemodynamic evaluation whenever there is discrepancy between the clinical picture and echocardiography. It is also indicated to evaluate coronary anatomy in patients at risk for coronary artery disease.

Dobutamine Echocardiography

- Indicated in patients with moderate aortic stenosis and LV dysfunction to predict the reversibility of LV dysfunction after AVR

SPECIAL TESTS

See Imaging Studies.

PATHOLOGY

- The aortic valve area must be reduced to one-fourth of its natural size before significant changes in the circulation occur.
- Aortic stenosis is graded based on the aortic valve area into mild ($>1.5\ cm^2$), moderate ($1.1–1.5\ cm^2$), severe (<0.75 to $1\ cm^2$), and very severe ($<0.75\ cm^2$).

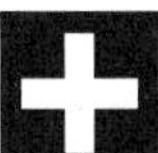

Treatment

GENERAL MEASURES

Prophylaxis against infective endocarditis and recurrent rheumatic fever, if applicable, is indicated.

SURGICAL MEASURES

Indications for Aortic Valve Replacement

- Symptomatic patients
  —AVR improves survival in patients with depressed as well as normal LV function.
  —Depressed LV function is secondary to either afterload mismatch or depressed contractility. In the latter, the improvement in the LV function and symptoms may not be complete.
- Asymptomatic patients
  —The risks of surgery and prosthetic valve complications outweigh the benefits of preventing sudden cardiac death and prolonged survival in asymptomatic patient. An exercise test is useful in those patients.
- Prophylactic AVR
  —Patients with severe AS undergoing coronary artery bypass grafting or other valve replacement should undergo AVR as well.
  —Patients with moderate AS may undergo AVR with similar surgeries.
  —This issue is controversial in patients with mild AS.

Aortic Balloon Valvotomy

- Percutaneous balloon dilatation offers little benefit for adults with calcific AS or with secondary calcification of a bicuspid aortic valve.
- This procedure is reserved for patients with serious severe comorbidity, patients requiring urgent noncardiac surgery, and as a bridge to AVR.

Medications

DRUG(S) OF CHOICE

AS is a mechanical problem, and medical treatment has no role in preventing the progression of the disease process. However, with the onset of LV systolic dysfunction, the use of intravenous inotropic agents may be advocated.

Contraindications

Vasodilators are relatively contraindicated in severe AS.

ALTERNATIVE DRUGS

N/A

Follow-up

PATIENT MONITORING

- Mild: annual history and physical examination and echocardiography every 5 years
- Moderate: More frequent visits and echocardiogram every 2 years
- Severe AS: yearly echocardiogram
- Echocardiogram should be performed if any change occurs in clinical findings.
- Patients should report any symptoms.

Prevention

Prophylaxis against infective endocarditis and recurrent rheumatic fever, if applicable, is indicated.

Complications

- Congestive heart failure
- Sudden cardiac death
- Atrial arrhythmias
- Infective endocarditis
- Systemic calcium embolism
- It can be associated with intestinal arteriovenous malformation.
- Prosthetic valve–related complications

EXPECTED COURSE AND PROGNOSIS

- Prognosis is similar to that for age-matched normal adults during the asymptomatic period.
- Development of symptoms is associated with a grave prognosis, showing a 2-year survival rate of <50% on medical therapy.

PATIENT EDUCATION

The development of symptoms in patients with AS is one of the cornerstones of the process of decision making. Thus, asymptomatic patients should report the onset of dyspnea, angina, or syncope.

Activity

Recommendations for physical activity are based on the clinical examination, with special emphasis on the hemodynamic severity of the stenotic lesion.

- Asymptomatic patients with mild AS: Physical activity is not restricted and patients can participate in competitive sports.
- Patients with moderate AS: They should avoid competitive sports that involve high dynamic and static muscular demands. Other forms of exercise can be performed after an exercise test with no ST segment changes or sustained arrhythmias.
- Patients with severe AS should be advised to limit their activity to relatively low levels.

Diet

- Low-salt diet

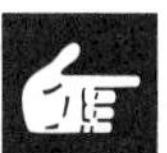

Miscellaneous

ICD-9-CM

424.1

BIBLIOGRAPHY

Bonow RO, Carabello B, de Leon AC Jr, et al. ACC/AHA guidelines for the management of patients with valvular heart disease: a report of the American College of Cardiology/American Heart Association Task Force on Practice Guidelines (Committee on Management of Patients with Valvular Heart Disease). *J Am Coll Cardiol* 1998;32:1486–1588.

Otto C. Aortic stenosis: clinical evaluation and optimal timing of surgery. *Cardiol Clin* 1998; 16:353–374.

Otto C. *Valvular heart disease,* 1st ed. Philadelphia: WB Saunders, 1999.

Rahimtoola SH. *Hurst's the heart,* 9th ed. New York: McGraw-Hill, 1998.

Authors: Amr El-Shafei, Steven Herrmann, Madhukar Gupta, and Bernard R. Chaitman

Aortic Stenosis, Supravalvular

Basics

DESCRIPTION

Supravalvular aortic stenosis is a congenital narrowing of the ascending aorta originating at the superior border of the sinus of Valsalva above the coronary artery ostia.

ETIOLOGY

Genetics

Can be nonfamilial, autosomal dominant, or sporadic. Linkage maps suggest that the gene is located on long arm of chromosome 7. Williams syndrome is both sporadic and familial and is often recognized in infancy.

Prevalence

- Rare

Age

- Often diagnosed in infancy when classic facial associations noted

CAUSES

- Congenital defect

RISK FACTORS

N/A

PREGNANCY

- Severe supravalvular stenosis may require repair prior to conception.
- Avoid dehydration during pregnancy.
- If symptoms of congestive heart failure develop in the presence of supravalvular stenosis, valvuloplasty or repair may be indicated with possible fetal demise.

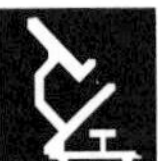

Diagnosis

DIFFERENTIAL DIAGNOSIS

- Valvular aortic stenosis, subvalvular aortic obstruction, hypertrophic obstructive cardiomyopathy

SIGNS AND SYMPTOMS

- Williams syndrome has classic associations with elfin faces (prominent forehead epicanthal folds, small nose bridge and mandible, and dental abnormalities), abnormalities in calcium metabolism, and mental retardation.
- Also associated with failure to thrive in infancy, inguinal hernias, constipation, colic, and hyperacusis, as well as narrowing of peripheral and pulmonary arteries.
- Older children may develop severe joint limitations.
- Adults with Williams syndrome generally have hypertension, urinary tract problems, and gastrointestinal defects.
- The familial forms of supravalvular aortic stenosis are associated with normal intelligence and can be seen with pulmonic stenosis.

LABORATORY PROCEDURES

- The ECG often show signs of left ventricular hypertrophy.
- Biventricular hypertrophy
- May be noted with coexisting pulmonic stenosis

IMAGING STUDIES

- In opposition to both valvular and subvalvular aortic stenosis, poststenotic dilation is rare on the chest radiograph.
- Sinus of Valsalva is dilated.
- Ascending aorta and arch appear normal on the chest film.

SPECIAL TESTS

- Echocardiography is the most helpful in diagnosis and localization of obstruction.
- The ratio of the sinotubular junction to aortic annulus is less than that in supravalvular stenosis.
- Cardiac catheterization is also valuable to measure the degree of hemodynamic abnormalities associated with the supravalvular stenosis.

PATHOLOGY

There are three types of supravalvular aortic stenosis:

- The most common form is a marked thickening of the aorta media, with disorganization of the media fibers forming a constricting ridge just proximal to the sinus of Valsalva. This is designated the hourglass type of supravalvular stenosis.
- The membranous type results from a fibrous membrane with a small central opening stretched across the aorta lumen.
- Rarely, the ascending aorta is hypoplastic, resulting in hypoplastic supravalvular aortic stenosis.
- Coronary arteries tend to be tortuous and dilated because of the high pressure proximal to the supravalvular stenosis with premature atherosclerosis.
- There are occasional thoracic aneurysms.

DIAGNOSTICS

- Physical examination shows an increased aortic valve closure sound secondary to increased pressure proximal to stenosis.
- Ejection murmur is common along the sternal border with thrill radiating to the jugular notch. Rarely, a diastolic murmur component may be heard if the supravalvular stenosis causes valvular leaflet fusion.
- Continuous systolic murmur may be heard with associated pulmonic stenosis.
- Blood pressure is frequently higher in the right arm as opposed to the left arm or legs.
- Disparity of pulses may be noted (Coanda effect).

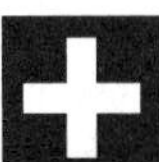

Treatment

GENERAL MEASURES

- Transcatheter balloon angioplasty may be effective.
- Surgical repair of supravalvular aortic stenosis is less favorable than valvular aortic stenosis.
- Aortotomy with excision of the fibrous obstruction is performed, often with a fabric prosthesis inserted into the area of the supravalvular narrowing to expand the lumen.
- The hypoplastic repair is challenging with high surgical mortality.

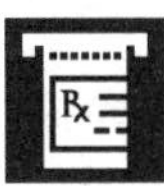

Medications

DRUG(S) OF CHOICE

N/A

Precautions

Avoid negative inotropic medications. Use diuretics and vasodilators cautiously.

ALTERNATIVE DRUGS

N/A

Follow-up

PATIENT MONITORING

Dependent on the severity of the hemodynamic abnormality:

- Severe obstruction should be monitored every 6–12 months, and mild obstruction every 2–5 years.
- A change in symptomatology demands immediate evaluation.

Complications

- Arterial hypertension, left ventricular hypertrophy

EXPECTED COURSE AND PROGNOSIS

Similar in respect to sudden cardiac death and risk of endocarditis and valvular aortic stenosis.

PATIENT EDUCATION

Endocarditis prophylaxis required.

Activity

Severe exercise and competitive sports should be discouraged.

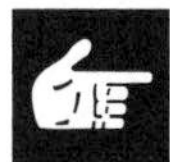

Miscellaneous

SYNONYMS

- Williams-Beuren syndrome

ICD-9-CM

747.22

See also: Aortic Stenosis; Congenital Heart Diseases

BIBLIOGRAPHY

Alexander RW, ed. *Hurst's the heart.* New York: McGraw-Hill, 1998.

Braunwald E, ed. *Heart disease: a textbook of cardiovascular medicine,* 5th ed. Philadelphia: WB Saunders, 1997.

Topol EJ, ed. *Textbook of cardiovascular medicine.* Philadelphia: Lippincott-Raven, 1998.

Authors: Steven Herrmann, Amr El-Shafei, Madhukar Gupta, and Bernard R. Chaitman

Arterial Embolism

Basics

DESCRIPTION

Occlusion of a cerebral artery resulting in stroke or transient ischemic attack (TIA) in 80% of patients, of a peripheral artery in 15%, or a visceral artery in ≤5% of patients

Systems Affected

- Cardiovascular

ETIOLOGY

Atherosclerosis has genetic implications.

EPIDEMIOLOGY

Incidence/Prevalence

Every year, 500,000 Americans develop new or recurrent stroke and 50,000 suffer TIAs.

- Incidence is higher in men >55 old.
- Stroke prevalence ranges from 1.1% to 2.2% in men and 0.8% to 1.9% in females.
- Prevalence is highest in non-Hispanic whites.
- Prevalence increases from 2% for age 50–59 to 12% for age ≥80.

Predominant Age

- Middle aged or older

Predominant Sex

- Men more than women

Age-Related Factors

- Pediatric: rare
- Geriatric: Incidence increases after age 50.

RISK FACTORS

Major embolic risk factors include:

- Atrial fibrillation: causes >50% of cases
- Prosthetic heart valves: 2%–4% embolism per year, highest for mitral valve prosthesis
- Aortic atheromatous disease: 12%–33% embolism over a 1- to 2-year period
- Anterior myocardial infarction: 30% incidence of left ventricular (LV) thrombus within first week and embolism of 5%–27% without anticoagulation
- Nonischemic cardiomyopathy: up to 30% prevalence of intracardiac thrombus and 14% embolism in normal sinus rhythm
- Aortic or cardiac surgery, aortic or arterial angiography, angioplasty, or intraaortic balloon pump insertion: embolism up to 12% and predominantly due to aortic atheroembolism
- Infective native or prosthetic valve endocarditis: 11%–44% embolism, highest in
  - —*Staphylococcus aureus* endocarditis or vegetations >10 mm
  - —Antiphospholipid syndrome up to 30% embolic risk

CAUSES

Ischemic stroke/TIA are caused by

- Intracerebral atherothrombosis or thromboembolism from cervicocephalic vessels in 60%
- Cardioembolism in 15% to 20%
- Lacunar infarcts in 20%
- Coagulopathy, vasculitis, migraine, or aortic dissection in 5%

PREGNANCY

- Increased incidence due to hypercoagulability.
- Oral contraceptives increase risk.

ASSOCIATED CONDITIONS

- Atrial fibrillation
- Prosthetic heart valves
- Infectious endocarditis
- Myocardial infarction
- Cardiomyopathy
- Vasculitis
- Cardiac surgery
- Mitral stenosis
- Left atrial myxoma
- Carotid and peripheral vascular disease

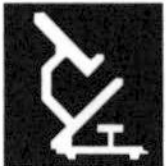

Diagnosis

DIFFERENTIAL DIAGNOSIS

- Intracranial/subarachnoid hemorrhage
- Hypoglycemia, drug overdose, seizures, or cerebral trauma if altered consciousness or coma
- Migraine, brain tumor, or subdural hematoma
- Infective/noninfective endocarditis, atrial myxoma, vasculitis, and hypercoagulability
- Primary aortic thrombosis occurs with severe aortoiliac atherosclerosis or aneurysm.

SIGNS AND SYMPTOMS

- Cerebral embolism
  - —Painless focal neurologic deficit with preserved consciousness that varies according to vascular occlusion distribution
- Ophthalmic artery
  - —Total or partial monocular blindness
- Anterior cerebral artery
  - —Contralateral weakness mainly of leg
- Middle cerebral artery (anterior branch)
  - —Contralateral motor and sensory loss of face, hand, arm, and nonfluent aphasia
  - —Posterior branch: contralateral hemisensory loss, homonymous hemianopsia and fluent aphasia
- Vertebrobasilar artery
  - —Binocular visual loss, quadriparesis, altered consciousness, ipsilateral cranial nerves or contralateral limbs, dysarthria, diplopia, vertigo, ataxia; impaired consciousness in hemorrhagic infarct, infarct-related seizure, intracranial hypertension, or brainstem involvement
- Cholesterol embolism
  - —Purple toe syndrome
  - —Acute nonoliguric renal failure
  - —Uncommonly, focal neurologic deficits, amaurosis fugax, or retinal emboli
  - —Rarely, mesenteric artery embolism
- Acute aortic occlusion
  - —Cold, pale, cyanotic or pulseless extremities, symmetrical weakness, loss of sensation, and areflexia
- Acute limb ischemia
  - —Severe pain in extremity, paresthesias, motor dysfunction, pulseless, and gangrene
- Splenic or renal infarct
  - —Left upper quadrant abdominal, shoulder pain and left pleural effusion; or flank pain, or gross or microscopic hematuria
- Antiphospholipid syndrome
  - —Young patient with embolism, thrombocytopenia, fetal loss, livedo reticularis, cardiolipin antibodies or lupus anticoagulant

LABORATORY PROCEDURES

- Complete blood and platelet count
- Prothrombin and partial thromboplastin time
- Serum electrolytes
- Blood glucose
- Renal and liver chemistries
- Fasting lipids
- Arterial blood gases if oxygen desaturation
- Serology or cardiolipin antibodies if vasculitis or antiphospholipid syndrome is suspected
- Erythrocyte sedimentation rate elevation, eosinophilia, and low complement levels in cholesterol embolism

Pathologic Findings

- Atherosclerosis, vascular occlusion
- Thromboembolia
- Organ infarction
- Vasculitis
- Endocarditis

IMAGING STUDIES

- Noncontrast CT
  - —Discriminates ischemic from hemorrhagic stroke
  - —Detects brain tumors or subdural hematoma
  - —Detects hypodensity suggestive of brain infarctions in 20% of TIAs
  - —Detects early edema, hydrocephalus, or hypodensities indicative of risk for hemorrhage
- Magnetic Resonance Imaging/Angiography (MRI/MRA)
  - —Most useful in patients with suspected brainstem or cerebellar infarctions
  - —Diffusion or perfusion MRI or MRI spectroscopy distinguishes infarct from ischemia.
  - —MRA best diagnostic value for intracranial and vertebrobasilar artery occlusions.
- Electrocardiography
  - —Detects myocardial infarction or arrhythmias.
- Color-Doppler Ultrasonography
  - —Method of choice for extracranial carotid and vertebral artery disease with 90% accuracy
- Transcranial Doppler Ultrasonography
  - —Assesses intracranial and vertebrobasilar arteries, or collaterals in carotid disease
- Angiography/Aortography
  - —Required for definition of severity/extent of carotid, vertebral and basilar artery disease in symptomatic patients with <70% carotid stenosis on ultrasonography or MRA
  - —Assesses severity of peripheral and aortic atherosclerosis and confirms aortic occlusion
- Echocardiography
  - —Can detect major cardioembolic substrates

—Saline contrast increases sensitivity for interatrial shunt in paradoxical embolism.
—TEE (transesophageal echocardiography) if equivocal or limited transthoracic echocardiogram or in young patients with embolism of undefined etiology

SPECIAL TESTS

- Cerebrospinal fluid exam in suspected infection or subarachnoid hemorrhage with negative CT
- Electroencephalography if seizures suspected

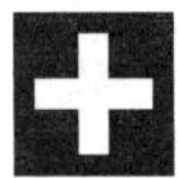

Treatment

GENERAL MEASURES

- Almost all patients are hospitalized.
- ECG monitoring for ≥24 hours
- In stroke patients, assure oxygenation, protect airways, and provide assisted ventilation if impaired consciousness.
- Keep NPO for at least first 24 hours.
- In stroke patients, do not treat hypertension aggressively unless severe (mean blood pressure of 130 mm Hg or systolic blood pressure >220 mm Hg), suspected hemorrhagic infarction, myocardial ischemia/infarction, hypertensive nephropathy, or aortic dissection. Keep systolic blood pressure just below 140 mm Hg or 160 mm Hg in those >60 years of age.
- Encourage mobilization after 24 hours
- Heparin s.c. or low-molecular-weight heparin to prevent DVT and pulmonary embolism
- Osmotherapy and hyperventilation if intracranial hypertension and clinical deterioration

SURGICAL MEASURES

- Primary prevention
  —In ascending aortic atheromatosis, change site of ortic cannulation
- Endarterectomy
  —Not better than aspirin for asymptomatic >50% carotid stenosis
- Secondary prevention
  —Elective carotid endarterectomy for symptomatic >70% carotid stenosis reduces ipsilateral stroke from 13.1%–16.8% to 2.5%–2.8% over a 2- to 3-year period.
- Immediate thromboembolectomy with aortic reconstruction or aortofemoral/axillofemoral bypass in aortic occlusion
- Primary angioplasty stent for aortoiliac, femoral, popliteal, or infrapopliteal artery occlusion. Alternatives include thrombolytics alone or followed by angioplasty stent or primary surgical revascularization.

Medications

DRUG(S) OF CHOICE

Primary Prevention

- Aspirin 325 mg/day: standard therapy for stroke/TIA prevention; up to 48% risk reduction, especially in men
- Warfarin (INR 2–3) in nonvalvular atrial fibrillation: reduces embolism from 5.8% to 2.6% per year (63% relative risk reduction)
- Aspirin reduces embolism from 6.3% to 3.6% (42% relative risk reduction).
- Heparin i.v. to 1.5–2.5 times baseline PTT, heparin s.c. 12,500 units every 12 hours, or warfarin (INR 2–3) reduces stroke rate from 3.8% to 0.8% in patients with anterior infarcts, LVEF <35%, or LV thrombus. Warfarin for 3–6 months is recommended.
- Long-term warfarin therapy (INR 2–3): in rheumatic mitral valve disease and atrial fibrillation; mitral stenosis and left atrial enlargement (>5.5 cm); before mitral valvuloplasty; nonischemic cardiomyopathy and atrial fibrillation, LVEF <35%, or LV thrombus; and mechanical heart valves (INR 2.5–3.5)

Secondary Prevention

- Aspirin 325 mg/day or ticlopidine 250 mg b.i.d. (if aspirin failure/intolerance) reduces recurrent nonfatal stroke, myocardial infarction, and vascular death by 14%–36%.
- Clopidogrel 75 mg/day if aspirin or ticlopidine intolerance
- Early heparin i.v. and lifelong anticoagulation are indicated after surgical correction of aortic occlusion.
- Thrombolytics (rtPA): beneficial when used within 3 hours of symptom onset in patients <77 years of age without cerebral infarct on CT, but this therapy awaits further studies
- Heparin i.v. in stroke/TIA lacks supportive data. Its early use may increase risk of hemorrhagic infarction.
- Antiplatelets or anticoagulants not beneficial for cholesterol embolism

Significant Possible Interactions

Warfarin interacts with many drugs.

ALTERNATIVE DRUGS

Lipid-lowering drugs in patients with high cholesterol levels.

Follow-up

PATIENT MONITORING

- Routine warfarin therapy.
- With ticlopidine therapy, complete blood count every 2 weeks for 3 months.

Prevention/Avoidance

- Detection/treatment of hypertension, hyperlipidemia, and diabetes mellitus
- Smoking cessation, weight reduction, and regular exercise
- Avoid/discontinue oral contraceptives.
- Enroll in rehabilitation programs.

Possible Complications

- Death
- Limb loss
- Incapacitation (stroke)
- Blindness
- Organ loss (i.e., kidney)

EXPECTED COURSE AND PROGNOSIS

- Stroke/TIA clinical course
  —The stroke risk after TIA is 4%–8% the first month, 12%–13% the first year, and 24%–29% in 5 years.
  —Patients with stroke/TIA related to carotid stenosis have a 7%–12% recurrent rate per year and 30%–35% within 5 years.
- Stroke/TIA mortality and morbidity
  —Mortality ranges from 26.8% to 52% in men and 22.7% to 39.9% in women.
  —Highest rates in black males and females, and in patients >65 years of age
  —Worst prognosis in those with basilar artery, internal carotid artery, or main stem middle cerebral artery occlusion (50%–75% die or have poor neurologic recovery)
  —Patients with cerebral edema or intracranial hypertension have a 10%–20% mortality rate during the first week.
  —DVT and pulmonary embolism account for a 10% mortality.
  —Pneumonia is also cause of death.
- Peripheral arterial embolism
  —Patients with cholesterol embolism have a 38%–80% mortality rate and those with aortic occlusion a 30%–40% operative mortality.
    - Coronary artery disease is the most important cause of death in elderly patients.

PATIENT EDUCATION

- Activity as tolerated
- Diet: Low fat, low cholesterol

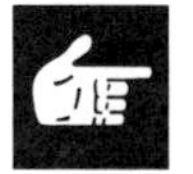

Miscellaneous

ICD-9-CM

434.1 Cerebral embolism
444.22 Peripheral artery embolism

BIBLIOGRAPHY

Braunwald E, ed. *Heart diseases. A textbook of cardiovascular medicine,* 5th ed. Philadelphia: WB Saunders, 1997.

Guidelines for the management of transient ischemic attacks. *Circulation* 1994;89:2950–2965.

Guidelines for the management of patients with acute ischemic stroke. *Circulation* 1994;90:1588–1601.

1997 Heart and Stroke Statistical Update, American Heart Association.

Topol EJ. *Textbook of cardiovascular medicine,* 1st ed. Philadelphia: Lippincott-Raven, 1998.

Author: Carlos A. Roldan

Arterial Hypertension

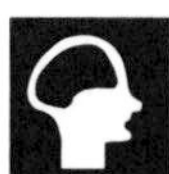

Basics

DESCRIPTION

Systolic blood pressure of 140 mmHg or greater, diastolic blood pressure of 90 mmHg or greater, or taking antihypertensive medication. These parameters are based on the level of blood pressure associated with the long-term risk of cardiovascular events.

EPIDEMIOLOGY

The prevalence of hypertension increases with the age of the population, such that 60% of U.S. adults 65–74 years of age have hypertension.

Race

- The prevalence of hypertension among blacks is greater at every age, and they tend to have more severe hypertensive disease with a higher mortality rate than whites.
- Among Americans 60 years or older: 60% of whites, 71% of blacks, and 61% of Mexican-Americans have hypertension.

Gender

Before menopause, hypertension is less common in women than in men.

ETIOLOGY

- In nearly 95% of patients with hypertension, there is no recognizable cause and it is referred to as "primary" hypertension.
  —Because blood pressure is determined by cardiac output and peripheral resistance, alteration in the factors that influence these parameters may precipitate hypertension, such as excessive sodium intake, stress, obesity, endothelium-derived factors, and genetic alterations.
- Secondary hypertension in which an identifiable secondary process precipitates hypertension includes the following possible causes:
  —Renal/renovascular disease
  —Endocrine disorders
  —Coarctation of the aorta
  —Neurologic disorders
  —Acute stress
  —Ethanol/drug use
  —Pregnancy-induced hypertension

Genetics

- Familial aggregation and twin studies confirm that hereditary plays a role and that genetic contributions are estimated to range from 30% to 60%.
- Hypertension appears to be polygenic and multifactorial with involvement of several genes.
- One linkage involves regions within or close to the angiotensinogen gene.

RISK FACTORS

- Obesity
- Sleep apnea
- Physical inactivity
- Alcohol intake
- Smoking
- Polycythemia vera or "pseudo-polycythemia vera"
- Hyperuricemia

PREGNANCY

Synonyms include preeclampsia, pregnancy-induced hypertension, and gestational hypertension.

- Preeclampsia is hypertension accompanied by proteinuria with or without abnormal coagulation, renal function, and liver function, which may progress to a convulsive phase and eclampsia.
- Occurs in 10% of first pregnancies in previously normotensive women
- Usually self-limited, rarely recurs in subsequent pregnancies
- Predisposing factors include increased age, black race, multiple gestations, concomitant renal or cardiac disease, and chronic hypertension.
- Clinical features include young age (<20 years), primigravida, >20 weeks of pregnancy, systolic blood pressure <160 mm Hg, edema, spasm and edema on funduscopic examination, proteinuria, and elevated plasma uric acid.
- Treatment includes modified bed rest, normal sodium intake, and antihypertensive medications if diastolic blood pressure exceeds 100 mm Hg. Antihypertensive therapy includes methyldopa and hydralazine. Angiotensin-converting enzyme (ACE) inhibitors are contraindicated.
- Cure is achieved with delivery.
- Excellent prognosis; does not cause hypertension nor is it a sign of latent hypertension

ASSOCIATED CONDITIONS

- Coronary artery disease/congestive heart failure, sudden death, arrhythmias
- Left ventricular hypertrophy
- Stroke/transient ischemic attacks
- Renal failure
- Retinopathy
- Carotid atherosclerosis
- Peripheral arterial disease

Diagnosis

CLINICAL DIAGNOSIS

Obtain the average of at least two blood pressure measurements taken at each of at least two visits after an initial screening visit, using standardized technique.

DIFFERENTIAL DIAGNOSIS

Secondary Hypertension

Because of the low frequency of secondary causes, be selective in screening and diagnostic tests. Reserve testing for the presence of features inappropriate for usual, uncomplicated primary hypertension, including:

- Onset at <20 or >50 years of age
- Extreme hypertension, particularly if refractory to standard treatment
- Accelerated or malignant hypertension
- Recent elevation of serum creatinine that is unexplained or reversibly induced by an ACE inhibitor
- Unprovoked hypokalemia
- Abdominal bruit
- Labile paroxysms of hypertension with headache, tachycardia, sweating, tremor
- Abdominal or flank mass
- Delayed/absent femoral pulses with lower blood pressure in the lower extremities
- Truncal obesity with purple striae

Isolated Systolic Hypertension

Defined as an elevated systolic pressure ≥140 mm Hg with normal diastolic pressure <90 mm Hg

- Increased pulse pressure indicates reduced vascular compliance in large arteries
- Accounts for more that half of the cases of hypertension in the elderly
- Increased risk of stroke, congestive heart failure, and coronary heart disease
- Elevated systolic blood pressure is a stronger risk factor for cardiovascular morbidity and mortality than elevated diastolic blood pressure

White Coat Hypertension

An excessive increase in blood pressure in response to the stress of being in the physician's office

- Particularly affects the systolic blood pressure
- Common in older women
- In the absence of target organ damage, if suspected, should obtain readings outside of the office with self-measurement or ambulatory monitoring

Pseudohypertension

Due to excessive vascular stiffness in which markedly calcified, sclerotic arteries do not collapse under the cuff, leading to spuriously high readings

Hypertensive Crisis

Involves clinical circumstances that require rapid blood pressure reduction to prevent or limit target organ damage, including encephalopathy, intracranial hemorrhage, unstable angina, acute myocardial infarction, acute left ventricular failure with pulmonary edema, acute aortic dissection, acute renal failure, and eclampsia. Hypertensive crisis can be categorized as follows:

- Hypertensive emergency that requires immediate reduction of blood pressure within 1 hour (e.g., encephalopathy, acute myocardial infarction, acute pulmonary edema, eclampsia)
- Hypertensive urgency in which blood pressure reduction is desirable within a few hours (e.g., optic disc edema, severe perioperative hypertension)

SIGNS AND SYMPTOMS

- Majority of patients are asymptomatic, for as long as 10–20 years
- Can present with symptoms of headache, tinnitus, syncope, angina, and dyspnea
- Common physical findings include prominent left ventricular apical impulse, fourth heart sound, funduscopic signs of arterial narrowing/arteriovenous nicking, hemorrhages, and exudates
- Look for other signs of target organ damage such as atherosclerosis and left ventricular failure.
- In hypertensive crisis: headache, confusion, somnolence/stupor, visual loss, focal neurologic deficits, seizure, coma, funduscopic hemorrhages/exudates, papilledema, and nausea/vomiting

LABORATORY PROCEDURES

- Urinalysis
- Chemical profile including creatinine, blood glucose, potassium, uric acid and lipids
- Optional tests include creatinine clearance, microalbuminuria, 24-hour protein, blood calcium, glycosylated hemoglobin, and thyroid-stimulating hormone.

IMAGING STUDIES

Echocardiography

- Not indicated in routine initial evaluation unless there is another specific indication; more sensitive and specific for identifying left ventricular hypertrophy than the electrocardiogram; too expensive for routine use

Chest X-ray

- Not indicated in routine evaluation

SPECIAL TESTS

- ECG
  - —Left ventricular hypertrophy, evidence of ischemic heart disease, arrhythmias
- Renin, catecholamines, and aldosterone are not recommended in the initial evaluation unless there are specific clinical clues to indicate them.
- Ambulatory blood pressure monitoring
  - —Correlates better with target organ involvement than office blood pressure measurement; may be useful in ruling out white coat hypertension, assessing abnormal nocturnal patterns in blood pressure, apparent drug resistance, and hypotensive symptoms with antihypertensive medication
  - —Not routine procedure in initial evaluation
- Additional studies may be necessary in the following conditions:
  - —Patients <15 years of age with hypertension; elderly patients with recent onset of moderate or moderate-severe hypertension
  - —Accelerated hypertension
  - —Worsening renal dysfunction
  - —Spontaneous hypokalemia
  - —Hypertension despite triple therapy including a diuretic
  - —Hypertension and symptoms of headache, unusual patterns of sweating and palpitations

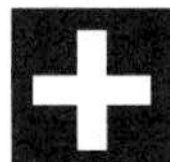

Treatment

GENERAL MEASURES

- Risk stratify patients according to severity of hypertension and presence of target organ damage, clinical cardiovascular disease, or cardiovascular risk factors in order to determine treatment strategy (see the Appendix for the table on Risk Stratification in Hypertensive Patients) as follows:
- Target organ damage includes those with:
  - —Heart diseases
    - Left ventricular hypertrophy
    - Angina or prior myocardial infarction
    - Prior coronary revascularization
    - Heart failure
  - —Stroke or transient ischemic attacks
  - —Nephropathy
  - —Peripheral arterial disease
  - —Retinopathy
- Life-style modification includes weight loss, sodium restriction, moderation of alcohol intake, physical activity, adequate intake of calcium/potassium, and magnesium

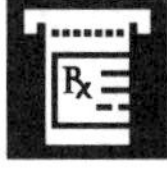

Medications

DRUG(S) OF CHOICE

- Unless another agent is indicated, a diuretic or beta-blocker should be chosen as the initial line of treatment.
- In certain clinical conditions, there are compelling indications for specific agents as initial treatment, such as ACE inhibitors in patients with diabetes with proteinuria, or heart failure.
- A second or third agent may be necessary if the response is inadequate after the full dose is given.

ADMISSION CRITERIA

- Hypertensive crisis

Follow-up

PATIENT MONITORING

- Most patients should be seen within 1–2 months after initiation of treatment to determine adequacy of blood pressure control.
- Once blood pressure stabilized, follow up at 3- to 6-month intervals.

EXPECTED COURSE AND PROGNOSIS

- Several trials have shown a 38% reduction in stroke morbidity/mortality, a 16% reduction in coronary heart disease events, and a 52% reduction in congestive heart failure occurrence.
- Lowering blood pressure in elderly hypertensive patients has resulted in a 37% reduction in stroke, a 25% reduction in transient ischemic attacks, a 30% reduction in myocardial infarctions, and a 54% reduction in occurrence of congestive heart failure

PATIENT EDUCATION

- Life-style modification as discussed above
- Medication compliance

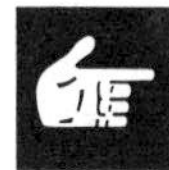

Miscellaneous

ICD-9-CM

401.9 Unspecified
401.1 Malignant

BIBLIOGRAPHY

Joint National Committee on Prevention, Detection, Evaluation and Treatment of High Blood Pressure and the National High Blood Pressure Education Program Coordinating Committee. The Sixth Report of the Joint National Committee on Prevention, Detection, Evaluation, and Treatment of High Blood Pressure. *Arch Intern Med* 1997;157:2413–2446.

Kaplan NM. System hypertension: mechanism and diagnosis. In: Braunwald E, ed. *Heart disease,* 5th ed. Philadelphia: WB Saunders, 1997:807–839.

Moser M. *Clinical management of hypertension,* 3rd ed. Professional Communication, Inc., 1998.

Author: Helene Glassberg

Arteriovenous Fistulas

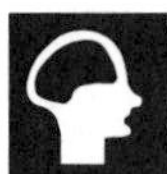

Basics

DESCRIPTION

Arteriovenous fistulas are direct connections between the arterial and venous blood supply bypassing the capillary bed.

- They may be found in the systemic, pulmonary and coronary circulation and are a rare cause of congestive heart failure and myocardial ischemia.
- They also can cause a variety of clinical problems, including cutaneous lesions, disfigurement and a mass effect causing local compression.

EPIDEMIOLOGY

The majority of arteriovenous fistulas are congenital. Fistulas also may occur after surgery or trauma.

- Reported incidence depends on varying definitions and local referral patterns
- Large arteriovenous fistulas (Knudson, n = 157)
  —Central nervous system 52%
  —Hepatic vascular tumors 39%
  —Pulmonary arteriovenous fistulas 9%
- Boston Children's Series 1973–1987 (Fyler, n = 31)
  —Coronary 45%
  —Cerebral 16%
  —Systemic 16%
  —Pulmonary 13%
  —Hepatic 10%

ASSOCIATED CONDITIONS

- Hereditary hemorrhagic telangiectasias
- Capillary-cavernous hemangiomas
- Klippel-Trenaunay-Weber Syndrome

ETIOLOGY

The causes of the congenital fistulas are unknown.

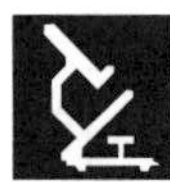

Diagnosis

DIFFERENTIAL DIAGNOSIS

- Large cerebral, hepatic or peripheral arteriovenous malformations (AVMs) can present shortly after birth with signs and symptoms of congestive heart failure.
- Tachycardia, tachypnea, hepatomegaly, and severe respiratory distress mimic heart failure due to other causes such as cardiomyopathy, and congenital heart lesions with large left-to-right shunts.
- Pulses are bounding, especially in the upper extremities, similar to findings in a patent ductus arteriosus, and often there is a differential in blood pressures between the arms and the legs, simulating a coarctation of the aorta.
- A bruit is typically heard over the fistula; therefore, auscultation of the head should be part of the physical examination in all newborns.

SIGNS AND SYMPTOMS

Intracranial Arteriovenous Fistulas

- These are commonly aneurysms of the vein of Galen but may be found in any vessel in the central nervous system.
- Clinical manifestations depend on the age of presentation.
- Birth to 1 month of age
  —Heart failure is the most common presenting sign and may be associated with a cranial bruit and rarely with hydrocephalus.
  —Severe symptoms may present in the first few hours of life
  —Because the shunt is mandatory and not dependent on pulmonary vascular resistance, right and left heart failure occur early.
  —Right ventricular failure is secondary to both volume loading from the AVM and pressure loading from the high pulmonary vascular resistance of the newborn period.
  —The early onset of heart failure seen in this lesion is in sharp contrast to intracardiac left-to-right shunts such as a ventricular septal defect, in which manifestations of heart failure are not seen until the pulmonary vascular resistance decreases associated with an increase in left-to-right shunting.
  —Rarely an AVM can be the cause of fetal hydrops.
- 1–12 months of age
  —Hydrocephalus is the most common presenting sign at this age. Heart failure (33%) and seizures (33%) also can occur.

Coronary Artery Fistulas

- Can occur between the coronary arteries and the atria, ventricles, and pulmonary artery
- Small fistulas
  —Usually asymptomatic but can present with a heart murmur, endocarditis, or ischemia later in life secondary to coronary steal
- Large fistulas
  —Can present with congestive heart failure in the newborn period.

Pulmonary Arteriovenous Fistulas

- Congenital
  —Hereditary hemorrhagic telangiectasia
- Acquired
  —Severe liver disease and cirrhosis
  —Following cardiopulmonary anastomosis (Glenn shunts)
- Clinical manifestations include dyspnea, cyanosis, clubbing, polycythemia, hemoptysis, and signs of embolic phenomenon including transient ischemic attacks, strokes, and cerebral abscesses.
- The heart examination is usually normal.

Hemangiomas

Hemangiomas are not true AVMs, but rather are vascular tumors of proliferating endothelial cells with capillary channels. These tumors are common in the first year of life and then usually undergo spontaneous involution. Occasionally they require treatment because of their unusual size or location.

- Small hemangiomas often are visible in the skin, usually follow a benign course, and resolve spontaneously.
- Large capillary cavernous hemangioma can present with serious or life-threatening complications secondary to:
  —Congestive heart failure due to increased volume
  —Respiratory compromise due to tracheal compression
  —Loss of vision due to invasion of the orbit
  —Kassbach-Merritt syndrome (rapidly enlarging hemangioma, thrombocytopenia, acute or chronic consumption coagulopathy)
- Hepatic hemangiomas most commonly are hemangioendotheliomas or cavernous hemangiomas. These may present in infancy, causing congestive heart failure or hepatomegaly and are often associated with hemangiomas of the skin.

PHYSICAL FINDINGS

- Intracranial arteriovenous fistulas
  —Tachypnea, tachycardia, and congestive heart failure
  —Pulses are usually bounding, especially in the upper extremities.
  —In patients with an intracranial aneurysm, bounding pulses in the arms and neck with decreased pulses in the lower extremities simulating a coarctation of the aorta have been reported.

IMAGING STUDIES

Intracranial Arteriovenous Fistulas

- Chest radiographs
  —Demonstrate cardiomegaly and increased pulmonary markings
- Echocardiography
  —Demonstrates normal intracardiac anatomy in most children
  —The degree of cardiac enlargement is proportional to the size of the fistula.
  —The presence of a large cerebral AVM can be suspected on echocardiography because of the increased size of the aorta, pulmonary artery, and superior vena cava.
  —The great vessels leading to the AVM are enlarged.
  —Doppler flow studies demonstrate abnormal retrograde diastolic flow patterns in the descending aorta.
  —Cranial ultrasonography will demonstrate the abnormal vessels in the majority of patients.
  —Cardiac catheterization is usually not necessary to establish the diagnosis of a cerebral AVM.

Coronary Artery Fistulas

- Echocardiography
  —Can localize the size and location
  —More precise localization by angiography is usually necessary to determine the extent of the lesion.

Pulmonary Arteriovenous Fistulas

- Echocardiography utilizing peripheral venous contrast techniques may be useful by identifying abnormal appearance of pulmonary arteries and veins.
- Catheterization demonstrates pulmonary venous desaturation in the affected segment
- Angiography demonstrates the rapid filling of the pulmonary vein in the affected segment.

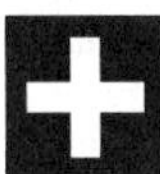

Treatment

GENERAL MEASURES

Intracranial Arteriovenous Fistulas

- Treatment consists of medical control of congestive heart failure and occlusion of the arteriovenous fistulas with embolization or surgical techniques depending on the size and location of the lesion.
- A variety of catheterization techniques using liquid adhesives, particulate agents, balloons, and coils can be used to achieve closure of the AVM.
- Optimal management uses a team approach combining neurosurgical, interventional, and pediatric disciplines.
- The use of these catheterization procedures can sometimes obviate or delay the need for neurosurgical procedures. Despite all measures, the prognosis is often poor.

Coronary Artery Fistulas

- Because the majority of these remain open, surgical treatment is usually required and may be life saving in those children with heart failure.
- Small to moderate fistulas are closed to prevent endocarditis and late myocardial ischemia.
- Tiny fistulas may close spontaneously.

Pulmonary Arteriovenous Fistulas

Pulmonary AVMs often can be treated successfully by coil embolization.

Hemangiomas

- Small hemangiomas usually require no treatment and undergo spontaneous regression.
- Large hemangiomas have been treated with steroids, cyclophosphamide, laser therapy, and interferon with variable rates of success.
- Surgical excision is difficult because of the lack of clear lines of demarcation between normal and abnormal tissue. Fortunately, these lesions often regress with age.

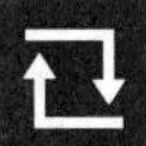

Follow-up

PATIENT MONITORING

- Patient follow-up depends on the size of the fistulas and the response to treatment.
- Children in heart failure require hospitalization to initiate management of heart failure and undergo closure of the fistulas.
- These children uniformly do poorly without treatment, and the success of treatment is dependent on the degree of closure of the AVM.
- Complete closure of the lesion is sometimes not possible, and partial closure can significantly decrease the degree of heart failure and allow the infant to grow and develop.
- Repeat attempts at closure can be undertaken when the child is older. In general, the overall prognosis for large AVMs in the central nervous system is guarded, although new catheter closure techniques are promising.
- The prognosis for hepatic hemangiomas most often is favorable, depending on the type of hemangioma. The prognosis for cardiac AVMs is usually excellent with optimal management.

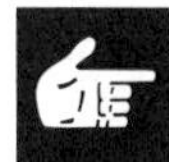

Miscellaneous

BIBLIOGRAPHY

Fyler DC. Aortopulmonary fistulas. In: Fyler DC, ed. *Nadas' pediatric cardiology.* Baltimore: Hanely & Belfus, 1992:707–714.

Knudson RP, Alden ER. Symptomatic arteriovenous malformations in infants less than 6 months of age. *Pediatrics* 1979;45:81–102.

McMahon WS. Arteriovenous fistulas. In: Garson A, Bricker JT, Fisher DJ, Neish SR, eds. *The science and practice of pediatric cardiology,* 2nd ed. Baltimore: Williams & Wilkins, 1998:1677–1688.

Musewe NN, Burrows PE, Culham JAG, Freedom RM. Arteriovenous fistulae: a consideration of extracardiac causes of congestive heart failure. In: Freedom RM, Benson LN, Smallhorn JF, eds. *Neonatal heart disease.* London: Springer-Verlag, 1992:759–772.

Preminger TJ, Perry SB, Burrows PE. Vascular anomalies. In: Emmanouilides GC, Riemenschneider TA, Allen HD, Gutgessel HP, eds. *Moss and Adams' heart disease in infants, children, and adolescents including the fetus and young adult,* 5th ed. Baltimore: Williams & Wilkins, 1995.

Authors: Thomas J. Starc and Welton M. Gersony

Atherosclerosis

Basics

DESCRIPTION

Inflammatory fibroproliferative response to insults to vascular endothelium

EPIDEMIOLOGY

- Leading cause of death in the United States and other developed countries (50%)
- 20% of all deaths worldwide (14 million/yr)
- Leading cause of death in men >35 years, and men and women >45 years
- Consumes at least 7.9% total health expenditure in industrialized countries
- Men are more commonly affected than women (4:1) until menopause, then similar incidence.
- Peak incidence for men is at 50–60 years of age; for women 60–70 years of age.

ETIOLOGY

Unknown; highly associated with risk factors; polygenic inheritance with tendency to clustering of risk factors within families

AGE-RELATED FACTORS

- Elderly: overall prognosis worse; more sensitive to side effects of medications
- Pediatrics: rare; consider homozygous familial hyperlipidemia or homocystinuria

RISK FACTORS

Traditional/Independent

- Age: men >45 years, women >55 years (postmenopausal without hormone replacement)
- Hypertension, even if treated
- Diabetes mellitus
- Family history of heart disease in primary relative: men <55 years, women <65 years
- Elevated LDL cholesterol
- Low HDL cholesterol
- Cigarette smoking

Nontraditional

- Physical inactivity
- Overweight (central obesity)
- Elevated homocysteine
- Elevated lipoprotein (a)
- Hypertriglyceridemia
- Increased C-reactive protein
- Increased fibrinogen, Factor VIII, Factor VII, plasminogen activator inhibitor type-1
- Syndrome X (insulin resistance)
- Angiotensin-converting enzyme DD genotype
- Passive smoking
- Increased small, dense LDL (pattern B)

PREGNANCY

- Rare; consider other causes of coronary artery disease: dissection, spasm, emboli and vasculitis

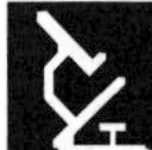

Diagnosis

DIFFERENTIAL DIAGNOSIS

N/A

SIGNS AND SYMPTOMS

- Coronary artery disease (CAD): often silent until angina or acute coronary syndrome [unstable angina, myocardial infarction (MI), or sudden death]
- Peripheral vascular disease: aneurysm, renal failure, hypertension, arterial ischemia
- Cerebrovascular disease: transient ischemic attacks, stroke, dementia

PATHOPHYSIOLOGY

- Response to injury hypothesis (most widely accepted)
- Fatty streak: type I injury secondary to blood flow pattern disturbance resulting in macrophage, lymphocyte, lipid accumulation (often begins in childhood); oxidized LDL major atherogenic lipid
- Fibrous plaque: type II injury secondary to release of growth factors, cytokines, vasoregulatory molecules from macrophages and platelets resulting in smooth muscle cell migration (vascular media to intima), proliferation (intima), platelet aggregation
- Thrombus formation: type III injury secondary to fissure in plaque resulting in lysis, growth of lesion, total occlusion of vessel
- Complicated lesion: calcified fibrous plaques containing central fatty necrosis with higher propensity for thrombotic process, plaque rupture

LABORATORY PROCEDURES

- Fasting lipid profile: consider serum homocysteine, lipoprotein (a), and C-reactive protein levels

IMAGING STUDIES

Noninvasive

- X-ray: calcification of coronary arteries and aorta as incidental finding
- Doppler ultrasonography: evaluates peripheral vessels, e.g., carotid artery stenosis, aortic abdominal aneurysms
- Electron beam CT: quantifies coronary artery calcification, which correlates with plaque burden, distribution; evolving clinical data
- MRI: direct assessment of arterial wall and plaque composition, not yet linked to clinical decisions

Invasive

- Angiography: gold standard
- Intravascular ultrasonography: evaluates lesion characteristics, stent patency; research tool, not widely available
- Transesophageal echocardiography: diagnoses atheromatous disease of the aorta

SPECIAL TESTS

- Risk stratification to determine management, prognosis
- Resting ECG commonly normal, may show infarction or ischemia; unreliable in left bundle branch block, Wolff-Parkinson-White syndrome, delayed intraventricular conduction
- Stress testing: exercise or pharmacologic (i.e., dipyridamole, adenosine, or dobutamine) for patients unable to exercise; indirectly detects obstructive disease, defines severity of ischemia; may help guide management decisions
- Myocardial perfusion imaging
  - —Thallium 201/technetium-99m: functional severity/marker for left ventricular dysfunction
  - —Stress echocardiogram: provides regional and functional assessment of stenosed coronary arteries
  - —Positron emission tomography scan: most sensitive/specific; low incidence of artifact; not widely available
- Radionucleotide angiography: evaluates left ventricular function if known CAD

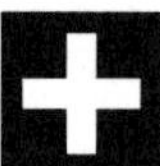

Treatment

GENERAL MEASURES

- Prevent event, disease progression by maximizing risk factor reduction.
- Stress reduction, tobacco cessation, dietary changes
- Risk stratify to determine medical management versus revascularization.
  - —Medical management: control symptoms, emphasis on secondary prevention
  - —Revascularization management
    - Angioplasty and stenting: major limitation is restenosis
    - Bypass graft: depends on location and severity

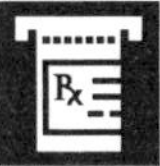

Medications

DRUG(S) OF CHOICE

Refer to Essential Hypertension; Coronary Atherosclerosis; Carotid Stenosis; Stroke; Congestive Heart Failure; Atrial Arrhythmias; Ventricular Arrhythmias; Chronic Renal Failure; Dissecting Aneurysm; Angina; Myocardial Infarction; Peripheral Vascular Disease; Arterial Thrombosis and Embolism.

Contraindications

Refer to manufacturer's literature.

Precautions

Refer to manufacturer's literature, also for interactions.

Follow-up

PATIENT MONITORING

- Patient symptoms, aggressive modification of risk factors

Prevention

- Primary prevention: Modify risk factors to prevent complications, progression of atherosclerosis.
  —Smoking cessation: risk equal to nonsmokers in 1–15 years
  —Hyperlipidemia: Management depends on LDL levels and other risk factors per National Cholesterol Education Program: target LDL <160 if 0–1 risk factors; LDL <130 if >2 risk factors; diabetics require LDL <100. HMG CoA inhibitors decrease coronary events with average to high cholesterol values. Combination therapy with other lipid-lowering agents may be used to optimize lipid profile.
  —Aspirin 325 mg orally daily
  —Hypertension: decrease diastolic BP to <85 mm Hg
  —Weight reduction/physical activity/diet: aerobic activity for 30 minutes at least three times per week; dietary therapy: American Heart Association Step I and Step II diets; improve hypertension, diabetes mellitus, and hyperlipidemia.
- Secondary prevention: Modify risk factors to prevent recurrent events.
  —Smoking cessation: reduces recurrence 50%
  —Hyperlipidemia: LDL goal <100; LDL goal <95 after coronary artery bypass grafting
  —Aspirin 80–325 mg orally daily; if contraindicated, clopidogrel, warfarin, or persantine alternative therapies
    - Hypertension: Decrease blood pressure to <140/90 mm Hg if no other risk factors, diastolic <80–85 mm Hg if diabetic.
    - Diabetes mellitus: Maintain fasting blood glucose <126 mg/dL and hemoglobin A1c <7%.
    - Beta-adrenergic blockers: Decrease mortality, treat arrhythmias, left ventricular failure, and further ischemia in post-MI patients
    - ACE inhibitors: Decrease mortality post-MI if started early, Rx systolic heart failure

Complications

- Arrhythmias, congestive heart failure, MI, renal failure, aortic dissection, stroke, peripheral vascular ischemia, sudden death

EXPECTED COURSE AND PROGNOSIS

Age and sex strong predictive risk factors for prognosis at onset of disease.

PATIENT EDUCATION

Activity

- Exercise program guided by physician

Diet

- Low-saturated fat, low-cholesterol, low-sodium American Heart Association step I and step II diets; possible benefit from Mediterranean diet, omega-3 fatty acids, antioxidants, vitamins E and C

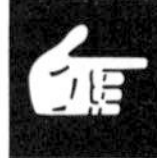

Miscellaneous

ICD-9-CM

414.01 Native coronary artery disease
414.00 CASHD, unspecified vessel
437.0 Cerebrovascular disease, arteriosclerotic
443.9 Peripheral vascular disease, unspecified

SYNONYMS

- Coronary artery disease
- Peripheral vascular disease
- Cerebral vascular disease

ORGANIZATIONS

- American Heart Association; phone 1-800-242-8721; http: www.americanheart.org
- American College of Cardiology; http: www.acc.org
- National Institutes of Health; http: www.nih.gov

See also: Myocardial Infarct, Angina, Peripheral Vascular Disease, Renal Failure, Arrhythmia (Atrial and Ventricular), Congestive Heart Failure, Stroke, Hypertension, Coronary Artery Disease, Dissecting Aneurysm

BIBLIOGRAPHY

Davies MJ. Pathology of coronary atherosclerosis. In: Alexander RW, Schlant RC, Fuster V, et al., eds. *Hurst's the heart,* 9th ed. New York: McGraw-Hill, 1998:1161–1173.

Hoeg JM. Evaluating coronary heart disease risk: tiles in the mosaic. *JAMA* 1997;227:1387–1390.

International Task Force for Prevention of Coronary Heart Disease. Coronary heart disease: reducing the risk. *Nutr Metab Cardiovasc Dis* 1998;8:212–271.

Maron DJ, Ridker PM, Pearson TA. Risk factors and the prevention of coronary heart disease. In: Alexander RW, Schlant RC, Fuster V, et al., eds. *Hurst's the heart,* 9th ed. New York: McGraw-Hill, 1998:1175–1195.

Ross R. The pathophysiology of atherosclerosis: a perspective for the 1990's. *Nature* 1993; 362:801–809.

Schlant RC, Alexander RW. Diagnosis and management of patients with chronic ischemic heart disease. In: Alexander RW, Schlant RC, Fuster V, et al., eds. *Hurst's the heart,* 9th ed. New York: McGraw-Hill, 1998:1275–1303.

Authors: Salem N. Sayar, Christine L. Nell, and Laurence S. Sperling

Athlete's Heart

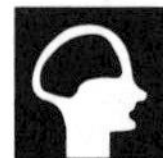

Basics

DESCRIPTION

Sustained exercise training induces adaptive changes in the cardiovascular system that allow for greater athletic performance. The major adaptations involve the heart, blood, and peripheral vascular system.

Heart

- Cardiac hypertrophy that is eccentric with predominant isotonic exercise and concentric with predominant isometric exercise
- Resting sinus bradycardia

Blood

Total blood volume increases due to proportional increases in red cells and plasma.

Peripheral Vascular System

Peripheral vascular capacitance increases, resulting in relative decreases in peripheral vascular resistance, allowing movement of a greater stroke volume without increases in systolic pressure.

Systems Affected

- Cardiovascular, hematopoietic

ETIOLOGY

Genetics

Adaptations to exercise and athletic ability may be partially determined by heredity.

Predominant Age

- Late adolescence to middle aged

Age-Related Factors

- Pediatric: Congenital heart disease predominates.
- Middle aged: Coronary artery disease dominates.

Predominant Sex

- Male more than female

CAUSES

- Regular, vigorous exercise training

RISK FACTORS

N/A

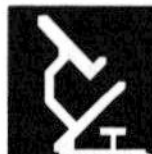

Diagnosis

DIFFERENTIAL DIAGNOSIS

- Abnormal bradyarrhythmias
- Pathologic ventricular hypertrophy
- Valvular heart disease
- Cardiomyopathy
- Coronary artery disease

SIGNS AND SYMPTOMS

- History of athletic training and prowess
- Orthostatic symptoms
- Athletic physique
- Sinus bradycardia
- Sinus arrhythmia
- Enlarged apical impulse
- Right ventricular lift
- Diastolic gallop sounds
- Systolic flow murmurs
- ECG: ventricular hypertrophy patterns (may mimic myocardial infarction), bradyarrhythmias
- Chest x-ray: cardiac enlargement

Pathologic Findings

- Ventricular hypertrophy

IMAGING STUDIES

- Chest x-ray: cardiac enlargement
- Echocardiography: Distinguish physiologic versus pathologic ventricular hypertrophy; identify valvular disease and cardiomyopathy.

SPECIAL TESTS

Exercise: Maximum oxygen uptake will identify exercise-trained individuals.

DIAGNOSTIC PROCEDURES

- If coronary artery disease is suspected, exercise testing with echo or radionuclide imaging may be indicated, or in some cases coronary angiography.
- Electrophysiologic testing may be required to distinguish pathologic rhythm disturbances from benign ones.
  —Tilt table testing may help elucidate the cause of dizziness or syncope encountered in an athlete.

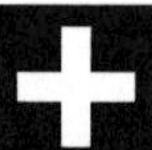

Treatment

GENERAL MEASURES

- Outpatient evaluation
- Distinguish normal physiologic changes from disease.
- Many cardiac diseases increase the risk of athletic activity:
  —Hypertrophic cardiomyopathy
  —Coronary artery anomalies or disease
  —Marfan's syndrome
  —Aortic valve disease
  —Complex congenital heart disease
  —Pulmonary hypertension
  —Mitral stenosis
  —Pulmonic stenosis

SURGICAL MEASURES

Corrective surgery for cardiac conditions may permit athletic activity.

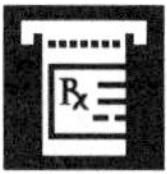

Medications

DRUG(S) OF CHOICE

- Depends on cardiac diseases
- Some performance-enhancing drugs have potential adverse effects on the heart, such as anabolic steroids and catecholamines.

Contraindications

Refer to manufacturer's profile of each drug.

Precautions

Athletically trained individuals are especially susceptible to drugs with vasodilator or heart rate–slowing properties such as alpha- and beta-blockers.

Significant Possible Interactions

Refer to manufacturer's literature.

ALTERNATIVE DRUGS

Occasionally athletic training will need to be stopped temporarily until a specific disease is treated with drugs that affect a response in the patient.

Follow-up

PATIENT MONITORING

- Occasionally the only way to distinguish normal physiology from disease is to cease exercise training and observe the patient.
- Sinus bradycardia and chamber enlargement usually regress significantly within weeks.

Prevention/Avoidance

Patients with certain cardiac diseases should have exercise activities limited to avoid sudden death or other serious consequences. Occasionally athletic competition can be allowed with successful drug, surgery, or device therapy (i.e., implantable defibrillator).

Possible Complications

- Sudden arrhythmic death
- Aortic dissection
- Precipitation of heart failure
- Syncope

EXPECTED COURSE AND PROGNOSIS

- Exercise-trained individuals are usually more healthy and live longer than sedentary individuals in the absence of significant cardiovascular disease.
- The combination of athletic activities and certain cardiovascular diseases can shorten life.

Activity

- Based on type of cardiac abnormality and the desired physical activity/sport

Diet

- Depends on cardiac conditions and training requirements

PATIENT EDUCATION

Important to describe risks of cardiac disease if patient desires participation in athletic activities.

Miscellaneous

ICD-9-CM

429.3 Athlete's heart

BIBLIOGRAPHY

Maron BJ, ed. The athlete's heart and cardiovascular disease. *Cardial Clin* 1997;15:345–513.

Maroon BJ, Mitchell JA. 26th Bethesda conference: recommendations for determining eligibility for competition in athletes with cardiovascular abnormalities. *J Am Coll Cardiol* 1994; 24:845–899.

Author: Michael H. Crawford

Atrial Fibrillation

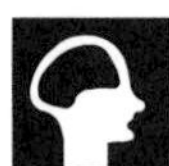

Basics

DESCRIPTION

Atrial fibrillation (AF) is the rapid, disorganized, and asynchronous contraction of atrial muscle.

- Characterized by the absence of clearly defined atrial complexes on the surface electrocardiogram
- AF increases cardiovascular mortality, total mortality following myocardial infarction, and stroke (17-fold if rheumatic heart disease)

EPIDEMIOLOGY

- Dependent on age and presence or underlying heart disease
- AF is increasingly frequent as population ages (0.02% prevalence among those 18–39 years of age; 11.6% among those >75 years of age)

ETIOLOGY

Usually related to one or more of the following:

- Hypertension
- Coronary artery disease
- Valvular heart disease
- Cardiomyopathy

Rare cases of familial AF have been reported.

RISK FACTORS

- For AF
  - —Hypertension
  - —Coronary artery disease
  - —Valvular heart disease
  - —Cardiomyopathy
- For stroke in association with AF
  - —Hypertension
  - —Congestive heart failure
  - —Diabetes
  - —Increasing age (>65 years)
  - —Left ventricular dysfunction, and increased left atrial dimension on echocardiogram
  - —Prior stroke or transient ischemic attack (TIA)

PREGNANCY

- May exacerbate arrhythmias in young women
- If AF occurs in concert with Wolff-Parkinson-White syndrome, regular reentrant tachycardias may be more frequent and can degenerate to AF.
- If there is underlying heart disease, pregnancy may either be dangerous or contraindicated. Warfarin is associated with congenital birth defects.

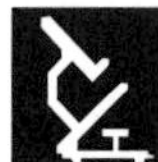

Diagnosis

DIFFERENTIAL DIAGNOSIS

- Atrial flutter (regular and irregular)
- Multifocal atrial tachycardia (irregular)
- Atrial tachycardia (regular)
- Atrioventricular (AV) reentrant and AV nodal reentrant tachycardias (regular)
- Junctional tachycardia (regular)

SIGNS AND SYMPTOMS

- None
- Palpitations
- Dyspnea
- Fatigue
- Congestive heart failure
- Angina
- Syncope
- Stroke

IMAGING STUDIES

- Cardiac catheterization and angiography if ischemia and/or coronary artery disease are suspected

SPECIAL TESTS

- ECG
- Ambulatory monitor (especially useful if AF paroxysmal)
- Echocardiogram to evaluate structural heart disease (myocardial and valvular)

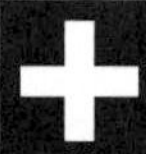

Treatment

GENERAL MEASURES

- Stroke is prevented by anticoagulation with warfarin.
- All patients >65 years of age, or younger if a risk factor for stroke is present (hypertension, diabetes, left ventricular hypertrophy, prior stroke or TIA, congestive heart failure), should be anticoagulated.
- Symptoms and quality of life can be improved either by controlling the ventricular response or by restoring sinus rhythm.
- The Atrial Fibrillation Follow-up Investigation of Rhythm Management (AFFIRM) Trial is designed to determine whether patients treated with a strategy to maintain sinus rhythm have better survival than those treated with a strategy only to control the ventricular response.
- The decision to cardiovert depends on an assessment of relative risks and benefits of the procedure.
  - —Benefits of restoring sinus rhythm include the possibilities of fewer symptoms related to AF and stopping anticoagulation.
  - —Associated with risks of proarrhythmia from antiarrhythmic drugs, bradycardia, and an increased chance for adverse drug reactions
- Rate control strategy may be less costly.
- Patients left in AF with a controlled ventricular response may have more symptoms, and certainly need continued anticoagulation.
- Either drugs or AV node ablation with pacemaker implantation can accomplish the goal of rate control.
- Conversion can be accomplished by drug therapy or by synchronized electrical cardioversion.
- Cardioversion should be immediate when there is hemodynamic instability, ongoing angina, or congestive heart failure.
- Rapid conduction over an accessory pathway in the Wolff-Parkinson-White syndrome is also an indication for emergent cardioversion. Patients with less severe signs or symptoms can be cardioverted electively.
- Certain patients should not be cardioverted, including those who are not anticoagulated (at least 3 weeks) when the duration of AF is unknown or >48 hours.
- Patients with an echocardiogram showing left atrial thrombus or a predictor of stroke (such as mitral stenosis) should be therapeutically anticoagulated for at least 3 weeks.
- People with frequent recurrences of AF despite multiple prior antiarrhythmic drug trials would not be anticipated to maintain sinus rhythm and therefore should not be converted.
- AF with a slow ventricular response carries a higher risk for cardioversion because sick sinus syndrome may be expected. For these people, rate support should be available at the time of shock delivery, for example, with a temporary or permanent transvenous pacemaker.
- New options for therapy to maintain sinus rhythm include the surgical Maze procedure

and the investigational catheter-based Maze procedure.
- Atrial defibrillators are in clinical trials.
- There are usually not restrictions on activity, and dietary recommendations are made as appropriate for underlying disease or syndrome such as diabetes, coronary artery disease, heart failure, and hypertension.

SURGICAL MEASURES

New, innovative therapies to manage AF include AV node ablation (or modification) and implantation of pacemaker (dual-chamber if AF paroxysmal), specialized atrial pacing techniques (dual-site and dual-chamber atrial-based pacing), cure with a Maze procedure (surgical or catheter-based), and the atrial implantable defibrillator.

Medications

DRUG(S) OF CHOICE

Rate Control

- Acutely: intravenous or oral beta-blocker (metoprolol, atenolol, esmolol) or calcium channel blocker (diltiazem, verapamil)
- Chronically: beta-blocker (metoprolol, atenolol, esmolol) or calcium channel blocker (diltiazem, verapamil)

Rhythm Control

- Acutely: ibutilide, procainamide, oral flecainide, or propafenone
- Chronically: quinidine, procainamide, disopyramide, propafenone, flecainide, sotalol, dofetilide or amiodarone
- QT-prolonging drugs contraindicated if history of Torsades de Pointes ventricular tachycardia

ADMISSION/DISCHARGE CRITERIA

- Patients can often be treated for AF on a completely outpatient basis.
- Criteria for admission include complications of AF such as:
  - —Uncontrolled ventricular response
  - —Heart failure or angina as a consequence of AF
  - —Initiation of antiarrhythmic drug therapy (especially those associated with proarrhythmia)
- Controversy exists as to who needs to be admitted for drug initiation, with considerations being:
  - —Age (and hence drug metabolism)
  - —Underlying heart disease
  - —Proarrhythmia potential

Follow-up

PATIENT MONITORING

- Anticoagulation followed with INR that should be 2–3 for optimal protection against embolization and minimization of risk for bleeding; start warfarin carefully
- Follow ECG and response to antiarrhythmic drugs, especially QT interval. Watch for ventricular proarrhythmia related to antiarrhythmic drug therapy.
- Assess ventricular rate control if left in AF with Holter or ambulatory monitoring.

EXPECTED COURSE AND PROGNOSIS

- Depends on age and population in question
- Young people with "lone" AF (no predisposing cause <65 years of age) have normal prognosis even without anticoagulation.
- Elderly patients with risk factor for stroke have risk ratio of >12 for stroke and death.
- AF can best be prevented by treating and preventing reversible risk factors (i.e., hypertension).

PATIENT EDUCATION

- Importance of anticoagulation and control of INR to prevent stroke
- Be vigilant for bleeding as consequence of anticoagulation, and proarrhythmia from antiarrhythmic drugs.

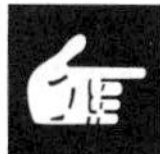

Miscellaneous

ICD-9-CM

427.31 Atrial fibrillation

BIBLIOGRAPHY

Cairns JA, Connolly SJ. Nonrheumatic atrial fibrillation—risk of stroke and role of antithrombotic therapy. *Circulation* 1991;84:469–481.

Cox JL, Jaquiss RDB, Schuessler RB, et al. Modification of the maze procedure for atrial flutter and fibrillation. *J Cardiovasc Surg* 1995;110: 485–495.

Feinberg WM, Blackshear JL, Laupacis A, et al. Prevalence, age distribution, and gender of patients with atrial fibrillation. *Arch Intern Med* 1995;155:469–473.

Gilligan DM, Ellenbogen KA, Epstein AE. The management of atrial fibrillation. *Am J Med* 1996;101:413–421.

Lêvy S, Maarek M, Coumel P, et al. Characterization of different subsets of atrial fibrillation in general practice in France—the ALFA Study. *Circulation* 1999;99:3028–3035.

Planning and Steering Committees of the AFFIRM Study for the NHLBI AFFIRM Investigators. Atrial Fibrillation Follow-up Investigation of Rhythm Management-the AFFIRM Study design. *Am J Cardiol* 1997;79:1198–1202.

Prystowsky EN, Benson DW, Fuster V, et al. Management of patients with atrial fibrillation. A statement for health care professionals from the Subcommittee on Electrocardiography and Electrophysiology, American Heart Association. *Circulation* 1996;93:1262–1277.

Wellens HJJ, Lau C-P, Lüderitz B, et al. Atrioverter: an implantable device for the treatment of atrial fibrillation. *Circulation* 1998;98:1651–1656.

Author: Andrew E. Epstein

Atrial Flutter

Basics

DESCRIPTION

Atrial flutter (Afl) is a reentrant tachycardia utilizing a circuit defined by the tricuspid annulus with the anterior free wall of the right atrium activated in the craniocaudal direction and the septum in the caudocranial direction.

- An isthmus between the inferior vena cava and the tricuspid annulus is the lower turnaround point; because it is narrow, it can be targeted for interruption by radiofrequency energy with subsequent cure of the arrhythmia.
- The atrial flutter circuit around the tricuspid annulus can support reentry in either the clockwise or counterclockwise direction.
  —Counterclockwise reentry around the tricuspid annulus is called typical, usual, or common atrial flutter and is characterized by negative (sawtooth) flutter waves in ECG leads II, III, and aVF. The flutter wave is positive in V1 and negative in V6.
  —Clockwise reentry around the tricuspid annulus is called unusual or uncommon atrial flutter and is characterized by positive flutter waves in ECG leads II, III, and aVF. These flutter waves often have a notch in the upstroke. The flutter wave is negative in V1 and positive in V6.
- The term *atypical AFl* has been used for not only isthmus-dependent clockwise AFl, but also atrial tachycardias not dependent on isthmus conduction.

EPIDEMIOLOGY

Prevalence

- Dependent on age and presence of underlying heart disease

Incidence

- Increases as the population ages
- Incidence may be up to 30% following open heart surgery.
- Common after surgery for congenital heart disease

ETIOLOGY

- Ideopathic
- Structural heart disease (including coronary and valvular heart disease and cardiomyopathy)
- Following open heart surgery
  —In children, atypical atrial flutters may use atrial incisions or prosthetic material (atrial septal defect patch) as an anatomic barrier around which reentry occurs.
- Usual, counterclockwise AFl may occur for the first time in patients treated with class IC antiarrhythmic drugs (i.e., flecainide, propafenone).
- AFls are often slowed by the IC antiarrhythmic drugs such that 1:1 atrioventricular (AV) conduction can occur leading to a faster ventricular response than at baseline when the AFl rate was faster but degree of AV block greater.

RISK FACTORS

- Following cardiac surgery
- Treatment with IC antiarrhythmic drugs for atrial fibrillation

PREGNANCY

- May exacerbate arrhythmias in young women
- If there is underlying heart disease, pregnancy may be either dangerous or contraindicated.
- Warfarin is associated with congenital birth defects such that risk-benefit ratio weighted against its use for AFl in this situation.

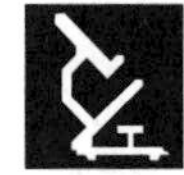

Diagnosis

DIFFERENTIAL DIAGNOSIS

- Atrial fibrillation (irregularly irregular, no flutter waves on ECG)
- Atrial tachycardia (regular)
- AV reentrant and AV nodal reentrant tachycardias (regular)
- Junctional tachycardia (rare, regular)
- Multifocal atrial tachycardia (irregular)

SIGNS AND SYMPTOMS

- None
- Palpitations
- Dyspnea
- Fatigue
- Congestive heart failure
- Angina

LABORATORY PROCEDURES

Check for hyperthyroidism.

IMAGING STUDIES

- Cardiac catheterization and angiography if coronary artery disease suspected

SPECIAL TESTS

- ECG is essential to establish diagnosis and determine if arrhythmia is amenable to ablative therapy (e.g., dependent on the isthmus discussed above).
- Ambulatory monitor (especially useful if paroxysmal)
- Echocardiogram to evaluate structural heart disease (myocardial and valvular)

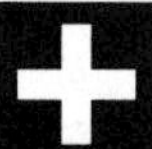

Treatment

GENERAL MEASURES

- The standard of therapy is slowing of the ventricular rate with drugs that block the AV node, followed by the administration of an antiarrhythmic drug (class I or III) to restore and maintain sinus rhythm.
- Conversion can be accomplished by drug therapy, electrical cardioversion, rapid atrial pacing (performed internally or via the esophagus), and most recently radiofrequency ablation. It is controversial as to the magnitude of risk for stroke attributable to AFl. Hence, the decision to anticoagulate is individual.

INTERVENTIONAL MEASURES

- Catheter ablation of AFl isthmus is curative in nearly 100% of patients if done by electrophysiologists skilled in the technique.
- For young patients and those who wish to avoid long-term drug dependency, it is the management of choice.

ADMISSION/DISCHARGE CRITERIA

- Often patients can be treated for AFl on a completely outpatient basis.
- Criteria for admission include complications of AFl such as an uncontrolled ventricular response, heart failure or angina as a consequence of AFl, and for the initiation of antiarrhythmic drug therapy, especially drugs that are associated with proarrhythmia.
- Controversy exists as to who needs to be admitted for drug initiation, with considerations being:
  —Age (and hence drug metabolism)
  —Underlying heart disease
  —Proarrhythmia potential

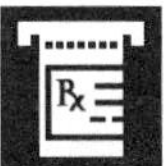

Medications

DRUG(S) OF CHOICE

Rate Control
- Acutely: intravenous or oral beta-blocker (metoprolol, atenolol, esmolol) or calcium channel blocker (diltiazem, verapamil)
- Chronically: beta-blocker (metoprolol, atenolol, esmolol) or calcium channel blocker (diltiazem, verapamil)

Rhythm Control

- Acutely: ibutilide, procainamide, oral flecainide, or propafenone
- Chronically: quinidine, procainamide, disopyramide, propafenone, flecainide, sotalol, or amiodarone
- QT-prolonging drugs are contraindicated if history of Torsades de Pointes ventricular tachycardia

Follow-up

PATIENT MONITORING

- If anticoagulation chosen
  —Follow INR, which should be 2–3 for optimal protection against embolization and minimization of risk for bleeding.
  —Start warfarin carefully.
- Follow ECG and response to antiarrhythmic drugs.
  —Watch for ventricular proarrhythmia related to antiarrhythmic drug therapy.
- Assess ventricular control if left in AFl with Holter or ambulatory monitoring.
- Bleeding as consequence of anticoagulation

EXPECTED COURSE AND PROGNOSIS

- Depends on age and population in question
- Patients with AFl in the absence of other diseases have a normal prognosis, and probably a very low risk for stroke.
- In contrast, patients with structural heart disease will have prognosis determined by their underlying disease.

PATIENT EDUCATION

- Importance of anticoagulation and control of INR to prevent stroke if anticoagulated
- Be vigilant for bleeding as a consequence of anticoagulation, and for proarrhythmia from antiarrhythmic drugs.

Diet

- Appropriate for underlying disease or syndrome such as diabetes, coronary artery disease, heart failure, and hypertension.

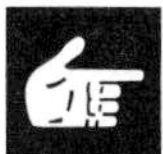

Miscellaneous

ICD-9-CM

427.32

BIBLIOGRAPHY

Cosio FG, Arribas F, López-Gil M, et al. Radiofrequency ablation of atrial flutter. *J Cardiovasc Electrophysiol* 1996;7:60–70.

Olshansky B, Wilber DJ, Hariman RJ. Atrial flutter—update on the mechanism and treatment. *PACE* 1992;15:2308–2335.

Windecker S, Kay GN, Epstein AE, et al. Atrial flutter. *Cardiac Electrophysiol Rev* 1997;1/2: 52–60.

Wood KA, Eisenberg SJ, Kalman JM, et al. Risk of thromboembolism in chronic atrial flutter. *Am J Cardiol* 1997;79:1043–1047.

Author: Andrew E. Epstein

Atrial Premature Beats

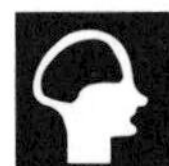

Basics

DESCRIPTION

Atrial premature beats or complexes (APCs) are early atrial systoles identified on the electrocardiogram by early P waves.

- The contour of the P wave may resemble sinus P waves, but it is usually different.
- They mimic sinus P waves when they arise near the sinus node, or close to it.
- When P waves occur very early, AV conduction may remain refractory such that the impulse is not propagated to the ventricles (blocked APC).
- Sometimes the P wave of an APC is difficult to identify because it falls in the T wave of the preceding QRS complex.

EPIDEMIOLOGY

APCs increase with aging. In the elderly, APCs are ubiquitous.

ETIOLOGY

- Often APCs have no particular cause, and are a function of aging.
- During times of stress and sympathetic stimulation
- Hyperthyroidism
- With myocardial infarction in >50% of patients
- In association with elevated atrial pressure and wall stress, for example left ventricular failure or cor pulmonale
- Alcohol, tobacco, and caffeine consumption
- Drug toxicity, e.g., digitalis toxicity

RISK FACTORS

- Structural heart disease with abnormalities of atrial structure or physiology, such as infiltrative diseases (amyloid), right or left ventricular failure, mitral or tricuspid insufficiency, following cardiac surgery, pericarditis

PREGNANCY

- Pregnancy may exacerbate frequency of APCs.
- Changes in intravascular volume and subsequent atrial wall stress may trigger stretch-induced atrial arrhythmias.

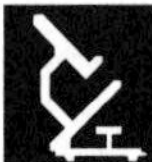

Diagnosis

DIFFERENTIAL DIAGNOSIS

- Junctional premature beats
- Wandering atrial pacemaker

SIGNS AND SYMPTOMS

- Usually none, but occasionally can be felt as palpitations.
- They may presage sustained supraventricular tachycardia, atrial fibrillation, and atrial flutter.

LABORATORY PROCEDURES

- None per se, except to test for hyperthyroidism
- Erythrocyte sedimentation rate if myocarditis or pericarditis suspected

SPECIAL TESTS

- ECG
- Event recorder
- Holter monitor
- Telemetry in hospital

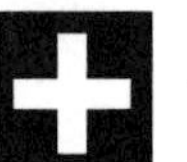

Treatment

GENERAL MEASURES

Usually no treatment is indicated or required.

ADMISSION/DISCHARGE CRITERIA

- Not applicable; patients are not admitted for APCs

Medications

DRUG(S) OF CHOICE

- If palpitations are a major complaint, beta-blockade or anxiolytics may be helpful.
- Beta-blockers
  —May decrease catecholamine stimulus, vigor of post-APC ventricular contraction, or timing of ventricular contraction, thereby improving symptoms
  —In otherwise healthy patients, adverse drug effects may be worse than symptoms resulting from the arrhythmia.
- Calcium channel blockers.

ALTERNATIVE DRUGS

Anxiolytic drugs may be helpful.

Follow-up

PATIENT MONITORING

- Virtually never needed
- If monitoring chosen, Holter monitor to quantify daily APC frequency and correlate symptoms with rhythm.
- Because drugs usually are not prescribed, proarrhythmia usually is not an issue.

EXPECTED COURSE AND PROGNOSIS

Normal; occasionally APCs may be a harbinger to atrial fibrillation, and may trigger reentrant supraventricular tachycardias.

PATIENT EDUCATION

- APCs are common and benign.
- Aggressive treatment with primary antiarrhythmic drugs may lead to morbidity and mortality in excess of that expected from APCs by themselves.
- Avoiding caffeine and other precipitating stimuli (alcohol, tobacco) may decrease APC frequency.
- Activity is usually not restricted, but rather encouraged.

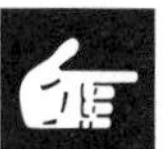

Miscellaneous

SYNONYMS

- Atrial premature complexes
- Atrial premature contractions

ICD-9-CM

427.61 Supraventricular premature beats

See also: Atrial Fibrillation, Atrial Flutter, Multifocal Atrial Tachycardia, Supraventricular Tachycardia.

BIBLIOGRAPHY

Braunwald E, ed. *Heart disease: a textbook of cardiovascular medicine.* Philadelphia: WB Saunders, 1997.

Author: Andrew E. Epstein

AV Block

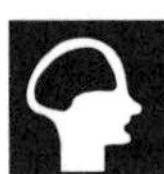

Basics

DESCRIPTION

- First-degree block is prolongation of the PR interval (<200 msec).
- Second-degree AV block is classified into two subcategories:
  - —Type I or Mobitz I second-degree atrioventricular (AV) block. Progressive prolongation of the PR interval before a blocked beat (Wenckebach block) usually is associated with a narrow QRS complex.
  - —Type II or Mobitz II second-degree AV block is the sudden loss of AV conduction without progressive prolongation of the PR interval before the blocked beat. Usually it is associated with a wide QRS complex.
- Advanced AV block refers to the block of two or more consecutive P waves.
- Third-degree AV block (complete heart block) is defined as absence of AV conduction.
  - —AV block can be of no or major clinical significance.
  - —Patients with abnormalities of AV conduction may be asymptomatic.
  - —Patients may experience serious symptoms related to bradycardia, ventricular arrhythmias, or both.
  - —Decisions regarding the need for a pacemaker are importantly influenced by the presence or absence of symptoms directly attributable to bradycardia.

EPIDEMIOLOGY

- Prevalence variable, depends on underlying structural heart disease, and increases with increasing age

ETIOLOGY

- Aging and fibrosis of AV conducting system
- No pathology if AV block is functional and related to drug therapy
- AV node and His-Purkinje system may be damaged due to myocardial infarction, impingement by calcium from aortic or mitral valve, or the development of fibrosis (Lev's and Lenegre's diseases).
- Aortic or mitral stenosis, especially following valve replacement. Because the mitral valve is close to the AV node, impaired AV conduction often is due to inflammation and resolves. The aortic valve, however, is close to the His-Purkinje system, and when AV block occurs as a consequence of aortic valve disease or surgery. AV block is usually permanent and pacing is required.
- Not a genetic disease, except in neuromuscular diseases with AV block such as myotonic muscular dystrophy, Kearns-Sayre syndrome, Erb's dystrophy (limb-girdle), and peroneal muscular atrophy

RISK FACTORS

- Structural heart disease

ASSOCIATED CONDITIONS

- Structural heart disease

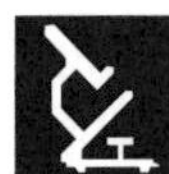

Diagnosis

DIFFERENTIAL DIAGNOSIS

- Junctional rhythm
- Concealed junctional extrasystoles
- When 2:1 AV block is present, the differentiation between Mobitz I and Mobitz II block is difficult because there is no progressive change in the PR interval that can be assessed.
  - —In general, 2:1 AV block with a narrow QRS is usually due to block in the AV node (e.g., Mobitz I) and 2:1 AV block with a wide QRS is usually due to block below the AV node (e.g., infra-Hissian, Mobitz II).
  - —Exceptions to these rules do occur.
  - —The importance of this distinction lies in the indication for pacing.

SIGNS AND SYMPTOMS

- None
- Lightheadedness
- Syncope
- Dyspnea, congestive heart failure
- Symptoms may be due to bradycardia itself, or to ventricular arrhythmias precipitated by bradycardia (e.g., Torsades de Pointes ventricular tachycardia).

LABORATORY PROCEDURES

Generally not applicable; drug level measurement (especially digitalis) is indicated if toxicity suspected.

IMAGING STUDIES

N/A

SPECIAL TESTS

- ECG most useful
- Ambulatory monitoring (Holter or telemetry)

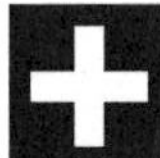

Treatment

GENERAL MEASURES

- For first-degree AV block and second-degree Mobitz type I AV block usually no treatment is recommended. These conduction disturbances are often the result of drug therapy and simply represent drug effects.
- Second-degree Mobitz type II AV block, especially if the QRS is wide, reflects infra-Hissian conduction disease, and permanent pacing is usually indicated.
- High-degree and third-degree AV block may be a consequence of drug therapy/toxicity, and a decision on pacing is made on the etiology.
- If a drug causing AV block is not essential, the drug can be stopped. If the drug is essential, permanent pacing is required to support the rate to allow drug administration.
- If there is drug toxicity, the rhythm should be supported by temporary pacing if needed while the toxicity resolves.

SURGICAL MEASURES

The indications for permanent pacing are outlined in the American College of Cardiology/American Heart Association Guidelines referenced below and include:

1. Third-degree AV block at any anatomic level associated with any one of the following conditions:
   a. Bradycardia with symptoms presumed to be due to AV block
   b. Arrhythmias and other medical conditions that require drugs that result in symptomatic bradycardia
   c. Documented periods of asystole >3.0 seconds or any escape rate <40 beats/min in awake, symptom-free patients
   d. After catheter ablation of the AV junction
   e. Postoperative AV block that is not expected to resolve
   f. Neuromuscular diseases with AV block such as myotonic muscular dystrophy, Kearns-Sayre syndrome, Erb's dystrophy (limb-girdle), and peroneal muscular atrophy
2. Second-degree AV block regardless of type or site of block, with associated symptomatic bradycardia
3. Asymptomatic third-degree AV block at any anatomic site with average awake ventricular rates of 40 beats/min or faster
4. Asymptomatic type II second-degree AV block

5. Asymptomatic type I second-degree AV block at intra- or infra-His levels found incidentally at electrophysiologic study for other indications
6. First-degree AV block with symptoms suggestive of pacemaker syndrome and documented alleviation of symptoms with temporary AV pacing
7. Marked first-degree AV block (>0.30 second) in patients with left ventricular dysfunction and symptoms of congestive heart failure in whom a shorter AV interval results in hemodynamic improvement, presumably by decreasing left atrial filling pressure

ADMISSION/DISCHARGE CRITERIA

If a patient has symptomatic AV block (especially third-degree or 2:1 AV block with a wide QRS, admission is warranted, usually for pacemaker implantation or treatment of drug toxicity.

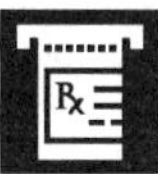

Medications

DRUG(S) OF CHOICE

There are no drugs that directly enhance AV conduction. If digitalis is toxic, Digibind antibody is indicated to inhibit digitalis effect on the heart.

Follow-up

PATIENT MONITORING

- For those without pacemakers, AV conduction should be systematically followed with ECGs or Holter monitors.
- Patients with pacemakers need telephone and intermittent face-to-face follow-up.
- Other than avoiding drug toxicity and preventing coronary artery disease, AV block is not preventable.

EXPECTED COURSE AND PROGNOSIS

- Variable and depends on underlying heart disease
- Patients with AV block have a worse prognosis than those with sinus node dysfunction, probably because the former have greater degrees of structural heart disease.
- Complications due to the AV block itself or to its treatment include syncope, injury, and occasionally death.

PATIENT EDUCATION

- Mostly related pacemaker follow-up in those with pacemakers. If drug toxicity is the cause, counsel to take measures to avoid further toxicity.
- If at risk for falls or syncope, counsel to avoid activities that put the patients or others in danger.

Activity

- Depends on hemodynamic consequences and underlying cause of AV block

Diet

- No specific diet

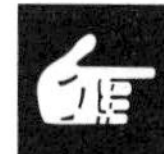

Miscellaneous

SYNONYM

- Heart block

ICD-9-CM

426.0 Atrioventricular block, complete
426.1 Atrioventricular block, other and unspecified
426.10 Atrioventricular block, unspecified
426.11 First-degree atrioventricular block
426.12 Mobitz (type) II atrioventricular block
426.13 Other second-degree atrioventricular block

BIBLIOGRAPHY

Braunwald E, ed. *Heart disease: a textbook of cardiovascular medicine.* Philadelphia: WB Saunders, 1997.

Gregoratos G, Cheitlin MD, Conill A, et al. ACC/AHA guidelines for implantation of cardiac pacemakers and antiarrhythmia devices: a report of the American College of Cardiology/American Heart Association Task Force on Practice Guidelines (Committee on Pacemaker Implantation). *J Am Coll Cardiol* 1998;31:1175–1206.

Author: Andrew E. Epstein

AV Nodal Reentrant Tachycardia (AVNRT)

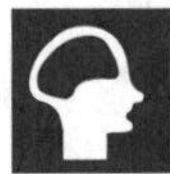

Basics

DESCRIPTION

Atrioventricular nodal reentrant tachycardia (AVNRT) is the most common paroxysmal, regular supraventricular tachycardia, accounting for greater than half of all cases referred for electrophysiologic study. The substrate for the arrhythmia is dual AV nodal pathway physiology.

EPIDEMIOLOGY

AVNRT is common. There is a 70% female predominance. Any age can be affected, but AVNRT usually presents at ages 30–50 years.

ETIOLOGY

There are at least two functionally distinct AV nodal conduction pathways:

- The fast pathway is characterized by fast conduction properties and a long refractory period.
- The slow pathway is characterized by slow conduction properties and a short refractory period.
- AVNRT usually begins with a premature atrial depolarization that blocks in the fast pathway since the latter has a long refractory period.
- The impulse then conducts through the slow pathway, and if the fast pathway recovers from depolarization, the impulse can reenter the fast pathway and conduct retrogradely to the atria. This completes the reentry circuit, which can repeat.
- Pathologic studies have shown a variety of changes, including entrapment, distortion, and division of the AV node, fibrosis, and even acute necrosis.
- Pathologic findings usually are described in electrical terms. Dual AV nodal pathway physiology is identified at electrophysiologic study.

PREGNANCY

Pregnancy not contraindicated, but supraventricular tachycardias may be more frequent and precipitated by pregnancy.

Diagnosis

DIFFERENTIAL DIAGNOSIS

- AV reentrant tachycardia that uses an accessory pathway in the retrograde direction
- Atrial tachycardia
- Atrial flutter with 2:1 AV conduction
- Junctional tachycardia

SIGNS AND SYMPTOMS

- Palpitations
- Pounding in the neck
- Dyspnea
- Dizziness
- Syncope
- Fatigue (sometimes related to drug therapy)
- Chest pain
- Diaphoresis

LABORATORY PROCEDURES

- Slow and fast AV nodal pathways are not clearly identifiable except at electrophysiologic study.

IMAGING STUDIES

N/A

SPECIAL TESTS

- ECG
  —Narrow QRS tachycardia either without identifiable P waves, or P waves immediately at the end of the QRS, sometimes seen as pseudo-R wave in lead V1 and/or pseudo-S waves in leads II or III
  —An atypical variety of AVNRT that uses the slow pathway in the retrograde direction has P waves in the second half of the ST segment (so-called long RP tachycardia).
- Electrophysiologic study, required if undergoing catheter ablation

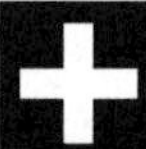

Treatment

GENERAL MEASURES

- Recording of 12-lead ECG during tachycardia is extremely important to help with diagnosis.
- If cured by catheter ablation, there is no long-term follow-up requirement.
- Due to the problems of long-term drug administration (adverse drug reactions, problem of multiple daily doses/noncompliance, and failure at some time over years of treatment), catheter ablation has emerged as one of the treatments, if not the treatment of choice, for recurrent AVNRT.
- The procedure can be performed safely with a low risk of AV block, and long-term is likely cost effective and improves quality of life compared with drug therapy, especially class IA and IC agents.
- For a single episode, a conservative approach may be adopted, including observation without drug therapy.
- If ablation is not performed, general medical follow-up is required. For acute management, cardioversion is almost never required because arrhythmia is very drug responsive.

SURGICAL MEASURES

Open heart surgery has been performed in the past, but this has been superseded by catheter ablation for cure.

ADMISSION/DISCHARGE CRITERIA

- Patients in general do not need to be admitted for AVNRT.
- If drug therapy is chosen, most antiarrhythmics can be started on an outpatient basis, especially because the risk for proarrhythmia is low in these patients with structurally normal hearts, and because drugs causing torsades de pointes ventricular tachycardia are usually not used for this disorder.
- After being seen by an electrophysiologist, a same-day ablation procedure can be arranged.

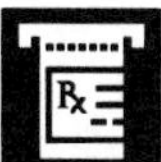

Medications

DRUG(S) OF CHOICE

Acute Management

- Adenosine (i.v.)
- Verapamil (i.v.)
- Esmolol (beta-blocker).

Chronic Management

- Calcium channel blocker (e.g., verapamil)
- Beta-blocker
- Class IC antiarrhythmic drugs (e.g., flecainide and propafenone)
- Digoxin may be helpful.

Precautions

- Watch for atrial fibrillation if adenosine used.
- Class IA drugs (quinidine, procainamide, disopyramide) limited due to adverse drug reactions.

Follow-up

PATIENT MONITORING

- Relates to treatment options, especially opportunity for cure with catheter ablation.

EXPECTED COURSE AND PROGNOSIS

- Excellent

PATIENT EDUCATION

- Although AVNRT can sometimes be precipitated by exercise and catecholamine increase, there are no specific recommendations regarding activity.
- Vagal maneuvers may terminate arrhythmia

Diet

There are usually no dietary restrictions.

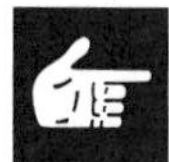

Miscellaneous

SYNONYMS

- PAT (paroxysmal atrial tachycardia); term now obsolete
- Junctional reentrant tachycardia
- Junctional reciprocating tachycardia
- Junctional tachycardia (this is a misnomer)

ICD-9-CM

427.0 Paroxysmal supraventricular tachycardia

BIBLIOGRAPHY

Ganz LI, Friedman PL. Supraventricular tachycardia. *N Engl J Med* 1995;332:162–173.

Kay GN, Plumb VJ. Selective slow pathway ablation (posterior approach) for treatment for atrioventricular nodal reentrant tachycardia. In: *Radiofrequency catheter ablation of cardiac arrhythmias: basic concepts and clinical applications.* Armonk, NY: Futura, 1994:171–203.

Jackman WM, Beckman KJ, McClelland JH, et al. Treatment of supraventricular tachycardia due to atrioventricular nodal reentry by radiofrequency catheter ablation of slow-pathway conduction. *N Engl J Med* 1992;327:313–318.

Author: Andrew E. Epstein

Brugada Syndrome

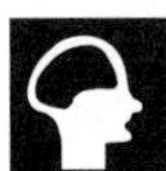

Basics

DESCRIPTION

- RBBB (right bundle branch block) and ST elevation in leads V1 and V2
- Risk of sudden death due to polymorphic ventricular tachycardia
- Half have inducible ventricular arrhythmia.

EPIDEMIOLOGY

The incidence and prevalence are unknown. It can be recognized in patients of any age.

ETIOLOGY

- Genetic abnormality of SCN5A and other genes
- Missense mutation: channel recovers from inactivation more rapidly than normal.
- Frameshift mutation renders channel nonfunctional, which increases dispersion of refractoriness and repolarization.
- Splice-donor mutation: consequences unknown

RISK FACTORS

- None

PREGNANCY

There is no contraindication to pregnancy. However, genetic counseling is recommended in view of the genetic cause and transmission of this disease.

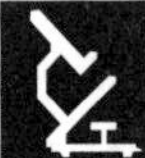

Diagnosis

DIFFERENTIAL DIAGNOSIS

- Simple RBBB
- Acute myocardial infarction (because of ST elevation)
- Left ventricular aneurysm
- Myocarditis
- Right ventricular infarction
- Duchenne muscular dystrophy
- Long QT syndrome (because of polymorphic ventricular tachycardia)
- Hypercalcemia
- Hyperkalemia
- Central and autonomic system abnormalities

SIGNS AND SYMPTOMS

- Syncope
- Cardiac arrest
- Asymptomatic

LABORATORY PROCEDURES

- No test available

IMAGING STUDIES

- Echocardiography to exclude cardiomyopathy
- Coronary angiography to exclude ischemia
- Ventriculography to exclude cardiomyopathy
- Cardiac MRI to exclude arrhythmogenic right ventricular dysplasia

SPECIAL TESTS

- ECG shows RBBB and ST elevation in leads V1 and V2.
- ECG abnormalities may be unmasked by flecainide or intravenous procainamide.
- Signal averaged ECG often shows late potentials, even in absence of r′ waves in right precordial leads.
- Ventricular arrhythmias provokable by programmed stimulation at electrophysiologic study
- Endomyocardial biopsies have been done to exclude arrhythmogenic right ventricular dysplasia.

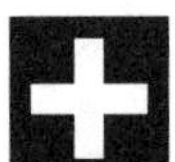

Treatment

GENERAL MEASURES

Because drug therapy is thought to be ineffective, implantation of an implantable cardioverter–defibrillator (ICD) is usually recommended, in symptomatic patients. The management of asymptomatic patients is controversial.

SURGICAL MEASURES

- None except implantation of an ICD

ADMISSION/DISCHARGE CRITERIA

- If the presentation of the Brugada syndrome is cardiac arrest, ICD implantation is recommended.
- If the syndrome is diagnosed incidentally, discussion about risk of disease (cardiac arrest) must be discussed. If ICD is desired, admission is then planned.
- If the patient presents with syncope and the ECG pattern of the Brugada syndrome is recognized, he or she should be hospitalized because recurrence may not spontaneously terminate.

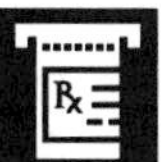

Medications

DRUG(S) OF CHOICE

- Drug therapy is apparently ineffective, including beta-blockers.
- Drugs that block transient outward current (I_{to}) current (i.e., quinidine and disopyramide) may be efficacious.

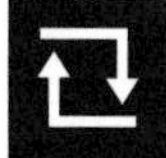

Follow-up

PATIENT MONITORING

- Once diagnosis is established, the patient should be seen by an electrophysiologist knowledgeable about Brugada syndrome.
- Syncope would be indication to initiate treatment (i.e., ICD).
- Avoid class I antiarrhythmic drugs that block I_{Na} more than I_{to} (i.e., procainamide and flecainide).

EXPECTED COURSE AND PROGNOSIS

- Guarded

PATIENT EDUCATION

- No intervention is known to prevent cardiac arrest. New drugs that selectively block I_{to} may be effective.
- Sudden death is a major risk of disease.
- Unknown if mental stress and alcohol are provocative factors

Activity

- No specific recommendations

Diet

- No special diet

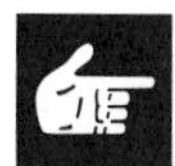

Miscellaneous

SYNONYMS

- None. Sudden unexpected death in Asian immigrants (also called pokkuri in Japan, bangungut in the Philippines, and lai tai in Thailand) are probably related.

ICD-9-CM

427.9 Cardiac dysrhythmia, unspecified

See also: Implantable Cardioverter-Defibrillator, Ventricular Fibrillation, Ventricular Tachycardia, Long QT Syndrome, Sudden Death

INTERNET RESOURCES

Internet site http://www.netvision.be/brugada

BIBLIOGRAPHY

Alings M, Wilde A. "Brugada" syndrome: clinical data and suggested pathophysiological mechanism. *Circulation* 1999;99:666–673.

Brugada J, Brugada P. Further characterization of the syndrome of right bundle branch block, ST segment elevation, and sudden cardiac death. *J Cardiovasc Electrophysiol* 1997; 8:325–331.

Gussak I, Antzelevitch C, Bjerregaard P, et al. The Brugada syndrome: clinical, electrophysiologic and genetic aspects. *J Am Coll Cardiol* 1999;33:5–15.

Authors: Andrew E. Epstein and John S. Strobel

Carcinoid Heart Syndrome

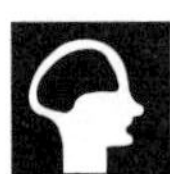

Basics

DESCRIPTION

Carcinoid is a tumor of Argentaffin cells. Carcinoid heart disease occurs with gastrointestinal carcinoid tumors that have metastasized to the liver or the lymph nodes.

ETIOLOGY

Prevalence

It occurs in approximately half of the patients with carcinoid syndrome; >50% develop valvular heart disease (VHD) congestive heart failure symptoms (late increased levels of serotonin).

CAUSES

The mechanism can be repeated chemical trauma from circulating serotonin and other vasoactive amines.

RISK FACTORS

N/A

PREGNANCY

N/A

Diagnosis

DIFFERENTIAL DIAGNOSIS

- Pheochromocytoma
- Panic attacks
- Cocaine abuse
- Causes of isolated right-sided heart failure (e.g., restrictive cardiomyopathy, primary pulmonary hypertension, etc.)

SIGNS AND SYMPTOMS

- Diagnosis of carcinoid heart disease is made by identifying the characteristic right-sided cardiac lesions via 2-D ECG in patients with histologically proven carcinoid disease.
- About 50% of patients with spread to the liver exhibit the syndrome of episodic flushing, bronchospasm, and diarrhea.
- It is usually diagnosed years after the diagnosis of metastatic carcinoid syndrome.
- The clinical picture depends on the valve involved: pulmonary stenosis (90%), tricuspid stenosis (42%), and tricuspid insufficiency (47%). Patients may present with restrictive cardiomyopathy.

LABORATORY PROCEDURES

N/A

SPECIAL TESTS

- Carcinoid syndrome is confirmed by increased levels of 5-hydroxyindoleacetic acid.

PATHOLOGY

- Gross pathology
  —The characteristic lesion is focal or diffuse white shiny endocardial plaque (endocardial fibroplasias) involving the endocardium of the right side of the heart.
    - The most extensive involvement is usually on the ventricular surface of tricuspid valve leaflets and on the arterial aspect of the pulmonic valve.
    - Left-sided heart lesion can develop in case of right-to-left shunt, which allows the amines to bypass the pulmonary circulation where amines can be metabolized, or with bronchial carcinoid tumor or pulmonary metastasis.

Histology

The plaques consist of smooth muscle cells and sparse collagen embedded in abundant acid mucopolysaccharide matrix with no elastic fibers.

IMAGING STUDIES

- Echocardiography
  —Shows leaflet thickening and chordal fusion
  —Doppler can demonstrate the presence and severity of valvular lesions.

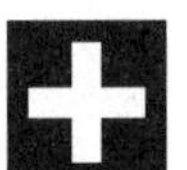

Treatment

GENERAL MEASURES

N/A

SURGICAL MANAGEMENT

Because right-sided heart failure is responsible for one-third of the deaths in patients with metastatic carcinoid, surgical management is an acceptable palliation for these compromised patients.

Indications

- Valvular dysfunction with congestive heart failure
- The patients most likely to benefit from surgery are those with worsening cardiac status despite an otherwise indolent course of metastatic carcinoid syndrome.
- The choice of the valve is a matter of surgeon preference; however, there is improved prognosis with mechanical valves.

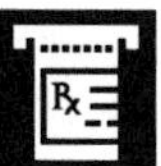

Medications

DRUG(S) OF CHOICE

- Medical therapy is ineffective.
- Somatostatin has been evaluated for use in carcinoid patients.

ALTERNATIVE DRUGS

- Hepatic artery embolization or ligation to control hepatic metastasis

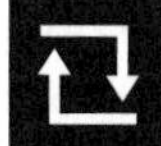

Follow-up

PATIENT MONITORING

N/A

EXPECTED COURSE AND PROGNOSIS

- In patients with metastatic carcinoid, half to 70% are expected to be alive at 5 years.
- With extensive hepatic metastasis, the median survival is about 3 years.
- Right-sided heart disease is reported as a cause of death in up to one-third of cases.

PATIENT EDUCATION

N/A

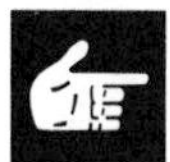

Miscellaneous

ICD-9-CM

259.2

BIBLIOGRAPHY

Bonow RO, Carabello B, de Leon AC Jr, et al. ACC/AHA guidelines for the management of patients with valvular heart disease: a report of the American College of Cardiology/American Heart Association Task Force on Practice Guidelines (Committee on Management of Patients with Valvular Heart Disease). *J Am Coll Cardiol* 1998;32:1486–1588.

Knott-Craig CJ, Schaff HV, Mullany CJ, et al. Carcinoid disease of the heart: surgical management of ten patients. *J Thorac Cardiovasc Surg* 1992;104:475–481.

Otto C. *Valvular heart disease,* 1st ed. Philadelphia: WB Saunders, 1999.

Authors: Amr El-Shafei, Steven Herrmann, Madhukar Gupta, and Bernard R. Chaitman

Cardiac Neoplasms

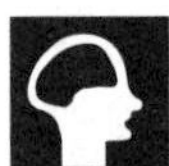

Basics

DESCRIPTION

Tumors and cysts of the heart or pericardium are relatively rare but have been detected more frequently since the introduction of echocardiography.

- Cardiac tumors secondary to metastatic disease are 16 to 40 times more common than primary cardiac tumors. However, identification of primary cardiac tumors is important because resection is likely to result in a cure.
- In contrast, resection of metastatic cardiac tumors is palliative at best.

Metastatic Cardiac Tumors

- 10% of malignant neoplasms metastasize to the heart; 10% of these metastases are clinically evident.
- Epicardium is the most common location.
- Carcinomatous invasion is more common than sarcomatous invasion.
- 85%–90% clinical dysfunction is related to pericardial involvement (effusion, neoplastic thickening).
- Tumors have been reported from every organ and of every tissue type except the central nervous system.
- Lung, breast, leukemia, and lymphoma are the most common metastatic malignancies.
- Highest percentage of cardiac metastases are melanomas (70%), leukemia, and lymphoma.
- Extension via direct (lung, breast, esophagus), retrograde lymphatic drainage (most carcinomas), venous extension (renal cell, hepatoma), and hematogenous (sarcoma, leukemia, lymphoma, melanoma)

Benign Cardiac Tumors

- Intracavitary neoplasms have the potential of producing a triad of obstruction, embolization, and constitutional symptoms.
- Myxoma most common, distribution as follows: left atrium (75%), right atrium (23%), and ventricular (2%)
- Rhabdomyoma most common in infants and children and usually multiple, ventricular, pedunculated masses
- Fibromas are most common in children; usually solitary and located in the intramural ventricular septum, and calcific deposits can be seen. Sudden death occurs in up to one-third due to conduction abnormalities.
- Lipomas may be extremely small or massive, may be located on valves, and sometimes are mistaken for pericardial cysts.
- Hemangiomas give tumor blush on angiography and may resolve spontaneously.

Malignant Cardiac Tumors

- Primary malignant cardiac neoplasms are almost always sarcomas.
- Local relapse in PCS (primary cardiac sarcoma) is relatively rare, and most patients die because of metastatic recurrence.
- Most frequent is angiosarcoma, which usually originates from right atrium and forms large quantity of vascular channels. Metastases occur in 66%–89% of cases, most commonly to the lung.
- Rhabdomyosarcoma is second most common primary malignancy and has no chamber predilection.
- Infrequent: fibrosarcoma, liposarcoma, and primary malignant lymphoma

Carcinoid Heart Disease

- Never primary and rarely metastasize but distinctive lesions often seen in the right heart
- Fibrous tissue deposits lacking elastic fibers seen on the ventricular aspect of the tricuspid valve leaflets and on the arterial aspect of the pulmonic valve leaflets, and to a lesser extent on the ventricular aspects of the mitral valve
- The development of carcinoid heart disease not related to duration of carcinoid symptoms
- Only condition to uniformly involve both tricuspid and pulmonic valve, most commonly tricuspid regurgitation and pulmonic stenosis

EPIDEMIOLOGY

Metastatic cardiac tumors are 16 to 40 times more common than primary tumors.

- Primary tumors of heart and pericardium have an incidence of 0.0001%–0.28% in autopsy series.
- In adults, almost half of all benign tumors are myxomas.
- The peak incidence for myxomas is in the sixth decade of life, and women account for 70% of cases. Malignant primary tumors comprised 25% and consisted of angiosarcomas (33%), rhabdomyosarcomas (20%), mesotheliomas (15%), and fibrosarcomas (10%).
- In infants and children, the most common cardiac tumor was the rhabdomyoma. Angiosarcoma and rhabdomyosarcoma are more frequent in men.
- Malignant tumors were rare in the pediatric age group, comprising less than 10% of all cardiac and pericardial neoplasms.

RISK FACTORS

- 10% of cardiac myxomas are familial (autosomal dominant) and are more likely to be multiple and located in the ventricular cavity.
- Carcinoid heart disease results from hepatic metastases from ileal, bronchial, or ovarian carcinoid.

ASSOCIATED CONDITIONS

- Familial myxomas associated with NAME (nevi, atrial myxoma, myxoid neurofibroma, and ephelides) and LAMB (lentigines, atrial myxoma, and ephelides) syndromes
- Rhabdomyoma associated with tuberous sclerosis in one-third of patients
- Fibromas may be associated with Gorlin's syndrome (basal cell nevus syndrome)
- Patients with cardiac hemangiomas also may have skin hemangiomas

Diagnosis

SIGNS AND SYMPTOMS

- All cardiac tumors can simulate more common types of cardiac disease
- The various signs and symptoms relate to tumor location
- Pericardial involvement is most common with metastatic disease, often presenting with signs and symptoms of tamponade.
- Intramyocardial neoplasms are often silent unless conduction disturbances present
- Left atrial masses often mimic mitral stenosis, including dyspnea, orthopnea, PND (paroxysmal nocturnal dypsnea), pulmonary edema, and hemoptysis.
- Right atrial or ventricular masses may produce right side congestive heart failure signs and symptoms, including peripheral edema, ascites, hepatomegaly, and prominent jugular venous *a* waves.
- A protodiastolic tumor plop murmur may result from right atrial tumors.
- Left ventricular masses frequently occur at the apex and are often clinically silent, but if large enough, can cause systolic murmur, chest pain, syncope, or heart failure.
- Myxomatous constitutional symptoms include fever, weight loss, Raynaud's syndrome, digital clubbing, and anemia.
- Rhabdomyomas may mimic pulmonic valve stenosis or present with ventricular obstruction, arrhythmias (including VT [ventricular tachycardia]), AV block, pericardial effusion, and sudden death.
- Angiosarcoma may produce a continuous precordial murmur due to vascular channels.

LABORATORY PROCEDURES

Elevated erythrocyte sedimentation rate, elevated white blood cell count, thrombocytopenia, and increased gamma globulins can be seen with myxomas.

PATHOLOGIC FINDINGS

- Carcinomatous metastases are usually visible on gross inspection, appearing as multiple small, discrete, firm nodules.
- Sarcomatous metastases are characterized by diffuse infiltration.
- Myxoma cell origin is unclear in endothelial-like cells that are elongated and spindle shaped with round nuclei and prominent nucleoli. Attachment usually atrial septum with stalk smaller than mass diameter. Microscopically, the myxoid matrix is composed of mucopolysaccharide.
- Rhabdomyomas are white to yellow-tan; microscopically they are circumscribed but not encapsulated and contain abundant glycogen.
- Calcific deposits are often seen in fibromas.

- Intramyocardial lipomas are encapsulated and usually small.
- Carcinoid tumors contain fibroblasts, myofibroblasts, and smooth muscle cells in collagen, not elastin.

IMAGING STUDIES

- Chest radiography is occasionally helpful (mostly for epicardial neoplasms, detection of calcified masses, or complications due to obstructive masses (i.e., pulmonary edema).
- ECG most common initial diagnostic modality
- TEE (transesophageal echocardiography) more sensitive than TTE (transthoracic echocardiography) and better approximates size, shape, and location as well as stalk attachment for intracardiac masses as well as mediastinal or extracardiac structures.
- Echocardiography is very useful in serial monitoring.
- CT is useful for diagnosis and often helpful in defining intramyocardial extension, but MRI provides clearer definition of tumor characteristics.
- Selective angiography techniques have been largely supplanted by noninvasive imaging but can be useful in detecting intracavitary filling defects as well as defining the vascular supply of the neoplasm.

SPECIAL TESTS

- Pericardiocentesis may provide a definitive cytologic analysis in addition to symptomatic relief of tamponade.
- Only in rare cases may an endomyocardial biopsy contribute to the diagnosis.

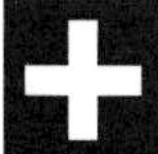

Treatment

GENERAL MEASURES

- Excision should be made early in primary tumors to prevent complications such as embolization or metastases.
- Treatment of secondary neoplasms is generally directed at underlying malignancy but may require surgical intervention if symptomatic.

SURGICAL MEASURES

- Pericardial tumor operative measures include biopsy, drainage, window, or resection.
- Intrapericardial tumors can sometimes be resected without cardiopulmonary bypass.
- Primary therapy for atrial myxoma, rhabdomyoma, fibroma, and lipoma is surgical resection.
- Partial excision should be considered only when it compromises valvular structure, coronary arteries, or the conduction system.
- Surgeon should be very careful regarding potential embolization.
- Total excision of hemangioma is usually not possible.
- Surgery for angiosarcoma and rhabdomyosarcoma is usually futile. After surgical excision, local relapse is relatively rare, but prognosis is poor due to metastatic disease.
- Right-sided valvular excision or replacement or valve commissurotomy or annuloplasty has been performed in some patients with carcinoid heart disease.

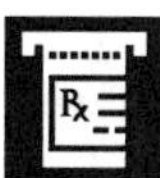

Medications

DRUG(S) OF CHOICE

- The role of adjuvant treatment in resected primary neoplasms (sarcomas) is controversial. In several series, the use of postoperative chemotherapy did not appear to improve survival, but isolated reports show prolonged survival after resection followed by adjuvant chemotherapy and radiation.
- Adjuvant chemotherapy seems advisable in a subset of patients with high mitotic rate tumors and adjuvant radiation with high-grade tumors at risk for metastases.

Follow-up

PATIENT MONITORING

- Noninvasive imaging is used to perform serial monitoring to determine size progression or detect recurrence following excision, most often with echocardiography.

EXPECTED COURSE AND PROGNOSIS

- Recurrences of atrial myxomas are rare, but if they occur, it is usually within a 4-year period
- Angiosarcoma and rhabdomyosarcoma carry extremely poor prognoses because their clinical course is rapid with diffuse metastases. Median survival ranges from 5 to 11 months in the different series.
- Patients with carcinoid heart disease have a similar life span following diagnosis compared with metastatic carcinoid without myocardial involvement.

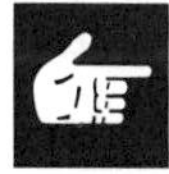

Miscellaneous

ICD-9-CM

Primary Neoplasms

215.9 Neoplasm, connective tissue, benign (myxoma, fibroma, lipoma, rhabdomyoma)
228.09 Heart hemangioma
171.9 Neoplasm, connective tissue, malignant, primary (angiosarcoma, rhabdomyosarcoma, others)

Secondary Neoplasms

Refer to ICD for specific primary neoplasm.

BIBLIOGRAPHY

Ceresoli G, Passoni P, Benussi S, et al. Primary cardiac sarcoma in pregnancy: a case report and review of the literature. *Am J Clin Oncol* 1999;22:460–465.

Majano-Lainez RA. Cardiac tumors: a current clinical and pathological perspective. *Crit Rev Oncogenesis* 1997;8:293–303.

McAllister HA Jr, Hall RJ, Cooley DA. Tumors of the heart and pericardium. *Curr Prob Cardiol* 1999;24:57–116.

Topol EJ. Cardiovascular medicine. Philadelphia: Lippincott Williams & Wilkins, 1998: 912–915.

Author: Christopher K. Dyke

Cardiac Surgery, Preoperative Assessment

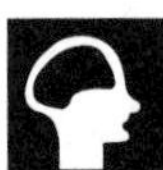

Basics

DESCRIPTION

Evaluation prior to coronary artery bypass graft (CABG) surgery, valve repair or replacement, repair of congenital heart disease, etc. Includes surgical procedures on or off pump, keyhole approach, or classic median sternotomy.

EPIDEMIOLOGY

367,000 patients underwent CABG surgery (255,000 men and 112,000 women) in 1996 according to the American Heart Association. 79,000 patients underwent valve surgery (41,000 men and 33,000 women) in 1996.

ETIOLOGY

- Pending underlying illness

RISK FACTORS

Clinical severity score based on 13 clinical variables can help predict mortality risk: low-risk score <3; high risk score ≥6.

Emergency surgery	6
Serum creatinine 1.6–1.8	1
≥1.9	4
Severe LV dysfunction (LVEF <35%)	3
Reoperation	3
Mitral regurgitation	3
Age 65–74	1
≥75	2
Prior vascular surgery	2
COPD	2
Anemia (Hct <35)	2
Aortic stenosis	1
Weight ≤65 kg	1
Diabetes not diet controlled	1
Cerebrovascular disease	1

LV, left ventricle; LVEF, left ventricular ejection fraction; COPD, chronic obstructive pulmonary disease; Hct, hematocrit
Adapted from Higgins, et al. Stratification of morbidity and mortality outcome by preoperative risk factors in coronary artery bypass patients. *JAMA* 1992;267:2344–2348.

PREGNANCY

Exclude presence in elective surgery in young women of childbearing age.

ASSOCIATED CONDITIONS

- Potentially increase morbidity/mortality (see chart above)

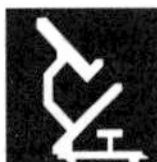

Diagnosis

DIFFERENTIAL DIAGNOSIS

None; diagnosis is established prior to surgery.

SIGNS AND SYMPTOMS

History

Pertinent findings include:

- Underlying pulmonary disease, dysrhythmias, renal insufficiency, liver dysfunction, peripheral vascular disease, previous cerbrovascular accident/baseline neurologic deficits, poor nutritional status, underlying infection, anemia/bleeding, poor family support.

Physical Examination

Pertinent findings:

- Dental caries, active upper respiratory tract infection (increase risk of endocarditis)
- Prior radical mastectomy contraindicates use of internal mammary artery (compromised thoracic blood supply).
- Aortic regurgitation worsens with cardiopulmonary bypass due to aortic jet.
- Intraaortic balloon pump is contraindicated with significant abdominal aortic aneurysm. Use is complicated by arterial insufficiency.
- Lower extremity venous varicosities may necessitate use of arm veins or only arterial conduits for bypass. No i.v. lines are placed in veins to be harvested.
- Tinea pedis increases risk local cellulitis.
- Carotid bruits increase the risk of perioperative cerebrovascular accident. Stenoses >75% diameter narrowed require staged or combined procedure.
- Baseline neurologic deficits may worsen postoperatively.

LABORATORY PROCEDURES

- Routine complete blood count, platelet count, prothrombin time/partial thromboplastin time, blood urea nitrogen, creatinine, potassium, magnesium, calcium, albumin, liver function tests, stool for occult blood, and urinalysis
- Pulmonary function tests and thyroid function tests if clinically indicated

IMAGING STUDIES

Pertinent data from cardiac catheterization and echocardiography include:

- Elevated left ventricular end-diastolic pressure
  - —May remain elevated postoperatively
  - —Requires adequate preload postoperatively
- Elevated right atrial pressure
  - —May reflect trucuspid or right ventricular dysfunction
  - —May require aggressive volume expansion postoperatively
- Elevated pulmonary artery diastolic pressure greater than pulmonary capillary wedge pressure
  - —Suspect fixed pulmonary vascular resistance.
  - —May require vigorous oxygenation and pulmonary vasodilator
- Ventricular systolic dysfunction
  - —Right ventricle: digoxin; perioperative supplemental oxygen to decrease pulmonary vascular resistance
  - —Left ventricle (LV): digoxin; afterload reduction with angiotensin-converting enzyme (ACE) inhibitors
- Mitral regurgitation: Afterload reduction with ACE inhibitors or i.v. nipride to maintain systolic pressure of 90–100 mm Hg (possible contraindications to nipride include severe aortic stenosis, significant cerebral or renal vascular disease). LV failure may occur postoperatively because the LV is conditioned to a low afterload state preoperatively.

SPECIAL TESTS

- Carotid Doppler for carotid bruits or diffuse atherosclerosis
- Intraoperative transesophageal echocardiogram used to safely cannulate aorta with aortic atherosclerotic disease

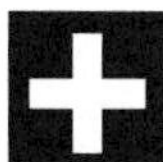

Treatment

GENERAL MEASURES

Dysrhythmia Prophylaxis

Correct electrolyte abnormalities (potassium 4.0–5.0 mEq/L and magnesium ≥2.0 mEq/L).

- Supraventricular tachyarrhythmias
- Beta-blocker prophylaxis recommended by some in absence of low ejection fraction, severe bronchospastic pulmonary disease, bradyarrhythmias
- Atrial fibrillation (A-fib)
- In normal sinus rhythm before surgery, continue antiarrhythmics until surgery.
  —A-fib, controlled ventricular response: Continue medication until surgery.
  —A-fib, uncontrolled rate: Control with beta-blockers or digoxin prior to surgery.

Ventricular Tachyarrhythmias

- Continue previous antiarrhythmics until surgery.
- Chronic amiodarone with lung disease: Consider holding drug 3 months preoperatively if no life-threatening rhythm.
- Automatic implantable cardiodefibrillators: Disable unit prior to surgery to minimize unnecessary shocks.

Bradyarrhythmias

- High-grade atrioventricular block (third-degree or type II second-degree): temporary transvenous pacer
- Permanent pacemaker
  —Document specifications, pacer dependency.
- Removal of Telectronics AccuFIX atrial J lead at atriotomy recommended due to history of retention wire fracture, protrusion
- Tricuspid valve replacement with mechanical prosthesis: Place permanent epicardial leads.
  —Intraoperatively: transvenous pacer wires contraindicated through tricuspid prosthesis

SURGICAL MEASURES

N/A

ADMISSION/DISCHARGE CRITERIA

N/A

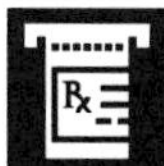

Medications

See above.

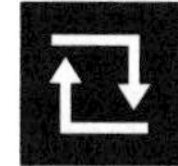

Follow-up

PATIENT MONITORING

- Not indicated preoperatively unless unstable

EXPECTED COURSE AND PROGNOSIS

- Operative mortality rates: isolated CABG 1%–2%, isolated aortic valve replacement 2%, isolated mitral valve replacement 6%

PATIENT EDUCATION

N/A

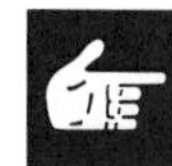

Miscellaneous

ICD-9-CM

414.0 Coronary artery disease
424.1 Aortic valve disease
394.9 Mitral valve disease, etc.

BIBLIOGRAPHY

Antman E. Medical management of the patient undergoing cardiac surgery. In: Braunwald E, ed. *Heart disease: a textbook of cardiovascular medicine,* 5th ed. Philadelphia: WB Saunders, 1997:1715–1740.

Higgins TL, Estafanous FG, Loop FD, et al. Stratification of morbidity and mortality outcome by preoperative risk factors in coronary artery bypass patients. *JAMA* 1992;267:2344–2348.

Morris DC, Clements SD, Hug CC. Management of the patient after cardiac surgery. In: Alexander RW, Schlant RC, Fuster V, eds. *Hurst's the heart,* 9th ed. New York: McGraw-Hill, 1998: 1489–1500.

Morris DC, St. Claire D Jr. Management of patients after cardiac surgery. *Curr Prob Cardiol* 1999;24:161–228.

Authors: Richard Chen and Jerre Lutz

Cardiac Surgery, Immediate Postoperative Management

Basics

DESCRIPTION

Pathophysiologic effects of cardiopulmonary bypass

- Fluid, electrolytes: increased extracellular fluid, total exchangeable sodium; decreased exchangeable potassium, elevated glucose levels
- Inflammatory response: From blood contact with synthetic surface of bypass equipment; inflammatory state results in platelet-endothelial cell interactions, vasospastic responses causing low-flow states in coronary circulation, and capillary leak syndrome.
- Transient depression ventricular function: from oxygen free radical production in response to reperfusion injury; depressed by 2 hours after cardiopulmonary bypass, worse at 4–5 hours, significant recovery by 8–10 hours, full recovery by 24–48 hours
- Hypothermia: predisposes to dysrhythmias, increases systemic vascular resistance (SVR), causes shivering, which increases oxygen consumption, impairs coagulation
- Respiratory insufficiency: secondary to alveolar dysfunction (atelectasis), decreased central respiratory drive (anesthetics), decreased respiratory muscle function (incisional pain), exacerbation underlying chronic obstructive pulmonary disease

See also the following tables in the Appendix:

- Risk Stratification Scoring System for Patients Undergoing Coronary Bypass Surgery
- Intravenous Drugs for Cardiac Surgical Patients: Pharmacologic Therapy
- Interpretation of Hemodynamic Patterns in Cardiac Patients
- Intravenous Positive Inotropic Agents

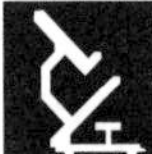

Diagnosis

DIFFERENTIAL DIAGNOSIS

N/A

SIGNS AND SYMPTOMS

N/A

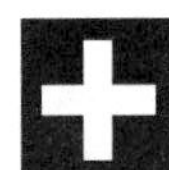

Treatment

GENERAL MEASURES

Postoperative Complications

Hypertension

- Present in most patients without left ventricular dysfunction secondary to increased peripheral vascular resistance from hypothermia

Low-Output Syndrome

Clinical features include:

- Cold extremities
- Systolic blood pressure (SBP) <90 mm Hg
  —Low output may be present with SBP >100 mm Hg when SVR is increased (>1,500 dyne-sec/cm^{-5}).
- Urine output <30 mL/h
- Cardiac index <2.0 L/min/m^2 (except in sepsis)
  —Strong relationship between early postoperative low cardiac index and probability of cardiac surgery death
  —Mixed venous O_2 saturation <50 (except in sepsis)
  —Acidosis
- Obtain hemodynamics with Swan-Ganz catheter, echocardiogram
- Categorize etiology: decreased preload, cardiogenic, sepsis, etc.

Perioperative Myocardial Infarction

- Symptoms unreliable
- Diagnose by ECG, creatine kinase-MB fraction troponin levels. Echocardiogram may be confirmatory, not routinely performed.
- No routine cardiac enzymes postoperatively unless hemodynamically unstable intraoperatively, new ECG changes

Dysrhythmias

- Supraventricular
  —Sinus tachycardia most common
  —Atrial fibrillation
    - 10%–30% occurrence postoperatively
    - Advanced age most important associated factor
    - Most common on postoperative day 2
    - 80% return to sinus rhythm within 1–3 days following digoxin or beta-blocker
    - i.v. diltiazem, esmolol for rate control
    - 10% require cardioversion
  —Atrial flutter
    - May convert to normal sinus rhythm using atrial epicardial pacing wires
    - Burst pacing: 15–30 seconds of 300–600 beats/min atrial rate
- Ventricular
  —Frequent ectopy (>6 beats/min) in first 12 hours postoperatively suggests ischemia.
    - Lidocaine for suppression often recommended by some (bolus 75 mg followed by 50 mg every 5 minutes for total of 225 mg or bolus 75 mg followed by 150 mg over 20 minutes)
  —Ventricular tachycardia
    - Most commonly due to revascularization in nonviable myocardium leading to reentry
    - Usually requires amiodarone to suppress or eliminate
    - Note: Wide complex tachycardia with rates of 250–300 beats/min suggests accessory pathway. Procainamide is the drug of choice for accessory pathway tachycardias with very fast rates.
- Bradyarrhythmias/conduction defects
  —Conduction defects in up to 45% of patients
  —Majority transient
  —Right bundle branch block most common conduction defect
  —Atrial fibrillation with slow ventricular response, sinus bradycardia, junctional rhythm less common
  —May support bradycardia with temporary atrial pacing (85–100 beats/min)
- Pulmonary
  —Most significant cause of morbidity after cardiopulmonary bypass
    - Atelectasis: common, 70% of patients
  —Decreased chest wall movement due to incisional pain
  —Decreased diaphragmatic excursion due to phrenic nerve damage may require up to six weeks for recovery and may be permanent.
  —Decreased central respiratory drive: anesthetics, analgesics
  —Exacerbation underlying chronic obstructive pulmonary disease
  —Pleural effusions, if large, may require repeat thoracentesis after chest tubes are removed.

—Postpump syndrome/capillary leak/adult respiratory distress syndrome
  • Early clues include diminished pulmonary compliance (determined from ventilator), increased arterial-alveolar gradient, clear chest x-ray, and increasing difficulty maintaining oxygenation
  • Supportive management includes positive end-expiratory pressure, minimization of wedge pressures with diuretics, and nutritional support

Infection

- Incisional
  - —Leg
    - 1% of patients
    - More common in obese women
  - —Sternal/mediastinitis
    - 2% of patients
    - Diabetics with bilateral IMA grafts at greatest risk
- Infective endocarditis
  - —Perioperative antibiotic prophylaxis beneficial
  - —CABG does not increase infection risk of abnormal native valves
  - —Prosthetic valve endocarditis rare, but serious

Neurologic

- Altered mental status
  - —Approximately 30% of patients
  - —Some patients note mild long-term cognitive disorders.
- Major cerebrovascular accident: 1%–2%
- Brachial plexopathy, ulnar nerve dysfunction
  - —Usually temporary
  - —May require up to 6 months for recovery

Anticoagulation: Prosthetic Valves

- Risk considerations for thromboembolism
  - —Type of valve (greater risk with mechanical than bioprosthetic)
  - —Valve location (greater risk with mitral than aortic)
  - —Presence of atrial fibrillation
  - —Left atrial size
  - —History of thromboembolism
  - —Presence of intracardiac thrombi
- Goal INR 2.5–3.5

SURGICAL MEASURES

Reexploration may be necessary with persistent, uncontrolled bleeding; suspected tamponade is secondary to thrombus formation.

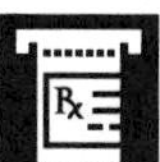

Medications

DRUG(S) OF CHOICE

- Reinstitute medications for comorbid diseases.
- Aspirin, lipid-lowering agents for CABG patients
- Infective endocarditis prophylaxis with valve disease
- Beta-blockers for atrial fibrillation prophylaxis
- Diltiazem for 1 month if radial artery graft used to prevent prevent spasm
- Diuretics transiently if volume overloaded

ADMISSION/DISCHARGE CRITERIA

- Hemodynamically stable, normal sinus rhythm or rate-controlled atrial fibrillation, able to ambulate and eat, adequate family support to provide basic needs

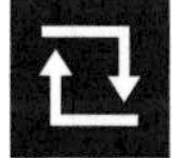

Follow-up

PATIENT MONITORING

First few weeks to months after discharge, physicians include cardiac surgeon, cardiologist, primary care provider. Patients are monitored for:

- Emotional/mental well being, attitude
- Healing at sternal, extremity wound sites
- Activity level/physical reconditioning
- Return of CBC indices to baseline

EXPECTED COURSE AND PROGNOSIS

Six weeks to several months is required to regain or improve exercise tolerance if postoperative course is uncomplicated. No driving and no lifting above 20 pounds are allowed for 4–6 weeks after sternotomy.

PATIENT EDUCATION

- Modify cardiac risk factors.
- Proper diet, types of activity, coping with stress

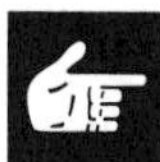

Miscellaneous

BIBLIOGRAPHY

Antman E. Medical management of the patient undergoing cardiac surgery. In: Braunwald E, ed. *Heart disease: a textbook of cardiovascular medicine,* 5th ed. Philadelphia: WB Saunders, 1997:1715–1740.

Higgins TL, Estafanous FG, Loop FD, et al. Stratification of morbidity and mortality outcome by preoperative risk factors in coronary artery bypass patients. *JAMA* 1992;267:2344–2348.

Morris DC, Clements SD, Hug CC. Management of the patient after cardiac surgery. In: Alexander RW, Schlant RC, Fuster V, eds. *Hurst's the heart,* 9th ed. New York: McGraw-Hill, 1998: 1489–1500.

Morris DC, St. Claire D Jr. Management of patients after cardiac surgery. *Curr Probl Cardiol* 1999;24:161–228.

Authors: Richard Chen and Jerre Lutz

Cardiac Transplantation, Pediatric

Basics

DESCRIPTION

Cardiac transplantation has become a common and rapidly expanding surgical option for children with end-stage heart disease.

EPIDEMIOLOGY

Incidence/Prevalence

Children comprise 10% of total cardiac transplants performed annually.

- By January 2000, the International Society for Heart and Lung Transplantation (ISHLT) Registry had recorded 4,671 heart transplants in children between birth and 18 years.
- Over half of children receiving transplants in the past 10 years were <5 years of age (average 400 children yearly).

ETIOLOGY

The two main indications for transplantation in pediatrics are cardiomyopathies and complex congenital heart disease (CHD).

- The predominant indication varies by age.
  - —In infants undergoing transplantation at <1 year of age, 75% have CHD.
  - —In the transition age (1–10 years), 40% of recipients have CHD and 50% myopathies.
  - —Cardiomyopathy is the indication for transplantation in 65% of adolescent recipients.
- Cardiomyopathies (in decreasing order of frequency)
  - —Dilated: idiopathic, adriamycin, familial, postmyocarditis
  - —Hypertrophic
  - —Restrictive
- CHD: 10%–20% of children with CHD might eventually benefit from transplantation in their lifetime.
  - —Primary operation: e.g., hypoplastic left heart syndrome, pulmonary atresia with intact septum and coronary sinusoids, and complex inoperable heterotaxy
  - —Previous biventricular repairs: poor function and/or valvar regurgitation when further repair too risky
  - —Palliated single ventricle: failed Fontans or if palliation untenable. Patients with failed Fontan physiology constitute a significantly expanding pretransplantation population.
- Death while waiting for transplant still approximates 30% in children, secondary to lack of donors.

PREGNANCY

Female heart transplant recipients can have successful pregnancies without apparent risk to the newborn from immunosuppressants.

- Hemodynamically the transplanted heart can tolerate pregnancy.
- There is some increased risk for rejection at the time of delivery.

ASSOCIATED CONDITIONS

Orthotopic cardiac transplantation is contraindicated in the presence of:

- Degenerative neurologic disease
- Pulmonary hypertension with pulmonary vascular resistance index >9 despite maximal therapy
- HIV infection
- End-stage renal, hepatic, or pulmonary disease, unless listed for the concomitant failed organ.

Diagnosis

DIFFERENTIAL DIAGNOSIS

The differential of complications in pediatric heart recipients relates to the cumulative side effects of immunosuppression or from ineffective immunosuppressive protection of the graft. Common major complications are:

- Rejection
- Infection
- Graft vasculopathy
- Posttransplantation lymphoproliferative disease (PTLD)
- End-organ toxicity of immunosuppressants

SIGNS AND SYMPTOMS

- Rejection: usually no significant cardiovascular symptoms, unless severe, presenting as heart failure and/or shock. Mild to moderate rejection may be accompanied by:
  - —Tachycardia or arrhythmia
  - —Gallop rhythm
  - —Enlarged tender liver
  - —Pericardial effusion
  - —Fever
  - —Malaise in older children, irritability in infants
  - —Abdominal complaints resembling gastroenteritis or "flu"
- Graft vasculopathy: Usually presenting late, may occur within first year. A form of chronic rejection. Symptoms depend upon severity. Patients will not experience angina. Common signs are
  - —Congestive heart failure (CHF) in absence of rejection
  - —CHF persisting following adequate rejection treatment
  - —Arrhythmia: atrial, ventricular or progressive heart block
  - —Syncope
  - —Sudden death

LABORATORY PROCEDURES

Common laboratory tests include monitoring of immunosuppressant levels, and potential toxic effects on bone marrow, kidney, and liver.

IMAGING STUDIES

The cardiac evaluation of recipients includes:

- Chest x-ray: A change in size of the cardiac silhouette may be the first objective evidence of rejection or pericardial effusion, particularly in long-term survivors.
- 2-D echocardiogram: Function is usually normal in transplanted hearts.
- Coronary angiograms: Serial angiograms are performed annually or biannually to evaluate graft vasculopathy. It is important to compare serial studies.
- Dobutamine stress echocardiogram: This modality is used to help define the presence of subtle graft vasculopathy not seen on angiography and to assess the functional severity of visible coronary disease.

SPECIAL TESTS

- ECG: Usually ECG shows sinus rhythm and residual nonconducted, native P waves from recipient sinus node. Findings indicative of rejection or coronary disease may or may not be present, including:
  - —Tachycardia
  - —Atrial or ventricular arrhythmias or progressive heart block
  - —Low voltage
  - —New Q waves or ST segment changes
- Endomyocardial biopsy: Right heart catheterization with endomyocardial biopsy is used by many centers on a routine decremental schedule postoperatively to evaluate for acute rejection.

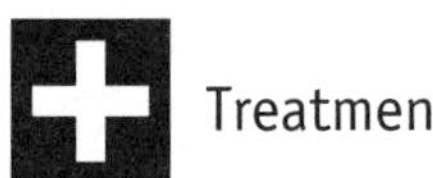

Treatment

GENERAL MEASURES

Medical management of heart recipients involves assessment of health of the graft and complications from immunosuppressant medications.

- Patients should receive endocarditis prophylaxis prior to dental work or invasive procedures.
- Care must be taken to avoid undue exposure to infectious diseases because the patient is on lifelong immunosuppression.
- Live viral vaccines are contraindicated.

SURGICAL MEASURES

Posttransplantation surgical intervention would include retransplantation, the only alternative for advanced transplant coronary disease. Indications for retransplantation include:

- Rapidly progressive graft arteriopathy with or without ischemia
- Stable arteriopathy with severe CHF
- Severe acute rejection unresponsive to therapy (outcome poor in this group)

ADMISSION/DISCHARGE CRITERIA

Posttransplantation admissions are usually for complications of immunosuppressant medications. Inadequate immunosuppression results in rejection or coronary artery disease. Overimmunosuppression may occur early postoperatively or following treatment for rejection and can result in admissions for infections or PTLD.

• Discharge criteria vary by diagnosis and treatment.
 —During the first year of follow-up, 51% of pediatric cardiac recipients did not require rehospitalization for illness.
  • Rejection hospitalization 13%
  • Infection hospitalization 10%
 —During the third posttransplantation year, 70% of children did not require hospitalization.
  • Rejection hospitalization 11%
  • Infection hospitalization 3%

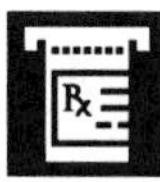

Medications

DRUG(S) OF CHOICE

Cardiac recipients are on multiple medications.

• Double or triple drug immunosuppression using combinations of
 —Cyclosporine
 —FK506
 —Azathioprine
 —Prednisone
 —Mycophenolate mofetil
 —Rapamycin
• Antihypertensive therapy (40%–60%)
 —Calcium channel blockers
 —Angiotensin-converting enzyme (ACE) inhibitors
• Cardiotonic therapy (digoxin, ACE inhibitors, diuretics) may be necessary transiently, at times following transplantation.
 —During recovery from prolonged rejection
 —CHF from coronary disease
 —Perioperative right heart failure
• Lipid-altering drugs (statins) are used by some centers.
 —Treatment of cyclosporine-induced hyperlipidemia
 —Possible additional immunosuppressant effect which may retard development of graft vasculopathy or prevent rejection

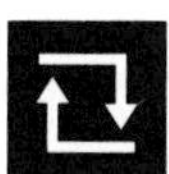

Follow-up

PATIENT MONITORING

Close routine outpatient follow-up is necessary at decreasing intervals for optimal survival. Transplant patients require lifelong monitoring of the graft and the chronic effects of the medications.

• Early postoperatively, the patient is seen frequently the first 3 months to adjust medications and monitor for infections, rejections, and rehabilitation.
• Later follow-up visits are centered on weaning immunosuppression to low maintenance levels, preventative care, and monitoring for complications.

EXPECTED COURSE AND PROGNOSIS

• The postoperative course in transplant recipients varies with degree of pretransplantation debilitation and morbidity. More stable children recover quickly with the addition of normal heart function.
• Actuarial survival in children has steadily improved with optimized therapy, making survival for decades seem likely. The Pediatric Registry of the ISHLT shows an excellent survival rates:
 —82% at 1 year and 79% at 4 years in children who underwent transplantation between 1995 and 1998
 —The conditional (surviving the first year posttransplantation) half-life for all pediatric recipients since 1982 is now >14 years.
• Causes of death in ISHLT Pediatric Registry:
 —Increased perioperative mortality (25%) in infants transplanted for CHD compared with older children with CHD or other infants with cardiomyopathy (10%).
 —Most common causes of death during the first year posttransplantation were acute rejection then infection.
 —Acute then chronic rejection (coronary disease) are the most common causes from 1 to 3 years posttransplantation.
 —Beyond 3 years posttransplantation, coronary disease is responsible for almost half of the deaths.
 —Malignancy remains an infrequent cause of death.
• Incidence of coronary disease in ISHLT Pediatric Registry:
 —10% at 2 years, 16% at 3 years
 —Rejection episodes in first year appear to be an indicator for subsequent events such as coronary disease and late mortality.
• Quality of life in ISHLT Pediatric Registry
 —For pediatric recipients who underwent transplantation from 1994 to 1998, >90% had no activity restrictions at 1 and 3 years of follow-up.
 —Growth spurts were reported in all age groups in the first year posttransplantation, with the exception of adolescents.
 —Growth appeared to be sustained in subsequent years in younger age groups.
 —All data show that children have a remarkable ability for rehabilitation to pursue a normal life-style following transplantation.

PATIENT EDUCATION

• Continuing education about the necessity for strict compliance with their immunosuppressant medications is required throughout their lives.
 —Significant, chronic noncompliance carries a 60% mortality risk.
 —Adolescent patients have a high incidence of noncompliance.
 —Previous compliance may wane with time from transplantation and age, so continued vigilance is required.
• The family and patient should be educated about signs and symptoms of rejection as well as infection precautions.
• There are no activity restrictions for transplant recipients; regular physical activity and exercise is advisable for rehabilitation.
• A low-fat healthful diet is recommended.
• There are numerous websites and support organizations for transplant recipients:
 —The United Network of Organ Sharing, which manages donor allocation, has extensive information available on transplantation programs across the United States.
 —The journal of ISHLT provides extensive information about transplantation research.

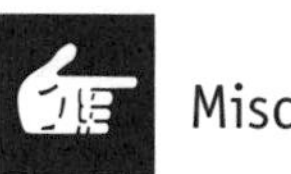

Miscellaneous

ICD-9-CM

V42.1 Cardiac transplantation

BIBLIOGRAPHY

Addonizio LJ. Cardiac transplantation during childhood. *Baillieres Clin Pediatr* 1996;4: 171–189.

Addonizio LJ, et al. Benefits and pitfalls of transplantation in children with congenital heart disease. In: Franco K, ed. *Pediatric cardiopulmonary transplantation.* Armonk, NY: Futura, 1997.

Boucek MM, et al. The Registry of the International Society of Heart and Lung Transplantation: third official pediatric report. *J Heart Lung Transplant* 1999:18:1151–1172.

Fricker FJ, Addonizio LJ, et al. Heart transplantation in children: indications. *Pediatr Transplant* 1999;3:333–342.

Webber SA. 15 Years of pediatric heart transplantation at the University of Pittsburgh: lessons learned and future prospects. *Pediatr Transplant* 1997;1:8–21.

Authors: Linda J. Addonizio and Welton M. Gersony

Cardiomyopathy, Dilated

Basics

DESCRIPTION

Dilatation of the ventricles with associated contractile dysfunction due to a variety of causes

- When an underlying disorder cannot be identified, dilated cardiomyopathy is referred to as idiopathic, often presumed to be of a viral etiology or on a genetic basis.

EPIDEMIOLOGY

- Approximately 5/100,000 new cases per year
- The incidence may be increasing.
- More common in men, African Americans
- Most common type of cardiomyopathy

ETIOLOGY

- Familial transmission occurs in 30% of cases.
- Usually autosomal dominant, although autosomal-recessive, X-linked recessive, and mitochondrial inheritance patterns have all been identified.
- Muscular dystrophies, such as Duchenne's
- Alcohol is another major cause, perhaps accounting for 30% of cases.
- Cocaine
- Infectious etiologies, particularly viral infections, are postulated to cause dilated cardiomyopathy. Coxsackie virus B has been linked with several cases of idiopathic dilated cardiomyopathy. HIV can cause such a cardiomyopathy.
- Peripartum cardiomyopathy occurs in about 1/4,000 births; autoimmune factors may be responsible.
- Uncontrolled tachycardia, such as atrial fibrillation or ventricular tachycardia
- Pheochromocytoma
- Thyroid disease (either hypo- or hyperthyroidism)
- Hemochromatosis and sarcoidosis are infiltrative cardiomyopathies, typically classified as restrictive, although in later stages, both can present as dilated cardiomyopathy.
- Acromegaly
- Chemotherapy with doxorubicin, bleomycin
- Hypertensive, ischemic, and valvular cardiomyopathies may present as dilated cardiomyopathy.
- Nutritional deficiencies (carnitine, selenium, thiamine)

RISK FACTORS

- Alcohol
- Family history of dilated cardiomyopathy
- Multiparity, advanced maternal age, African American (for peripartum cardiomyopathy)

PREGNANCY

- Peripartum cardiomyopathy is a dilated cardiomyopathy that occurs in the last trimester of pregnancy or in the 6 months following pregnancy.
- Repeat pregnancy is not advised, particularly if left ventricular function has not normalized since the initial pregnancy.
- Women with peripartum cardiomyopathy whose ejection fractions have returned to normal have subsequently had successful pregnancies without development of clinical heart failure.
- Dobutamine echocardiography of women with recovered resting ventricular function often still shows impaired contractile reserve.

ASSOCIATED CONDITIONS

- Depends on the etiology
- Pulmonary or systemic emboli

Diagnosis

DIFFERENTIAL DIAGNOSIS

- Other causes of congestive heart failure

SIGNS AND SYMPTOMS

- Dyspnea on exertion, at rest
- Paroxysmal nocturnal dyspnea
- Orthopnea
- Cough
- Fatigue
- Chest pain
- Lower extremity edema
- Hepatomegaly, pulsatile liver
- Ascites
- Palpitations
- Pulmonary rales
- S3
- S4
- Apical impulse laterally displaced
- Jugular venous distention
- Murmur of mitral and/or tricuspid regurgitation
- Pulsus alternans

LABORATORY PROCEDURES

- Hyponatremia is common in advanced heart failure.
- Thyroid function tests
- Iron, ferritin, and iron saturation levels (for hemochromatosis)
- Urine and serum protein electrophoresis (for amyloidosis)
- ECG may show sinus tachycardia. Left bundle branch block is not unusual. Ventricular arrhythmias, especially nonsustained ventricular tachycardia, are common.

IMAGING STUDIES

- Chest x-ray reveals cardiomegaly.
  - —Pulmonary congestion may be present.
- Echocardiography reveals a dilated left ventricle with global hypokinesis.
  - —Segmental wall motion abnormalities can be present and do not necessarily imply the presence of coronary artery disease.
  - —Usually all four cardiac chambers are enlarged.
  - —Mural thrombi may be observed in the ventricles.
  - —Atrioventricular regurgitation secondary to annular dilatation is common.

SPECIAL TESTS

- Coronary arteriography
  - —Typically would be normal, other than in ischemic cardiomyopathy.
  - —This test should be performed if there is clinical suspicion of coronary artery disease
- Right heart catheterization
  - —In the decompensated patient, reveals a high wedge pressure, an elevated systemic vascular resistance, and a low cardiac output
- Endomyocardial biopsy
  - —Formerly a popular procedure for routine diagnosis of dilated cardiomyopathy, but is now discouraged unless a specific etiology is being considered
  - —In cases with a high suspicion of giant cell myocarditis, biopsy is generally performed prior to initiation of empiric immunosuppressive therapy.
- Cardiopulmonary exercise stress testing
  - —Can objectively assess a patient's functional capacity and can be used to determine the need for heart transplantation

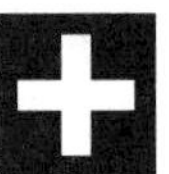

Treatment

GENERAL MEASURES

- Low-salt diet
- Free water restriction
- Cardiac rehabilitation to strengthen peripheral muscles.

SURGICAL MEASURES

- Transplantation is an excellent option for end-stage disease, with symptoms refractory to medical therapy.
- Implantable cardioverter–defibrillator therapy is being studied for patients with nonsustained ventricular tachycardia.
- Biventricular pacing is being studied as a method of improving hemodynamic function.
- Implantable left ventricular assist devices appear to have a role as a bridge to tranplantation, and are being investigated as stand-alone therapy.

ADMISSION/DISCHARGE CRITERIA

- Many exacerbations of congestive heart failure can be managed as an outpatient with frequent telephone contact.
- Intravenous diuresis is possible on an outpatient basis in certain circumstances.
- Admission is advisable for any sudden change in symptomatology or for aggressive diuresis.
- Discharge is possible once a patient is converted to oral medications.
- Home intravenous inotropic therapy is possible for relief of symptoms, but may be associated with worse outcomes.

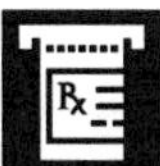

Medications

DRUG(S) OF CHOICE

- Angiotensin-converting enzyme (ACE) inhibitors at adequate doses; contraindicated in pregnancy
- Hydralazine and nitrates for patients intolerant to ACE inhibitors
- Possibly angiotensin receptor blockers for patients intolerant to ACE inhibitors or in addition to ACE inhibitors; contraindicated in pregnancy
- Beta-blockers unless in pulmonary edema
- Diuretics for symptoms of edema or pulmonary congestion
- Digoxin for symptom control, especially if atrial fibrillation is present
- Amiodarone for ventricular arrhythmia
- Warfarin for treatment of thrombi or atrial fibrillation; contraindicated in pregnancy
- Intravenous immune globulin may have a role in peripartum cardiomyopathy, although it does not appear to be beneficial in idiopathic dilated cardiomyopathy.

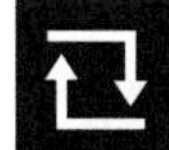

Follow-up

PATIENT MONITORING

- Some have recommended echocardiographic screening of family members with idiopathic dilated cardiomyopathy, even in the absence of symptoms, given the high incidence of familial cardiomyopathy.
- Routine echocardiography, in the absence of worsening symptoms, although frequently performed, is not recommended.

EXPECTED COURSE AND PROGNOSIS

- Symptomatic patients who are referred to a tertiary care center have a 50% 5-year mortality rate.
- Right ventricular dilatation portends a more ominous prognosis.
- A lower ejection fraction is associated with a higher risk of mortality in populations of patients with heart failure; it is less predictive of outcome in an individual.
- Peripartum cardiomyopathys show significant improvement within 6 months in almost half of all women who develop this disorder.
- Heart transplantation has been successfully used in peripartum cardiomyopathy that does not improve with time or medical measures, although the risk of early rejection episodes may be higher.
- Alcoholic cardiomyopathy is largely reversible with complete abstinence.
- Arrhythmias are common.
- Thromboembolic events may occur.

PATIENT EDUCATION

- Patients should weigh themselves daily and report any sudden increase to their doctor.
- Avoid alcohol and tobacco.
- Restrict sodium intake.

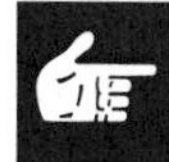

Miscellaneous

ICD-9-CM

428.0 Failure, heart, congestive
425.4 Cardiomyopathy, dilated
674.8 Cardiomyopathy, postpartum

BIBLIOGRAPHY

Bozkurt B, Villaneuva FS, Holubkov R, et al. Intravenous immune globulin in the therapy of peripartum cardiomyopathy. *J Am Coll Cardiol* 1999;34:177–180.

Dec GW, Fuster V. Idiopathic dilated cardiomyopathy. *N Engl J Med* 1994;331:1564–1575.

Homans DC. Peripartum cardiomyopathy. *N Engl J Med* 1985;312:1432–1437.

Lampert MB, Lang RM. Peripartum cardiomyopathy. *Am Heart J* 1995;130:860–870.

Rickenbacher PR, Rizeq MN, Hunt SA, et al. Long-term outcome after heart transplantation for peripartum cardiomyopathy. *Am Heart J* 1994;127:1318–1323.

Rodkey SM, Ratliff NB, Young JB. Cardiomyopathy and myocardial failure. In: Topol EJ, ed. *Comprehensive cardiovascular medicine.* Philadelphia: Lippincott-Raven, 1998:2591–2593.

Sun JP, James KB, Yang XS, et al. Comparison of mortality rates and progression of left ventricular dysfunction in patients with idiopathic dilated cardiomyopathy and dilated versus nondilated right ventricular cavities. *Am J Cardiol* 1997;80:1583–1587.

Tajik AJ, Murphy JG. Dilated cardiomyopathy. In: Murphy JG, ed. *Mayo Clinic cardiology review.* Philadelphia: Lippincott Williams & Wilkins, 2000:445–454.

Wynne J, Braunwald E. The cardiomyopathies and myocarditides. In: Braunwald E, ed. *Heart disease: a textbook of cardiovascular medicine, 5th ed.* Philadelphia: WB Saunders, 1997:1407–1414.

Authors: Deepak L. Bhatt and Gary S. Francis

Cardiomyopathy, Hypertrophic

Basics

DESCRIPTION

Massive hypertrophy of the ventricle results in a dynamic outflow tract obstruction.

- Also called idiopathic hypertrophic subaortic stenosis and hypertrophic obstructive cardiomyopathy (HOCM)

EPIDEMIOLOGY

- Familial hypertrophic cardiomyopathy is inherited as an autosomal-dominant trait with variable penetrance.
- Apical hypertrophic obstructive cardiomyopathy is a variant that is found more often in Japan than in other parts of the world.

ETIOLOGY

- Several chromosomal abnormalities due to multiple mutations have been identified that are responsible for hypertrophic cardiomyopathy.
- Mutations in the genes for cardiac myosin heavy chain, troponin T, and alpha tropomyosin are some that have been discovered, and there will likely be more.

RISK FACTORS

- Family history of HOCM

PREGNANCY

- High risk, especially in the postpartum period, where blood and fluid loss can lead to exacerbation of the outflow tract gradient

ASSOCIATED CONDITIONS

- Arrhythmias

Diagnosis

DIFFERENTIAL DIAGNOSIS

- Athlete's heart
- Hypertensive cardiomyopathy, especially in the elderly
- Amyloid
- Aortic stenosis

SIGNS AND SYMPTOMS

- "Spike and dome" contour of the carotid pulse
- S2 paradoxically split
- Harsh systolic murmur along the left sternal border, increases with Valsalva maneuver or in beat after a premature ventricular contraction
- Systolic thrill
- Pulmonary rales
- Mitral regurgitation murmur
- S4
- S3
- Double or triple apical impulse
- Dyspnea on exertion, and at rest
- Syncope
- Chest pain
- Palpitations

LABORATORY PROCEDURES

- ECG reveals a large amount of voltage across the precordium.
- T-wave inversion also may be present in the precordial leads.
- Atrial and ventricular arrhythmias may be present, as may septal Q waves.

IMAGING STUDIES

- Chest x-ray may reveal cardiac enlargement.
- 2-D echocardiography is the cornerstone of diagnosis.
  —Left ventricular hypertrophy is present, classically asymmetric septal hypertrophy.
  —However, other patterns of hypertrophy exist, such as predominant apical hypertrophy.
  —There is systolic anterior motion of the mitral valve and associated mitral regurgitation.
  —Left ventricular systolic function is hyperdynamic.
  —The cavity size is not enlarged.
- Doppler interrogation reveals a gradient across the outflow tract that increases with the Valsalva maneuver or inhalation of amyl nitrate.

SPECIAL TESTS

- Left ventriculography shows cavity obliteration.
  —In mid-ventricular obstruction, a spade-shaped left ventricle is classic.
- Coronary arteriography typically reveals normal coronary arteries in young patients. Older patients may have coexistent coronary artery disease. Prominent septal perforators may be present, which may display systolic compression from the thickened septum.
- Genetic testing is not routinely recommended; many different mutations have been identified, with varying natural histories.

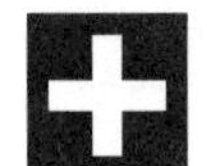

Treatment

GENERAL MEASURES

Adequate hydration; avoid volume depletion.

SURGICAL MEASURES

- Septal myectomy can successfully reduce the outflow tract gradient and improve symptoms.
- More recently, percutaneous transluminal septal ablation has been accomplished with localized alcohol injection into the first or second septal perforator in order to selectively destroy septal tissue.
- Dual-chamber pacing has been used as a means to reduce outflow tract gradient and improve symptoms, but results have been mixed.

ADMISSION/DISCHARGE CRITERIA

- As for heart failure of any etiology

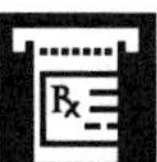

Medications

DRUG(S) OF CHOICE

- Antibiotic prophylaxis for procedures that may lead to bacterial endocarditis
- Avoid positive inotropes such as digoxin.
- Beta-blockers are first-line therapy.
- Calcium channel blockers such as verapamil and diltiazem can be useful; watch for excessive vasodilation, which can be detrimental.
- Disopyramide, due to its negative inotropic effects, can be useful, but anticholinergic side effects, such as urinary retention in men, can limit its tolerability.

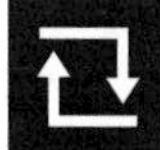

Follow-up

PATIENT MONITORING

- As for heart failure of any etiology

EXPECTED COURSES AND PROGNOSIS

- Earlier reports of these patients were from referral centers and suggested a high incidence of sudden death.
- More contemporary analyses suggest that the risk of sudden death, while elevated, is not as high as previously believed.
- Risk of sudden death is increased in patients with malignant ventricular arrhythmias or a family history of sudden death, and is more common in children.
- Hypertrophic cardiomyopathy is the most common identified cause of sudden cardiac death in the young athlete. Competitive sports participation is contraindicated.

PATIENT EDUCATION

- Avoid dehydration; maintain adequate volume intake.
- No participation in competitive sports

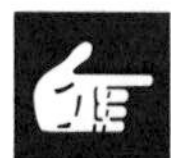

Miscellaneous

ICD-9-CM

428.0 Failure, heart, congestive
425.1 Cardiomyopathy, hypertrophic obstructive

BIBLIOGRAPHY

Miller DH, Borer JS. The cardiomyopathies: a pathophysiologic approach to therapeutic management. *Arch Intern Medicine* 1983;143:2157–2162.

Rodkey SM, Ratliff NB, Young JB. Cardiomyopathy and myocardial failure. In: Topol EJ, ed. *Comprehensive cardiovascular medicine.* Philadelphia: Lippincott-Raven, 1998:2593–2594.

Tajik AJ, Murphy JG. Hypertrophic and restrictive cardiomyopathies. In: Murphy JG, ed. *Mayo Clinic cardiology review.* Philadelphia: Lippincott Williams & Wilkins, 2000:455–482.

Wynne J, Braunwald E. The cardiomyopathies and myocarditides. In: Braunwald E, ed. *Heart disease: a textbook of cardiovascular medicine,* 5th ed. Philadelphia: WB Saunders, 1997:1414–1426.

Authors: Deepak L. Bhatt and Gary S. Francis

Cardiomyopathy, Pediatric

Basics

DESCRIPTION

Cardiomyopathy (CM) is defined as disease of the heart muscle with histologic or morphologic myocardial abnormality resulting in decreased compliance of the ventricle. The left ventricle (LV) is usually affected or there may be biventricular involvement. There are primary cardiomyopathies of unknown origin or secondary, when disease is a result of another known systemic disorder. The World Health Organization/International Society and Federation of Cardiologists adopted this empiric division in 1995.

The three main types of primary CM are classified morphologically:

- Dilated: LV dilation; poor systolic function; disproportionately thin free wall and septal thickness; loss of myocytes, fibrosis
- Hypertrophic: left and/or right ventricular hypertrophy, concentric or asymmetric, involving septum; LV volume normal or reduced; normal systolic, abnormal diastolic function; massive myocyte hypertrophy and fiber disarray with increased connective tissue
- Restrictive: restrictive filling, low diastolic volume of either ventricle; near normal systolic function and wall thickness; fibrosis of myocardium, endocardial rigidity

EPIDEMIOLOGY

Estimates of incidence of CM vary widely according to type and age group. There is no bias to age, race or sex.

- Idiopathic dilated CM accounts for >90% of all cardiomyopathies seen in childhood:
  - National Heart, Lung, and Blood Institute Workshop: 2–8 cases/100,000 over all age groups
  - Mayo Clinic Study: 36.5 cases/100,000 over all age groups
  - Baltimore-Washington Infant Study: 1/10,000 live births (this incidence includes all forms of neonatal CM)
- Hypertrophic CM
  - Mayo Clinic Study: 2.5 cases/100,000
  - Iceland Echocardiographic Study: 33 cases/100,000
- Restrictive CM: rare; includes contracted form of endocardial fibroelastosis (EFE)

ETIOLOGY

- Dilated CM may be idiopathic (unknown etiology), familial/genetic, viral and/or autoimmune, alcoholic/toxic, or associated with other disease.
- Hypertrophic CM may be sporadic, associated with syndromes or more commonly familial, with autosomal-dominant pattern and wide variability of penetrance.
  - 60% of families have more than one case.
  - The 14q1 chromosome is a major locus.
- Restrictive CM may be idiopathic or associated with infiltrative disease (amyloidosis, hypereosinophilia).

RISK FACTORS

None for idiopathic; some risk factors for specific etiologies are listed above.

PREGNANCY

Risk for pregnancy depends on degree of ventricular dysfunction and/or heart failure.

- Symptomatic patients with dilated CM and all patients with hypertrophic CM are at increased risk for mortality and for cardiovascular decompensation during pregnancy.

ASSOCIATED CONDITIONS

Primary cardiomyopathies by definition have no associated conditions. In the specific cardiomyopathies, >100 associated diseases have been identified.

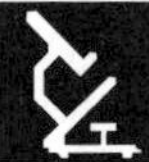

Diagnosis

DIFFERENTIAL DIAGNOSIS

The differential diagnosis of idiopathic CM is one of exclusion.

- Diagnostic focus should center on establishing an etiology that might be curable.
- Examples of treatable causes of dilated CM are carnitine deficiency or other metabolic disorders, arrhythmia, toxic reactions, and inflammatory diseases.
- Usually there is no difficulty diagnostically in distinguishing dilated CM from either hypertrophic or restrictive forms.

SIGNS AND SYMPTOMS

Symptoms depend on the morphologic type of CM and degree of impairment of ventricular muscle.

Dilated CM

Initial symptoms range from exercise intolerance to overt congestive heart failure (CHF) as a consequence of poor systolic function.

- Respiratory distress, chronic cough, frequent "upper respiratory infections"
- Easy fatigability (during feeding with infants)
- Abdominal complaints, pain, nausea, vomiting
- Failure to thrive, growth failure
- Signs of CHF: tachycardia, tachypnea, gallop rhythm, hepatomegaly, diminished perfusion
- Murmur of mitral incompetence may be heard with severe LV dilatation

Hypertrophic CM

Termed "the great masquerader," because signs and symptoms usually result in a false diagnosis of other diseases. Symptoms vary in intensity depending on the extent and distribution of the hypertrophy. They result from high filling pressures (diastolic dysfunction), low cardiac output from LV outflow tract (LVOT) obstruction, or angina. Obstruction may occur at rest or with provocation.

- Increased fatigability, exercise intolerance
- Cough, breathlessness, "asthma"
- Chest pain
- Syncope or dizziness
- Sudden death
- Murmur and examination related to hemodynamic state:
  —Outflow obstruction: double or triple apical LV impulse and medium pitch systolic ejection murmur (increases with Valsalva maneuver)
  —Nonobstructive form: only nonspecific ejection murmur
- Atrial or ventricular arrhythmias

Restrictive CM

Presentation varies with age and degree of diastolic impairment:

- In newborn, CHF common with respiratory distress and low output
- Pronounced growth retardation in young children
- Abdominal pain or GI complaints
- Dyspnea on exertion, dry cough, "asthma" are seen in older children.
- Hepatomegaly, ascites, and peripheral edema in older children with more chronic course.
- Atrial arrhythmias, predominantly fibrillation and flutter
- Thromboembolism secondary to above
- Third heart sound, prominent apical impulse, increased jugular venous pressure

IMAGING STUDIES

Evaluations establish diagnosis and treatment effectiveness.

- Chest x-ray: Enlarged heart
  —Dilated CM: larger, more globular shape, pulmonary edema or congestion, left atrium dilated
  —Hypertrophic CM: cardiomegaly greater in infants than older children, unless end stage
  —Restrictive CM: biatrial dilatation, pulmonary venous pattern, ventricular enlargement not prominent
- Echocardiography: provides definitive diagnosis of three morphologic types, rules out other abnormalities (e.g., anomalous coronary or subaortic membrane)
  —Dilated CM: thin-walled, globular LV, low fractional shortening, mitral insufficiency and/or mural thrombi in late stages, both ventricles can be affected
  —Hypertrophic CM: very thick septum, free wall, near obliteration of LV cavity, normal to hyperdynamic function, systolic anterior motion of mitral leaflet, and/or LVOT obstruction with measurable Doppler gradient
  —Restrictive CM: massive biatrial enlargement, normal to small-sized somewhat hypertrophied ventricles, normal systolic function with abnormal diastolic function
- Angiocardiography: only indicated if unable to visualize coronary arteries by echocardiography or to rule out discrete aortic obstruction
- MRI: useful to rule out constrictive pericarditis

SPECIAL STUDIES

- Electrocardiogram: Varying patterns of LV hypertrophy with nonspecific left precordial inversion or flattening of T waves and sometimes deep Q waves. Abnormalities specific to each form:
  —Dilated: ventricular, atrial arrhythmias; in EFE very tall QRS voltage present in all precordial and limb leads
  —Hypertrophic: 90% abnormal ECG with a wide variety of patterns; infants often have paradoxic right ventricular hypertrophy; cannot discriminate LVOT obstruction or risk for sudden death by ECG; atrial fibrillation or ventricular tachycardia
  —Restrictive: biatrial enlargement, right ventricular enlargement in infants, atrial arrhythmias or progressive heart block
- Cardiac catheterization
  —Dilated CM: Rule out myocarditis by endomyocardial biopsy, evaluate hemodynamic efficacy of medical therapy and need for transplantation.
  —Hypertrophic CM: evaluation for arrhythmias and possible surgical relief of obstruction
  —Restrictive CM: Rule out constrictive pericarditis (dip and plateau pressure tracing present in both, LV end-diastolic pressure greater than right ventricular end-diastolic pressure favors restrictive). Pulmonary hypertension with rapidly increasing resistance is seen frequently and earlier in restrictive types but not in hypertrophic type.

Cardiomyopathy, Pediatric

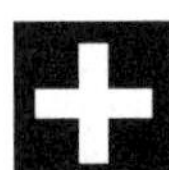

Treatment

GENERAL MEASURES

Medical management involves control of CHF and arrhythmias and potential prevention of progression of disease. In asymptomatic patients continued reevaluation is warranted.

- A tailored cardiotonic regimen for patients with CHF is optimal.
- To prevent thromboembolism, warfarin anticoagulation is advised if atrial fibrillation, ejection fraction $<20\%$, and/or mural thrombus is present.
- Endocarditis prophylaxis is only necessary with concomitant valvular abnormality.
- Influenza and pneumococcal vaccines are advisable with significant cardiovascular compromise.

SURGICAL MEASURES

- Hypertrophic CM: excision of muscular LVOT or right ventricular outflow tract obstruction can relieve symptoms.
- Hypertrophic CM: resolution of symptoms with release of coronary stenosis by myocardial bridging
- Implantable defibrillators help prevent outpatient sudden death when ventricular arrhythmias are significant in hypertrophic CM.
- When maximal medical therapy fails, cardiac transplantation should be considered.

ADMISSION/DISCHARGE CRITERIA

- Children can present in severe CHF or shock at time of diagnosis with dilated CM.
  - —After stabilization and discharge, admissions are for acute pulmonary edema or transient low output or progression of disease.
- Patients with hypertrophic CM usually do not require admission except for life-threatening arrhythmia or if end stage.
- Restrictive patients can have episodic increase in CHF symptoms, and with rising pulmonary vascular resistance index will need transplantation sooner than dilated patients to avoid need for lung transplantation as well.

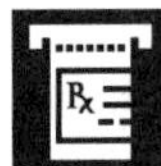

Medications

DRUG(S) OF CHOICE

Presentation can vary from mild CHF to shock. Patients should be placed on bed rest initially, with fluid restriction until stabilized.

Dilated CM

CHF treatment should be tailored and maximized. Some of these agents may be needed in other types of CM in later stages.

- Digoxin
- Angiotensin-converting enzyme (ACE) inhibitors
- Diuretics such as furosemide, thiazides,
- Spironolactone may be added to maintain potassium levels (caution when adding to ACE inhibitor).
- Beta-adrenergic blockers may result in significant improvement, but should only be administered cautiously, under direct care of experienced cardiologist.
- If outpatient management is unsuccessful, intravenous inotropic agents and vasodilators may be necessary for stabilization; in extreme cases, ventilatory support or LV assist devices may be needed.
- Arrhythmia management: isolated or even frequent premature ventricular beats do not warrant the addition of an antiarrhythmic unless:
  - —Episodes of ventricular tachycardia with syncope are featured: amiodarone
  - —Implantable defibrillator is a better option for malignant rhythms

Hypertrophic CM

Treatment usually is focused on minimizing outflow obstruction, myocardial relaxation, and arrhythmia (see above).

- Calcium channel blockers may alleviate symptoms and questionably prevent progression of disease.
- Beta-blocker therapy may decrease ectopic beats while controlling heart rate and LV compliance.
- If CHF occurs, cardiotonics may be necessary. Caution is needed when using diuretics in hypertrophic or restrictive CM.

Restrictive CM

No specific medications. Children most often need anticongestive measures, which can share the same danger as with hypertrophic patients.

Follow-up

PATIENT MONITORING

- Close outpatient follow-up of all patients with CM is necessary to detect progression of disease and to tailor their medications.
- Frequency of visits will depend on cardiac disability and instability. Progress can be evaluated by periodic:
  - —Exercise testing: to determine VO_{2max} in dilated patients, and level of inducible ischemia in hypertrophic CM
  - —Holter monitoring: to detect malignant arrhythmias or progressive heart block
  - —Cardiac catheterization: pretransplant hemodynamic testing and progression of PVRI

EXPECTED COURSE AND PROGNOSIS

The prognosis varies with the type of CM.

Dilated CM

The course is highly variable, with some children surviving many years but a significant number lost in the first year after diagnosis.

- Survival ranges from 40% to 90% at 1 year.
- CHF symptoms despite therapy is a poor prognostic sign.
- LV ejection fraction is not predictive of course.
- Elevated LV end-diastolic pressure >25 mm Hg: mortality 46% at 1 year, 68% at 5 years
- Low serum sodium correlated with poor outcome

Hypertrophic CM

Course depends on age at presentation.

- Infant survival dismal with CHF; transplant should be considered.
- Most diagnosed after age 12 years are stable for years.
- 3%–6% annual mortality rate; 5-year survival 80%
- Progressive disease, especially during rapid somatic growth
- Sudden death during exercise most common in adolescents
- No predictive variables for sudden death in children
- If late CHF or unmanageable symptoms develop, transplantation is indicated.

Restrictive CM

Rare, but course is accelerated, with most deaths occurring in young childhood, either sudden or from advancing CHF. May have a period of well-being after initial CHF symptoms, when pulmonary resistance increases. Transplantation should be considered early.

PATIENT EDUCATION

- Patients with CHF and their family should be educated about:
  —Importance of low-salt diet
  —Adequate rest, but graded regular exercise important (cardiac rehabilitation based on the severity of compromise)
  —Importance of routine follow-up and compliance with medications
  —Signs and symptoms of disease progression and arrhythmias
- Hypertrophic CM: strenuous physical exercise and stress should be avoided.

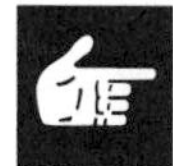

Miscellaneous

ICD-9-CM

425.4 Primary cardiomyopathy
425.9 Secondary cardiomyopathy

INTERNET RESOURCES

There are numerous websites and support organizations for patients with heart failure. Many AHA sites exist, but most are geared to older adolescents or adults.

- www.healthlinkusa.com
- www.searchwebmd.com
- www.americanheart.org

BIBLIOGRAPHY

Addonizio LJ. Cardiac transplantation in childhood cardiomyopathies. *Prog Pediatr Cardiol* 1992;1:72–80.

Benson LN, Freedom RM, et al., eds. Cardiomyopathies of childhood: part II. *Prog Pediatr Cardiol* 1992;14:1–80.

Garson A Jr, et al. *The science and practice of pediatric cardiology,* 2nd ed. Baltimore: Williams & Wilkins, 1998.

Lewis AB, Chabot M. Outcome of infants and children with dilated cardiomyopathy. *Am J Cardiol* 1991;68:365–369.

Wiles HB, et al. Prognostic features of children with idiopathic dilated cardiomyopathy. *Am J Cardiol* 1991;68:1372–1376.

Authors: Linda J. Addonizio and Welton M. Gersony

Cardiomyopathy, Restrictive

Basics

DESCRIPTION

Infiltration of the myocardium by one of several disease processes leads to severe impairment of diastolic filling of the ventricle.

- Rarely is any specific cause found.
- Needs to be distinguished from constrictive pericarditis (not easy), which may respond to pericardiectomy
- Even a small increase in ventricular volume can lead to a substantial increase in intracavitary pressures.
- Systolic function is normal until the terminal stages of the disease.

EPIDEMIOLOGY

- Most forms are uncommon in the United States.
- Least common class of cardiomyopathy
- There are certain rare familial forms of restrictive cardiomyopathy.

ETIOLOGY

- Amyloidosis
- Sarcoidosis
- Hemochromatosis
- Scleroderma
- Fabry's disease
- Glycogen storage disorders
- Gaucher's disease
- Hurler's disease
- Endomyocardial fibrosis
- Loffler endocarditis
- Endocardial fibroelastosis
- Carcinoid
- Radiation
- Metastatic cancer
- After heart transplantation; also, with rejection

RISK FACTORS

- Depends on etiology

PREGNANCY

- Not advisable in symptomatic restrictive cardiomyopathy

ASSOCIATED CONDITIONS

- Atrial fibrillation
- Pleural effusions
- Thromboembolism
- Hypercalcemia, kidney stones (in sarcoid)
- Diabetes (in hemochromatosis)

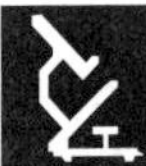

Diagnosis

DIFFERENTIAL DIAGNOSIS

- Constrictive pericarditis, which can appear clinically identical in terms of symptoms and physical examination findings
- Other causes of right-sided heart failure

SIGNS AND SYMPTOMS

- Exertional dyspnea
- Fatigue
- Edema
- Hepatomegaly, pulsatile liver
- Ascites
- JVD (jugular venous distension), with rapid x and y descents
- Kussmaul's sign (increase in JVP [jugular venous pressure] with inspiration)
- S3, right- or left-sided
- S4 (uncommon)
- Cutaneous flushing, diarrhea, bronchoconstriction (with carcinoid syndrome)
- Anterior uveitis (sarcoid)
- Erythema nodosum (tender red nodules in sarcoid)

LABORATORY PROCEDURES

- In hemochromatosis, serum ferritin levels are markedly elevated, along with iron levels and transferrin saturation.
- The angiotensin-converting enzyme level may be elevated with sarcoidosis, although it can be within the normal range.
- Eosinophilia is associated with eosinophilic heart disease.
- Urinary 5-hydroxyindoleacetic acid levels are elevated in carcinoid.
- ECG may show various degrees of conduction block.

IMAGING STUDIES

- Chest x-ray is notable for absence of cardiomegaly
  —Pulmonary congestion and pleural effusions may be present.
  —Bilateral hilar lymphadenopathy may be seen with sarcoid.
- Doppler tracings reveal marked impairment of diastolic function.
  —In contrast with constrictive pericarditis, there is no significant respiratory variation in mitral and tricuspid inflow patterns.
  —The mitral inflow pattern shows a high E-to-A ratio and a short deceleration time. The pulmonary venous flow reveals a blunted systolic waveform.
  —Systolic function may be well-preserved, except at terminal stages.
  —Atria are dilated, with the ventricles of normal size.
  —Apparent hypertrophy, due to infiltration, may occur.
  —Left ventricular aneurysms may be seen in sarcoid.
- Thallium 201 imaging may show patchy perfusion defects in sarcoidosis.
- Gallium 67 scanning may show abnormal uptake in sarcoidosis, although the test is rather nonspecific.

SPECIAL TESTS

- Right heart catheterization usually reveals a dip and plateau (square root sign) in ventricular pressure.
- Left and right ventricular pressures are not interdependent, unlike constrictive pericarditis (in which right ventricular pressure increases with inspiration while left ventricular pressure decreases).
- The atrial pressure tracing may have an M or W waveform, due to rapid x and y descents.
- Endomyocardial biopsy can point to the specific cause, and it can reliably diagnose anthracycline toxicity.
- CT scanning and MRI can help differentiate restrictive cardiomyopathy from constrictive pericarditis, although both entities can coexist.

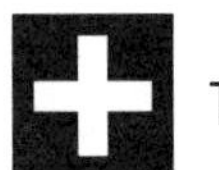

Treatment

GENERAL MEASURES

- As for heart failure of any cause

SURGICAL MEASURES

- Heart transplantation is the only effective long-term therapy for most restrictive cardiomyopathies.
- Sarcoid and amyloid can recur in the transplanted heart.
- Electrical cardioversion can be used for atrial fibrillation.
- Permanent pacemakers may be implanted for advanced heart block or symptomatic bradyarrhythmias.
- Implantable cardioverter–defibrillators may be used for ventricular arrhythmias.

ADMISSION/DISCHARGE CRITERIA

- Same as for other etiologies of congestive heart failure

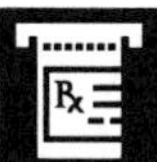

Medications

DRUG(S) OF CHOICE

- Diuretics are useful to treat pulmonary congestion, but overly aggressive diuresis can lead to a marked decline in cardiac output.
- Beta-blockers and calcium channel blockers can both be deleterious.
- Digoxin is useful to treat any coexistent atrial fibrillation. It can lead to toxicity at lower than usual doses in amyloidosis.
- Amiodarone can be used for treatment of atrial fibrillation.
- Chelation therapy with desferrioxamine or phlebotomy may be useful in restrictive cardiomyopathy due to hemochromatosis.
- Steroid therapy can treat sarcoidosis successfully.
- Warfarin therapy is indicated in the presence of thrombi or atrial fibrillation.

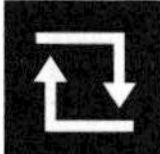

Follow-up

PATIENT MONITORING

- As for other etiologies of heart failure

EXPECTED COURSE AND PROGNOSIS

- The prognosis is generally poor.
- Involvement of the conduction system can lead to advanced heart block and sudden death or to ventricular arrhythmias. This is of particular concern in amyloid and sarcoid.

PATIENT EDUCATION

- Daily weights with reporting of any significant increase or loss

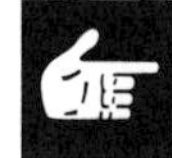

Miscellaneous

ICD-9-CM

428.0 Failure, heart, congestive
425.4 Cardiomyopathy, restrictive
135 [425.8] Cardiomyopathy, sarcoidosis

BIBLIOGRAPHY

Klein AL, Scalia GM. Diseases of the pericardium, restrictive cardiomyopathy and diastolic dysfunction. In: Topol EJ, ed. *Comprehensive cardiovascular medicine.* Philadelphia: Lippincott-Raven, 1998:669–735.

Kushwaha SS, Fallon JT, Fuster V. Restrictive cardiomyopathy. *N Engl J Med* 1997;336: 267–276.

Newman LS, Rose CS, Maier LA. Sarcoidosis. *N Engl J Med* 1997;336:1224–1234.

Shammas RL, Movahed A. Sarcoidosis of the heart. *Clin Cardiol* 1993;16:462–472.

Sharma OP, Maheshwari A, Thaker K. Myocardial sarcoidosis. *Chest* 1993;103:253–258.

Tajik AJ, Murphy JG. Hypertrophic and restrictive cardiomyopathies. In: Murphy JG, ed. *Mayo Clinic cardiology review,* Philadelphia: Lippincott Williams & Wilkins, 2000:455–482.

Wynne J, Braunwald E. The cardiomyopathies and myocarditides. In: Braunwald E, ed. *Heart disease: a textbook of cardiovascular medicine,* 5th ed. Philadelphia: WB Saunders, 1997:1426–1434.

Authors: Deepak L. Bhatt and Gary S. Francis

Carotid Sinus Syndrome

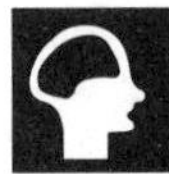

Basics

DESCRIPTION

One of the neurally mediated syncopal syndromes characterized by bradycardia and/or hypotension in response to carotid sinus pressure

EPIDEMIOLOGY

Incidence/Prevalence

- Data unavailable

Predominant Age

- More common in the elderly

RISK FACTORS

- Unknown

PREGNANCY

N/A

ASSOCIATED CONDITIONS

- Coronary and carotid atherosclerosis

ETIOLOGY

- Uncertain

Possible Mechanisms

- Increased acetylcholine release
- Increased responsiveness to acetycholine
- Hypersensitive baroreceptors
- Failure of baroreceptor feedback mechanisms
- Dissociation between the afferent signals arising from the sternomastoid muscles and the carotid sinus
- Abnormalities of the carotid sinus receptors and the medullary cardiovascular centers have all been suggested as possible mechanisms.

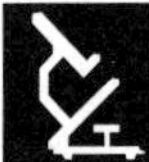

Diagnosis

DIFFERENTIAL DIAGNOSIS

- Sick sinus syndrome
- Atrioventricular block secondary to conduction tissue disease
- Tachyarrhythmias
- Vasovagal syndromes
- Postural hypotension
- Aortic stenosis
- Seizure disorders
- Transient ischemic attacks
- Falls due to neuromuscular or musculoskeletal disorders

SIGNS AND SYMPTOMS

- Dizziness
- Lightheadedness
- Falls
- Syncope

LABORATORY PROCEDURES

N/A

IMAGING STUDIES

N/A

SPECIAL TESTS

- Carotid sinus pressure (CSP)
  - —Check for carotid bruits first.
  - —A cardioinhibitory response is defined as ventricular asystole of >3 seconds and a vasodepressor response as a 50 mm Hg or more decrease in systolic blood pressure without associated bradycardia, or a 30 mm Hg or more decrease with reproduced symptoms. Most patients have varying combinations of both responses.
  - —Correlating asystole with the patient's symptoms is important because carotid sinus hypersensitivity (>3-second pause) can be present in about 4% of the healthy elderly population.
  - —CSP should be determined both supine and upright with continuous ECG and blood pressure monitoring.
  - —The bradycardia may be only relatively inappropriate to the severity of hypotension.
- Tilt table testing, ambulatory ECG monitoring, electroencephalography, vascular studies and electrophysiologic studies may be required to exclude other causes of syncope.

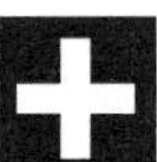

Treatment

GENERAL MEASURES

- Avoid tight collars, neckties and sudden head turning.
- Avoid vasodilator (e.g., calcium channel blockers) and vagomimetic (e.g., digoxin) medications.
- Elastic support hose may help.

Pacing

Dual-chamber pacing prevents bradycardia. However, patients often remain symptomatic from the vasodilatory component, which is more difficult to treat. Rate-drop response pacing (bradycardia triggers relatively rapid pacing for a few minutes) might blunt the hypotensive response.

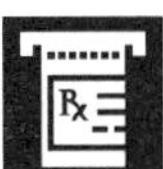

Medications

DRUG(S) OF CHOICE

- Beta-blockers, disopyramide, serotonin reuptake inhibitors (fluoxetine, sertraline), vasoconstrictors (midodrine), and sodium-retaining drugs (fludrocortisone) have been tried.
- Response varies, and large-scale clinical trials are lacking.

ALTERNATIVE DRUGS

In severe cases not responding to pacing or pharmacologic measures, radiation therapy or surgical denervation of the carotid sinus may be required.

Follow-up

PATIENT MONITORING

- If a pacemaker is implanted, evaluate after 1 week, then at 1 month, and every 6 months thereafter.
- Many patients have associated carotid and coronary atherosclerosis, which require monitoring.

Complications

- Injuries related to syncope/falls
- Rarely, sudden death from asystole

EXPECTED COURSE AND PROGNOSIS

Frequency of symptoms is variable, and the severity will depend on the extent of the vasodilatory response.

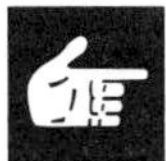

Miscellaneous

ICD-9-CM

337.0 Carotid body or sinus syndrome

BIBLIOGRAPHY

Benditt DG. Neurally mediated syncopal syndromes: pathophysiological concepts and clinical evaluation. *Pacing Clin Electrophysiol* 1997;20:572–584.

Benditt DG, Fahy GJ, Lurie KG, et al. Pharmacotherapy of neurally mediated syncope. *Circulation* 1999;100:1242–1248.

Benditt DG, Sutton R, Gammage MD, et al. Clinical experience with Thera DR rate-drop response pacing algorithm in carotid sinus syndrome and vasovagal syncope. The International Rate-Drop Investigators Group. *Pacing Clin Electrophysiol* 1997;20:832–839.

Braunwald E, ed. *Heart disease: a textbook of cardiovascular medicine,* 5th ed. Philadelphia: WB Saunders, 1997.

Jeffreys M, Wood DA, Lampe F, et al. The heart rate response to carotid artery massage in a sample of healthy elderly people. *Pacing Clin Electrophysiol* 1996;19:1488–1492.

Author: Benoy J. Zachariah

Cerebrovascular Disease

Basics

DESCRIPTION

- Stroke: The sudden onset of focal neurologic deficit resulting from either infarction or hemorrhage within the brain.
- Transiet ischemic attack (TIA): The sudden onset of focal neurologic deficit, usually resulting from atherothrombosis or embolism, which completely resolves within 24 hours

EPIDEMIOLOGY

Incidence/Prevalence

- Cerebrovascular disease affects 0.2%–0.3% of the U.S. population each year.
- 731,000 strokes occur annually in the United States; there are 4 million stroke survivors.
- Cerebrovascular disease is the third leading cause of death in the United States.

Predominant Age

- Over 65

Predominant Sex

- Men are affected more than women.

ETIOLOGY

Ischemic Stroke

- Carotid atherosclerosis with *in situ* thrombosis or artery-to-artery embolism
- Cardiogenic embolus: mitral valve disease (especially stenosis), atrial fibrillation, myocardial infarction (MI), left ventricular (LV) aneurysm, cardiomyopathy, prosthetic valves, endocarditis
- Hypercoagulable states: antiphospholipid antibodies, oral contraceptives, Factor V Leiden mutation; deficiency of protein C, protein S, and antithrombin III
- Hemoglobinopathies
- Carotid dissection
- Cerebral venous thrombosis
- Vasculitis
- Drugs: cocaine, amphetamines

Intracranial Hemorrhage

- Hypertension
- Anticoagulation, antiplatelet, and fibrinolytic treatment
- Vascular malformations: atrioventricular (AV) malformation, angiomas, berry aneurysm
- Amyloid angiopathy
- Trauma

RISK FACTORS

Ischemic Stroke

- Age
- Hypertension
- Smoking
- Diabetes mellitus
- Hyperlipidemia
- Hyperhomocysteinemia
- Family history
- Coronary artery disease

PREGNANCY

N/A

ASSOCIATED CONDITIONS

- Coronary artery disease
- Peripheral vascular disease.

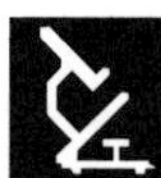

Diagnosis

DIFFERENTIAL DIAGNOSIS

- Demyelinating disease
- Postictal paralysis
- Tumor
- Abscess
- Encephalitis
- Metabolic disturbances (especially hypoglycemia)
- Migraine
- Psychogenic weakness

SIGNS AND SYMPTOMS

- Headache, seizures, altered sensorium
- Carotid territory: aphasia, hemiplegia, hemianesthesia, hemianopia, neglect, confusion, amnesia, monocular blindness, paralysis of gaze, and difficulty in reading, writing, and calculating
- Vertebrobasilar territory: vertigo, ataxia, diplopia, nystagmus, quadrantanopia, dysarthria, facial weakness, dysphagia, Horner's syndrome, hemiplegia, hemianesthesia

LABORATORY PROCEDURES

- CBC, glucose, electrolytes, urinalysis, ABG (atrial blood gas), INR, partial thromboplastin time (PTT), ECG, chest x-ray

IMAGING STUDIES

- CT scan (emergent study of choice)
- MRI/magnetic resonance angiography
- Carotid ultrasonography
- Transthoracic or transesophageal echocardiography
- Cerebral and vertebral angiography

SPECIAL TESTS

- Anticardiolipin antibodies and lupus anticoagulant
- Assays for protein C and S
- Antithrombin III
- Factor V Leiden mutation
- Hemoglobin electrophoresis
- Holter monitor

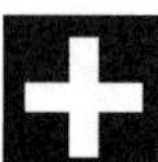

Treatment

ISCHEMIC STROKE

- Rapid evaluation for possible thrombolysis is essential.
  - —Intravenous tissue plasminogen activator (t-PA 0.9 mg/kg, 10% as a bolus and the remainder over 1 hour) administered within 3 hours of ischemic stroke onset improves functional outcome without an increase in overall mortality, despite an increase in the incidence of intracerebral hemorrhage.
  - —A large infarct, as evidenced by extensive neurologic deficits or early changes on CT scan, predict an increased risk of bleeding.
  - —A CT scan to exclude hemorrhage is mandatory prior to treatment.
  - —Strict inclusion and exclusion criteria have been defined.
  - —Intravenous thrombolysis more than 3 hours after symptom onset is not beneficial and is probably harmful.
  - —Intraarterial thrombolysis might be an option up to 6 hours after symptom onset; further research studies are awaited.
  - —Patients who have received t-PA should not be given i.v. heparin, aspirin, ticlopidine, clopidogrel, or coumadin for 24 hours.
  - —ASA therapy at presentation is not a contraindication for thrombolysis.
- Heparin: Intravenous heparin use is controversial, and although widely used, it does not decrease stroke severity. It may prevent recurrent embolic strokes and may be useful in hypercoagulable states. If used, heparin should be started without a bolus at 15 to 18 units/kg/h; target PTT is 1.5 times control. Massive hemispheric stroke and PTT more than twice control predispose to hemorrhagic transformation. Heparinoids have not shown any benefit.
- Antiplatelet agents: ASA 300–325 mg/day provides a modest benefit in preventing early stroke recurrence when used in acute ischemic stroke; whether it decreases stroke severity is uncertain. No other antiplatelet agents have been tested in acute ischemic stroke.
- Cerebral edema (peaks 3–5 days after onset) should be treated with mannitol or intubation with hyperventilation.
- Seizure prophylaxis with phenytoin for patients with large infarcts

GENERAL MEASURES

- Admit patient to stroke unit if possible: patients have fewer complications and better outcomes.
- Monitor cardiac rhythm for 48 hours.
- Blood pressure is often elevated at presentation; most experts recommend against acutely lowering the blood pressure because autoregulation is often defective and stroke severity may be worsened.
  - —Hypertension should be treated if there is ongoing cardiac ischemia, severe (systolic blood pressure >220 mm Hg, diastolic

>120 mm Hg) or malignant hypertension, aortic dissection, and in those receiving t-PA. Blood pressure should be gradually lowered to 170 to 180 mm Hg systolic and 95 to 100 mm Hg diastolic.
—Angiotensin-converting enzyme inhibitors and beta-blockers (including labetolol) are the preferred agents.

- If patients are immobile, they should have deep venous thrombosis (DVT)/PE (pulmonary embolism) prophylaxis.
- Institute feeding early. Patients with dysphagia should be fed through a soft feeding tube and should have gastrostomy early if dysphagia persists.
- Hyperglycemia and fever worsen outcome and should be treated aggressively.

INTRACRANIAL HEMORRHAGE

- Admit to intensive care.
- Ensure airway protection and adequate oxygenation.
- Hypertension should be treated aggressively.
- Intracranial pressure (ICP) monitoring for patients with suspected elevated ICP, deteriorating level of consciousness, Glassgow coma score <9.
- Reduce elevated ICP with mannitol or hyperventilation. Neuromuscular paralysis and barbiturate coma are other options; keep ICP <20 mm Hg and cerebral perfusion pressure >70 mm Hg.
- Ventricular drains for patients with hydrocephalus
- Seizure prevention with phenytoin
- Surgical evacuation of the hematoma for patients with cerebellar hemorrhage (emergent), subdural or epidural hemorrhages, associated structural lesions such as an aneurysm, AV malformations (if surgically accessible and likely to have a good outcome), and in young patients with large lobar hemorrhage who are deteriorating

GENERAL MEASURES

- DVT prophylaxis with compression boots
- Early institution of feeding
- Physical therapy, speech therapy, and occupational therapy as soon as possible

Follow-up

PATIENT MONITORING

- Should be individualized
- Concomitant coronary artery disease (CAD) and PVD (peripheral vascular disease) are common and should be addressed.

Prevention of Ischemic Stroke

- Control hypertension: target blood pressure is <140/90 mm Hg.
- Nonvalvular atrial fibrillation: warfarin for those at high risk (history of hypertension, diabetes, heart failure, prior TIA or stroke, age >60 years); ASA 325 mg/day for low-risk patients
- Hyperlipidemia: For those with CAD and hyperlipidemia and no prior stroke, lipid lowering with statins reduces stroke risk. Treatment is also recommended for stroke patients with hyperlipidemia and following carotid endarterectomy, even if they do not have an h/o CAD. Whether lipid lowering should be attempted for stroke prevention in patients without an h/o CAD or stroke is unclear; these patients may need to be treated for CAD prevention anyway.
- Smoking is a significant risk factor for a first stroke, recurrent stroke, and restenosis following carotid endarterectomy. Cessation reduces risk of recurrent stroke by about half.
- Diabetes: Tight control reduces the risk of microvascular complications. A beneficial effect on ischemic stroke has not been conclusively demonstrated.
- Antiplatelet agents
  —ASA reduces stroke risk following TIAs, ischemic stroke, and carotid endarterectomy; 81 mg/day is as effective as higher doses.
  —Ticlopidine 250 mg b.i.d. or Clopidogrel 75 mg/day (fewer side effects) is indicated for those who cannot take ASA.
  —The optimal treatment for recurrent stroke despite ASA is unclear; options include the addition of warfarin, clopidogrel, or dipyridamole. A recent study found combined ASA 25 mg and sustained-release dipyridamole 200 mg twice daily to be better than ASA or didyridamole alone. ASA does not offer significant protection against a first ischemic stroke in low-risk patients.
- Warfarin reduces stroke risk following MI or a first ischemic stroke; it is recommended for patients who cannot have an antiplatelet agent and for 3–6 months following a large anterior wall MI.
- Carotid endarterectomy: Indicated for patients with TIAs or nondisabling stroke and 70%–99% ipsilateral stenosis. Symptomatic patients with 50%–69% stenosis and asymptomatic patients with a life expectancy of >5 years who have >60% stenosis have a modest reduction in stroke incidence.
- Carotid angioplasty/stenting: appears to benefit symptomatic patients with significant carotid stenosis, but role has not yet been well defined
- The optimal preventive strategy for symptomatic patients with ascending aortic arch atheroma or patent foramen ovale is uncertain. Most experts recommend anticoagulation with warfarin.
- Postmenopausal hormone replacement probably does not reduce risk of stroke.

Prevention of Intracranial Hemorrhage

- Control hypertension.
- Careful monitoring of anticoagulated patients
- Careful selection of patients for anticoagulation and thrombolytic therapy when these are indicated
- Avoid heavy alcohol use.
- Increase consumption of fruits and vegetables (recommendation based on epidemiologic data).

EXPECTED COURSE AND PROGNOSIS

- Ischemic stroke: One-third die within a year, one-third remain permanently disabled, and one third make a reasonable recovery.
- Intracranial hemorrhage: 35%–50% die within a month (half of them in the first 2 days); 20% live independently at 6 months.
- Complications
  —Death
  —DVT/PE
  —Hemorrhagic transformation of ischemic strokes
  —Pneumonia
  —Decubiti
  —Residual neurologic deficits
  —Contractures

PATIENT EDUCATION

Organization

- National Stroke Association, 96 Inverness Dr E # I, Englewood, CO 80112

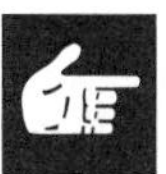

Miscellaneous

ICD-9-CM

436 Disease, cerebrovascular acute
431 Hemorrhage, cerebral
435.9 TIA

BIBLIOGRAPHY

Adams HP Jr, Brott TG, Crowell RM, et al. Guidelines for the management of patients with acute ischemic stroke. A statement for healthcare professionals from a special writing group of the Stroke Council, American Heart Association. *Stroke* 1994;25:1901–1914.

Adams HP Jr, Brott TG, Furlan AJ, et al. Guidelines for thrombolytic therapy for acute stroke: a supplement to the guidelines for the management of patients with acute ischemic stroke. A statement for healthcare professionals from a special writing group of the Stroke Council, American Heart Association. *Stroke* 1996; 27:1711–1718.

Alberts MJ. Diagnosis and treatment of ischemic stroke. *Am J Med* 1999;106:211–221.

Broderick JP, Adams HP Jr, Barsan W, et al. Guidelines for the management of spontaneous intracerebral hemorrhage: a statement for healthcare professionals from a special writing group of the Stroke Council, American Heart Association. *Stroke* 1999;30:905–915.

Forbes CD. Secondary stroke prevention with low-dose aspirin, sustained release dipyridamole alone and in combination. ESPS Investigators. European Stroke Prevention Study. *Thrombosis Res* 1998;92(suppl 1):1–6.

Gorelick PB, Sacco RL, Smith DB, et al. Prevention of a first stroke: a review of guidelines and a multidisciplinary consensus statement from the National Stroke Association. *JAMA* 1999;281:1112–1120.

Author: Benoy J. Zachariah

Chagas' Disease and the Heart

Basics

DESCRIPTION

Multiple clinical syndromes including acute Chagas' disease and chronic Chagas' disease, both resulting from infection with the protozoan parasite *Trypanosoma cruzi*

- Multiple presentations including acute and chronic myocarditis with potentially devastating effects on conduction, myocyte function, and myocardial architecture.
- Acute Chagas' myocarditis demonstrates focal myocytolytic necrosis and degeneration with an intense mononuclear infiltrate and parasitism of myofibers.
- An intermediate clinically silent phase exists of up to 10–30 years.
- Chronic Chagas' heart disease, however, presents with focal and diffuse chronic fibrosing myocarditis with accompanied lymphomononuclear infiltrate and no evidence of active parasitism.
- Destruction of the parasympathetic nervous system and loss of cardiac innervation is always seen.

Case Definition Criteria for Diagnosis

- History of residence where Chagas' disease is endemic, unequivocally positive serologic test for *T. cruzi,* clinical syndrome compatible with Chagas' heart disease, no evidence of another cardiac disorder to account for findings

EPIDEMIOLOGY

Natural reservoirs of *T. cruzi* from the central United States to southern Argentina are thought to be the source.

- Estimated 15–20 million people infected worldwide with >65 million people at risk of infection
- Countries with highest incidence: Brazil, Argentina, Chile, Bolivia, and Venezuela
- Most common cause of dilated cardiomyopathy and significant cause of cardiovascular death in endemic countries
- *T. cruzi* infection acquired in the United States is almost nonexistent. However, it is estimated that approximately 400,000 infected immigrants reside in the United States.

ETIOLOGY

The parasite is transmitted to humans via bloodsucking insects of the Reduviidae family (assassin bugs) through contaminated feces at the site of the blood meal. It is also possibly congenitally transmitted in chronic maternal infection or through blood transfusion.

RISK FACTORS

- Geographic prevalence, rural substandard housing secondary to facilitation of Reduviid breeding

ASSOCIATED CONDITIONS

Chronic manifestations include megadisease of the esophagus or colon.

Diagnosis

DIFFERENTIAL DIAGNOSIS

- Toxoplasmosis, viral myocarditis (Coxsackie, HIV, cytomegalovirus), postpartum cardiomyopathy, alcoholic cardiomyopathy, endomyocardial fibrosis, ischemic cardiomyopathy, idiopathic cardiomyopathy, toxic cardiomyopathy (anthracycline, cobalt, etc.), neuromuscular dystrophies, hemochromatosis, amyloidosis, sarcoidosis, Kawasaki disease, arrhythmogenic cardiomyopathy, Lyme carditis, eosinophilic myocarditis

SIGNS AND SYMPTOMS

Acute Chagas' Disease and Myocarditis

- Only 1% develop clinically evident acute myocarditis.
- Incubation period lasts at least 1 week.
- Localized erythema and induration at site of bite (chagoma), fever, generalized lymphadenopathy, hepatosplenomegaly, chest pain/discomfort (ischemic or atypical in quality), tachycardia, arrhythmia/palpitations, local periorbital swelling (Romana's sign)

Chronic Chagas' Disease and Cardiomyopathy

- Chronic cardiac involvement in 30%–60%
- Fatigue, arrhythmia/palpitations, sudden death, dizziness/presyncope, chest pain/discomfort (ischemic or atypical in quality), shortness of breath, dyspnea on exertion, orthopnea, paroxysmal nocturnal dyspnea, lower extremity edema, transient ischemic attacks/stroke, thromboembolic phenomena, chagasic megaesophagus (dysphagia, regurgitation), chagasic megacolon (constipation, abdominal pain, obstruction)

LABORATORY PROCEDURES

- Gold standard is xenodiagnosis (culture using actual insect vector), not commonly used.
  - —Examine buffy coat of blood for motile trypanosomes in acute disease.
- Serologic testing mainstay of chronic clinical diagnosis
  - —IgG antibodies to *T. cruzi* trypomastigote antigens
  - —Antibodies appear within 3–6 weeks of infection and remain for life.
  - —Titer does not correlate with severity of infection.

IMAGING STUDIES

- 2-D Doppler echocardiography or angiography
  - —Hallmark finding of marked segmental ventricular wall motion abnormalities (hypokinesis or akinesis)
  - —Narrow neck aneurysm involving localized area of left ventricular (LV) apex with normal surroundings (50% of patients)
  - —May resemble segmental changes of ischemic cardiac disease; LV or apical thrombus

SPECIAL TESTS

- ECG
  - —Traditional mainstay of diagnosis of Chagasic cardiac involvement.
  - —Involvement of conduction system ubiquitous with cardiac involvement
  - —Characteristically right bundle branch block or left anterior fascicular block signifies underlying myocarditis.
  - —Complete heart block, atrioventricular conduction abnormalities, and ectopy can be seen. Left bundle branch block is uncommon.
  - —Abnormalities resembling myocardial infarction or ischemia may be prominent in advanced disease.

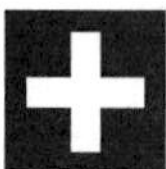

Treatment

GENERAL MEASURES

- Antitrypanosomal therapy exists for acute Chagas' disease (active parasitemia) with evidence for cure and prevention of development of sequelae of chronic manifestations.
- Patients with negative serology after treatment of acute disease can be considered cured.
- Management of chronic cardiomyopathy primarily supportive to treat and prevent complications of congestive heart failure, thromboembolism, arrhythmogenic events, and cardiac conduction abnormalities

SURGICAL MEASURES

- No specific measures exist for Chagas' disease.

ADMISSION/DISCHARGE CRITERIA

- No specific indications

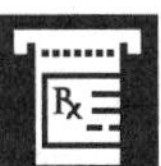

Medications

DRUG(S) OF CHOICE

- Nifurtimox 10 mg/kg/day in three doses for up to 60–120 days and benzimidazole 5 mg/kg/day for up to 60 days act as trypanosomal antimetabolic agents.
  —Drugs available from Centers for Disease Control
  —For use only in acute Chagas' disease; transfusion-acquired disease; reactivation in immunosuppressed patients
- Supportive regimens identical to those for congestive heart failure, arrhythmic events, and thromboembolism

Contraindications

- Potential mutagenicity in children

Precautions

- Refer to manufacturer's profile.
- GI toxicity for nifurtimox
- Leukopenia and polyneuritis side effects for both regimens

Follow-up

PATIENT MONITORING

- Periodic clinical evaluation in addition to relevant testing (ECG, echocardiography) to monitor for signs of cardiac disease

EXPECTED COURSE AND PROGNOSIS

- No treatment proven to halt progressive myocardial damage in chronic Chagasic cardiomyopathy
- Overall mortality best predicted by LV function
- Strong predictors for mortality include LV dilatation, presence of aneurysm, and development of heart disease at an early age.

PATIENT EDUCATION

N/A

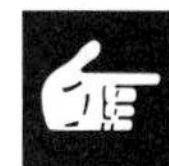

Miscellaneous

ICD-9-CM

422.90 Acute myocarditis, unspecified
425.4 Idiopathic cardiomyopathy
429.0 Myocarditis, unspecified

BIBLIOGRAPHY

Alexander RW, et al., eds. *Hurst's the heart,* 9th ed. New York: McGraw-Hill, 1998.

Hagar JM, Rahimtoola SH. *Chagas' heart disease. Curr Probl Cardiol* 1995;20:827–924.

Rossi MA, Bestetti RB. The challenge of chagasic cardiomyopathy. *Cardiology* 1995;86:1–7.

Author: Chandan Devireddy

Chemotherapy and the Heart

Basics

DESCRIPTION

- Anthracycline-induced cardiomyopathy
  —Cardiomyopathy secondary to chemotherapy is most commonly associated with doxorubucin (adriamycin), but also has been reported with other anthracycline agents such as daunorubicin and epirubicin, as well as the anthraquinone agent mitoxantrone.
- Myocardial ischemia
  —Abnormal vasoreactivity and spasm have been reported primarily with 5-fluorouracil therapy, but also with vinblastine, vincristine, cisplatin, bleomycin, and interleukin-2 administration.
- Dysrhythmia
  —Rhythm disturbances may occur in the context of anthracycline-induced cardiomyopathy, but ventricular and supraventricular tachycardias also have been described independently with interferon administration.
  —Taxol also has been associated with bradycardia and heart block.

Systems Affected

- Cardiac

ETIOLOGY

Incidence/Prevalence

The overall incidence of anthracycline-induced cardiomyopathy in the United States is approximately 2.2%.

Predominant Age

Rates are higher at extremes of patient age, in elderly patients over 70 years of age, and in pediatric patients under 15 years of age.

Predominant Sex

Men are affected as often as women.

CAUSES

- Anthracycline-induced myocardial necrosis is due to direct membrane lipid damage and local free radical production. Vasospasm can occur with 5-fluoro-uracil and other agents.

ASSOCIATED CONDITIONS

- Anemia

Age-Related Factors

- Pediatric: frequent
- Geriatric: frequent
- Others: less common

RISK FACTORS

In addition to age, the following risk factors increase the incidence of anthracycline-induced cardiomyopathy by as much as eight- to tenfold:

- Increased cumulative dose
  —The incidence of cardiomyopathy with doxorubucin adminstration at doses <400 mg/m^2 is approximately 0.12%.
  —The incidence increases to 7% at 550 mg/m^2, and escalates sharply at higher doses.
  —It has been reported at 18%–30% at doses above 700 mg/m^2.
  —Therefore, 550 mg/m^2 is considered to be the upper limit for doxorubicin administration in most clinical scenarios.
- Rapid schedule of administration
  —Less cardiotoxicity has been reported when doxorubicin infusion is prolonged over 48–96 hours than when compared with standard 1- to 2-hour infusions.
  —This may be due to lower peak plasma concentration of drug.
- Other underlying heart disease
  —Anthracycline-induced cardiomyopathy is more common in the presence of preexisting heart diseases, particularly those that increase left ventricular wall stress.
  —These include hypertensive heart disease, hypertensive obstructive cardiomyopathy, aortic stenosis, or other forms of underlying cardiomyopathy.
- Concomitant therapy for malignancy
  —Radiation therapy through a portal that includes the heart (such as mediastinum, breast, or lung) has been shown to substantially increase the risk of developing anthracycline-induced cardiomyopathy.
- Other chemotherapeutic agents, such as concomitant administration of cyclophosphamide or mitomycin C chemotherapy, may increase the risk of developing cardiomyopathy, although available data are somewhat variable.

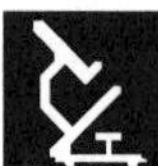

Diagnosis

DIFFERENTIAL DIAGNOSIS

At presentation, anthracycline-induced cardiomyopathy may be clinically indistinguishable from other other etiologies of cardiac dysfunction in the cancer patient, including:

- Underlying cardiovascular disease, which may have been previously subclinical, including atherosclerosis, hypertensive heart disease, valvular heart disease, myocarditis or viral, alcoholic or idiopathic cardiomyopathy.
- Other cardiac complications of malignancy
  —Metastatic or primary tumor involvement of the pericardium or myocardium.
  —Obstruction of venous inflow (SVC or IVC [superior or inferior vena cava] syndrome)
    - Radiation-induced pericardial, myocardial, or coronary artery disease
    - Dysrhythmia secondary to other drugs or metabolic abnormalities
    - Other adverse drug effects

SIGNS AND SYMPTOMS

Heart failure due to anthracycline-induced cardiotoxicity is clinically indistinguishable from other etiologies of biventricular heart failure.

- Symptoms
  —Fatigue
  —Exercise intolerance
  —Dyspnea
  —Paroxysmal nocturnal dyspnea
  —Orthopnea
  —Edema
  —Palpitation, syncope, or presyncope
- Physical findings
  —Resting tachycardia
  —Jugular venous distention
  —S3 gallop
  —Pulmonary congestion
  —Peripheral edema
- ECG abnormalities are nonspecific and may be transient.
  —Sinus tachycardia
  —ST- or T-wave changes
  —Premature ventricular contractions or other dysrhythmia
  —Decreased voltage
  —QT interval prolongation
- Chest x-ray
  —Cardiac enlargement
  —Pulmonary vascular plethora
  —Kerley B lines
  —Pleural effusions

Clinical Manifestations

- Acute toxicity occurs either during or immediately after treatment (even a single cycle of drug).
  —Acute toxicity is rare and is most commonly manifested as a transient ECG abnormality or dysrhythmia.
  —However, it can present as myocarditis, pericarditis, fulminant cardiac failure or even sudden death.
- Chronic toxicity most commonly occurs within 1 year of treatment but also may occur after a prolonged asymptomatic interval, sometimes even years later.
- Asymptomatic reduction in LV systolic function is the most common manifestation of chronic anthracycline-induced cardiomyopathy.
  —The criteria for asymptomatic cardiomyopathy are an absolute decrease in left ventricular ejection fraction (LVEF) of >10% or a decline in LVEF to 50% when previously normal.
- Less commonly, anthracycline-induced cardiomyopathy may present as overt clinical congestive heart failure.

LABORATORY PROCEDURES

- Anemia

Pathologic Findings

- Cardiac necrosis

IMAGING STUDIES

- Radionuclide ventriculography
  —Reduced LVEF
- Echocardiography
  —Biventricular enlargement
  —Abnormal systolic function: reduced LVEF and fractional shortening, most commonly without segmental wall motion abnormality
  —Abnormal diastolic function: endocardial thickening and Doppler evidence of prolonged isovolumic relaxation
  —Stress imaging to assess enhancement of LV contractility with exercise may add sensitivity to either radionuclide or echocardiographic imaging.

SPECIAL TESTS

N/A

DIAGNOSTIC PROCEDURES

- Endomyocardial biopsy
  —Best method for absolute quantitation of cardiac damage and may be used to guide decisions about subsequent anthracycline dosing
  —Cardiac muscle involvement may be patchy, so multiple right ventricular specimens should be obtained when possible.
  —Pathology reveals swelling of sarcoplasmic reticulum and mitochondria, myofibrillar dropout, vacuole formation,and frank myocyte necrosis.
  —Pathologic severity is graded on a scale of 0–3, with biopsy grade >1.5 considered a contraindication to continuing anthracycline therapy.

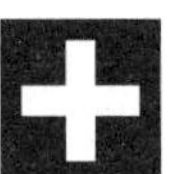

Treatment

GENERAL MEASURES

- Unless overt congestive heart failure occurs, patients can be managed as outpatients.
- Treatment for documented anthracycline-induced cardiomyopathy
  —Anthracycline administration should be discontinued
- Baseline screening should include:
  —History and physical examination
  —ECG
  —Chest x-ray
  —Assessment of left ventricular function by echocardiography or radionuclide ventriculography

SURGICAL MEASURES

Selected patients with severe anthracycline-induced cardiomyopathy who have achieved cure from malignancy might be considered acceptable candidates for cardiac transplantation.

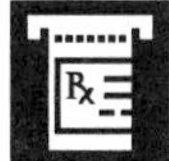

Medications

DRUG(S) OF CHOICE

- There is no specific therapy for athracycline-induced cardiomyopathy.
- Treatment of heart failure, myocardial ischemia, and arrhythmias would be the same as for other etologies of these conditions.
- Anthracycline dose limitation
  —Total cumulative doxorubicin dose should be limited to less than 550 mg/m^2.
  —Total cumulative doxorubicin dose should be limited to less than 350 mg/m^2 for patients receiving radiation therapy.

Follow-up

PATIENT MONITORING

- Serial monitoring for patients receiving doxorubicin chemotherapy can be performed using radionuclide ventriculography or echocardiographic assessment of left ventricular systolic function.
- Follow-up LVEF assessment should be performed at least 3 weeks after a given dose, before consideration of subsequent dose administration.
- Guidelines for the frequency of follow-up are as follows:
  —Patients with normal baseline LVEF (>50%)
  —Repeat assessment of left ventricular function after 200–300 mg/m^2 and again after 450 mg/m^2 or after 400 mg/m^2 in patients with other risk factors for cardiomyopathy.
  —Repeat assessment before every dose after 400–450 mg/m^2
  —Discontinue doxorubicin when LVEF falls by >10% or absolute LVEF is less than 50%.
- Patients with moderately reduced baseline LVEF (30%–50%)
  —Repeat assessment of LVEF before every dose
  —Discontinue doxorubicin when LVEF falls by >10% or absolute LVEF is less than 30%.

Prevention/Avoidance

- Care should be taken in dosing strategies for patients with baseline LV dysfunction and for patients with other risk factors for cardiotoxicity.
- Patients with severely reduced baseline LVEF (<30%) should not receive doxorubicin chemotherapy.
- Pharmacologic cardioprotectants
  —Dexrazoxane, an iron-chelating agent that reduces free radicle production, has recently been approved for use in patients with metastatic breast cancer receiving >300 mg/m^2 of doxorubicin.
  —Other free-radical scavenger or antioxidant agents may play an important role in the prevention of anthracycline-induced myocyte injury in the future. These agents have shown promise in early clinical trials and in animal models.

Possible Complications

- Cardiac death, persistent heart failure

EXPECTED COURSE AND PROGNOSIS

- Prognosis is poorer in patients who develop overt congestive heart failure, with reported mortality rates as high as 43%.
- Outcomes in patients with congestive heart failure are improved with conventional medical therapy.
- Reversal of even severe cardiac dysfunction has been reported.

PATIENT EDUCATION

- American Cancer Society

Activity

- As tolerated

Diet

- Low sodium

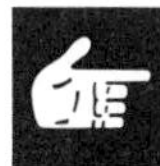

Miscellaneous

ICD-9-CM

425.9 + 909.5 Cardiomyopathy

See also: Heart Failure, Myocardial Ischemia

BIBLIOGRAPHY

Schwartz RG, et al. Congestive heart failure and left ventricular dysfunction complicating doxorubicin therapy: seven year experience using serial radionuclide angiocardiography. *Am J Med* 1987;82:1109–1118.

Shan K, et al. Anthracycline-induced cardiomyopathy. *Ann Intern Med* 1996;125:47–58.

Topol EJ, ed. *Textbook of cardiovascular medicine.* Philadelphia: Lippincott-Raven, 1998.

Author: Sarah M. Vernon

Cheyne-Stokes Respirations

Basics

DESCRIPTION

Also referred to as cyclic respiration or periodic breathing

- Characterized by cyclic variations in minute ventilation
- Periods of hyperpnea alternate with periods of hypopnea and apnea. Sleep is interrupted with frequent arousals. These arousals usually occur during early non-REM sleep (stages 1 and 2), resulting in reduced REM sleep.
- Commonly occurs in patients with congestive heart failure (CHF) and neurologic disorders (cerebral hemorrhage infarct or embolism, meningitis, trauma, tumor)
- Can also be seen with lactic acidosis, diabetic ketoacidosis, and uremic coma
- Mechanism responsible is unclear: however, several theories have been proposed.

System(s) Affected

- Respiratory, cardiovascular

Pediatric

- Can be seen in premature and full-term infants

EPIDEMIOLOGY

Incidence/Prevalence

- 40%–50% of patients with chronic CHF, 25% of cases of cerebral embolism, and 10% of cerebral infarcts

Predominant Sex

- Males are affected more than females.

CAUSES

The mechanism responsible is unknown. Cheyne-Stokes respirations may be due to instability in ventilatory control and feedback systems. Factors contributing this may include:

- Hypoxemia
- Circulatory delay
- Reduced blood gas buffering capacity
- Abnormal central and peripheral receptors
- Increased sympathetic activity

RISK FACTORS

Predisposing disorders such as:

- CHF
- Neurologic disorders
- Renal failure
- High altitude
- Narcotics

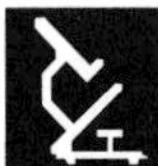

Diagnosis

DIFFERENTIAL DIAGNOSIS

- Obstructive sleep apnea
- Ataxic breathing
- Neurogenic hyperventilation
- Neurogenic hypoventilation

SIGNS AND SYMPTOMS

- History of one of the following:
  —CHF
  —Neurologic disorder (cerebral hemorrhage, infarct or embolism, meningitis, tumor, trauma)
  —Renal failure/uremic coma
  —Acidosis (lactic acidosis, diabetic ketoacidosis)
- Most common signs and symptoms
  —Daytime sleepiness
  —Fatigue
  —Paroxysmal nocturnal dyspnea
  —Snoring
  —Witnessed apnea
  —Dyspnea
  —Orthopnea

LABORATORY PROCEDURES

Blood gas may reveal a respiratory alkalosis.

SPECIAL TESTS

Polysomnography can verify diagnosis and rule out obstructive sleep apnea.

DIAGNOSTIC PROCEDURES

Polysomnogram can verify diagnosis and rule out obstructive sleep apnea.

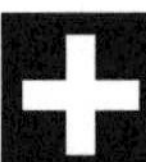

Treatment

GENERAL MEASURES

- The severity of the patient's underlying disorder (i.e., CHF, stroke) usually determines the level of care required.
- Treatment includes treatment of any associated disorder, particularly treatment of CHF.
- Other beneficial therapy may include:
  —Oxygen or continuous positive airway pressure
  —Respiratory stimulants such as theophylline and acetazolamide have been used.

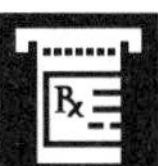

Medications

DRUG(S) OF CHOICE

- Possible benefit from respiratory stimulants such as theophylline and acetazolamide

Contraindications

- Narcotics

Precautions

Refer to manufacturer's profile of each drug:

- Theophylline: may increase risk of arrhythmias
- Acetazolamide: causes a metabolic acidosis

Significant Possible Interactions

Many drugs can affect theophylline levels.

Follow-up

EXPECTED COURSE/PROGNOSIS

- In patients with Cheyne-Stokes respiration there is increased mortality if a respiratory alkalosis exists.
- In patients with CHF the development of Cheyne-Stokes respiration is associated with increased mortality that is independent of left ventricular function.

PATIENT EDUCATION

Activity

Physical training may increase exercise tolerance and decrease abnormal ventilation.

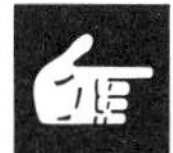

Miscellaneous

SYNONYMS

- Periodic breathing or cyclic respiration

BIBLIOGRAPHY

Crystal RG, West JB, Weibel ER, et al. *The lung.* Philadephia: Lippincott Raven, 1997.

George RB, Matthay MA, Light RW, et al. *Chest medicine: essentials of pulmonary and critical care medicine,* 3rd ed. Baltimore: Williams & Wilkins, 1995.

Baum GL, Crapo JD, Celli BR, et al. *Textbook of pulmonary medicine,* 6th ed. Philadelphia: Lippincott-Raven, 1998.

Wilcox I, McNamara SG, Wessendorf T, et al. Prognosis and sleep disordered breathing in heart failure. *Thorax* 1998;53(suppl 3):33–36.

Quaranta AJ, D'Alonzo GE, Krachman SL. Cheyne-Stokes respiration during sleep in congestive heart failure. *Chest* 1997;111:467–473.

Piepoli MF, et al. Aetiology and pathophysiological implications of oscillatory ventilation at rest and during exercise in chronic heart failure. Do Cheyne and Stokes have an important message for modern-day patients with heart failure? *Eur Heart J* 1999;20:946–953.

Authors: Richard Mascolo and Gerard P. Aurigemma

Clubbing

Basics

DEFINITION

Clubbing is a bulbous enlargement of the distal phalanges due to connective tissue proliferation. Concurrent with this proliferation is an increase in the number of capillaries and formation of arteriovenous aneurysms in these regions. These changes occur largely in the dorsal aspect of the fingers and toes and usually are painless.

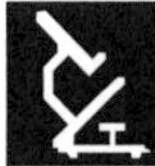

Diagnosis

SIGNS AND SYMPTOMS

- The normal angle between the fingernail and the nail base is approximately 160 degrees and has a firm feeling on palpation. As clubbing progresses, the angle between the nail and its base increases to 180 degrees (and sometimes more) as the nail base becomes swollen and edematous.
- The nail base in the individual with clubbing has a spongy or swollen feeling on palpation. The nail itself may have a convex appearance in advanced clubbing, although this should not be confused with the curved nails sometimes seen in normal individuals. An important distinguishing feature is that the normal nail will have a preserved angle between the nail and its base, whereas the truly clubbed individual will not.
- The diagnosis of clubbing is made solely by physical examination. The softening of tissue at the nail base can be felt on palpation. The skin around the cuticle is noted to take on a smooth and shiny appearance. Although quantification of clubbing has been accomplished using various techniques, including plaster casts and "shadowgrams" of the digital profile, the methods have not replaced bedside diagnosis in standard clinical practice.

EPIDEMIOLOGY

- Clubbing may be idiopathic, hereditary, or acquired and is associated with a number of conditions. Among cardiac causes are those associated with central cyanosis such as congenital heart disease with right-to-left shunting. Examples include:
  - —Tetrology of Fallot
  - —Tricuspid atresia
  - —Transposition of the great vessels
- In these patients, clubbing typically develops after 2 or 3 years of central cyanosis. Pulmonary diseases associated with clubbing include:
  - —Cystic fibrosis
  - —Pulmonary arteriovenous shunts
  - —Bronchiectasis
  - —Primary or metastatic lung cancer
  - —Lung abscess
  - —Mesothelioma
- Clubbing is relatively rare in COPD and suggests the presence of bronchiectasis or bronchogenic carcinoma.
- Clubbing without cyanosis may be seen in patients with endocarditis, a number of gastrointestinal diseases including inflammatory bowel disease (both Crohn's disease and ulcerative colitis), and end-stage liver disease.
- Usually clubbing is symmetric, although occasionally unilateral clubbing has been associated with aneurysms of the subclavian or inominate arteries.
- Rarely, clubbing may be associated with hyperthyroidism and periostitis of the long bones (thyroid acropachy).
- This association occurs in approximately 1% of patient's with Grave's disease, and may develop months to years after the resolution of the hyperthyroidism.

CLINICAL MANIFESTATIONS AND COMPLICATIONS

- Clubbing may occur as part of a spectrum of musculoskeletal manifestations referred to as hypertrophic osteoarthropathy (HOA).
  - —HOA is characterized by digital clubbing, periosteal bone formation, arthritis, and neurovascular changes of the hands and feet, including chronic erythema, paresthesias, and increased sweating.
  - —HOA may occur as a familial form beginning in childhood or as a secondary form, related to any of the diseases mentioned above.
  - —HOA is most frequently diagnosed after the patient presents with persistent pain in the extremities. Bony tenderness due to periostitis may be elicited on palpation of the shafts of the long bones.
  - —The skeletal findings in HOA consist of periosteal elevation and new bone formation, seen primarily in the distal phalanges and long bones.
  - —Synovial involvement also may lead to pain and swelling of the knees ankles, wrists and elbows.
  - —Occasionally, other joints such as the shoulders, clavicles, and temporomandibular joints also may be involved.
  - —There may be mononuclear infiltration in adjacent soft tissue. Connective tissue proliferation occurs in the nail bed, giving rise to clubbing, which is seen in virtually all patients.
- The etiology and pathogenesis of HOA remain unclear.
  - —Neurogenic and humoral theories have both been advanced.
  - —The neurogenic theory postulates that bony and soft tissue proliferation may somehow be related to increased vagal tone because many of the conditions associated with HOA involve organs innervated by the vagus.

—In support of this theory is the observation that vagotomy sometimes leads to a resolution of symptoms.
—The humoral theory states that a circulating substance normally removed by the lungs is allowed into systemic circulation, causing the manifestations of HOA.
—A number of mediators have been suggested, but none have been proven.
- Primary HOA (Touraine-Soulente-Gole syndrome) develops slowly in puberty, is inherited in an autosomal-dominant fashion with variable expression, and is more common in boys than in girls.
—There is marked thickening of the distal extremities as well as clubbing, leading to a spadelike appearance to the hands.
—The face often has a leonine appearance that may mimic acromegaly. Symptoms of bone and joint pain may not occur until 20–30 years from the onset of the disease.
- Secondary HOA is more common than primary HOA and accompanies many of the cardiac and pulmonary diseases discussed above.
—HOA may precede the accompanying manifestations of the primary disorder by several months.
—Joint manifestations may be very painful and most commonly involve the metacarpophalangeal and metatarsophalangeal joints, as well as the wrists, ankles, and knees.
—HOA may occur in as many as 5%–10% of pulmonary-related malignancies and may progress particularly rapidly in cases of bronchogenic carcinoma.
—Symptoms of HOA may precede pulmonary manifestations when there is underlying lung cancer. Full-blown HOA may occur with cyanotic congenital heart disease, but is less common than clubbing alone.
—Blood tests are normal in patients with HOA with the exception of a mild increase in the erythrocyte sedimentation rate.
—Joint effusions are small and most commonly noninflammatory when they occur. Periosteal elevation that occurs in the disease produces a characteristic appearance on radiographs of long bones.
—Bone scan imaging detects areas of increased osteoblastic activity and may identify periostitis before it is apparent clinically or on plain films.
—HOA is frequently confused with rheumatoid arthritis.
—The presence of clubbing is an important clue to the diagnosis. HOA-associated effusions are noninflammatory, as attested to by the absence of rheumatoid factor or antinuclear antibodies.

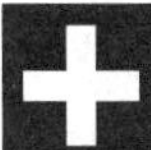

Treatment

- Vagotomy has provided relief of symptoms in some patients with HOA.
- Nonsteroidal antiinflammatory agents also have shown some benefit.
- Most fundamental to the treatment of both clubbing and HOA, however, is the identification and care of the underlying disorder with which they are associated.
- Both may regress or resolve with identification and proper therapy of the related condition.

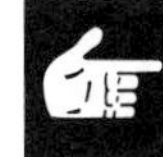

Miscellaneous

BIBLIOGRAPHY

Hansen-Flaschen J, Nordberg J. Clubbing and hypertrophic osteoarthropathy. *Clin Chest Med* 1987;8:287–299.

Braunwald E, Gilliland B. In: *Harrison's principles and practice of internal medicine,* 13th ed. New York: McGraw-Hill, 1994:182–183, 1705–1706.

Braunwald E. In: *Heart disease.* Philadelphia: WB Saunders, 1997.

Fishman A. In: *Pulmonary diseases and disorders.* New York: McGraw-Hill, 1988:352–354.

Authors: Peter Kringstein and Gerard P. Aurigemma

Congenital Heart Diseases, Adult

Basics

DESCRIPTION

Congenital cardiac lesions are categorized into cyanotic and acyanotic types. These groups are subdivided into patients who have had palliative or corrective cardiac surgery or interventional cardiac catheterization and those who have never had intervention. The most common defects, among patients who are most likely to survive to adulthood are:

- Adult patients with cyanotic heart disease who may have survived without corrective surgery/interventional catheterization
  - —Eisenmenger's syndrome
  - —Ebstein's anomaly
  - —Balanced complex lesions with adequate pulmonary blood flow and normal pulmonary artery pressure (e.g., tetralogy of Fallot with moderate pulmonary stenosis)
- Adult patients with cyanotic heart disease who have had surgery/interventional catheterization who may remain cyanotic
  - —Status post fenestrated Fontan procedure with right-to-left shunt
  - —Glenn alone
  - —Arterial shunt
- Adult patients with acyanotic congenital heart disease who have not had surgery/interventional catheterization
  - —Atrial septal defect (ASD)
  - —Small, medium-sized ventricular septal defect (VSD) with left-to-right shunt
  - —Bicuspid aortic valve
  - —Coronary artery fistula
  - —Sinus of Valsalva aneurysm
  - —Partial anomalous pulmonary venous return
  - —Mild pulmonary stenosis
  - —Idiopathic dilatation of the pulmonary trunk
  - —Primary pulmonary hypertension
  - —Congenitally corrected transposition
  - —Quadricuspid aortic valve
  - —Mild subaortic stenosis
  - —Mild supraaortic stenosis
  - —Mitral valve prolapse
  - —Marfan's syndrome
  - —Situs inversus and dextrocardia
- Adult patients with acyanotic congenital heart disease who have had surgery/interventional catheterization
  - —Aortic valve disease, valvotomy or replacement, Ross procedure
  - —Pulmonary stenosis, valvotomy
  - —ASD
  - —VSD
  - —Fontan surgery for complex congenital heart disease
  - —Transposition of great arteries, atrial redirection, or arterial switch
  - —Tetralogy of Fallot
  - —Aortopulmonary window
  - —Anomalous origin of left coronary artery from the pulmonary trunk
  - —Vascular ring
  - —Patent ductus arteriosus, surgical division or transcatheter occlusion
  - —Total anomalous pulmonary venous connection
  - —Truncus arteriosus, right ventricular to pulmonary artery conduit, right ventricular outflow tract patch
  - —Ebstein's anomaly, tricuspid valve repair or replacement, accessory pathway ablation, foramen closure
  - —Cor triatriatum
  - —Coarctation of the aorta
  - —Mitral valve disease, valvotomy or replacement
  - —Hypoplastic left heart syndrome, Norwood procedure

EPIDEMIOLOGY

Incidence/Prevalence

The prevalence of adults with residual congenital heart defects requiring follow-up is increasing as the number of patients who have had corrective or palliative surgery has increased and survival improves.

ETIOLOGY

- The cause of most congenital heart disease is unknown; thought to be multifactorial.
- An increasing number of cases are known to be genetic, among the most common: Holt-Oram syndrome with autosomal-dominant transmission of an ASD; Williams syndrome with supravalvular aortic stenosis; and Down's syndrome with atrioventricular (AV) canal defects.
- Approximately 2% of cases are environmental (e.g., congenital rubella syndrome).
- Genetic counseling should be provided for all potential parents with congenital heart disease, both male and female.

PREGNANCY

- Patients with cyanosis are at high risk of early spontaneous abortion.
- Elevated pulmonary vascular resistance from Eisenmenger's syndrome or primary pulmonary hypertension is a contraindication to pregnancy.
- Patients with Marfan's syndrome and some patients with bicuspid aortic valve are at risk for aortic rupture.
- Patients with severe aortic stenosis are at high risk for complications.
- Patients with aortic coarctation are at risk for aortic rupture and cerebral hemorrhage as well as increased fetal risk of compromised placental blood supply.
- Management of pregnant women with prosthetic valves is a difficult issue. The 1998 AHA/ACC guidelines for the management of valvular heart disease recommend warfarin until the 35th week of pregnancy, then i.v./s.c. heparin. Risk of warfarin embryopathy is approximately 3.4%. Data suggest that a warfarin dose of $\leq$5 mg/day lowers risk of fetal complications. Heparin is more difficult to regulate and is associated with a greater risk of thromboembolism in the mother.

ASSOCIATED CONDITIONS

N/A

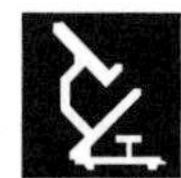

Diagnosis

DIFFERENTIAL DIAGNOSIS

N/A

SIGNS AND SYMPTOMS

History

Depending on the underlying lesion, patients may have one or more of the following:

- History of murmur in childhood
- History of palliative surgery in early infancy
- History of corrective surgery in early infancy or childhood
- History of arrhythmia
- History of endocarditis

Cyanotic Secondary to Uncorrected Cardiac Defect

- Effort-induced dyspnea
- Increased cyanosis with exercise
- Effort induced fatigue

Cyanotic Secondary to Pulmonary Vascular Disease (Eisenmenger's Syndrome)

- Hemoptysis (late)
- Decrease in intensity of childhood murmur
- Palpable P2, right ventricular heave
- Clubbing of fingers and toes, perioral cyanosis, hypertrophic osteopathy

Acyanotic

- Range from asymptomatic to significant limitation of activities of daily living with symptoms at rest secondary to heart failure.

LABORATORY PROCEDURES

Cyanotic

- Hemoglobin/hematocrit elevated secondary to elevated erythropoietin levels (hemoglobin 16–23 g, hematocrit 55–80)
- Platelet count low to markedly reduced
- Blood urea nitrogen/creatinine may be elevated.
- Uric acid elevated secondary to inappropriately low renal excretion

Acyanotic

- Depends on the nature of the underlying lesion

IMAGING STUDIES

Chest x-ray

- Cyanotic secondary to pulmonary vascular disease
  - —Decreased pulmonary blood flow

—Prominent pulmonary arteries at the hilum with rapid tapering
—Enlarged right ventricular silhouette
—Acyanotic
—Depends on the underlying lesion

Transthoracic Echo (2-D)

- Color flow imaging for
  —Following the course of arteries and veins
  —Detecting small atrial or ventricular septal defects
  —Detecting small aortic-to-pulmonary connections
  —Delineating stenotic and regurgitant lesions
- Doppler studies for identification and quantification of
  —Valvular, supravalvular, and subvalvular stenosis
  —Valvular regurgitation
  —Extracardiac and intracardiac conduit obstructions
  —Pulmonary and systemic venous stenoses
  —Septal defects
  —Surgical shunts

Transesophageal Echo

- Evaluate anatomic areas not easily demonstrated by transthoracic echo.
- Monitor therapeutic interventions in the cardiac catheterization laboratory.
- Intraoperative imaging during cardiac surgery

Cardiac Catheterization

- Primary diagnostic tool to evaluate coronary artery atherosclerotic disease
- Evaluate ventricular filling pressures.
- Delineate patterns of collateral blood flow.
- Delineate pulmonary anatomy.

SPECIAL TESTS

- Cardiovascular/pulmonary anatomy
- MRI
- Magnetic resonance angiography
- Arrhythmia
  —Holter
  —Event monitor
  —Electrophysiology study
- Functional capacity and cardiac ischemia
- Standard Bruce protocol exercise stress testing
- Thallium and sestamibi nuclear stress testing

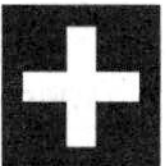

Treatment

GENERAL MEASURES

- Nonchemotherapeutic prophylaxis for endocarditis
- Meticulous oral hygiene, skin and nail care

SURGICAL MEASURES

Indications for operation in adults with congenital heart disease include:

- Repair of primary congenital heart defect: ASD, aortic stenosis, pulmonary stenosis, Ebstein's anomaly, coarctation of the aorta, tetralogy of Fallot, etc.
- Inevitable reoperation: bioprosthetic heart valve, extracardiac conduit
- Residual defects after repair: mitral valve regurgitation and/or subvalvular aortic stenosis after AV canal defect repair
- New/recurrent defects after corrective surgery: subaortic stenosis recurrence, pulmonary regurgitation after repair of tetralogy of Fallot
- Staged repair of complex defect: Fontan procedure
- Late complications: infective endocarditis
- Patient with acquired heart disease: coronary atherosclerotic disease
- Uncorrectable congenital heart disease: heart or heart/lung transplant
- Insertion of permanent pacemaker and/or defibrillator
- Mapping and ablation of arrhythmias

ADMISSION/DISCHARGE CRITERIA

- Symptomatic arrhythmia for drug treatment or electrophysiology study (ablation or intracardiac defibrillator placement)
- Exacerbation of congestive heart failure
- Surgery or interventional/diagnostic cardiac catheterization
- Endocarditis
- Cerebral abscess or stroke in cyanotic patient

Medications

DRUG(S) OF CHOICE

- Patients with left-sided ventricular dysfunction benefit from established medical therapy for congestive heart failure (digoxin, angiotensin-converting enzyme inhibitor, diuretic, beta-blockade).
- Prior to dental work or invasive procedures patients must receive endocarditis prophylaxis.
- Phlebotomy recommended for secondary erythrocytosis only if patient is significantly symptomatic with hematocrit of $>65\%$
- Iron repletion in cyanotic patients who are iron deficient (close monitoring of hematocrit required as blood counts may increase quickly with iron therapy)
- Colchicine for treatment of gouty arthritis in cyanotic patients
- Anticoagulation and chronic pulmonary vasodilator therapy for primary pulmonary hypertension
- Avoid aspirin and other antithrombotic medications in patients with Eisenmenger's syndrome because these patients are at an increased risk of bleeding.
- Antiarrhythmic therapy

Follow-up

PATIENT MONITORING

- Close regular visits with both primary care physician and a cardiologist trained in congenital heart disease. The frequency of visits would depend on the functional class of the patient and the expected natural history of the congenital cardiac lesion.

EXPECTED COURSE AND PROGNOSIS

- Depends on the severity of the underlying lesion

PATIENT EDUCATION

- The patient must be educated as to the particular risks and limitations of his or her type of congenital heart disease.
- The degree of exercise that is safe for an individual patient depends on the nature of the underlying congenital lesion. Lesions that are at least moderate risk for strenuous exercise:
  —Aberrant coronary artery that crosses between the aorta and the right ventricular outflow track
  —Greater than moderate coarctation of the aorta, Marfan's syndrome, or bicuspid aortic valve with aortic root dilatation (patients should especially avoid isotonic exercise)
  —Moderate to severe aortic stenosis
  —Moderate to severe pulmonary stenosis
  —Balanced tetralogy of Fallot

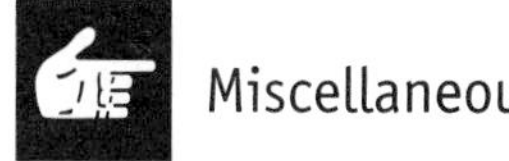

Miscellaneous

BIBLIOGRAPHY

Bonnow RO, Carabello B, de Leon AC Jr, et al. ACC/AHA guidelines for the management of patients with valvular heart disease: a report of the American College of Cardiology/American Heart Association Task Force on Practice Guidelines (Committee on the Management of Patients with Valvular Heart Disease). *J Am Coll Cardiol* 1998;5:1486–1582.

Deanfield JE, Gersh BJ, Warnes CA, et al. Congenital heart disease in adults. In: Alexander RW, Schlant RC, Fuster V, eds. *The heart.* New York: McGraw-Hill, 1998:1995–2031.

Perloff JK. Congenital heart disease in adults. In: Braunwald E, ed. *Heart disease,* 5th ed. Philadelphia: WB Saunders, 1998:963–987.

Perloff JK, Child JS. *Congenital heart disease in adults,* 2nd ed. Philadelphia: WB Saunders, 1998.

Authors: Deborah R. Gersony and Welton M. Gersony

Congenital Valvar Aortic Stenosis

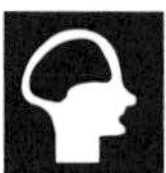

Basics

DESCRIPTION

Congenital aortic stenosis is characterized by narrowing of the aortic valve orifice, leading to left ventricular hypertrophy, and in the most severe form predisposing the patient to exercise intolerance and myocardial dysfunction.

- Pathologic abnormalities described include fusion of the valve leaflets leading to a unicuspid or bicuspid valve, or more rarely, fusion of normal tricuspid leaflets.
- The valve leaflets are often thickened due to the turbulence of flow across the area, which may lead to calcification in later life.

EPIDEMIOLOGY

The incidence of congenital valvar aortic stenosis is 2–4/10,000 live births, occurring in 3%–6% of children with congenital heart disease.

- It is more common among boys, with a male to female ratio of 4:1.
- Aortic stenosis has two modes of presentation: the majority of patients present in infancy or early childhood with an asymptomatic heart murmur; neonates with critical aortic stenosis present with severe congestive heart failure shortly after birth secondary to severe obstruction and left ventricular dysfunction.

ETIOLOGY

Aortic stenosis is rarely associated with a chromosomal abnormality.

- Valvar aortic stenosis has been described in 18% of patients with Turner's syndrome (XO).
- In patients with multiple congenital anomalies, rare reports of associated chromosomal deletions have been described.

RISK FACTORS

N/A

PREGNANCY

The presence of significant aortic stenosis is a risk factor for adverse outcome during pregnancy due to the increased cardiac demands of the fetus.

- Adequate relief of aortic stenosis should be achieved prior to pregnancy whenever possible.
- Patients with severe aortic stenosis have undergone balloon valvuloplasty during pregnancy, with care to limit radiation exposure.

ASSOCIATED CONDITIONS

Cardiac anomalies occur in approximately 20% of cases and include ventricular septal defect, coarctation of the aorta, subaortic stenosis, hypoplastic left ventricle, mitral valve abnormalities, and other complex lesions.

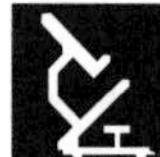

Diagnosis

DIFFERENTIAL DIAGNOSIS

The differential diagnosis of the asymptomatic child with a murmur of the left ventricular outflow tract obstruction includes subaortic stenosis, valvar aortic stenosis, and supravalvar aortic stenosis.

SIGNS AND SYMPTOMS

Signs

Unlike congenital heart defects characterized by volume overload or cyanosis, significant disease can be present in the absence of symptoms.

- Murmur at the base of the heart, radiating to the jugular notch, carotid vessels, and apex
- Suprasternal notch thrill, even in mild aortic stenosis
- Valve click at the cardiac apex in mild to moderate stenosis
- Left ventricular heave and a thrill at the base of the heart are felt in moderate-severe stenosis.

Symptoms

Symptoms are related to decreased cardiac output and/or myocardial ischemia and present only with moderate to severe obstruction. In general, symptoms are a late manifestation.

- Exercise intolerance
- Exertional dyspnea
- Angina
- Syncope
- Palpitations

Critical Aortic Stenosis of the Neonate

- Congestive heart failure
- Low cardiac output
- Pulmonary edema
- Patent ductus arteriosus augments cardiac output via flow from the right ventricle to the aorta.

LABORATORY PROCEDURES

In the neonate with critical aortic stenosis, evaluation of renal and hepatic function should be performed to assess the adequacy of cardiac output.

IMAGING STUDIES

- ECG
  —Electrocardiographic abnormalities including left ventricular hypertrophy, left ventricular strain and ischemic changes with exercise are an indication of the severity of the obstruction, but occasionally severe stenosis may have a relatively benign ECG.
- Echocardiography
  —Optimal method of evaluating aortic valve anatomy and hemodynamics
  —The instantaneous gradient across the valve can be estimated from the velocity of blood flow measured by continuous-wave Doppler, but overestimation is not unusual.
  —Left ventricular hypertrophy can be quantitatively assessed and aortic insufficiency can be documented by color flow Doppler.
- Cardiac catheterization
  —Cardiac catheterization is not indicated to establish the diagnosis of valvar aortic stenosis in the majority of patients.
  —Catheter assessment of the aortic valve gradient may be necessary in patients when symptoms are out of proportion to the predicted echocardiographic gradient.

SPECIAL TESTS

Exercise testing can be carried out with caution in the patient with moderate aortic stenosis to assess symptomatology and the degree of hemodynamic compromise due to left ventricular outflow obstruction.

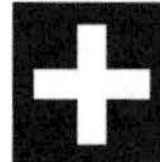

Treatment

GENERAL MEASURES

- Aortic stenosis is a progressive disease that requires close monitoring for signs of increasing obstruction and left ventricular hypertrophy.
- Antibiotic prophylaxis against bacterial endocarditis should be administered according to the recommendations of the American Heart Association.
- Recommendations for participation in recreational and competitive sports are guided by the echocardiographically estimated valve gradient, the degree of left ventricular hypertrophy, and the presence of symptoms such as exertional dyspnea, chest pain, syncope, or exercise intolerance.

(See the Appendix for the table on Activity Recommendations in Patients with Congenital Aortic Stenosis.)

Indications for Intervention

- Echocardiographic estimation of the gradient across the aortic valve of >70 mm Hg, usually in conjunction with at least moderate left ventricular hypertrophy by echocardiography or ECG
- In children with lesser echocardiographic findings and symptoms, cardiac catheterization may be indicated to determine hemodynamics.
- If the gradient at catheterization is ≥60 mm Hg, balloon valvuloplasty is indicated in infants, children, and young adults.
- Balloon valvuloplasty may be indicated in patients with a gradient of <60 mm Hg who have significant ventricular hypertrophy or symptoms of exercise intolerance and/or myocardial insufficiency.

INTERVENTION

Relief of aortic stenosis can be achieved by:

- Transcatheter balloon valvuloplasty
- Surgical aortic valvotomy
- Aortic valve replacement

Balloon Valvuloplasty

- Procedure of choice for relief of moderate to severe aortic stenosis in infants and children
- Although effective in the majority of patients, balloon valvuloplasty may be complicated by aortic insufficiency.
- Aortic valve replacement may be required following balloon valvuloplasty if severe aortic insufficiency occurs.
- In patients who develop restenosis of the aortic valve following valvuloplasty, repeat valvuloplasty cannot be performed if significant aortic insufficiency is present.

Surgical Valvotomy

- May be performed as a primary procedure in the severely compromised neonate with critical aortic stenosis as circulatory support via cardiopulmonary bypass is provided prior to relieving the obstruction.
- In older children and adults, direct visualization of the aortic valve at surgery also may be necessary to relieve stenosis in certain types of aortic valve morphology, especially calcific, that are unresponsive to balloon valvuloplasty.

Aortic Valve Replacement

- Can be performed using a prosthetic mechanical valve, a bioprosthesis, such as an aortic allograft or porcine valve, or a pulmonary autograft (the Ross operation)
- The procedure of choice for aortic valve replacement for children at many centers is the Ross operation.
  —The native aortic and pulmonary valves are excised, and the pulmonary valve is inserted into the aortic root.
  —A pulmonary or aortic homograft is used to reestablish continuity between the right ventricle and the main pulmonary artery.
  —The use of the native pulmonary valve to replace the stenotic aortic valve obviates the need for chronic anticoagulation and affords the potential for growth.
  —The incidence of restenosis of the neoaortic valve is low, although valve replacement has been necessary in the setting of significant neoaortic insufficiency.
  —In patients with right ventricular outflow tract obstruction, replacement of a right ventricular to pulmonary artery homograft usually is necessary within 10 years, but following the Ross operation, the homograft may last longer because it is positioned anatomically in a nonhypertrophied right ventricle.
- Aortic valve replacement also can be performed using a mechanical valve or a bioprosthetic valve.
  —In adult patients, mechanical valves, such as the St. Jude's prosthetic valve, offer excellent relief of stenosis for up to 15–20 years.
  —Replacement may be necessary for recurrent stenosis or paravalvar leak.
  —Chronic anticoagulation is necessary to prevent complications of thromboembolism.
  —In infants and small children, mechanical valve use is limited by the lack of growth, which necessitates earlier valve replacement.
  —Chronic anticoagulation can be more difficult to regulate in pediatric patients and carries a greater risk of bleeding in children learning to ambulate.
- Aortic valve replacement with a bioprosthetic valve is rarely indicated because the failure rate is high.
  —A bioprosthetic valve may be used in patients in whom chronic anticoagulation may be contraindicated, such as young women who are planning pregnancy.

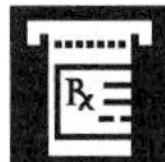

Medications

DRUG(S) OF CHOICE

- Medical therapy is not indicated in the asymptomatic patient with valvar aortic stenosis.
- In neonates with critical aortic stenosis, aggressive medical therapy is required to stabilize the patient, including mechanical ventilation, correction of acidosis, and inotropic support.
- Prostaglandin E_1 may be used to maintain ductal patency and augment systemic output via the right ventricle prior to intervention.

Follow-up

PATIENT MONITORING

- Although balloon valvuloplasty and surgical valvotomy result in significant relief of obstruction in 80%–90% of patients, valvar aortic stenosis is a progressive disease, with 50% of patients requiring further intervention within 10 years after initial therapy.
- If obstruction recurs, balloon valvuloplasty or valvotomy should be performed, however, if unsuccessful or contraindicated, surgical intervention is indicated.

Critical Aortic Stenosis in Infants

- The mortality rate in newborns with critical aortic stenosis is 12%–30%, due to the presence of significant left ventricular systolic and diastolic dysfunction.
- Restenosis is common after surgical or catheter relief of obstruction in the neonatal period, with 20% of survivors requiring further intervention within 5 years of their initial procedure.
- Nevertheless, long-term survival and quality of life has improved markedly in recent years.

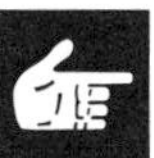

Miscellaneous

ICD-9-CM

746.3

BIBLIOGRAPHY

American Heart Association. Prevention of Bacterial Endocarditis: Recommendations by the American Heart Association. *JAMA* 1997;277:1794–1801.

Congenital valvar aortic stenosis. In: Kirklin JW, Barratt-Boyes BG, eds. *Cardiac surgery,* 2nd ed. New York: Churchill Livingstone, 1993:1196–1212.

Graham TP, Bricker JR, James FW, et al. 26th Bethesda Conference. Recommendations for determining eligibility for competition in athletes with cardiovascular abnormalities. Task Force 1: Congenital Heart Disease. *J Am Coll Cardiol* 1994;24:845–889.

McCrindle BW for the VACA registry investigators. Independent predictors of immediate results of percutaneous balloon aortic valvotomy in childhood. *Am J Cardiol* 1996;77:286–293.

Mosca RS, Iannettoni MD, Schwartz S, et al. Critical aortic stenosis in the neonate. *J Thorac Cardiovasc Surg* 1995;109:147–154.

Ross DN. Replacement of aortic and mitral valves with pulmonary autograft. *Lancet* 1967;2:956–958.

Shim D, Lloyd T, Beekman RH. Usefulness of repeat balloon aortic valvuloplasty in children. *Am J Cardiol* 1997;79:1141–1143.

Authors: Daphne T. Hsu and Welton M. Gersony

Cor Pulmonale

Basics

DESCRIPTION

Right ventricular dilatation and hypertrophy due to pulmonary hypertension that results from an underlying pulmonary parenchymal or vascular disorder

- Symptoms are predominantly related to right ventricular failure.
- Chronic cor pulmonale is most frequently due to chronic obstructive pulmonary disease (COPD).
- Acute cor pulmonale is associated with pulmonary thromboembolism.

PATHOPHYSIOLOGY

In the setting of lung disease, pulmonary hypertension develops as a result of increased resistance to blood flow, whether due to a significant loss of the total cross-sectional area of the pulmonary circulation or vasoconstriction of the pulmonary vessels.

- Reduction in the cross-sectional area of the pulmonary vascular bed may occur due to capillary destruction (emphysema), vascular obstruction (pulmonary embolism), or intimal thickening (primary pulmonary hypertension).
- In patients with underlying lung disease, the major stimuli for vasoconstriction are hypoxemia and acidosis.
- Increased blood viscosity in patients with severe hypoxemia who develop a compensatory increase in hematocrit also may increase resistance to flow and contribute to the development of pulmonary hypertension.

Systems Affected

- Cardiopulmonary

EPIDEMIOLOGY

Incidence/Prevalence

The true prevalence of cor pulmonale is difficult to estimate.

- However, because it is associated with common forms of pulmonary disease, it is encountered regularly in both the outpatient and inpatient settings.
- After age 50, cor pulmonale is the third most frequent form of cardiac disease after coronary artery atherosclerosis and hypertensive heart disease.
- It may play a role in up to 10%–30% of hospital admissions for heart failure.

Predominant Age

- Increases with advancing age

Age-Related Factors

- Pediatric: unusual
- Geriatric: common

PREGNANCY

N/A

ASSOCIATED CONDITIONS

- COPD
- Pulmonary embolus
- Primary pulmonary hypertension
- Restrictive lung disease
- Infiltrative lung disease
- Thoracic cage dysfunction

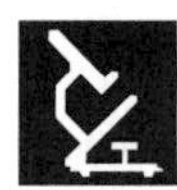

Diagnosis

SIGNS AND SYMPTOMS

- The presence of underlying pulmonary disease is usually clinically evident. Therefore, many patients complain of cough, sputum production, and dyspnea.
- Patients with acute cor pulmonale due to pulmonary embolism also may complain of chest pain, which is usually pleuritic in nature.
- Symptoms related to right ventricular failure include:
  —Fatigue due to low cardiac output
  —Dependent edema
  —Abdominal pain (right upper quadrant) due to liver engorgement
  —Anorexia and bloating
  —Exertional syncope

Physical Examination

- Cyanosis/hypoxemia
- Distended neck veins with prominent a and v waves.
- Right ventricular (parasternal) heave
- Right ventricular S3
- Holosystolic murmur at left lower sternal border that increases with inspiration (tricuspid regurgitation)
- Loud pulmonary component of the second heart sound
- Ascites
- Pitting edema

ETIOLOGY

- Essentially any disease of the lung parenchyma or vasculature, if severe enough, can cause pulmonary hypertension and eventually right ventricular failure.
- The most common cause is COPD.
- Other causes include:
  —Pulmonary embolism
  —Cystic fibrosis
  —Infiltrative diseases (sarcoidosis, idiopathic pulmonary fibrosis)
  —Processes affecting thoracic cage movement (sleep apnea, kyphoscoliosis, neuromuscular disease)

DIFFERENTIAL DIAGNOSIS

- All of the above symptoms and findings may be present in patients with biventricular failure of any cause.
- The presence of left-sided cardiac disease must be excluded before making the diagnosis of cor pulmonale.
- Shares some features with constrictive pericarditis, restrictive cardiomyopathy, and mitral stenosis
- Presence of advanced lung disease in a patient with symptoms and physical findings of right ventricular dysfunction makes the diagnosis of cor pulmonale most likely.

LABORATORY PROCEDURES

- Patients with advanced lung disease may manifest hypoxemia and hypercapnia on arterial blood gas (ABG) testing.
- In acute cor pulmonale due to pulmonary embolism, a widened alveolar to arterial (A-a) oxygen gradient will be present on the ABG.

Pathologic Findings

- Right ventricular hypertrophy
- Pulmonary vascular disease

SPECIAL TESTS

- ECG findings differ with respect to the acute and chronic forms of cor pulmonale and depending on whether or not obstructive airway disease is present.
- ECG is relatively insensitive for the detection of right ventricular hypertrophy.
- In general, the ECG should be examined for the following:
  —Right atrial enlargement (P waves >2.5 mm in leads II, III, and aVF or >1.5 mm in leads V1 or V2)
  —Right axis deviation >110 degrees
  —Incomplete right bundle branch block
  —RSR′ or qR pattern in lead V1
  —S1, Q3, T3 pattern
  —ST segment depression with or without T-wave inversion in the right precordial leads (V1 to V3)
  —R/S ratio in V6 of <1
  —Low-voltage QRS
- Chest x-ray
  —Hyperinflation/diaphragmatic flattening
  —Enlarged central pulmonary arteries
  —Peripheral oligemia
  —Loss of the retrosternal airspace secondary to right heart enlargement

IMAGING STUDIES

- Echocardiography
  —The echocardiogram can provide detailed structural and physiologic information.
  —The size and systolic function of the right ventricle can be assessed, as can regurgitation of the tricuspid and pulmonic valves.
  —If tricuspid regurgitation is present, its velocity can be used in the modified Bernoulli equation to obtain an estimate of right ventricular systolic pressure.

—This can then be added to an estimate of mean right atrial pressure (based on the size of the inferior vena cava and its response to respiration) to obtain an estimate of the pulmonary artery systolic pressure.
—An additional important function of the echocardiogram is to rule out significant left ventricular dysfunction, left-sided valvular disease, or congenital heart disease as potential causes of pulmonary hypertension.

DIAGNOSTIC PROCEDURES

- Cardiac catheterization
  —Right heart catheterization provides a direct measure of pulmonary artery pressure.
  —The diagnosis of cor pulmonale is supported by the finding of significant pulmonary hypertension with a normal pulmonary capillary wedge pressure.
  —The diagnosis of cor pulmonale can usually be made on the basis of the clinical picture, ECG, and echocardiographic findings.
  —Occasionally right heart catheterization is helpful, especially when the echocardiographic images are suboptimal.

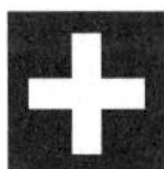

Treatment

GENERAL MEASURES

- Hospitalization if hemodynamically unstable or hypoxic
- The main thrust of therapy for cor pulmonale should be directed at improving the status of the underlying pulmonary disorder.
  —Superimposed infections should be aggressively treated.
  —Supplemental oxygen therapy to correct hypoxia has been proven to improve survival.
  —Oxygen therapy results in a decrease in pulmonary artery pressure and pulmonary vascular resistance.
  —The progression of pulmonary hypertension may be halted or slowed.
  —In studies that compared duration of therapy, the greatest reduction in mortality was seen when oxygen was administered 24 h/day.
- Supplemental oxygen should be prescribed for patients with a PaO_2 of <55 mm Hg.
- Other measures
  —Periodic phlebotomy to maintain a hematocrit of $<55\%$ reduces blood viscosity and improves pulmonary blood flow.

SURGICAL MEASURES

- Markedly symptomatic patients with chronic cor pulmonale due to recurrent episodes of pulmonary thromboembolism may benefit from pulmonary thromboendarterectomy. This is a high-risk procedure that has limited clinical application.

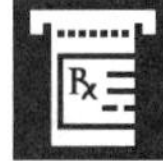

Medications

DRUG(S) OF CHOICE

- Bronchodilators
  —By relieving bronchoconstriction, gas exchange is improved, which has a beneficial effect on hypoxia-mediated vasoconstriction.
- Warfarin
  —For patients with a thromboembolic etiology
  —Recurrent thromboembolism while on anticoagulation may call for placement of an inferior vena cava filter.
- Diuretics
  —Relieve fluid retention but have no documented positive effect on pulmonary hemodynamics in the absence of left ventricular failure.

Contraindications

Refer to manufacturer's profile on each drug.

Precautions

Refer to manufacturer's profile on each drug.

Significant Possible Interactions

Refer to manufacturer's profile on each drug.

ALTERNATE DRUGS

N/A

Follow-up

PATIENT MONITORING

- Arterial oxygen saturation should be monitored periodically.
- INR needs to be periodically assessed in patients on warfarin.
- Renal function should be periodically assessed in patients on diuretics.

Prevention/Avoidance

Smoking is the most important modifiable risk factor.

Possible Complications

Atrial arrhythmias are the most common nonpulmonary complication. Recurrences of atrial fibrillation and difficulty restoring sinus rhythm are found in patients with significant right atrial dilatation.

EXPECTED COURSE AND PROGNOSIS

- The prognosis is closely related to the etiology and severity of the underlying lung disease and the degree of pulmonary hypertension.
- Patients with COPD who develop cor pulmonale have a 50% chance of surviving for 2–3 years, although this may be improved with oxygen therapy.

Activity

- Restricted if right heart failure or hypoxia is present

Diet

- Low sodium if right heart failure or hypoxia is present

PATIENT EDUCATION

N/A

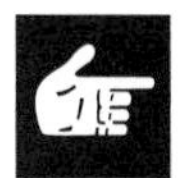

Miscellaneous

ICD-9-CM

415.0 Acute cor pulmonale
416.9 Chronic cor pulmonale

BIBLIOGRAPHY

Braunwald E. *Heart disease: a textbook of cardiovascular medicine,* 5th Ed. Philadelphia: WB Saunders, 1997.

Murphy J. *Mayo Clinic cardiology review.* Armonk, NY: Futura, 1997.

Author: Bryan J. Reynolds

Cushing's Syndrome

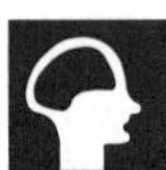

Basics

DESCRIPTION

A combination of clinical features and biochemical abnormalities that occur as a result of excessive tissue exposure to cortisol

EPIDEMIOLOGY

Incidence/Prevalence

The incidence of endogenous Cushing's syndrome (CS) in the United States is estimated to be 13 million per year. Exogenous CS from therapeutic use of glucocorticoids is even more common.

Predominant Age

- Varies with the cause of CS
  - —Pituitary (corticotroph) adenoma: 25–40 years
  - —Ectopic adrenocorticotrophic hormone (ACTH) secretion: >40 years
  - —Adrenal carcinoma: bimodal age distribution with peaks in childhood/adolescence and late in life.
  - —Adrenal adenoma: around 35 years

Predominant Sex

- Varies with the cause of CS
  - —Adrenal adenomas, adrenal carcinomas, and corticotroph adenomas are four to six times more common in women than in men.
  - —Ectopic ACTH secretion is more common in men than women (may change as more women develop lung cancer, the most common cause of ectopic ACTH secretion).

Predominant Race

- None

ETIOLOGY

- Exogenous (iatrogenic or factitious): CS secondary to use of high-dose glucocorticoids (most common cause of CS)
- Endogenous
  - —ACTH (corticotropin)-dependent: adrenal activation caused by excessive ACTH
    - Pituitary corticotroph adenoma (80%): Cushing's disease (CD)
    - Ectopic ACTH secretion (20%): most commonly associated with small cell lung carcinoma; less commonly with intrathoracic carcinoids, pancreatic carcinoid or islet cell tumors, pheochromocytoma, neuroblastoma, ganglioma, paraganglioma, medullary carcinoma of the thyroid
    - Ectopic corticotropin-releasing hormone (CRH)/corticotroph hyperplasia, corticotroph carcinomas very rare
  - —ACTH-independent: Adrenal activation apart from ACTH
    - Adrenal adenoma (40%–50%)
    - Adrenal carcinoma (40%–50%)

RISK FACTORS

N/A

PREGNANCY

- May be difficult to make the diagnosis of CS during pregnancy because of physical and biochemical changes that are common in both conditions (hypertension, glucose intolerance, weight gain, fatigue, striae, increased serum cortisol, increased urine free cortisol)
- Maternal CS is associated with increased rates of premature delivery and stillbirth.
- Maternal and fetal outcomes are better if hypercortisolism is treated.
- Use of ketoconazole is contraindicated in pregnancy.

ASSOCIATED CONDITIONS

- Affective disorders
- Opportunistic infections
- Perforated viscus
- Renal calculi

Diagnosis

DIFFERENTIAL DIAGNOSIS

- Glucocorticoid resistance: compensatory increases in ACTH and excessive glucocorticoid production
- Pseudo-Cushing's syndrome: mild glucocorticoid excess of unclear pathophysiology seen in affective disorders, renal failure, chronic alcoholism, withdrawal from alcohol, hypoglycemia, strenuous exercise (urine free cortisol threefold normal)
- Many signs/symptoms of CS are common in the general population (hypertension, obesity, mood changes, menstrual irregularities).

SIGNS AND SYMPTOMS

Signs

- Obesity: increased fat deposition in abdomen, face (moon facies), supraclavicular or temporal fossae, dorsocervical area ("buffalo hump")
- Hypertension: Present in 80%–90% of patients. Consider the diagnosis in patients with hypertension who are <40 years of age, especially if blood pressure is difficult to control.
- Plethora
- Hirsutism
- Striae: purple, >1 cm in diameter, usually over the abdomen
- Thin skin
- Ecchymoses after minimal trauma
- Proximal muscle wasting and weakness with preservation of distal strength
- Edema
- Acne
- Female balding
- White blood cell count ≥11,000/mm^3
- Hypokalemic metabolic alkalosis
- Elevated triglyceride, LDL, HDL levels
- Reduced thyroid-stimulating hormone, luteinizing hormone, follicle-stimulating hormone levels
- ECG abnormalities
- Accelerated atherosclerosis
- Osteopenia on x-ray

Symptoms

- Weight gain
- Fatigue
- Decreased libido
- Impotence
- Menstrual changes/infertility
- Mood changes
- Impaired concentration or memory
- Insomnia
- Easy bruising
- Poor wound healing
- Fractures
- Headache, backache, abdominal pain

LABORATORY PROCEDURE

- Establish the diagnosis of CS:
  - —24-hour urine for creatinine, free cortisol on 3 consecutive days (as an outpatient); or
  - —Low-dose dexamethasone suppression test
    - 2-day dexamethasone suppression test: Administer 0.5 mg dexamethasone every 6 hours for eight doses. Urine free cortisol (UFC) levels >10 μg (>28 μmol) per 24 hours or urinary 17-hydroxycorticosteroid values >2.5 mg (6.9 μmol) per 24 hours indicate the presence of CS; or
    - Overnight dexamethasone suppression test: Administer 1 mg dexamethasone at 11 p.m. or midnight. If plasma cortisol levels at 8 a.m. are >5 μg/dL (>138 nmol/L), CS is likely present.
    - If UFC is up to fourfold elevated, exclude pseudo-CS states:
      - —Midnight plasma cortisol: Evening nadir is preserved in patients with pseudo-CS but not in those with CS.
      - —Dexamethasone-CRH test: In pseudo-CS, plasma cortisol levels are low (<1.4 μg/dL) after administration of dexamethasone and remain low when CRH is given soon after. In patients with CS, levels are higher than this.
      - —Insulin tolerance test: Plasma cortisol levels increase in response to insulin-induced hypoglycemia in patients with pseudo-CS but not in patients with CS.
      - —Administration of naloxone releases less CRH (and therefore less ACTH and cortisol) in patients with CS than in those with pseudo-CS.
- Determine if CS is ACTH-dependent or ACTH-independent:
  - —Measurement of ACTH by radioimmunoassay
    - Levels <5 to 10 pg/mL suggest ACTH-independent (primary adrenal) CS
    - Levels >15 to 20 pg/mL suggest ACTH-dependent CS
- If ACTH-dependent, determine the source of excess ACTH secretion:
  - —High-dose dexamethasone suppression test

• 2-day: Administer 2 mg dexamethasone every 6 hours for eight doses with measurement of UFC or urine cortisol metabolites. Suppression of UFC by more than 90% of mean basal values or suppression of 17-hydroxysteroid excretion by more than 64% is suggestive of a pituitary source of excess ACTH secretion (CD).
• Overnight: Dexamethasone, 8 mg, is administered at 11 p.m., and plasma cortisol is measured between 7 a.m. and 8 a.m. that morning and the next morning. A decrease in plasma cortisol by ≥50% is suggestive of CD

—Metyrapone stimulation test
• Metyrapone blocks the conversion of 11-deoxycortisol to cortisol, leading to a decrease in plasma cortisol, increase in ACTH secretion by the pituitary, increase in plasma 11-deoxycortisol, and urinary 17-hydroxycorticosteroid concentrations.

—CRH stimulation test
• Corticotropinomas retain responsivity to CRH, whereas noncorticotroph tumors do not respond to CRH.

—Bilateral inferior petrosal sinus sampling
• Consider performing this test if the results of two or more noninvasive tests are inconsistent.

IMAGING STUDIES

• Not useful for making the diagnosis of CS and should be used only for localization of tumors
• If the patient has ACTH-independent CS, thin-section CT or MRI of the adrenal glands should be performed.
• If the patient has ACTH-dependent CS with ACTH secretion that cannot be suppressed with dexamethasone, chest CT or MRI should be performed.
• If the patient has CD, high-resolution CT or MRI of the sella turcica should be performed to determine the location of the adenoma and to locate bony landmarks prior to transsphenoidal surgery.

SPECIAL TESTS

See laboratory procedures above.

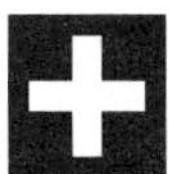

Treatment

GENERAL MEASURES

• Hypertension and cardiovascular disease should be assessed and treated prior to surgery.
• Impaired glucose tolerance should be treated with insulin.
• For iatrogenic CS, weaning and eventual discontinuation of glucocorticoid ingestion should be attempted. If this is not possible, a change in dose may improve symptoms of CS.

SURGICAL MEASURES

• Directed toward resection of abnormal tissue (ACTH- or cortisol-producing)
• Most ACTH-producing nonpituitary tumors are not resectable; bilateral adrenalectomy is a possible therapeutic approach in these cases.

ADMISSION/DISCHARGE CRITERIA

• Outpatient management except for complications or surgery

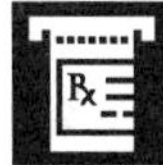

Medications

DRUG(S) OF CHOICE

• Second-line therapies for patients who cannot safely undergo surgery or for those with occult or metastatic tumors
• Used in conjunction with radiation therapy for CD for patients who are not candidates for surgery
• Agents that modulate CRH or ACTH release
—Bromocriptine (dopamine agonist)
—Cyproheptadine (antiserotonergic agent)
—Ritanserin (antiserotonergic agent)
—Valproic acid (blockade of hypothalamic GABA reuptake)
—Octreotide (somatostatin analogue)
• Agents that inhibit steroidogenesis
—Mitotane
—Trilostane
—Metyrapone
—Aminoglutethamide
—Ketoconazole
—Etomidate
• Agent that binds competitively to the glucocorticoid receptor and inhibits the action of the endogenous ligand
—RU 486

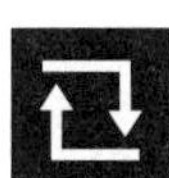

Follow-up

PATIENT MONITORING

• Most patients have underlying suppression of the hypothalamic–pituitary–adrenal axis that is unmasked after surgical correction of CS.
• Once routine postoperative supraphysiologic doses of glucocorticoids have been tapered off, patients should have morning serum cortisol and daily UFC measured for 3 days.
• If these levels are persistently low, physiologic replacement doses of hydrocortisone should be initiated and continued until recovery of the adrenal axis.
• Recovery of the adrenal axis can be assessed by evaluation of the patient's signs and symptoms and by the cortisol response to synthetic ACTH; initial testing should be done at 6 to 9 months postoperatively.
• After pituitary surgery, patients should have serum osmolality, serum sodium, and urine output monitored, because diabetes insipidus is a potential complication.
• After bilateral adrenalectomy, patients will need lifelong glucocorticoid replacement as well as mineralocorticoid replacement.

EXPECTED COURSE AND PROGNOSIS

• The life expectancy of patients with nonmalignant causes of CS has improved significantly with effective surgical and medical treatments, antibiotics, antihypertensive agents, lipid-lowering agents, and glucocorticoids.
• The life expectancy of patients with malignant causes of CS varies depending on the type of tumor.
• Recurrence of CS after surgical resection varies depending on the cause. It is common with adrenal carcinoma, rare with adrenal adenoma, and relatively uncommon with pituitary adenoma.

PATIENT EDUCATION

• Patients should wear an identification bracelet that notes the requirement for glucocorticoids.
• Patients should be aware of the importance of compliance with the daily dose of glucocorticoids and the signs and symptoms of adrenal insufficiency.
• Patients should be aware of the need to increase the oral dose of glucocorticoids for fever, nausea, and diarrhea and of the need for parenteral administration of glucocorticoids and medical evaluation for emesis, trauma, or severe medical stress.

ORGANIZATIONS

• National Adrenal Diseases Foundation (NADF), 505 Northern Boulevard, Great Neck, NY 11021; (516)487-4992
• Cushing's Support and Research Foundation, 65 East India Row, Suite 22-B, Boston, MA 02110

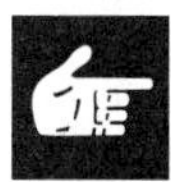

Miscellaneous

ICD-9-CM

255.0

BIBLIOGRAPHY

Kaplan NM. Systemic hypertension: mechanisms and diagnosis. In: Braunwald E, ed. *Heart disease,* 5th ed. Philadelphia: WB Saunders, 1997:829.

Nieman L, Cutler GB. Cushing's syndrome. In: Degroot LJ, ed. *Endocrinology,* 3rd ed. Philadelphia: WB Saunders, 1995:1741–1769.

Orth DN. Cushing's syndrome. *N Engl J Med* 1995;332:791–803.

Williams GH, Lilly LS, Seely EW. The heart in endocrine and nutritional disorders. In: Braunwald E, ed. *Heart disease,* 5th ed. Philadelphia: WB Saunders, 1997:1896.

Author: Deborah L. Ekery

Defibrillators, Implantable

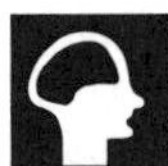

Basics

DESCRIPTION

Implantable device designed to terminate ventricular tachycardia and fibrillation. Implantable cardioverter–defibrillators (ICDs) are usually implanted in the pectoral region much like a pacemaker, and are connected to the heart by at least one electrode wire in the ventricle and sometimes one in the atrium. ICDs can not only treat ventricular tachycardia (VT) and ventricular fibrillation (VF) but also function as pacemakers for bradycardia. Newer devices are able to defibrillate the atrium when atrial fibrillation is present. The indications for ICD implantation are outlined in the American College of Cardiology/American Heart Association Guidelines referenced below and include:

- Cardiac arrest due to VF or VT not due to a transient or reversible cause
- Spontaneous sustained VT
- Syncope of undetermined origin with clinically relevant, hemodynamically significant sustained VT or VF induced at electrophysiologic study when drug therapy is ineffective, not tolerated, or not preferred
- Nonsustained VT with coronary disease, prior myocardial infarction (MI), left ventricular (LV) dysfunction, and inducible VF or sustained VT at electrophysiologic study that is not suppressible by a class I antiarrhythmic drug
- Cardiac arrest presumed to be due to VF when electrophysiologic testing is precluded by other medical conditions
- Severe symptoms attributable to sustained ventricular tachyarrhythmias while awaiting cardiac transplantation
- Familial or inherited conditions with a high risk for life-threatening ventricular tachyarrhythmias such as long QT syndrome or hypertrophic cardiomyopathy
- Nonsustained VT with coronary artery disease, prior MI, and LV dysfunction, and inducible sustained VT or VF at electrophysiologic study
- Recurrent syncope of undetermined etiology in the presence of ventricular dysfunction and inducible ventricular arrhythmias at electrophysiologic study when other causes of syncope have been excluded

EPIDEMIOLOGY

- Over 50,000 new ICDs are implanted each year.
- The devices are implanted in appropriate candidates irrespective of age.
- Most common cause of heart disease in the United States is atherosclerosis. Thus, most patients with ICDs (about 80%) have underlying coronary artery disease. ICD implantation in small individuals, especially children, may be limited by size.

PREGNANCY

- Possible especially with pectorally implanted devices
- Underlying heart disease, however, may be a relative contraindication (e.g., valve disease, cardiomyopathy).
- Some diseases that are genetically transmitted (long QT syndrome, hypertrophic cardiomyopathy) require counseling before pregnancy, irrespective of ICD implantation.

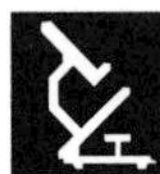

Diagnosis

DIFFERENTIAL DIAGNOSIS

- Not applicable because ICDs are not diseases, but rather a treatment

SIGNS AND SYMPTOMS

N/A

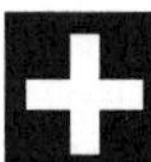

Treatment

GENERAL MEASURES

See Follow-up section below.

SURGICAL MEASURES

ICDs are now implanted in an electrophysiology laboratory.

ADMISSION/DISCHARGE CRITERIA

Depends on clinical situation. Often patients are discharged the day following ICD implantation. Whether discharge is delayed depends on the particular clinical situation. For example, some patients need additional drug therapy for their arrhythmias, or therapy for concomitant comorbid conditions such as heart failure.

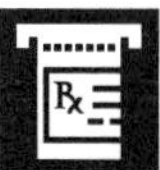

Medications

DRUG(S) OF CHOICE

- Drugs can sometimes be used with ICDs to:
  —Decrease the frequency of arrhythmia occurrence
  —Slow the rate of VT so that antitachycardia pacing can be more effective
  —Treat other arrhythmias, such as atrial fibrillation
  —Treat concomitant diseases, such as coronary artery disease and heart failure (e.g., beta-blockers, nitrates, aspirin, angiotensin-converting enzyme inhibitors, etc.)

Precautions

The initiation of antiarrhythmic drugs must be undertaken with caution. Electrophysiologic evaluation of the ICD is often indicated after drug initiation because these agents can slow VTs to below the programmed ICD detection rate (so that the arrhythmia is not identified) and/or increase the defibrillation threshold (rendering defibrillation ineffective).

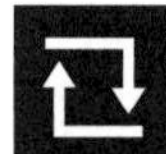

Follow-up

PATIENT MONITORING

- Follow-up is generally performed by an electrophysiologist.
- Unlike pacemakers that can be checked over the telephone, ICDs at this point in time must be checked in person.
- Multiple shocks. This is a medical emergency and can be due either to repetitive VT or VF, a supraventricular arrhythmia exceeding the ICD tachycardia detection rate, or to device/lead malfunction. Multiple shocks are poorly tolerated by patients and can lead to psychological distress. A posttraumatic stress disorder-like syndrome can occur in some of these patients.
- Other complications of ICD therapy include infection, bleeding, lead fracture, and device failure.

EXPECTED COURSE AND PROGNOSIS

- Variable and depends on frequency of arrhythmia recurrence, and the underlying heart disease
- In general, patients with worse left ventricular function have worse prognoses. ICDs are very effective in preventing death due to VT or VF, but do not change the natural history of other diseases.

PATIENT EDUCATION

- Patients should be instructed to avoid activities that could place themselves or others in danger if syncope were to occur, recalling that ICDs do not prevent arrhythmias but only treat them when they occur.
- Driving is controversial.
  —An American Heart Association statement in conjunction with the North American Society of Pacing and Electrophysiology (NASPE) says that patients with VT regardless of whether or not an ICD is implanted should not drive for 6 months following an arrhythmia event.
  —If a patient has been doing well without arrhythmia recurrence and has VT or VF recurrence, driving is again prohibited for another 6 months.

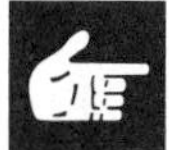

Miscellaneous

SYNONYMS

- Automatic implantable defibrillator (AICD): AICD is a trademark name of ICDs made by Guident, Inc. Because AICDs were the first ICDs available, the term is sometimes used generically.
- Atrioverter: New term for atrial defibrillators to treat atrial fibrillation

BIBLIOGRAPHY

The AVID Investigators. A comparison of antiarrhythmic drug therapy with implantable defibrillators in patients resuscitated from near-fatal sustained ventricular arrhythmias. *N Engl J Med* 1997;337:1576–1583.

Epstein AE, Miles WM, Benditt DG, et al. American Heart Association Medical/Scientific Statement. Personal and public safety issues related to arrhythmias that may affect consciousness: implications for regulation and physician recommendations. *Circulation* 1996;94:1147–1166.

Gregoratos G, Cheitlin MD, Conill A, et al. ACC/AHA guidelines for implantation of cardiac pacemakers and antiarrhythmia devices: a report of the American College of Cardiology/American Heart Association Task Force on Practice Guidelines (Committee on Pacemaker Implantation). *J Am Coll Cardiol* 1998;31:1175–1206.

Pinski SL, Trohman RG. Implantable cardioverter-defibrillators: implications for the nonelectrophysiologist. *Ann Intern Med* 1995;122:770–777.

Author: Andrew E. Epstein

Dermatomyositis

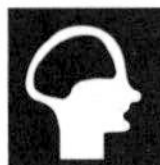

Basics

DESCRIPTION

Dermatomyositis (DM) is an inflammatory muscle disease similar to polymyositis. Both are characterized by symmetric muscle weakness, but specific cutaneous manifestations or rash also accompany DM. Potential cardiovascular manifestations include myocarditis; pericarditis; conduction abnormalities, including bundle branch blocks and complete heart block (CHB); congestive heart failure (CHF); coronary artery vasculitis (rare); and mitral valve prolapse.

- Most CV conditions are secondary to inflammatory injury of cardiac myocytes with subsequent fibrosis.
- Specifically, the pericardium, myocardium, and conduction system may be involved. For example, CHF results from left ventricular (LV) diastolic dysfunction imparted by myocardial fibrosis and pericardial constriction.
- Electrical conduction abnormalities are due largely to fibrosis of the myocardial conduction system.
- The incidence and significance of these lesions in terms of prognosis has not been well studied.

Systems Affected

- Cardiovascular, skeletal muscle, skin

ETIOLOGY

Incidence/Prevalence

Prevalence in the hospitalized population in the United States is 5/1,000,000. ECG abnormalities are detected in 72%, myocarditis in 30%, and pericardial effusion in 5%–25%.

Predominant Age

DM is bimodal (child and adulthood). Cardiac manifestations are more common in older patients or those with a longer duration of DM.

Predominant Sex

- Female

Predominant Race

- Black

CAUSES

- Inflammatory injury of cardiac myocytes and the conduction system

RISK FACTORS

N/A

Diagnosis

DIFFERENTIAL DIAGNOSIS

Patients with DM may present with various syndromes of cardiovascular dysfunction as described above.

- More common causes of these conditions, e.g., coronary artery disease (CAD) and myocardial ischemia leading to CHF or CHB, must be excluded.
- Diagnosis can be difficult because a patient with DM can present with symptoms similar to those of a patient with CAD, with ECG changes, with focal wall motion abnormalities on echocardiogram, and with elevated cardiac enzymes.
- Myocarditis may be associated with other connective tissue diseases, including systemic lupus erythematosus or scleroderma.

SIGNS AND SYMPTOMS

Patients typically are asymptomatic from a cardiovascular perspective.

- Cardiovascular manifestations usually are encountered in the setting of active skeletal muscle involvement.
- Patients may present with conduction abnormalities or arrhythmias and their attendant signs, symptoms, and complications.
- They also may present with myocarditis and pain mimicking angina.
- CHF is a possible presenting syndrome.
- LV dysfunction may be present, but the degree of dysfunction may or may not correlate with the degree of DM activity.

LABORATORY PROCEDURES

- Creatinine kinase and myocardial band fraction (CK-MB)
  - —Serum levels of CK are almost always elevated in DM patients with active myopathy, sometimes accompanied by elevations in serum aldolase.
  - —CK-MB also may be elevated due to significant skeletal myopathy, with no cardiac involvement.
  - —Myocarditis should be considered if CK-MB is >3%.

PATHOLOGIC FINDINGS

- Myocardial biopsy reveals myocardial necrosis, loss of cross-striations, and conduction system fibrosis.
- Postmortem examination: fibrinous pericarditis has been rarely reported as an incidental finding at autopsy.

SPECIAL TESTS

- ECG
  - —No findings specific to DM have been described.
  - —Some ECG abnormalities may be observed in up to 53% of patients with DM, including nonspecific ST- and T-wave abnormalities, ECG evidence for LV hypertrophy (with or without a history of hypertension), and conduction abnormalities.
- Ambulatory ECG
  - —Most common abnormalities are premature ventricular contractions.

IMAGING STUDIES

- Echocardiography
  - —LV diastolic dysfunction
  - —Hyperdynamic LV (ejection fraction >75%)
  - —Focal wall motion abnormalities
  - —MVP
  - —Septal/endocardial fibrosis
  - —Pericardial effusion
- Nuclear perfusion scan
  - —Thallium scintigraphy may reveal areas of hypoperfusion that correlate with regions of myocarditis and not ischemia.
  - —These perfusion defects may resolve with steroid therapy.

DIAGNOSTIC PROCEDURES

- Cardiac catheterization: Coronary angiography is usually normal. Rarely is vasculitis seen.
- Myocardial biopsy: see above.

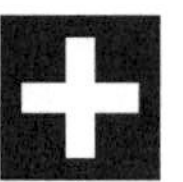

Treatment

GENERAL MEASURES

- Routine cardiac evaluation in patients with DM has been advocated by some, although this is controversial.
- At the least, noninvasive measures should be considered, including ECG and echocardiography.
- Cardiac catheterization should be performed if CAD is suspected or cannot be safely excluded. At that time, myocardial biopsy may be considered.

SURGICAL MEASURES

N/A

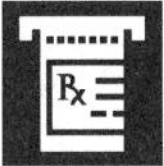

Medications

DRUG(S) OF CHOICE

- Corticosteroids and other immunosuppressants such as methotrexate, azathioprine, and cytoxan
  —Steroid therapy can lead to resolution of ECG changes, perfusion defects by thallium scintigraphy, and regional wall motion abnormalities.
  —Usual dosing is prednisone 60–80 mg daily for 6–8 weeks.
  —Further immunosuppressive therapy should be directed by a rheumatologist experienced with the other agents listed above; however, these other medications have not been shown to be effective when prednisone has failed.

Precautions

Complications associated with long-term steroid use include osteopenia, hyperglycemia, immunosuppression, adrenal suppression, weight gain, truncal obesity, myopathy, fluid retention, avascular necrosis, gastrointestinal complaints, and skin changes.

Significant Possible Interactions 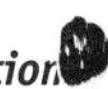

- Variable

Alternative Drugs

- Methotrexate
- Azathioprine
- Cytoxan

Follow-up

PATIENT MONITORING

- No specific guidelines
- Serial noninvasive monitoring may be warranted, including CK-MB and echocardiography, especially for patients with known cardiovascular involvement.

Possible Complications

- See below.

EXPECTED COURSE AND PROGNOSIS

- The presence of cardiac manifestations is the most important factor associated with a poor prognosis in DM.
- CHF is considered the greatest negative outcome predictor of the various cardiovascular manifestations.
- Degree of CK-MB elevation also may correlate directly with poor outcomes; the highest levels of CK-MB are seen in CHF.

PATIENT EDUCATION

Organizations

- Muscular Dystrophy Association, USA National Headquarters, 3300 E. Sunrise Drive, Tucson, AZ 85718; (800)572-1717; http://www.mdausa.org/home.html
- Myositis Association of America, 755 Cantrell Ave, Suite C, Harrisonburg, VA 22801; (540)433-7686; http://www.myositis.org/
- National Institute of Arthritis & Musculoskeletal & Skin Diseases, Building 31, Room 4C05, Bethesda, MD 20892-2350; (301)496-8188; http://www.nih.gov/niams/
- National Organization for Rare Disorders (NORD), P.O. Box 8923, New Fairfield, CT 06812-1783; (800)999-6673

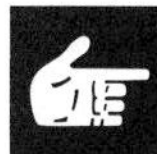

Miscellaneous

ICD-9-CM

710.3 Dermatomyositis (acute) (chronic)

See also: Congestive heart failure; Complete heart block

BIBLIOGRAPHY

Askari AD. The heart in polymyositis and dermatomyositis. *Mount Sinai J Med* 1988;55: 479–482.

Dalakas M, Bohan A, eds. *Polymyositis and dermatomyositis.* Boston: Butterworth, 1988:26, 177.

Gonzalez-Lopez L, et al. Cardiac manifestations in dermato-polymyositis. *Clin Exp Rheumatol* 1996;14:373–379.

Hochberg ML, et al. Adult onset polymyositis/dermatomyositis: an analysis of clinical and laboratory features and survival in seventy-six patients with a review of the literature. *Semin Arthritis Rheumatism* 1986;15:168–178.

Tami LF, Bhasin S. Polymorphisms of the cardiac manifestations in dermatomyositis. *Clin Cardiol* 1993;16:260–264.

Author: James A. Kong

Digitalis Toxicity

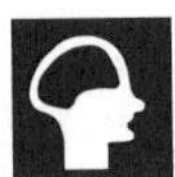

Basics

DESCRIPTION

Although the role of the cardiac glycoside therapy has been the subject of debate, the drug is generally accepted as effective treatment for heart failure due to systolic dysfunction and rate control in atrial fibrillation. A common complication of digoxin therapy is toxicity, which in its mildest form may go unrecognized and in its severest form can be fatal.

EPIDEMIOLOGY

Incidence/Prevalence

The incidence and severity of digoxin intoxication has decreased significantly with the introduction of digoxin assays in 1969.

- Occurs in 4%–15% of patients at some point during therapy
- Mortality with current day treatment of digoxin intoxication is 5%–24%.

ETIOLOGY

Digoxin toxicity is frequently seen in the clinical setting of advancing age, renal insufficiency, drug interaction, diuretic use, or accidental/deliberate overdose.

RISK FACTORS

A number of risk factors influence an individual's sensitivity to cardiac glycosides.

- Advanced age: Diminished glomerular filtration rate; comorbid cardiac conditions
- Renal failure: Prolongs the drug half-life; increases serum concentrations; reduces volume of distribution
- Thyroid status: Hypothyroidism prolongs the half life of digoxin.
- Pulmonary disease: Hypoxemia and respiratory failure increases arrhythmogenesis.
- Underlying heart disease
  —Preexisting conduction and automaticity abnormalities
  —Cardiac amyloid and ischemic cardiomyopathy increase sensitivity to digoxin.
  —Heart failure reduces volume of distribution.
- Hypochlorhydria (gastric pH >7 in older patients and those on H_2 blockers): Reduces gastric metabolism and nonrenal clearance of digoxin
- Electrolyte abnormalities
  —Hypokalemia: Increases binding of digoxin to the sodium pump, causing sensitization of the myocardium to the effects of digoxin and exacerbation of arrhythmias
  —Hyperkalemia: Further depolarization of myocardial conduction tissue potentiates condition abnormalities.
  —Hypomagnesemia: Causes hypokalemia
  —Hypercalcemia: Increases ventricular automaticity, exacerbation of arrhythmias
- Pharmacokinetic interactions (see the Appendix for the table on Effect on Digoxin Concentration).

PREGNANCY

- Digoxin crosses the placenta, and fetal umbilical cord venous blood levels of the drug are similar to maternal blood levels.
- Digoxin is a Pregnancy Category C drug, and thus should only be given to a pregnant woman if absolutely needed.

ASSOCIATED CONDITIONS

See Risk Factors.

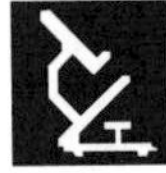

Diagnosis

DIFFERENTIAL DIAGNOSIS

Arrhythmias identical to those of digoxin intoxication also can be caused by primary heart disease, drugs other than digoxin, and a variety of extracardiac factors.

SIGNS AND SYMPTOMS

The features of digoxin toxicity are nonspecific and can be divided into cardiac and noncardiac.

Cardiac

Digitalis is known to induce every known arrhythmia. Although there is no single ECG abnormality that is pathognomonic of digitalis excess, the combination of enhanced automaticity and impaired conduction is the hallmark of toxicity.

- Enhanced automaticity: ectopic rhythms, nonparoxysmal junctional tachycardia, premature ventricular contractions (PVCs), ventricular tachycardia (VT), ventricular fibrillation (VF), accelerated escape, and atrioventricular (AV) dissociation
- Abnormal conduction: sinoatrial (SA) nodal arrest, SA block, AV block, exit block
- Combination (rare but highly suggestive): fascicular tachycardia, bidirectional VT, and alternating right- and left-axis deviation
- Most common: PVC's, atrial tachycardias with block, and nonparoxysmal junctional tachycardia

Noncardiac

ECG signs of toxicity may be preceded by noncardiac manifestations such as:

- Gastrointestinal: anorexia, nausea, vomiting
- Neurologic: confusion, agitation, anxiety, lethargy, headaches, and nightmares
- Ophthalmologic: visual disturbances, usually described as halos around bright objects
- Renal: renal dysfunction

LABORATORY PROCEDURES

Digoxin plasma level concentration has limited clinical value and may be useful only to confirm clinical signs of toxicity.

- Digoxin is rapidly absorbed with a peak serum concentration within 1.5–6 hours after ingestion.
- The therapeutic range of serum digoxin is considered 0.8–2.0 ng/mL.
- Overt digitalis toxicity tends to emerge at two- to threefold higher serum concentration than the target, but it must always be remembered that a substantial overlap of serum levels exists among patients who exhibit signs and symptoms of intoxication.
- Patients can manifest toxic symptoms at below therapeutic range.
- Hyperkalemia is often seen in massive overdoses and results from extracellular redistribution of potassium because of inhibition of the Na^+K^+ATPase pump.

IMAGING STUDIES

N/A

SPECIAL TESTS

N/A

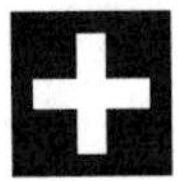

Treatment

GENERAL MEASURES

The key to successful treatment of digoxin toxicity is early recognition that an arrhythmia or other signs and symptoms may be related to intoxication.

- Supportive Care
  —Minor ECG changes (first-degree AV block, accelerated AV junctional pacemaker, atrial fibrillation with slow ventricular response, ectopy) can be treated by temporary discontinuation of the drug, monitoring, and future dose adjustment.
  —Conduction abnormalities (sinus bradycardia, sinus arrest, exit block, and second- and third-degree AV block) may respond to atropine or require temporary cardiac pacing.

—Treat conditions that increase the likelihood of digitalis intoxication: myocardial ischemia, hypovolemia, hypoxemia, acidosis, renal impairment.
—Activated charcoal within 4 hours of overdose may be very effective.
- Electrolyte management
  —Hypokalemia: Potassium levels should be kept >4 mM/L. Potassium supplementation even in the setting of normal serum potassium is useful for atrial and AV junctional or ectopic rhythms. Parenteral potassium may be beneficial for severe arrhythmias such as VT but should only be given under close monitoring.
  —Hyperkalemia: Associated with a worse prognosis and can precipitate complete heart block. May be an indication for digoxin-specific Fab antibody fragments.
  —Hypocalcemia: Calcium supplementation should be avoided because it may act to increase automaticity and predispose to life-threatening ventricular arrhythmias.
- Antiarrhythmics
  —Lidocaine or phenytoin may be beneficial for suppressing life-threatening arrhythmias. Both have little or no adverse effect on cardiac conduction.
  —Quinidine and procainamide should be avoided due to their suppression of AV conduction and proarrhythmic effects.
- Electrical cardioversion
  —Great caution should be used in treating atrial and ventricular arrhythmias with direct current cardioversion due to the increased sensitivity of the digoxin toxic myocardium, and the propensity to develop further arrhythmias.
- Hemodialysis is ineffective in the treatment of digoxin toxicity.

SURGICAL MEASURES

N/A

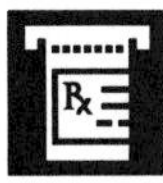

Medications

DRUG(S) OF CHOICE

Digoxin-Specific Fab Antibody Fragments

- Most effective treatment available
- High affinity and specificity for cardiac glycosides; have been shown to reverse digoxin toxicity and reduce the risk of death.
- 80% will have complete resolution, 10% improve, and 10% may not respond
- Indications:
  —Ventricular tachyarrhythmias
  —Symptomatic bradycardia, second- or third-degree AV block
  —Progressive hyperkalemia
  —Serum level >10 ng/mL
  —Total ingestion >10 mg
- Dosage: Each 40-mg vial of Fab fragment neutralizes 0.6 mg of digoxin. Determine "drug load" of digoxin using either plasma concentration or amount ingested.
  —Drug load = [serum level (ng/mL) × volume of distribution (5.6 L/kg) × weight (kg)]/1000 or
  —Drug load = amount ingested (mg) × digoxin bioavailability (0.8)
  —Fab dose (mg) = drug load (mg) × 64 (based on equimolar dose of Fab [MW = 50 daltons] to digoxin [MW = 781 daltons]
- Dose should be infused over 15–30 minutes.
- Improvement in signs and symptoms occur within 40 minutes.
- Digoxin-Fab fragment complexes are cleared from the system via renal excretion.
- Total serum digoxin levels are no longer meaningful following administration of Fab fragments, but free digoxin levels may be obtained and can be helpful.
- Common adverse side effects include hypokalemia and exacerbation of CHF.
- Anaphylaxis, serum sickness, and febrile reactions are potential complications, especially with repeated administrations.

ADMISSION/DISCHARGE CRITERIA

- Most patients with clinical signs or symptoms of digoxin intoxication should be admitted to the hospital.
- They should be closely monitored for arrhythmia until the symptoms of toxicity have resolved and serum digoxin concentrations are in the therapeutic range.

Follow-up

PATIENT MONITORING

- Cardiac monitoring should be considered and intensive care may be required in all patients with signs and symptoms of digoxin intoxication or in suspected overdose cases.
- In cases where cardiac toxicity is limited to ectopic beats or first-degree AV block, temporary drug withdrawal may be all that is needed.

EXPECTED COURSE AND PROGNOSIS

Several factors have been associated with a worse prognosis and higher overall mortality.

- Elderly
- Male
- Underlying heart disease
- Hyperkalemia

PATIENT EDUCATION

Prevention of digoxin toxicity is enhanced by taking the following measures:

- Discuss and emphasize the importance of proper dosing with patients.
- Awareness of drug-drug interactions
- Avoid use of drug in high-risk patients.
- Consider digitoxin, which is metabolized by the liver, in patients with renal disease.

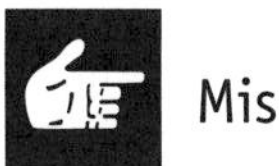

Miscellaneous

ICD-9-CM

972.1

BIBLIOGRAPHY

Kelly RA, Smith TW. Recognition and management of digitalis toxicity. *Am J Cardiol* 1992; 69:1086–1196.

Borron SW, Bismuth C, Muszynski J. Advances in the management of digoxin toxicity in the older patient. *Drugs Aging* 1777;10:18–33.

Hauptman PJ, Kelly RA. Digitalis. *Circulation* 1999;99:1265–1270.

Author: Jarvis W. Lambert

Ehlers-Danlos Syndrome and the Heart

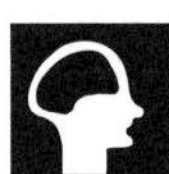

Basics

DESCRIPTION

Ehlers-Danlos syndrome (EDS) is a heterogeneous group of heritable connective tissue disorders characterized by varying degrees of skin elasticity, joint hyperextensibility, and cutaneous fragility classified as types I to X.

- Cardiovascular (CV) manifestations (based mainly on case reports of types I–IV, with little prospective survey data):
  - —Aortic dilatation (more common in Marfan's syndrome)
  - —Bicuspid aortic valve
  - —Pulmonic root dilatation
  - —Pulmonic stenosis
  - —Mitral valve prolapse (MVP)
  - —Tricuspid valve prolapse
  - —Ventricular or atrial septal defects
  - —Sinus of Valsalva ectasia or aneurysm
  - —Myocardial infarction due to coronary artery dissection (rare)
  - —Type I and especially type IV: spontaneous rupture of large/medium-sized arteries and viscera (e.g., gravid uterus)
- Cardiac manifestations are less common and peripheral vascular effects are more common in type IV EDS, presumably due to the paucity of type III collagen in the heart.
- CV effects may be present in the absence of obvious external manifestations of EDS.

Systems Affected

- Cardiovascular (including peripheral vasculature), skin, visceral organs

ETIOLOGY

Genetics

The most common EDS types are autosomal dominant/recessive; few, rare types are sex-linked. The pattern of CV effects is unknown.

Incidence/Prevalence

In the United States:

- EDS occurs in 1/5,000 births, types I–III are most common (90%).
- In one series, the presence of congenital CV manifestations in a hospitalized population was as high as 47%.
- Prevalence in the general population is unknown.

Predominant Age

- Congenital to adult

PREGNANCY

Women with Ehlers-Danlos type IV are of increased risk of vascular rupture and, therefore, pregnancy may be hazardous. Careful consideration and counseling are warranted.

CAUSES

EDS type IV is due to a defect of type III collagen. Underlying biochemical defects of other types are unknown.

RISK FACTORS

N/A

Diagnosis

DIFFERENTIAL DIAGNOSIS

Similar aortic vessel and aortic valve disease may be observed in Marfan's syndrome. In cases of congenital heart disease or great vessel dilatation, consider EDS.

SIGNS AND SYMPTOMS

- Asymptomatic to acute CV decompensation from structural heart disease or arterial/visceral rupture
- Severe cases may have hemorrhage leading to death.
- The most common presentations are referable to underlying valvulopathy or shunt, with chest pain, dyspnea, and/or congestive heart failure.
- Severe valvulopathy (e.g., mitral regurgitation, aortic insufficiency) and aortic dissection have been reported.

LABORATORY PROCEDURES

Molecular techniques may identify collagen defects, although these tests are not routinely available. In general, diagnostic biochemical tests are unavailable.

PATHOLOGIC FINDINGS

- As for the particular lesions noted above

SPECIAL TESTS

- No pathognomonic findings for ECG are described.
- Conduction delays, chamber hypertrophy, etc., secondary to cardiac structural defects have been described.

IMAGING STUDIES

- Echocardiography may reveal findings characteristic of the lesions mentioned above, including valvular abnormalities.
- Structural and functional chamber abnormalities associated with these particular valvulopathies also may be seen.
- Progression of disease may be followed by echocardiography or nuclear cardiography.

DIAGNOSTIC PROCEDURES

Cardiac catheterization may be indicated for evaluating valvular disease or for preoperative or medical management. Peripheral vascular lesions may require angiography in some cases (e.g., for preoperative management).

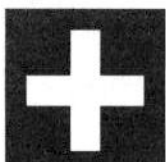

Treatment

GENERAL MEASURES

- Screening echocardiography for patients with EDS, particularly types I and II
- Appropriate antibiotic prophylaxis for valvular disease (e.g., MVP)
- Especially in patients with EDS types I and IV, who are at risk for spontaneous rupture of blood vessels and viscera
  - —Avoid contact sports and heavy physical activity.
  - —Handle invasive procedures with care due to the risk of scar formation, bleeding, dissection, and arterial rupture.
  - —Administer anticoagulants (including antiplatelet agents) cautiously.
  - —Avoid intramuscular and intravenous therapies if possible.
  - —Control hypertension.

SURGICAL MEASURES

- Often met with unsatisfying results, surgical therapy is directed toward valvular replacement or repair of arterial dissection or rupture.
- Although successful aortic valve replacements have been reported, surgery is complicated by variable wound healing and widened scars, wound dehiscence, and failure of tissue-graft unions.
- Bleeding may be excessive.

ADMISSION/DISCHARGE CRITERIA

Asymptomatic or mildly symptomatic CV abnormalities may be evaluated on an outpatient basis. Hemodynamic instability should be evaluated and treated emergently.

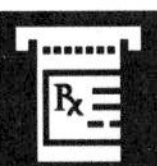

Medications

DRUG(S) OF CHOICE

Vitamin C, despite its importance in collagen synthesis, has little efficacy in the treatment of EDS.

Precautions

- Antiplatelet therapy as above

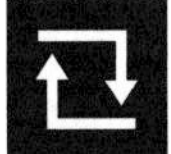

Follow-up

PATIENT MONITORING

- Objective evaluation of cardiac function, either with echocardiography or nuclear cardiography
- Referring a patient for surgery should follow conventional guidelines for treatment of valvular abnormalities, while considering the patient's clinical status and symptoms.
- Potential for progression of CV abnormalities, especially in cases of congenital abnormalities, is an important factor, weighed against the risks of surgery in EDS.

Activity

Some patients with EDS should avoid strenuous activity or contact sports.

EXPECTED COURSE AND PROGNOSIS

Variable.

- Those with EDS type IV have a shorter life expectancy, usually surviving to only the fourth decade, due to the catastrophic nature of their CV abnormalities.

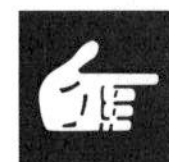

Miscellaneous

ICD-9-CM

756.83 Ehlers-Danlos syndrome

See also: Marfan's syndrome

PATIENT EDUCATION

Organizations

- Ehlers Danlos National Foundation, 6399 Wilshire Blvd., Suite 510, Los Angeles, CA 90048; (323)651-3038; http://www.ednf.org/ The Foundation publishes a quarterly newsletter, *Loose Connections.*
- National Institute of Arthritis & Musculoskeletal & Skin Diseases, Building 31, Room 4C05, Bethesda, MD 20892-2350; (301)496-8188; http://www.nih.gov/niams/

BIBLIOGRAPHY

Ades LC, et al. Myocardial infarction resulting from coronary artery dissection in an adolescent with Ehlers-Danlos syndrome type IV due to a type III collagen mutation. *Br Heart J* 1995;74:112–116.

Antani J, Srinivas HV. Ehlers-Danlos syndrome and cardiovascular abnormalities. *Chest* 1973; 63:214–272.

Dolan AL, et al. Clinical and echocardiographic survey of the Ehlers-Danlos syndrome. *Br J Rheumatol* 1997;36:459–462.

Leier CV, et al. The spectrum of cardiac defects in the Ehlers-Danlos syndrome, types I and III. *Ann Intern Med* 1980;92:171–178.

Pyeritz RE. Cardiovascular manifestations of the heritable disorders of connective tissue. *Prog Med Genet* 1983;5:191–301.

Shohet I, et al. Cardiovascular complications in the Ehlers-Danlos syndrome with minimal external findings. *Clin Genet* 1987;3:148–152.

Steinmann B, et al. *Connective tissue and its heritable disorders.* New York: Wiley-Liss, 1993:351–407.

Author: James A. Kong

Eisenmenger Syndrome

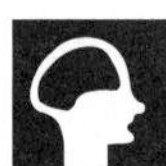

Basics

DESCRIPTION

- Pulmonary vascular obstructive disease secondary to congenital heart disease (i.e., Eisenmenger syndrome) develops after a period of left-to-right shunting with increased pulmonary flow and elevated pulmonary pressure.
- Shear stress on pulmonary arterioles creates medical and intimal proliferation and increasing pulmonary vascular obstruction.

Systems Affected

- Cardiovascular

ETIOLOGY

Genetics

Although there are no genetic data for Eisenmenger syndrome, an immunogenetic predisposition is suggested by HLA typing and an increased incidence of autoimmune abnormalities in Eisenmenger syndrome patients.

- The Eisenmenger physiology begins in infancy in patients with posttricuspid defects: ventricular septal defects of all types, single ventricles, and aortopulmonary communications (patent ductus arteriosus, aortopulmonary windows, and large surgical shunts).
- It is uncommon in patients with pretricuspid defects (e.g., atrial septal defects of all types, sinus venosus defects, common atrium), but when it occurs, it does so most often during adult life.

Incidence/Prevalence

In the United States:

- Maximal estimate of incidence of pulmonary vascular obstructive disease in uncorrected congenital heart disease is 32%.
- The incidence is approximately equal in males and females for posttricuspid defects. When the disease occurs in adults, there appears to be an increased incidence among female patients, with Eisenmenger syndrome associated with an atrial septal defect (similar to the increased incidence in females with primary pulmonary hypertension).
- Although pulmonary vascular obstructive disease has been reported in children under 2 years of age with posttricuspid defects, it is uncommon except with Down syndrome and certain cyanotic heart diseases associated with pulmonary arterial hypertension (e.g., truncus arteriosus, transposition of the great vessels-ventricular septal defect, etc.).

Predominant Sex

- More females than males

RISK FACTORS

- High altitude
- Complicated neonatal history (e.g., spontaneous pneumothorax) may trigger maintenance of high pulmonary vascular tone after birth.
- Family history of pulmonary vascular disease
- Autoimmune abnormalities (possibly)

PREGNANCY

- Pregnancy is associated with significant risk to fetus and mother. Spontaneous abortion occurs in 20%–40%, premature delivery in 50%, and term delivery in only 25%. At least 30% of infants have intrauterine growth retardation; 8%–28% die perinatally. The maternal mortality rate is 45%.
- Pregnant patients with the Eisenmenger syndrome should be advised to have an elective abortion without delay.

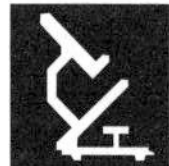

Diagnosis

DIFFERENTIAL DIAGNOSIS

- Precapillary pulmonary vascular disease
  - —Lung disease
  - —Collagen vascular disorders
  - —Chronic thromboembolic disease
  - —Primary pulmonary hypertension (including portal hypertension, HIV infection, and toxin/drug exposure)
- Postcapillary pulmonary vascular disease (e.g., pulmonary venous hypertension)
  - —Left-sided heart disease (e.g., pulmonary venous obstruction)
  - —Cor triatriatum
  - —Mitral stenosis
  - —Left ventricular dysfunction

SIGNS AND SYMPTOMS

- Natural history
  - —Failure to thrive and congestive heart failure (due to large left-to-right shunt) spontaneously improves as pulmonary vascular resistance increases.
- Most common signs and symptoms
  - —Exercise intolerance
  - —Syncope
  - —Chest pain
  - —Hemoptysis
  - —Congestive heart failure
  - —Squatting
  - —Central cyanosis
  - —Digital clubbing
- Other signs and symptoms
  - —Normal jugular venous pressure
  - —Normal or small peripheral arterial pulse pressure
  - —Right ventricular lift
  - —Increased pulmonary closure with variable splitting of the second heart sound
  - —Pulmonary ejection click
  - —Pulmonary ejection murmur or left sternal border systolic murmur
  - —High-pitched protodiastolic murmurs of pulmonary valve insufficiency at the left sternal border
  - —Third heart sound

LABORATORY STUDIES

- Hemoglobin normal to increased

PATHOLOGIC FINDINGS

- Progressive pulmonary vascular changes (Heath-Edwards classification grade I–VI)
  - —Medial hypertrophy
  - —Intimal proliferation
  - —Intimal fibrosis
  - —Plexiform lesions
  - —Dilatation lesions
  - —Necrotizing arteritis

IMAGING STUDIES

- ECG
  - —Right axis deviation
  - —Right ventricular hypertrophy with or without strain
- Chest x-ray
  - —Right ventricular enlargement on lateral projection
  - —Enlarged central pulmonary arteries
  - —Normal to decreased pulmonary vascular markings peripherally.

SPECIAL TESTS

- Echocardiography (2-D)
  - —Normal to decreased right ventricular function
  - —Dilated right heart
  - —Right ventricular hypertrophy
  - —Flattened to posterior bowing of the interventricular and interatrial septae
  - —Bidirectional shunting or right-to-left shunting via defects
- Cardiac catheterization
  - —Increased pulmonary vascular resistance
  - —Pulmonary arterial hypertension
  - —Bidirectional shunt or right-to-left shunt via the pretricuspid or posttricuspid defects

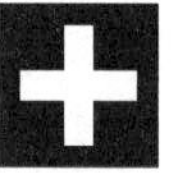

Treatment

SURGICAL MEASURES

- Prevention: early correction in infancy of unrestrictive ventricular septal defect(s) or other posttricuspid communications
- "Corrective cardiac surgery" in older children and adults if pulmonary vasoreactivity is demonstrated with acute vasodilator drug testing, e.g. inhaled citric oxide, intravenous prostacyclin, i.v. adenosine
  - —If a patient with elevated pulmonary vascular resistance is considered for surgery, with the increased risk of postoperative pulmonary hypertensive crises, short-term pulmonary vasodilator therapy (e.g., inhaled nitric oxide or prostacyclin) in the perioperative pe-

riod may be needed to treat acute pulmonary hypertensive crises.
—Consideration of creating a "palliative atrial septal defect" during corrective cardiac surgery also may be indicated.

- Palliative atrial septostomy may be helpful in selected patients with advanced pulmonary vascular obstructive disease, intractable right heart failure, and/or recurrent syncope who previously underwent surgical repair of their congenital heart defects.
- Transplantation
  —Heart/lung, single lung, bilateral lung, and living related lung transplantation have all been performed successfully for patients with pulmonary vascular disease, although the long-term outlook remains unknown with 1-, 3-, and 5-year survival rates with lung transplantation for pulmonary vascular disease currently 64%, 56%, and 48%, respectively (United Network of Organ Sharing 1998).

GENERAL MEASURES

- Aggressive antibiotic therapy for significant upper respiratory tract infections
- Antipyretic therapy for febrile illnesses
- Dietary and/or medical therapy for constipation to prevent Valsalva maneuvers from precipitating abrupt decreases in cardiac output
- Yearly flu vaccine and pneumonia vaccine as indicated
- Supplemental oxygen with airplane flying to prevent alveolar hypoxia from exacerbating the underlying pulmonary vascular disease by hypoxic pulmonary vasoconstriction

Precautions

- Avoidance of circumstances or substances that may aggravate the pulmonary vascular disease, e.g., exercise should be guided by symptoms and exposure to high altitude may worsen pulmonary arterial hypertension by producing hypoxic-induced pulmonary vasoconstriction due to alveolar hypoxia
- Dehydration (e.g., from physical activity, environmental effects, diarrhea, etc.) can precipitate a significant decrease in cardiac output and should be prevented or treated if it occurs.
- Although airplane travel is generally safe, supplemental oxygen therapy may be advisable. Pregnancy, oral contraceptives, and appetite suppressants should be avoided.
- Patients with Eisenmenger syndrome who become pregnant are at increased risk of sudden death both within the course of delivery and immediately postpartum.
- Phlebotomy with replacement of fluid (e.g., plasma or albumin) is helpful in cyanotic congenital heart disease in which severe hypoxemia has evoked a large increase in red blood cell mass. Caution is required to avoid depletion of iron stores and to avoid reduction of the circulating blood volume.

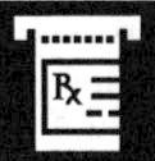

Medications

DRUG(S) OF CHOICE

- Oxygen/digitalis/diuretics
  —Supplemental oxygen with sleep may slow the progression of polycythemia; ambulatory supplemental oxygen may improve exercise capacity.
  —Digitalis and diuretics may be beneficial for patients with severe right ventricular failure, although excessive diuresis can lead to a decrease in cardiac output in patients who are highly preload dependent.
- Anticoagulation
  —Anticoagulation has been demonstrated to improve survival in patients with primary pulmonary hypertension, although its usefulness in patients with Eisenmenger syndrome is unknown.
- Vasodilator therapy
  —Although chronic vasodilator therapy (e.g., oral calcium channel blockade or intravenous prostacyclin) has been shown to improve quality of life, hemodynamics, exercise capacity, and survival in patients with primary pulmonary hypertension, its long-term effects in patients with Eisenmenger syndrome is unknown.

Follow-up

PATIENT MONITORING

- Close regular visits for assessment of signs/symptoms to serially optimize chronic medical/surgical therapeutic regimen

EXPECTED COURSE AND PROGNOSIS

- The natural history of Eisenmenger syndrome demonstrates a wide spectrum of variability, although the overall survival is significantly better than with primary pulmonary hypertension.
- This wide variability suggests that the immunogenetic predisposition demonstrated in primary pulmonary hypertension also may play a significant role in the development of Eisenmenger syndrome.
- Overall 80% 5-year and 40% 20-year survival rates have been reported with Eisenmenger syndrome versus a 2- to 3-year mean survival after diagnosis in primary pulmonary hypertension.
- This underscores the need to individualize therapeutic options for patients based on risk/benefit considerations of the various therapeutic modalities currently available.

PATIENT EDUCATION

Organization

- Pulmonary Hypertension Association, P.O. Box 463 Ambler, PA 19002; phone: 1-800-748-7274

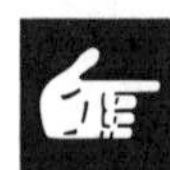

Miscellaneous

ICD-9-CM

416.0 Primary pulmonary hypertension

BIBLIOGRAPHY

Barst RJ. Recent advances in the treatment of pulmonary artery hypertension. *Pediatr Clin North Am* 1999;46:331–345.

Barst RJ. Clinical management of patients with pulmonary hypertension. In: Allen HD, Gutgesell HP, Clark EB, et al., eds. Moss and Adams' heart disease in infants, children and adolescents, 6th ed. Baltimore: Lippincott Williams & Wilkins, 2001.

O'Fallon WM, Weidman WH, eds. Long-term follow-up of congenital aortic stenosis, pulmonary stenosis and ventricular septal defect—report from the Second Joint Study on the Natural History of Congenital Heart Defects. *Circulation* 1993;87(suppl):1–126.

Wood P. The Eisenmenger syndrome or pulmonary hypertension with reversed central shunt. *BMJ* 1958;2:701–709, 755–762.

Young D, Mark H. Fate of the patient with Eisenmenger syndrome. *Am J Cardiol* 1971;28:658–669.

Authors: Robyn J. Barst and Welton M. Gersony

Endocardial Cushion Defects

Basics

DESCRIPTION

Atrioventricular (AV) canal defects include a spectrum of anomalies caused by maldevelopment of the endocardial cushions.

- Three major potential hemodynamic disturbances contribute to the pathophysiology, natural history, and medical and surgical management of these lesions.
- The relative effects of interatrial shunting, interventricular shunting, and AV valve function will determine the general course of patients with uncomplicated AV canal defects.
- The term *complete atrioventricular canal defect* refers to a heart with both significant ventricular and atrial components, whereas *partial atrioventricular canal defect* refers to a predominant primum atrial defect, cleft mitral valve, or restrictive or no ventricular shunting.
- *Unbalanced canal defect* refers to hearts with a right or left dominant ventricle.
- These are often associated with hypoplasia or atresia of one side of the common AV valve.

EPIDEMIOLOGY

- AV canal defects occur in 4%–5% of patients diagnosed with congenital heart disease.
- Among patients with Down's syndrome, 40%–50% will have congenital heart disease, and among those, approximately 40% will have AV canal defects.

ETIOLOGY

Genetics

- Complex AV canal defects with hypoplasia of one ventricle and/or variable degrees of pulmonic stenosis are associated with heterotaxy syndromes.
- Families in which several members had AV canal defects not associated with trisomy 21 have been described.

RISK FACTORS

N/A

PREGNANCY

- Fetal diagnosis of AV canal defects is readily made on the four-chamber view of the fetal heart alone.
- Identifying features include absence of primum atrial septum, loss of the offsetting of the mitral valve above the tricuspid valve at the crux of the heart, and an inlet ventricular septal defect.
- The relative size of the atrial and ventricular septal defects, the size of the left and right ventricles, and the degree of AV valve insufficiency, if any, should be specifically evaluated.
- Currently, no specific *in utero* management other than prenatal counseling is available for this diagnosis.

ASSOCIATED CONDITIONS

Associated cardiac anomalies include straddling, stenosis, or atresia of part of the AV valve, often associated with hypoplasia of a ventricular chamber. Occasionally, complete AV canal defects are seen in combination with tetralogy of Fallot.

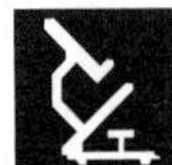

Diagnosis

DIFFERENTIAL DIAGNOSIS

- Patients with mainly atrial shunting may present similarly to patients with isolated secundum atrial septal defects.
- If a restrictive ventricular septal defect is present, a left sternal border pansystolic murmur may be dominant, suggesting an isolated ventricular septal defect.
- Complete AV canal defects may present similarly to moderate to large ventricular septal defects.

SIGNS AND SYMPTOMS

- Patients with mainly atrial shunting are generally recognized following detection of a cardiac murmur on routine pediatric evaluation.
- The examination is similar to that noted in patients with isolated secundum atrial septal defects (systolic pulmonic flow murmur with fixed wide splitting of S2), often with the additional finding of an apical blowing systolic murmur of mitral regurgitation.
- A low-pitched diastolic rumble may be appreciated at the mitral area. Patients with complete AV canal defects are usually symptomatic by 4–6 weeks of life.
- Those noted to have earlier signs of congestive heart failure in the first or second week often have significant AV valve regurgitation.
- This occurs in up to 20% of patients. Failure-to-thrive tachypnea, tachycardia, and poor feeding are common presenting symptoms.
- Physical examination also may reveal a pulmonary flow murmur, fixed splitting of the S2, a blowing systolic murmur of AV valve regurgitation, and often a mid-diastolic low-pitched rumble.
- When the ventricular septal defect is unrestrictive, it often does not generate a prominent separate systolic murmur.

LABORATORY PROCEDURES

The ECG usually shows a right ventricular conduction delay pattern, and PR interval prolongation may be present. A left superior QRS axis is almost always noted.

IMAGING STUDIES

- The diagnosis of all variants is readily confirmed on 2-D echocardiography.
- Occasionally, a dilated coronary sinus secondary to a left superior vena cava can be identified incorrectly as a primum atrial septal defect.
- Careful visualization of the intact primum septum (anterior to the coronary sinus) and tracing of the course of the left superior vena caval connection help differentiate this possibility.
- Color flow Doppler is helpful in estimating the degree of mitral regurgitation.
- Searching for evidence of increased right ventricular pressure (ventricular hypertrophy, septal orientation, and Doppler estimation of pressure on the basis of tricuspid regurgitation) is important in the echocardiographic assessment of these defects.
- In complete AV canal defects, attention should be directed to the morphology and attachments of the AV valve leaflets, and estimating the sizes of the right and left ventricles.
- These observations are important in determining the type of surgical management.

SPECIAL TESTS

Generally, cardiac catheterization is unnecessary in uncomplicated cases, unless pulmonary vascular disease or associated cardiac lesions such as tetralogy of Fallot are suspected.

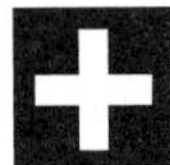

Treatment

GENERAL MEASURES

- Medical intervention in the form of inotropes, afterload reduction, or diuretics are usually not indicated in the group of asymptomatic patients with partial AV canal defects.
- Endocarditis prophylaxis is required in the presence of AV valve regurgitation.
- Most patients with complete AV canal defects require inotropic and diuretic therapy in the first weeks to months of life to control symptoms of congestive heart failure and improve feeding intake and weight gain.
- Often it is difficult to determine the primary cause of poor feeding in the setting of patients with Down's syndrome who may be feeding poorly because of noncardiac issues despite optimal medical management.

SURGICAL MEASURES

- Surgical repair in partial AV canal patients is indicated when there is a clear-cut defect identified and clinical or echocardiographic evidence of cardiac chamber dilatation.
- The timing of repair is elective and similar to that for closure of isolated secundum atrial septal defects.
- The majority of defects should be closed by 2–5 years of age.
- Patients with trivial defects can be followed medically.
- Surgical repair in complete AV canal patients is indicated in the setting of severe symptoms resistant to medical therapy or failure to thrive.
- Patients who are well controlled with adequate weight gain on medical therapy nevertheless should undergo complete repair prior to 4 or 5 months of age to avoid irreversible pulmonary vascular disease.
- Relatively early repair is particularly important in the large subgroup of patients with Down's syndrome.
- This group has been shown to have a greater degree of elevation of pulmonary vascular resistance in the first year of life and may have more rapid progression to fixed pulmonary obstructive disease than children with normal chromosomes.

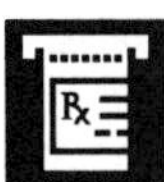

Medications

DRUG(S) OF CHOICE

Early management involves close observation until signs of congestive heart failure appear, when digoxin and diuretic therapy will most likely be necessary to control symptoms.

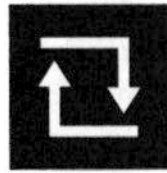

Follow-up

PATIENT MONITORING

- Close regular visits for assessment of adequacy of weight gain and or signs of congestive heart failure

EXPECTED COURSE AND PROGNOSIS

- Results of surgical repair of primum atrial septal defects and partial AV canal defects have been excellent, with a mortality rate of <1% and a reoperation rate of <3%.
- Late death after surgery is rare, reported in 0%–4% of patients.
- The overall long-term survival of patients with primum atrial septal defect following repair was found to match that of the general population.
- Residual interatrial communication rarely occurs.
- Left AV valve regurgitation is the major cause of late morbidity in all forms of AV canal defects.
- In partial canal repair follow-up studies, the incidence of significant regurgitation requiring reoperation ranges from 7% to 10% of patients.
- Subaortic stenosis is noted in fewer than 5% of postoperative patients.
- The early postoperative mortality rate following repair of complete AV canal defects has been reduced from approximately 20% to 25% in the past to 3%–4% in the current era.
- Strong risk factors for early death included postoperative pulmonary hypertensive crisis, immediate postoperative severe left AV regurgitation, and double-orifice left AV valve.
- Improved surgical skills, postoperative care of small infants, and management of perioperative pulmonary hypertension are undoubtedly responsible for the notable decline in early mortality.
- Intraoperative transesophageal echocardiography has been noted to favorably alter surgical treatment in some patients by detecting inadequate repair in the operating room.
- Heart block, residual ventricular septal defect, left ventricular outflow tract obstruction, and mitral valve dysfunction are potential long-term complications that must be considered in patients following repair of complete AV canal defects.
- Although heart block and residual ventricular septal defect are uncommon in the current era, left ventricular outflow tract obstruction and mitral insufficiency continue to be significant long-term issues.
- Persistent elevation of pulmonary vascular resistance may be an issue in some patients, especially if surgical correction was delayed, or pulmonary vascular resistance was marginal at the time of surgery.
- Reoperation for residual mitral regurgitation, recently has been reported at rates varying from 2% to 10%.

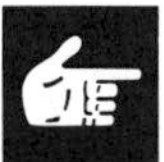

Miscellaneous

BIBLIOGRAPHY

Castaneda AR, Jonas RA, Mayer JE, et al. Atrioventricular canal defects. In: *Cardiac surgery of the neonate and infant.* Philadelphia; WB Saunders, 1994:167–186.

Feldt RH, Porter CJ, Edwards WD, et al. Atrioventricular septal defects. In: Adams FH, Emanouilides GC, Riemenschneider TA, et al. *Heart disease in infants, children and adolescents.* Baltimore: William & Wilkins, 1989:704–723.

Kirklin JW, Barrat-Boyes BG. Atrioventricular canal defect. In: *Cardiac surgery.* New York: Churchill Livingston, 1993:693–749.

Laks H, Pearl JM. Primum atrial septal defect. *Semin Thorac Cardiovasc Surg* 1997;9:2–7.

Pearl JM, Laks H. Intermediate and complete forms of atrioventricular canal. *Semin Thorac Cardiovasc Surg* 1997;9:8–20.

Permut LC, Mehta V. Later results and reoperation after repair of complete and partial atrioventricular canal defect. *Semin Thorac Cardiovasc Surg* 1997;9:44–54.

Authors: Howard D. Apfel and Welton M. Gersony

Endocarditis

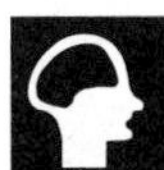

Basics

DESCRIPTION

Endocarditis is a disease caused by a microbial infection of the endothelial lining of the heart. Vegetations are characteristic, with involvement of heart valves and possibly endocardium. Endocarditis is classified by several definitions:

- Acute bacterial endocarditis (ABE): aggressive course usually caused by highly virulent organisms such as *Staphylococcus aureus* with diagnosis usually made in less than 2 weeks; often affects normal heart valves
- Subacute bacterial endocarditis (SBE): indolent course over weeks to months caused by low virulence organisms such as viridans streptococci; usually develops on previously abnormal valves
- Early prosthetic valve endocarditis (PVE): infection of an artificial heart valve within the first 2 months after surgery
- Late prosthetic valve endocarditis: infection 2 months after valve implantation
- Nonbacterial thrombotic endocarditis (NBTE): any endocardial sterile vegetation (wide spectrum of presentations)

EPIDEMIOLOGY

Incidence is estimated at 1.6–6.0 cases/100,000 person-years in developed countries. In intravenous (i.v.) drug users alone the incidence is estimated at 11.6/100,000 person-years.

ETIOLOGY

Most patients who develop infective endocarditis have a preexisting cardiac condition.

- NBTE: Endothelial damage leads to platelet aggregation and deposition with fibrin deposition and development of sterile thrombotic vegetations.
- ABE/SBE: Microbes probably colonize preexisting NBTE or even directly invade endothelium in the case of ABE. Microbial adherence is a crucial factor for selection of organisms that colonize the endocardium.
- Valves normally involved (downstream side of high/low-pressure valves): mitral > aortic > tricuspid > pulmonary
- Valves involved in i.v. drug abusers: tricuspid > mitral = aortic > pulmonary
- Patients secondarily develop embolic phenomena from friability of vegetation and immune complex damage secondary to humoral reaction to bacterial proliferation in vegetation.

Causative Agents

- ABE: *S. aureus, Hemophilus influenzae, Neisseria gonorrhoeae, Streptococcus pneumoniae, Enterococcus* species
- SBE: alpha-hemolytic streptococci (viridans), *Streptococcus bovis* (group D Strep), enterococcal species, HACEK group (*Haemophilus aphrophilus, Actinobacillus actinomycetemcomitans, Cardiobacterium hominis, Eikenella corrodens, Kingella kingae*), *S. aureus*
- Early PVE: *S. aureus, Staphylococcus epidermidis,* gram-negative rods, *Aspergillus* species
- Late PVE: alpha-hemolytic streptococci (viridans), enterococcal species, *S. epidermidis, Aspergillus* species
- Intravenous drug abusers: *S. aureus, Pseudomonas aeruginosa,* other gram-negative rods, enterococcal species, *Candida* species

RISK FACTORS

Conditions predisposing to development of endocarditis:

- High risk: prosthetic heart valves, previous endocarditis, cyanotic congenital heart disease, preexisting rheumatic heart disease, acquired valvular disease, aortic valve disease, mitral regurgitation with or without stenosis, ventricular septal defect, patent ductus arteriosus, coarctation of aorta
- Intermediate risk: mitral valve prolapse with regurgitation, pure mitral stenosis, tricuspid disease, pulmonary valve disease, asymmetric septal hypertrophy, degenerative valve disease, intracardiac prosthetic implants (nonvalvular), intracardiac catheters
- Other factors: i.v. drug abuse, arteriovenous shunt for hemodialysis, creation of persistent portals of entry (wounds, catheters), perinatal infective complications

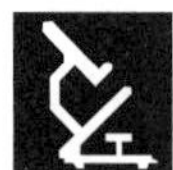

Diagnosis

DIFFERENTIAL DIAGNOSIS

Pneumonia, pleurisy, meningitis, brain abscess, stroke, malaria, acute pericarditis, vasculitis, disseminated intravascular coagulation, rheumatic fever, osteomyelitis, tuberculosis, intraabdominal infection, glomerulonephritis, salmonellosis, brucellosis, myocardial infarction, atrial myxoma, occult malignancies, septic pulmonary infarction, fever of unknown origin

SIGNS AND SYMPTOMS

- Fever (low-grade or severe if acute)
- Chills, rigors, night sweats
- Pallor, malaise, anorexia, weight loss
- New or prominent murmur (also may be absent)
- Myalgias, arthralgias, back pain
- Focal neurologic signs (embolic phenomenon or meningeal reaction)
- Delirium or headache
- Chest pain, dyspnea, cough, hemoptysis
- Flank pain, hematuria, left upper quadrant pain (evidence of distal emboli or immune complex glomerulonephritis)
- Cold painful extremity
- Splenomegaly
- Petechiae (Roth's spots if retinal)
- Osler's nodes (tender erythematous extremity nodules)
- Janeway lesions (flat nontender red spots)
- Splinter hemorrhages (linear, subungual)
- Clubbing of digits
- Rales, gallops

Diagnostic Criteria

Duke Endocarditis Service Criteria for diagnosis of infective endocarditis: two major criteria, or one major and three minor criteria, or five minor criteria

Major Criteria

- Typical microorganism for infective endocarditis from two separate blood cultures (viridans strep, strep bovis, HACEK group, community-acquired *S. aureus,* or enterococci in absence of primary focus), or persistently positive blood culture, defined as recovery of a microorganism consistent with infective endocarditis from blood cultures drawn more than 12 hours apart, or all or a majority of four positive with first and last drawn 1 hour apart
- Positive echocardiogram for infective endocarditis
  - —Oscillating intracardiac mass, on valve or supporting structures, or in the path of regurgitant jet or on implanted material, in the absence of an alternative anatomic explanation, or abscess, or new partial dehiscence or prosthetic valve, or new valvular regurgitation (increase or change in preexisting murmur not sufficient)

Minor Criteria

- Predisposing heart conditions or i.v. drug use
- Fever (>38.0°C)
- Vascular phenomena: major arterial emboli, septic pulmonary infarcts, mycotic aneurysm, intracranial hemorrhage, conjunctival hemorrhages, Janeway lesions
- Immunologic phenomena: glomerulonephritis, Osler's nodes, Roth's spots, rheumatoid factor
- Microbiologic evidence: positive blood culture but not meeting major criterion as previously defined or serologic evidence of active infection with organism consistent with infective endocarditis
- Echocardiogram: consistent with infective endocarditis but not meeting major criterion as previously defined

LABORATORY PROCEDURES

- Blood cultures (draw three separate samples first day)
- Complete blood count (anemia and leukocytosis possible)
- Elevated erythrocyte sedimentation rate in 90%
- Elevated C-reactive protein
- Urinalysis (microscopic hematuria in 50%)
- Rheumatoid factor positive in 35%–50% of SBE
- Special serology tests (*Coxiella, Bartonella*)

IMAGING STUDIES

- Echocardiography crucial for diagnosis
- Transthoracic echo with color flow Doppler sensitivity for detection of vegetation is 60%–75%.
- Transesophageal echo more sensitive (>95%), especially with mitral involvement, abscesses, valve perforation, rupture of sinus of Valsalva; echo also helpful with ventricular function
- Cardiac catheterization: Depending on age of patient, catheterization may be necessary for coronaries when surgery of valve is considered.
- Radionuclide studies: No technique justified for detection of vegetations
- Chest x-ray: Evaluate for signs of congestive heart failure (CHF), septic emboli, widening of aorta (mycotic aneurysm)

SPECIAL TESTS

ECG: Disturbance of conduction may suggest extension of infection into myocardium from abscess formation. It also may reveal embolic phenomena causing myocardial ischemia.

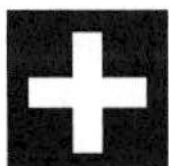

Treatment

GENERAL MEASURES

- Eliminate offending organism as soon as possible.
- Determine if surgical intervention is necessary and when is the best time to perform.
- Treat symptoms (CHF, embolic phenomena, immune complex phenomena).
- Adjust length of treatment to patient's presentation and offending organism (usually 4–6 weeks).

SURGICAL MEASURES

Major Indications

- Moderate or severe heart failure not responding to medical treatment, valvular obstruction, periannular or myocardial abscess, prosthetic valve dehiscence, persistent bacteremia despite appropriate antibiotics, fungal infection

Relative Indications

- Recurrent emboli, staphylococcal and gram-negative infections, persistent fever despite treatment, vegetations enlarging despite treatment

ADMISSION/DISCHARGE CRITERIA

Patients with suspected endocarditis should be hospitalized for i.v. antibiotics with option for home parenteral treatment in selected cases for remainder of duration.

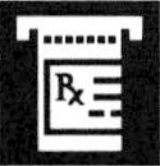

Medications

DRUG(S) OF CHOICE

Antibiotics

- Bactericidal antibiotics are drugs of choice secondary to inadequate host defense within vegetation.
- Be suspicious for emerging drug-resistant organisms.
- Penicillin-sensitive streptococci (viridans): penicillin G 4 million units every 6 hours i.v.
- Penicillin-resistant streptococci: penicillin G 4 million units i.v. every 4 hours plus gentamicin 1.0 mg/kg every 12 hours i.v., or vancomycin 15 mg/kg i.v. every 12 hours
- Enterococci: penicillin G 18–30 million units/day i.v. plus gentamicin 1 mg/kg i.v. every 8 hours, or ampicillin 12 g/day i.v. plus gentamicin 1 mg/kg i.v. every 8 hours, or vancomycin 15 mg/kg i.v. plus gentamicin 1 mg/kg i.v. every 8 hours
- Staphylococci (no prosthetic material): nafcillin 2 g i.v. every 4 hours, or vancomycin 15 mg/kg i.v. every 12 hours if methicillin resistant
- Staphylococci (prosthetic material): nafcillin 2 g i.v. every 4 hours and gentamicin 1.0 mg/kg i.v. every 8 hours, or vancomycin 15 mg/kg i.v. every 12 hours plus gentamicin 1 mg/kg i.v. every 8 hours and rifampin 300 mg orally every 8 hours if methicillin resistant
- HACEK group: ceftriaxone 2 g i.v. once daily
- *P. aeruginosa:* Extended-spectrum penicillin or third-generation cephalosporin or imipenem plus aminoglycoside

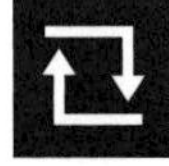

Follow-up

PATIENT MONITORING

Inpatient monitoring and diligent observation if treated as outpatient

EXPECTED COURSE AND PROGNOSIS

- Fatal unless treated; median time from onset of symptoms to death in untreated SBE is 6 months.
- Median time from onset of symptoms to death in untreated ABE is <4 weeks. Adverse prognostic factors include central nervous system complications, CHF, renal failure, culture-negative disease, gram-negative or fungal infection, prosthetic valve infection, and abscesses of myocardium or valve ring.
- Favorable prognostic factors include youth, early diagnosis and treatment, mitral valve prolapse infection, and penicillin-sensitive SBE infection. Rates of cure depend on classification of endocarditis and microbiologic diagnosis, from 98% cure in native valve viridans strep SBE to <1% cure in fungal infection of prosthetic valves.

PATIENT EDUCATION

- Prophylaxis: Most cases of endocarditis are not attributable to an invasive procedure. Determine the risk posed by the preexisting cardiac lesion and inherent risk posed by the procedure itself.
- High risk: Prosthetic heart valves, previous history endocarditis, complex cyanotic congenital heart disease, surgically constructed systemic pulmonary shunts or conduits
- Moderate risk: Most other congenital cardiac malformations, acquired valvar dysfunction, hypertrophic cardiomyopathy, mitral valve prolapse with valvar regurgitation and/or thickened leaflets
- Procedures for which prophylaxis is recommended: Dental procedures with significant bleeding from hard or soft tissues, and surgical procedures involving respiratory, intestinal, or genitourinary mucosa
- Standard general prophylaxis: Amoxicillin 2.0 g orally 1 hour before procedure only

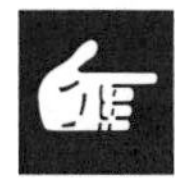

Miscellaneous

ICD-9-CM

421.0 Acute and subacute bacterial endocarditis
421.9 Acute endocarditis, unspecified
424.9 Endocarditis, valve unspecified, unspecified cause

BIBLIOGRAPHY

Alexander RW, et al., eds. *Hurst's the heart,* 9th ed. New York: McGraw-Hill, 1998.

Dajani AS, et al. Prevention of bacterial endocarditis: recommendations by the American Heart Association. *Circulation* 1997;96: 358–366.

Fauci AS, et al., eds. *Harrison's principles of internal medicine,* 14th ed. New York: McGraw-Hill, 1998.

Author: Chandan Devireddy

Eosinophilic Heart Disease

Basics

DESCRIPTION

Patients are occasionally seen with striking eosinophilia and cardiomyopathy.

- The eosinophilia can persist for many years before the cardiomyopathy appears.
- The major cause of death and disability is progressive, restrictive heart disease.
- The contents of the eosinophil can be toxic to many organs, including the heart, but it is not clear if this is the mechanism of cardiac fibrosis.
- In 1936, Löffler recognized the association of eosinophilia, constrictive cardiomyopathy, a thickened endomyocardium, and intraventricular mural thrombus.
  - —This disorder is now considered part of a continuum of disease that has been termed hypereosinophilic syndrome (HES).
  - —More than 75% of patients with HES have severe heart failure.

EPIDEMIOLOGY

- HES tends to occur between the ages of 20 and 50 years.
- Occasionally it occurs in children.
- The incidence is unknown, but hypereosinophilic heart disease is relatively uncommon.
- Multiple organs may be involved.
- Men tend to have more myocardial involvement.

ETIOLOGY

- The mechanism of HES and subsequent organ involvement (including heart) is unknown.
- HES patients develop multiple organ damage.
- The eosinophils may have decreased granules and abnormal cytoplasmic inclusions.
- Eosinophils are attracted to a region of the heart (i.e., the endocardium), apparently in response to foreign antigenic stimulus.
- It is not clear if the eosinophilic contents are actually toxic to the myocardium.
- Clinical picture and underlying pathology differ from acute eosinophilic necrotizing myocarditis and drug-related hypersensitivity myocarditis.
- Extent of organ infiltration does not appear to explain the amount of organ dysfunction.

RISK FACTORS

- None known

PREGNANCY

N/A

ASSOCIATED CONDITIONS

Major organ involvement includes the heart, lungs, gastrointestinal tract, liver, urinary bladder, central and peripheral nervous system, skin, spleen, lymph nodes, and vasculature.

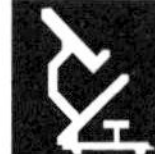

Diagnosis

DIFFERENTIAL DIAGNOSIS

- Patient must have sustained blood eosinophilia $>1{,}500/\text{mm}^3$ present for longer than 6 months.
- The amount of eosinophilia may vary from 20% to 90%.
- Other etiologies for eosinophilia must be absent, including parasitic infections and allergic disease.
- Other restrictive or infiltrative cardiomyopathies such as amyloidosis and sarcoidosis should be excluded.

SIGNS AND SYMPTOMS

- Elevated venous pressure
- Heart is not dilated.
- Mitral and tricuspid regurgitation
- Systemic embolization
- Hepatosplenomegaly
- Dyspnea
- Cough
- Fatigue
- Ascites
- Peripheral edema

LABORATORY PROCEDURES

- Eosinophils may have decreased number of granules and vacuolation of the cytoplasm.
- Anemia and thrombocytopenia may be present.
- Myelodysplastic features such as increased vitamin B_{12} levels, abnormal leukocyte alkaline phosphatase, and cytogenic abnormalities are sometimes present.

IMAGING STUDIES

- An echocardiogram should be performed and will show restricted diastolic filling.
- It will usually demonstrate marked thickening of the walls of both ventricles, a pattern suggestive of infiltrative cardiomyopathy, and mural thrombus.

SPECIAL TESTS

- Electron microscopy of eosinophils is sometimes performed.
  - —Eosinophils have large, round, and homogeneously electron-dense cytoplasmic inclusions.
  - —The inclusions are usually larger than normal, mature granules.

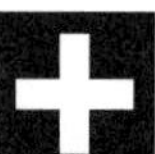

Treatment

GENERAL MEASURES

- Eosinophilic heart disease may be reactive, although some cases of HES are believed to be leukoproliferative.
- Prognosis is poor, with a mean survival from diagnosis of about 9 months.
- Occasionally there is prolonged survival for decades.
- When there is organ involvement such as cardiac disease, a short course of prednisone may sometimes suppress the eosinophilia.
- 38% of patients respond well to prednisone and 31% respond partially to prednisone.
- Patients unresponsive to prednisone may respond to hydroxyurea.
- Vincristine has helped an occasional patient, as has interferon-α and cyclosporine.
- Pheresis does not seem to help.
- Supportive therapy for heart failure including diuretics may be helpful.
- Both anticoagulation and antiplatelet agents have been administered to reduce thromboembolic events.

SURGICAL MEASURES

- Mitral and tricuspid valve replacement or repair have been performed with benefit in occasional patients.
- Patients receiving mechanical valves have experienced thrombosis of the valves.
- If valve replacement is contemplated, a bioprosthesis should be used.
- Rarely, mitral and tricuspid stenosis can occur, and valve replacement may be helpful.

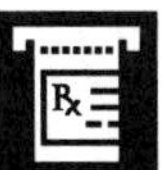

Medications

DRUG(S) OF CHOICE

- As for restrictive cardiomyopathy of any cause

Follow-up

PATIENT MONITORING

Patients need careful, regular follow-up by the cardiologist and hematologist, especially if chemotherapy is used.

EXPECTED COURSE AND PROGNOSIS

Prognosis for restrictive cardiomyopathy is very poor.

PATIENT EDUCATION

- As for restrictive cardiomyopathy of any cause

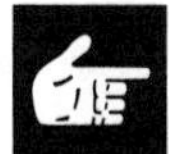

Miscellaneous

ICD-9-CM

428.0 Failure, heart, congestive

BIBLIOGRAPHY

Parillo JE. Heart disease and the eosinophil. *N Engl J Med* 1990;323:1560–1561.

Solley GO, Maldonado JE, Gleich GJ, et al. Cardiomyopathy with eosinophilia. *Mayo Clin Proc* 1976;51:697–708.

Weller PF, Bubley GJ. The idiopathic hypereosinophilic syndrome. *Blood* 1994;83:2759–2779.

Authors: Gary S. Francis and Deepak L. Bhatt

Fabry's Disease and the Heart

Basics

DESCRIPTION

Glycosphingolipid metabolism is disordered due to deficiency of the lysosomal enzyme alpha-galactosidase A.

- This deficiency leads to intracellular accumulation of the glycolipid ceramide trihexoside.
- Angiokeratoma corporis diffusum universale is another name for this disease.

EPIDEMIOLOGY

- Occurs in 1/40,000 births

ETIOLOGY

- X-linked, with full expression in males and only partial expression in females
- Several possible mutations; some atypical forms, due to partial gene deletions and point mutations, lead to isolated myocardial disease that presents later in life
- Women typically have either no symptoms or mild disease; skin lesions and corneal deposits may be present.

RISK FACTORS

N/A

PREGNANCY

Prenatal diagnosis is possible.

ASSOCIATED CONDITIONS

- Kidney failure
- Hypertension (due to renal involvement)

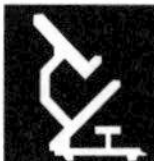

Diagnosis

DIFFERENTIAL DIAGNOSIS

- Other causes of cardiomegaly such as amyloidosis and hypertrophic obstructive cardiomyopathy

SIGNS AND SYMPTOMS

- Fever
- Purple skin lesions (angiokeratoses)
- Corneal opacities
- Paresthesias
- Edema
- Mitral valve prolapse
- Cardiomegaly
- Hypertension
- Vasospastic angina, myocardial infarction, mitral regurgitation
- Renal failure

LABORATORY PROCEDURES

- Decreased alpha-galactosidase A activity in leukocytes
- Lipid vacuoles in the cytoplasm of myocardial cells
- On ECG, left ventricular hypertrophy (LVH), atrial fibrillation, conduction abnormalities, and ventricular ectopy are seen. Short PR interval may be seen.

IMAGING STUDIES

- Chest x-ray
  - —Shows cardiomegaly, aortic root dilatation
- Echocardiography
  - —Shows massive LVH and LV dilatation
  - —Mitral valve prolapse and aortic root dilation also may occur.
- Doppler reveals diastolic dysfunction.

SPECIAL TESTS

- Cardiac catheterization typically reveals normal coronary arteries.
- Endomyocardial biopsy can make the diagnosis.

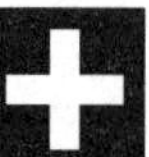

Treatment

GENERAL MEASURES

- Dialysis

SURGICAL MEASURES

- Renal transplantation

Medications

DRUG(S) OF CHOICE

- As for heart failure of any etiology

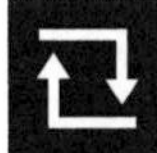

Follow-up

PATIENT MONITORING

- As for heart failure of any etiology

EXPECTED COURSE AND PROGNOSIS

- Cardiac and renal failure in the third and fourth decade of life
- Increased risk of stroke

PATIENT EDUCATION

- As for heart failure of any etiology

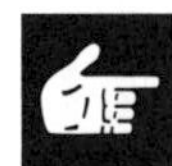

Miscellaneous

ICD-9-CM

272.7 Fabry's disease (angiokeratoma corporis diffusum)
428.0 Failure, heart, congestive

BIBLIOGRAPHY

Wynne J, Braunwald E. The cardiomyopathies and myocarditises. In: Braunwald E, ed. *Heart disease: a textbook of cardiovascular medicine,* 5th ed. Philadelphia: WB Saunders, 1997:1430.

Rodkey SM, Ratliff NB, Young JB. Cardiomyopathy and myocardial failure. In: Topol EJ, ed. *Comprehensive cardiovascular medicine.* Philadelphia: Lippincott-Raven, 1998:2604–2606.

Bleiden LC, Moller JH. Cardiac involvement in inherited disorders of metabolism. *Prog Cardiovasc Dis* 1974;26:615–631.

Authors: Deepak L. Bhatt and Gary S. Francis

Foramen Ovale

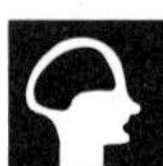

Basics

DESCRIPTION

The foramen ovale is an opening in the midportion of the interatrial septum, in the developing fetus, at the junction of the septum primum and septum secundum.

- A flaplike membranous portion of the septum primum covers this opening. *In utero,* the high right atrial pressure allows right-to-left shunting of blood and delivery of oxygenated blood to the unborn fetus.
- Normal changes in the intracardiac pressures with elevation of the left atrial pressure after delivery of the infant results in the flaplike membrane closing the foramen ovale such that no shunting of blood can occur.
- Fusion of the membrane with permanent closure of the foramen normally occurs in the majority of people. Patency of the foramen ovale does occur and has been associated with unexplained stroke.

Systems Affected

- Cardiovascular and cerebrovascular

Incidence

A patent foramen ovale (PFO) is present in 10%–20% of the general population by autopsy series. Patency may be related to conditions where there are abnormal intracardiac pressures.

- Specifically, congenital heart disease or other conditions associated with high right atrial pressure may predispose people to maintenance of patency of the foramen ovale and may result in right-to-left shunting.
- Patients with unexplained stroke have a higher incidence of PFO (up to 50%). This may be due to paradoxical embolus—a venous embolus passing through the PFO and causing an arterial embolic event—but there may be other mechanisms as well.

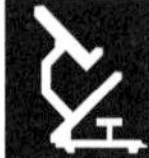

Diagnosis

DIFFERENTIAL DIAGNOSIS

- For patients with interatrial shunting, the differential would include an atrial septal defect (ASD) or atrial septal aneurysm (ASA).
- Echocardiography should be able to differentiate a PFO from an ASD or an associated ASA.
- For patients with unexplained stroke and no interatrial shunting, mitral valve prolapse, mitral annular calcification, valvular vegetations, aortic atherosclerotic plaque, atrial and ventricular thrombus, and left atrial myxoma have been associated.

SIGNS AND SYMPTOMS

- No specific signs or symptoms are associated with an isolated PFO with no shunting of blood.
- Unexplained stroke should lead to an evaluation of a cardiac source of embolus, including PFO.
- In conditions where the right atrial pressure is high and significant right-to-left shunting of blood occurs through a PFO, symptoms of dyspnea and fatigue with associated hypoxia may be present.
- In severe hypoxia, clubbing, cyanosis and erythrocytosis may occur.
- Findings seen with an ASD, such as wide, fixed splitting of the second heart sound and right ventricular conduction delay, have not been clearly associated with a PFO.
- ECG with an isolated PFO is generally normal.

IMAGING STUDIES

- Echocardiography is the diagnostic test of choice for identifying a PFO.
- PFO may be found, incidentally, during an echocardiogram obtained for other reasons.
- Transesophageal echocardiography (TEE) is superior to transthoracic echo (TTE) in identification of PFO and differentiation of ASD or ASA from a PFO. Both 2-D and color flow Doppler are used for PFO evaluation. Injection of agitated saline with both TEE and TTE improves the sensitivity for the diagnosis of PFO.
- Having a patient cough or perform a Valsalva maneuver during agitated saline contrast injection also increases the sensitivity for identification of PFO.
- Patients with unexplained stroke should undergo echocardiography as part of the workup, with the ordering physician specifically requesting a saline contrast study with and without Valsalva maneuver.
- If a TTE is nondiagnostic, TEE should be considered.

Specific Echo Findings of Patent Foramen Ovale

- Thinning of the interatrial septum
- Atrial septal aneurysm may be present.
- Color flow Doppler demonstration of interatrial shunting
- Pulsed Doppler through the interatrial septum may demonstrate shunting.
- Calculation of a shunt ratio can be performed when significant shunting is present.
- Right atrial and/or left atrial enlargement may occur with significant shunting.
- Saline contrast study with the presence of microbubbles in the left heart within three to five cardiac cycles is consistent with intracardiac shunting.
- Saline contrast study may require a Valsalva maneuver to diagnose PFO.
- Workup for a deep venous thrombosis should be performed in patients with a PFO and a cerebral ischemic event. Further testing of patients with unexplained stroke and a PFO also may include cardiac catheterization to determine the shunt size, as well as intracardiac pressures.

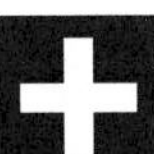

Treatment

GENERAL MEASURES

- In asymptomatic patients with the incidental finding of a PFO, no specific treatment is indicated.
- In patients with unexplained stroke and the finding of a PFO, treatment options include antiplatelet therapy, anticoagulation therapy, transcatheter closure, and surgical closure.
- Currently there is no consensus as to which treatment is most effective.

SURGICAL MEASURES

- In patients with an unexplained stroke and PFO, surgical closure has been performed with a low incidence of complications and recent studies reporting no serious complications.
- Residual shunting and recurrent stroke or transient ischemic attack has been reported after surgical closure, with one study reporting a 35% incidence of recurrent events in a group of patients over the age of 45 and zero recurrent events in patients under the age of 45.
- Catheter-based closure devices have been deployed with low complication rates, but the experience with this is relatively new.
- Incidence of residual shunting and recurrent cerebral ischemic events has been as high as 10%.

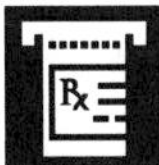

Medications

DRUG(S) OF CHOICE

- In patients with an unexplained stroke and PFO, antiplatelet therapy with aspirin has been associated with a higher recurrence rate of stroke or transient ischemic attack than in patients treated with anticoagulant therapy with coumadin, but other studies have shown no statistical difference.
- The consideration of potential bleeding risk on coumadin needs to be considered when deciding on treatment. Overall, the available data suggest that the recurrence rate of cerebral ischemic events is relatively low (0%–4%) in individuals treated medically with antiplatelet therapy alone or in combination with short-term anticoagulant therapy.
- If a deep venous thrombus is present, anticoagulant therapy would be indicated.

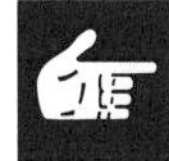

Miscellaneous

BIBLIOGRAPHY

Bogousslavsky J, Devuyst G, Nendaz M, et al. Prevention of stroke recurrence with presumed paradoxical embolus. *J Neurol* 1997;244:71–75.

Gin FG, Huckel VF, Pollick C, et al. Femoral vein delivery of contrast medium enhances transthoracic echocardiography detection of patent foramen ovale. *J Am Coll Cardiol* 1993;22: 1994–2000.

Haussmann D, Mugge A, Becht I, et al. Diagnosis of patent foramen ovale by transesophageal echocardiography and association with cerebral and peripheral embolic events. *Am J Cardiol* 1992;70:668–672.

Homma S, Di Tullio MR, Sacco RR, et al. Surgical closure of patent foramen ovale in cryptogenic stroke patients. *Stroke* 1997;28:2376–2381.

Lechat PH, Mas JL, Lascault G, et al. Prevalence of patent foramen ovale in patients with stroke. *N Engl J Med* 1988;318:1148–1152.

Mas JL, Zuber M. Recurrent cerebrovascular events in patients with patent foramen ovale, atrial septal aneurysm, or both and cryptogenic stroke or transient ischemic attack. *Am Heart J* 1995;30:1083–1088.

Siostrzonek P, Zangeneh M, Gossinger H, et al. Comparison of transesophogeal and transthoracic echocardiography for the detection of patent foramen ovale. *Am J Cardiol* 1991;68: 1247–1249.

Authors: Christopher Abadi and Gerard P. Aurigemma

Heart Failure

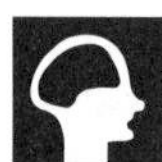

Basics

DESCRIPTION

Heart failure is a clinical syndrome characterized by signs and symptoms of exertional dyspnea due to structural and/or functional heart failure.

- Virtually any form of heart disease can lead to heart failure.
- There are many secondary manifestations: fatigue, circulatory congestion, edema, muscle wasting, etc.

EPIDEMIOLOGY

- Heart failure is one of the most common and important clinical problems in cardiology.
- An estimated 5 million people in the United States have heart failure, and it is believed to be present in 10% of patients over the age of 65 years.
- Coronary disease is present in about 60%–65% of patients with heart failure.
- It is a serious disorder with a poor prognosis.

ETIOLOGY

- There are as many etiologies of heart failure as there are types of heart disease.
- The most common etiologies of heart failure in the United States are coronary artery disease and hypertension.
- Valvular heart disease, dilated cardiomyopathy, left ventricular hypertrophy, and abnormal diastolic function are common etiologic factors.

RISK FACTORS

Risk factors for the development of heart failure include hypertension, coronary artery disease, previous myocardial infarction, left ventricular hypertrophy, diabetes mellitus, hyperlipidemia, cigarette smoking, and obesity.

PREGNANCY

- Pregnancy can sometimes be accompanied by heart failure.
- Stress of delivery can precipitate acute heart failure in patients who are predisposed to have heart failure (i.e., mitral stenosis, congenital heart disease).
- In general, pregnancy is contraindicated or is to be strongly discouraged in patients with heart failure or who are at risk to develop heart failure.

ASSOCIATED CONDITIONS

Numerous associated conditions occur with heart failure, including renal insufficiency, peripheral vascular disease, cerebral vascular disease, arrhythmias, pneumonia, uncontrolled diabetes mellitus, hyperthyroidism, and volume overload, among others.

Diagnosis

DIFFERENTIAL DIAGNOSIS

- Any cause of breathlessness, such as chronic obstructive lung disease or asthma
- It is sometimes difficult to distinguish the cause of shortness of breath in patients who have chronic obstructive lung disease and heart failure.

SIGNS AND SYMPTOMS

- Exertional dyspnea
- Fatigue
- Cough
- Edema
- S3
- Rales
- Elevated jugular venous pressure

LABORATORY PROCEDURES

- ECG
- Chest x-ray
- CBC
- Blood urea nitrogen
- Serum creatinine
- Thyroid function tests, in some cases

IMAGING STUDIES

- Imaging studies are critical to the diagnosis of heart failure because they help to distinguish systolic dysfunction from diastolic dysfunction.
- Echocardiography should be performed in virtually every new patient with the diagnosis of heart failure.
- The echocardiogram provides information regarding cardiac size and function, and valuable information regarding valvular stenosis and incompetence.

SPECIAL TESTS

- Occasionally, patients undergo metabolic exercise testing with measurement of total body oxygen consumption.
- Although myocardial biopsy is not routinely performed, it is useful in selected patients in whom infiltrative cardiomyopathy or inflammatory myocarditis is being considered.

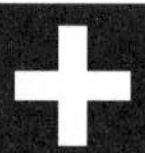

Treatment

GENERAL MEASURES

- Sodium restriction, continued physical activity (including modest or recreational dynamic exercise), avoidance of isometric exercise, careful and frequent follow-up by a physician knowledgeable about heart failure
- Fluid restriction is rarely necessary unless there is concomitant hyponatremia, provided that salt restriction is strictly maintained.
- Most patients are advised to follow a 2-g/day low-sodium diet.

SURGICAL MEASURES

- Surgical measures are growing in importance.
- A patient with advanced heart failure may sometimes benefit from left ventricular assist devices or volume reduction surgery, such as the Dor procedure.
- In some cases, coronary artery bypass surgery has improved left ventricular performance remarkably.
- Heart transplantation is the ultimate palliative therapy.

ADMISSION/DISCHARGE CRITERIA

- Patients should be admitted to the hospital for:
  - —Respiratory distress
  - —Acute pulmonary edema
  - —Desaturated blood that is not due to underlying lung disease
  - —Concomitant medical illnesses that are poorly controlled or need treatment, such as diabetes mellitus, rapid atrial fibrillation, pneumonia, syncope, or demonstrate refractoriness to standard therapy
- Patients with anasarca who are unable to comply with medical therapy should be considered for hospitalization.
- The average hospital stay for heart failure is 5–7 days.
- Patients can usually be safely discharged when there is obvious clinical improvement, reduction in weight, and the ability to ambulate in the hospital without obvious difficulty.

Medications

DRUG(S) OF CHOICE

- Medications include angiotensin converting enzyme (ACE) inhibitors, β-adrenergic blockers, loop diuretics, and digoxin.
- Cornerstones of therapy are the ACE inhibitors and the β-blockers.
- Nearly every patient will require a loop diuretic, usually taken once a day.
- For patients with advanced heart failure who have no associated renal insufficiency, spironolactone 12.5–25 mg is sometimes prescribed.

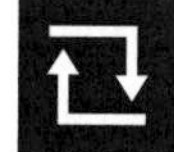

Follow-up

PATIENT MONITORING

- Follow-up for patients with heart failure is extremely important.
- Patients discharged from the hospital should be seen in 1–2 weeks and every 1–3 months thereafter.

EXPECTED COURSE AND PROGNOSIS

- The course of heart failure may wax and wane, with some patients demonstrating prolonged stability and others requiring frequent hospitalization.
- The prognosis generally is poor, with an annual mortality rate that varies from 9% to 12%.

PATIENT EDUCATION

- Patient education is critical.
- Patients should be informed about the natural history of their disease, the prognosis, and should have ample information regarding their medications and how to use them.

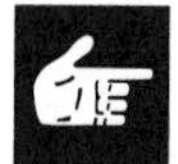

Miscellaneous

ICD-9-CM

428.0 Failure, heart, congestive

BIBLIOGRAPHY

Francis GS. Congestive heart failure. In: *Stein's internal medicine,* 5th ed. St. Louis: CV Mosby, 1998:156–175.

Francis GS. Congestive heart failure. In: Rake RE, ed. *Conn's current therapy.* Philadelphia: WB Saunders, 1998:292–296.

Francis GS. Pathophysiology of the heart failure syndrome. In: Topol EJ, ed. *Textbook of cardiovascular medicine.* Philadelphia: Lippincott-Raven, 1998:2179–2303.

Authors: Gary S. Francis and Deepak L. Bhatt

Heart Transplantation

Basics

DESCRIPTION

Heart transplantation entails the surgical implantation of a recently explanted heart from a brain-dead human, for severely symptomatic heart failure.

- In the absence of significant symptoms, transplantation should not be performed, even if ventricular function is markedly impaired.
- There are many contraindications, and due to donor shortage, patients must be rigorously screened.

EPIDEMIOLOGY

- Over 4,000 patients are currently on the waiting list for heart transplantation in the United States.
- Over 2,300 heart transplants were performed in 1998.

ETIOLOGY

- Heart transplantation is used for end-stage heart failure of almost any cause.
- Dilated cardiomyopathy is the most frequent indication.
- Reversible etiologies, such as alcoholic cardiomyopathy, should be sought.
- Furthermore, spontaneous improvement may occur in the first 6 months after initial presentation with many cardiomyopathies.

RISK FACTORS

- Heart transplantation is contraindicated in severe, fixed pulmonary hypertension.
- Although it is increasingly being performed for older patients, advanced age is a relative contraindication for transplantation.
- Severe, long-standing diabetes with end-organ damage is a contraindication.
- Social support and psychological stability are requisites.

PREGNANCY

- Has been successful in patients who have undergone heart transplantation

ASSOCIATED CONDITIONS

- Immunosuppressive therapy predisposes to infections (including unusual ones) and skin cancers.
- Hypertension, renal insufficiency
- Hyperlipidemia
- Coronary artery disease (i.e., allograft vasculopathy)

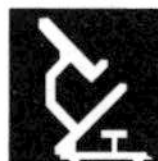

Diagnosis

DIFFERENTIAL DIAGNOSIS

N/A

SIGNS AND SYMPTOMS

- Fever, even low-grade, can signify infection or rejection.
  - —Rejection
  - —Fatigue
  - —Dyspnea
  - —Pericardial rub
  - —Supraventricular arrhythmias

LABORATORY PROCEDURES

- ECG may show dual sinus node activity (from donor and recipient atria).
- Typical ECG shows an incomplete right bundle branch block.
- Blood cultures, sputum Gram stain, and culture if infection is suspected

IMAGING STUDIES

With rejection, echocardiography may show pericardial effusion and myocardial edema, reflected as increased ventricular wall thickness.

SPECIAL TESTS

- Cardiopulmonary stress testing is useful to decide upon the need for transplantation in outpatients.
- Endomyocardial biopsy is mandatory if rejection is suspected.
  - —Allows grading of the degree of rejection
  - —Helps guide immunosuppressive therapy

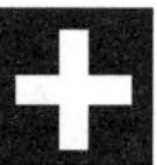

Treatment

GENERAL MEASURES

N/A

SURGICAL MEASURES

N/A

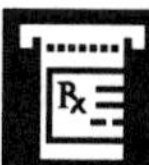

Medications

DRUG(S) OF CHOICE

- Immunosuppressants
  —Cyclosporine, azathioprine, prednisone, tacrolimus (FK506), mycophenolate mofetil, OKT3
- Antihypertensives are usually necessary due to the hypertensive effects of cyclosporine.
- Cholesterol-lowering medications
  —Pravastatin is the preferred statin
  —Increased risk of rhabdomyolysis with concomitant cyclosporine
- Atropine may not be effective for bradyarrhythmias, due to denervation of the transplanted heart.
- Trimethoprim/sulfamethoxazole for *Pneumocystis carinii* prophylaxis
  —Monthly inhaled pentamidine is a less effective alternative for patients who are allergic to sulfa drugs.

ADMISSION/DISCHARGE CRITERIA

Suspicion of rejection or infection is usually an indication for admission.

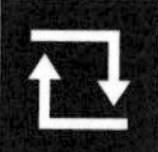

Follow-up

PATIENT MONITORING

- Yearly endomyocardial biopsies to monitor for rejection
- Yearly coronary angiography, potentially accompanied by intravascular ultrasonography, is recommended to monitor for transplant vasculopathy.
- Dobutamine stress echocardiography also appears to have powerful prognostic ability and may be a means to noninvasively assess the presence of vasculopathy.
- Female patients should have routine 6-month Pap smears to monitor for human papilloma virus-induced cervical dysplasia.

EXPECTED COURSE AND PROGNOSIS

- 1-month survival rate is 93%.
- 1-year survival rate is 85%.
- 3-year survival rate is 76%.
- Infection with bacteria, viruses, fungi, or protozoa
- Human papilloma virus infection can lead to cutaneous warts or to cervical cancer.
- Rejection most commonly occurs in the first 3 months posttransplantation.
- Transplant vasculopathy can be problematic because there is no established therapy.
  —Many cardiologists increase the level of immunosuppression when vasculopathy is detected.
  —Angina is often absent due to denervation of the transplanted heart, even in the presence of significant arterial obstruction.
  —The coronary vasculopathy is diffuse and not typically amenable to angioplasty.
  —Vasculopathy can progress rapidly and is a cause of sudden death.
  —Transplant vasculopathy remains the major cause of late mortality.
  —Retransplantation has been performed successfully, but has a much higher associated mortality.
- Skin cancers (squamous cell carcinoma, basal cell carcinoma, keratoacanthomas) are common.
- Lymphoma
- Osteoporosis (secondary to steroids)

PATIENT EDUCATION

- Regular skin self-examinations
- Use sunscreen (minimum SPF of 15).
- Report fevers.

Organizations

- United Network for Organ Sharing: www.unos.org

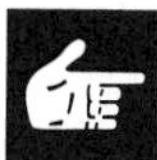

Miscellaneous

ICD-9-CM

428.0 Failure, heart, congestive
996.83 Transplanted heart: failure, infection, rejection

BIBLIOGRAPHY

Spes CH, Klauss V, Mudra H, et al. Diagnostic and prognostic value of serial dobutamine stress echocardiography for noninvasive assessment of cardiac allograft vasculopathy: a comparison with coronary angiography and intravascular ultrasound. *Circulation* 1999;100:509–515.

Smith JA, McCarthy PM, Sarris GE, et al. *The Stanford manual of cardiopulmonary transplantation.* Armonk, NY: Futura, 1996.

Shumway SJ, Shumway NE. *Thoracic transplantation.* Cambridge, MA: Blackwell, 1995.

Authors: Deepak L. Bhatt and Gary S. Francis

High-Output Heart Failure

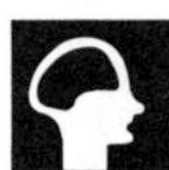

Basics

DESCRIPTION

The symptoms of high-output heart failure are associated with an increased cardiac output as opposed to the typical decreased cardiac output.

EPIDEMIOLOGY

- Extremely rare, especially in the United States

ETIOLOGY

- Chronic anemia
- Arteriovenous fistulas
- Osler-Weber-Rendu disease (hereditary hemorrhagic telangiectasia)
- Hyperthyroidism
- Paget's disease
- Thiamine deficiency (beriberi)
- Multiple myeloma
- Pregnancy
- Albright's syndrome (fibrous dysplasia)
- Obesity
- Glomerulonephritis
- Cor pulmonale
- Polycythemia vera
- Carcinoid syndrome

RISK FACTORS

- Depends on the etiology

PREGNANCY

- Not advisable until the underlying condition has been corrected
- Pregnancy itself can be associated with a high-output state, rarely leading to failure.

ASSOCIATED CONDITIONS

- Peripheral neuropathy with beriberi

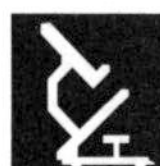

Diagnosis

DIFFERENTIAL DIAGNOSIS

- An elevated cardiac output secondary to conditions such as fever must be distinguished from true high-output heart failure.

SIGNS AND SYMPTOMS

- Wide pulse pressure
- Tachycardia
- Brisk carotid upstroke
- S3, S4
- Branham's sign (reduction in heart rate during manual compression of an arteriovenous fistula)
- Edema

LABORATORY PROCEDURES

- Hemoglobin, thyroid function tests, thiamine levels
- Elevated alkaline phosphatase in Paget's disease

IMAGING STUDIES

Echocardiography can help assess left ventricular function.

SPECIAL TESTS

- Right heart catheterization reveals elevated cardiac output and low systemic vascular resistance.
- Oxygen extraction is increased and the arterial-mixed venous O_2 difference is decreased.

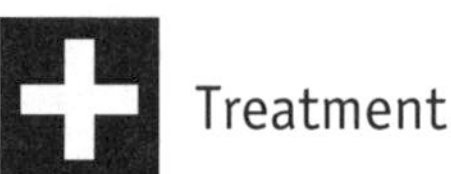

Treatment

GENERAL MEASURES

- Correction of underlying cause if possible

SURGICAL MEASURES

N/A

ADMISSION/DISCHARGE CRITERIA

- As for heart failure of any etiology

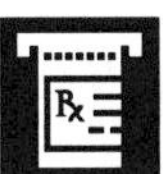

Medications

DRUG(S) OF CHOICE

- In cases of beriberi, thiamine replacement is critical.
- Diuretics and digoxin also may be useful.
- Beta-blockers may be used judiciously in hyperthyroidism.

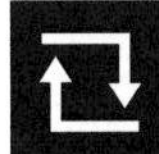

Follow-up

PATIENT MONITORING

- As for heart failure of any etiology

EXPECTED COURSE AND PROGNOSIS

The underlying condition must be treated before any improvement in symptoms.

PATIENT EDUCATION

- As for heart failure of any etiology

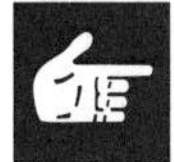

Miscellaneous

ICD-9-CM

428.0 Failure, heart, congestive
265.0 [425.7] Cardiomyopathy, beriberi
242.9 [425.7] Cardiomyopathy, thyrotoxic

BIBLIOGRAPHY

Braunwald E, Colucci WS, Grossman W. Clinical aspects of heart failure: high-output heart failure. In: Braunwald E, ed. *Heart disease: a textbook of cardiovascular medicine,* 5th ed. Philadelphia: WB Saunders, 1997:460–462.

Authors: Deepak L. Bhatt and Gary S. Francis

Hurler's Syndrome and the Heart

Basics

DESCRIPTION

Hurler's syndrome is one of the family of mucopolysaccharidosis diseases in which there is a deficiency of lysosomal enzymes involved in degrading glycosaminoglycans.

ETIOLOGY

Genetics

- Autosomal recessive, localized to chromosome 22 (22q11)

Prevalence

- Approximate incidence is 1/40,000.

Age

- Usually diagnosed in infancy

CAUSES

Deficiency of alpha-L-iduronidase

RISK FACTORS

N/A

PREGNANCY

Screening is not routinely performed in pregnancy.

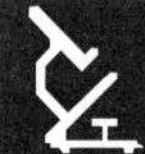

Diagnosis

DIFFERENTIAL DIAGNOSIS

- Scheie's syndrome
- Hunter's syndrome
- Hurler-Scheie syndrome
- Sanfilippo's A-D syndromes
- Morquio's syndrome
- Maroteaux-Lamy syndrome
- Sly's syndrome

SIGNS AND SYMPTOMS

- Infants with Hurler's syndrome usually present in the first year of life with severe mental retardation, hepatosplenomegaly, skeletal deformities, and corneal clouding.
- Patients usually die of obstructive airway symptoms and respiratory infection.
- Cardiac involvement includes early coronary artery disease and infarction, pulmonary hypertension, valvular involvement including mitral and aortic insufficiency, and psuedohypotrophic cardiomyopathy.

LABORATORY PROCEDURES

- High concentrations of both heparin and dermatan sulfate in the urine suggestive evidence of biochemical defect

SPECIAL TESTS

- Leukocyte DNA analysis and demonstration of lack of alpha-L-iduronidase in white cells.

PATHOLOGY

- Deficiency of alpha-L-iduronidase results in the increase of both heparin and dermatan sulfate in the interstitium.
- The increase in undegraded glycosaminoglycans results in abnormal tissue function.

IMAGING STUDIES

N/A

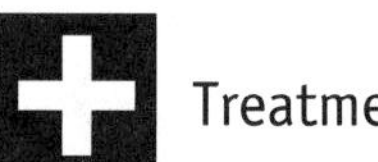

Treatment

GENERAL MEASURES

- Bone marrow transplantation has been suggested, but no data on this are available.
- Genetic replacement remains a possibility.

Medications

DRUG(S) OF CHOICE

- None

ALTERNATIVE DRUGS

N/A

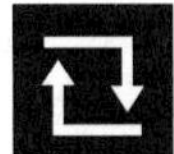

Follow-up

PATIENT MONITORING

- None

Prevention

- None

EXPECTED COURSE AND PROGNOSIS

Most patients die before age 10.

PATIENT EDUCATION

Activity

- Limited

Diet

- No restrictions

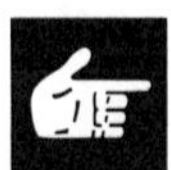

Miscellaneous

SYNONYMS

- Mucopolysaccharidoses
- MPS IH

ICD-9-CM

277.5

See also: Scheie's syndrome; Hunter's syndrome; Hurler-Scheie syndrome; Sanfilippo's syndrome; Morquio's syndrome; Sly's syndrome.

BIBLIOGRAPHY

Alexander RW, ed. *Hurst's the heart.* New York: McGraw-Hill, 1998.

Berkrow R, ed. *The Merck manual,* 16th ed. Rahway, NJ: Merck Research Laboratories, 1992.

Braunwald E, ed. *Heart disease: a textbook of cardiovascular medicine,* 5th ed. Philadelphia: WB Saunders, 1997.

Topol EJ, ed. *Textbook of cardiovascular medicine.* Philadelphia: Lippincott-Raven, 1998.

Authors: Steven Herrmann, Amr El-Shafei, Madhukar Gupta, and Bernard R. Chaitman

Hyperaldosteronism, Primary

Basics

DESCRIPTION

- Increased levels of the hormone aldosterone due to adrenal overproduction
- Hyperaldosteronism is an important, treatable cause of secondary hypertension.

EPIDEMIOLOGY

Prevalence

- In unselected patients with hypertension: 1%–2%

Age

- Majority of cases occur in middle age (30–50 years).
- Glucocorticoid-remediable aldosteronism is noted in childhood.

Sex

- Aldosteronomas are twice as common in women.
- Idiopathic aldosteronism is more common in men.

ETIOLOGY

Causes

- Adrenocortical adenoma (aldosteronoma), also known as Conn's syndrome
- Idiopathic aldosteronism (bilateral cortical hyperplasia)
- Unilateral or primary hyperplasia
- Glucocorticoid-remediable aldosteronism
- Adrenal carcinomas
- Ectopic aldosterone-producing tumor

Genetics

A genetic form of aldosteronism, called glucocorticoid-remediable aldosteronism, is inherited as an autosomal-dominant trait.

PREGNANCY

N/A

ASSOCIATED CONDITIONS

See Differential Diagnosis.

Diagnosis

CLINICAL DIAGNOSIS

Primary aldosteronism should be considered in patients with persistent hypokalemia without edema in the setting of normal sodium intake and the absence of potassium-wasting diuretics.

- Diastolic hypertension without edema
- Hyposecretion of renin that fails to increase due to volume depletion
- Hypersecretion of aldosterone that does not suppress to volume loading

DIFFERENTIAL DIAGNOSIS

- Secondary aldosteronism (high renin)
- Adrenal tumor (multiple corticoid hormone production)
- Bartter's syndrome
- Licorice ingestion (due to glycyrrhizinic acid inhibition of 11β-hydroxysteroid dehydrogenase)
- Deoxycorticosterone-producing adenomas
- Defect in cortisol biosynthesis
- Liddle's syndrome (autosomal-dominant inherited condition due to defect in beta subunit of sodium channel)

SIGNS AND SYMPTOMS

- Asymptomatic
- Diastolic hypertension
- Headache
- Polyuria, nocturia, and polydipsia
- Muscle cramps
- Serious muscle weakness, paresthesia, tetany, or paralysis resulting from profound hypokalemia can be prominent
- ECG may show prominent U waves, cardiac arrhythmias, and premature depolarizations.
- Edema usually absent

LABORATORY PROCEDURES

- Spontaneous hypokalemia with metabolic alkalosis and serum sodium level at the high end of the normal range or hypernatremia
- Isolated hypokalemia (may be <3 mM/L)
- Hypomagnesemia
- Overnight urine concentration tests show failure to concentrate urine.
- Urine pH is neutral to alkaline (due to excessive ammonium and bicarbonate secretion to compensate for metabolic alkalosis).
- Plasma renin levels distinguish primary aldosteronism (low renin) from secondary aldosteronism (high renin).
- Plasma and urinary aldosterone levels

IMAGING STUDIES

- CT scan of abdomen
- Scintigraphy with radiolabeled iodocholesterol or 6-β ^{131}I iodomethyl-19-norcholesterol after dexamethasone suppression; the uptake of tracer is increased in patients with aldosteronoma and absent in those with idiopathic aldosteronism and usually also in those with adrenal carcinoma.

SPECIAL TESTS

- A plasma aldosterone level of <8.5 ng/dL (240 picomoles/L) at the end of saline infusion (performed in the morning) rules out all types of primary aldosteronism.
- Urinary aldosterone excretion of less than 14 μg in 24 hours after sodium loading rules out primary aldosteronism (except for the glucocorticoid-remediable type).
- Plasma aldosterone response to postural change:
  - —Normal response: two- to fourfold increase after 2–3 hours of upright posture
  - —Hyperaldosteronism: decrease in levels after upright posture
- Percutaneous transfemoral bilateral adrenal vein catheterization may be used to localize the affected side (up to two- to threefold increase of plasma aldosterone on affected side).

PATHOLOGY

- Aldosteronomas are usually small (<2 cm in diameter), are benign, and have a golden yellow color on their cut surfaces.
- Bilateral micronodular or macronodular adrenal hyperplasia is seen in idiopathic aldosteronism.
- Adrenal carcinomas
  - —Larger than the more common, benign aldosteronomas
  - —Often produce other adrenal hormones (although they also can secrete only aldosterone)
  - —May show evidence of local invasion or distant metastasis

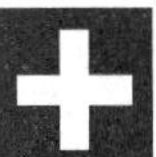

Treatment

GENERAL MEASURES

Dietary sodium restriction may be effective in combination with spironolactone.

SURGICAL MEASURES

- Patients with aldosteronoma are best treated with removal of the adrenal tumor.
- After surgery, hypertension diminishes markedly or resolves in the majority of these patients.

ALTERNATE DRUGS

- Other antihypertensive agents, such as calcium channel blockers or angiotensin-converting enzyme (ACE) inhibitors
- Triampterine and amiloride are also used.
- Glucocorticoid-remediable aldosteronism can be treated with low doses of a glucocorticoid.

ADMISSION/DISCHARGE CRITERIA

- Admission with telemetry monitoring may be indicated for severe hypokalemia.
- Admission for diagnostic workup may be appropriate.
- Surgical removal of adrenal tumor requires inpatient hospitalization; laparoscopic removal may shorten hospital stay.

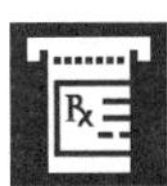

Medications

DRUG(S) OF CHOICE

- Spironolactone

Contraindications

- Chronic renal failure

Precautions

- Gastrointestinal symptoms, fatigue, impotence, rash, and gynecomastia

Interactions

- Potential hyperkalemia if used with ACE inhibitor or potassium supplements

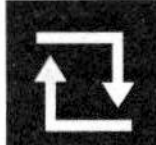

Follow-up

PATIENT MONITORING

- Blood pressure
- CT scans for follow-up of adrenal carcinoma

EXPECTED COURSE AND PROGNOSIS

- Complications
  —Stroke and cardiac disease secondary to hypertension
  —Metastatic complications in those with carcinoma
  —Side effects of medication in patients not surgically treated
- Prognosis
  —Surgery is usually curative.
  —Medical therapy is often successful, but it is limited in men due to side effects of spironolactone (e.g., gynecomastia).
  —With idiopathic bilateral hyperplasia, surgery is only indicated if medical therapy is not effective in preventing serious hypokalemia.

PATIENT EDUCATION

For patients on medical therapy, instruction regarding dietary sodium intake is important.

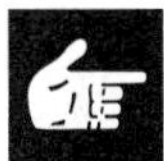

Miscellaneous

ICD-9-CM

255.1 Primary hyperaldosteronism

BIBLIOGRAPHY

Ganguly A. Current concepts: primary aldosteronism. *N Engl J Med* 1998;339:1828–1834.

Williams GH, Dluhy RG. Diseases of the adrenal cortex. In: Fauci AS, et al. *Harrison's principles of internal medicine,* 14th ed. New York: McGraw-Hill, 1998:2035–2057.

Author: Daniel T. Price

Hyperlipidemia

Basics

DESCRIPTION

- Primary or secondary disorders of cholesterol and triglyceride (TG) metabolism resulting in elevated atherosclerotic cardiovascular disease risk: coronary, cerebrovascular, and peripheral vascular disease
- Total cholesterol >200 mg/dL confers increased risk
- Total cholesterol >240 mg/dL confers high risk

EPIDEMIOLOGY

- Elevated cholesterol and cardiovascular disease risk has been firmly established in multiple primary and secondary prevention trials.
- 2% decrease coronary artery disease (CAD) risk for each 1% decrease total cholesterol

ETIOLOGY

- Most patients have a primary or familial disorder of lipid metabolism.
- Secondary causes
  - —Diet rich in saturated fatty acids
  - —Obesity
  - —Diabetes mellitus, type II
  - —Nephrotic syndrome
  - —End-stage renal disease
  - —Hypothyroidism
  - —Cushing's syndrome
  - —Chronic liver disease
  - —Drugs (excessive alcohol, isotretinoin, thiazide diuretics, beta-blockers, estrogens, glucocorticoids, cyclosporine)

RISK FACTORS

See secondary causes above under Etiology.

PREGNANCY

- May cause secondary hypertriglyceridemia
- HMG-CoA reductase inhibitors contraindicated

ASSOCIATED CONDITIONS

See secondary causes above under Etiology.

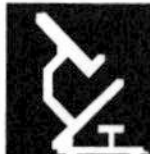

Diagnosis

DIFFERENTIAL DIAGNOSIS

N/A

SIGNS AND SYMPTOMS

- Angina/myocardial infarction
- Cerebrovascular accident
- Claudication
- Arterial bruits
- Xanthelasmas/xanthomas

LABORATORY PROCEDURES

- Total cholesterol, HDL, very low density lipoprotein (VLDL), and triglyceride (TG) measured directly
- Calculated LDL = total cholesterol − (HDL + VLDL + 0.2 × TG)

IMAGING STUDIES

N/A

SPECIAL TESTS

- Lipoprotein(a) controversial

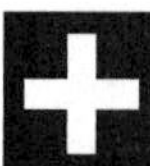

Treatment

GENERAL MEASURES

- Start therapy in hospital after myocardial infarction, unstable coronary syndrome, or revascularization.
- Treatment goals
  - —No CAD and fewer than two risk factors: LDL <160 mg/dL
  - —No CAD and two or more risk factors: LDL <130 mg/dL
  - —CAD: LDL <100 mg/dL
  - —Diabetes mellitus: LDL <100 mg/dL

SURGICAL MEASURES

N/A

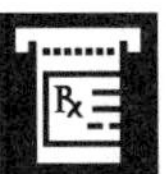

Medications

DRUG(S) OF CHOICE

- HMG-CoA reductase inhibitors (statins)
  —Lovastatin (Mevacor), simvastatin (Zocor), pravastatin (Pravachol), fluvastatin (Lescol), atorvastatin (Lipitor)
  —Usual dose: varies for each agent
  —Expected effect: 25%–40% decrease in LDL, 5%–10% increase in HDL
  —Common side effects: hepatocellular dysfunction, myositis, lens opacification
- Nicotinic acid (niacin)
  —Usual dose: 50 mg with meals, gradually increased to 1–2 g with meals
  —Expected effect: 25% decrease in LDL, 75% decrease in VLDL, 20%–40% increase in HDL
  —Common side effects: cutaneous flushing, nausea, abdominal discomfort
- Bile acid sequestrants
  —Cholestyramine (Questran) and colestipol (Colestid)
  —Usual dose: 4–5 g mixed with fluid, taken with meals
  —Expected effect: 15%–30% decrease in LDL
  —Common side effects: nausea, abdominal discomfort, constipation, indigestion, decreased absorption of other medications (warfarin, thiazides, thyroxine, digitalis, phenobarbital, tetracycline)
- Fibric acid derivatives
  —Gemfibrozil (Lopid)
  —Usual dose: 600 mg twice daily
  —Expected effect: 10%–20% decrease in LDL, 10%–20% increase in HDL, up to 50% decrease in TG
  —Common side effects: nausea, abdominal discomfort, potentiates effect of warfarin

ADMISSION/DISCHARGE CRITERIA

- N/A: ambulatory care

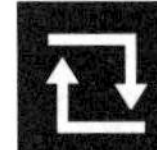

Follow-up

PATIENT MONITORING

- Check lipid panel 4–6 weeks after institution or change in therapy.
- Desirable lipid profiles on stable therapy; monitor yearly.
- Liver function tests after 12 weeks with HMG-CoA reductase inhibitors and niacin

EXPECTED COURSE AND PROGNOSIS

See Epidemiology above.

PATIENT EDUCATION

Diet

Minimize dietary fats, meats, eggs; emphasize fiber, fruit, vegetables, low-fat dairy.

AHA Step One Diet

- Total calories to achieve/maintain ideal weight
- Cholesterol <300 mg/day
- Total fat $\leq 30\%$ of calories
  —Saturated fat 8%–10% of calories
  —Polyunsaturated fat up to 10% of calories
  —Monounsaturated fat up to 15% of calories
- Carbohydrates 55% or more of calories
- Protein ~15% of calories

AHA Step Two Diet

- Involve registered dietician.
- Total calories to achieve/maintain ideal weight
- Cholesterol <200 mg/day
- Total fat $\leq 30\%$ of calories
  - Saturated fat 7% or less of calories
  - Polyunsaturated fat up to 10% of calories
  - Monounsaturated fat up to 15% of calories
  - Carbohydrates 55% or more of calories
  - Protein ~15% of calories

Organizations

- American Heart Association, 7272 Greenville Ave., Dallas, TX 75231

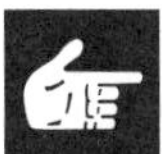

Miscellaneous

ICD-9-CM

272.0 Pure hypercholesterolemia
272.1 Pure hyperglyceridemia
272.2 Mixed hyperlipidemia

INTERNET SITES

- American Heart Association: www.americanheart.org
- American College of Cardiology: www.acc.org
- DrKoop.com: www.drkoop.com
- National Cholesterol Education Program: rover.nhlbi.nih.gov/chd

BIBLIOGRAPHY

Expert Panel on Detection, Evaluation, and Treatment of High Blood Cholesterol in Adults. Summary of the Second Report of the National Cholesterol Education Program (NCEP) Expert Panel on Detection, Evaluation, and Treatment of High Blood Cholesterol in Adults (Adult Treatment Panel II). *JAMA* 1993;269:3015–3023.

Havel RJ, Rapaport E. Drug therapy: management of primary hyperlipidemia. *N Engl J Med* 1995;332:1491–1498.

Authors: Thomas M. Guest and Nanette K. Wenger

Hyperthyroid Heart Disease

Basics

DESCRIPTION

Cardiac manifestations are among the earliest as well as the most consistent features of hyperthyroidism, including increased contractility and high-output state.

- Myocardial ischemia (with or without coronary artery disease) can occur secondary to coronary vasospasm and increased oxygen consumption.
- High-output congestive heart failure (CHF; 5% of cases occur in absence of cardiac disease)
- Worsening of CHF in those with cardiac disease
- Stimulation of atrial fibrillation
- Cardiac effects of thyroid hormone
  —Triiodothyronine (T_3) alters cardiac function by regulation of cardiac-specific genes (stimulatory). This increases contractility and cardiac work.
  —T_3 decreases peripheral vascular resistance through a direct extranuclear effect on arterial smooth muscle cells.
  —T_3 and thyroxine (T_4) indirectly affect the cardiovascular system by stimulating metabolism.

Systems Affected

- Cardiovascular, endocrine

ETIOLOGY

Genetics

Genetics play an important role in Graves' disease.

- Increased frequency of haplotypes HLA-B8 and -DRw3 in white patients
- Increased frequency of haplotype HLA-Bw36 in Japanese patients
- Increased frequency of haplotype HLA-Bw46 in Chinese patients

Incidence/Prevalence

Thyroid disease becomes more common with advancing age.

- Graves' disease is especially common in the third and fourth decades of life and affects 0.02%–0.4% of the U.S. population.
- Graves' disease is more frequent in women (4:1 to 10:1).
- Graves' disease has a strong familial predisposition.

Predominant Age

- Young adults and the elderly

Predominant Sex

- Females affected more than males

CAUSES

- The most common causes of hyperthyroidism are Graves' disease, toxic multinodular goiter, and toxic adenoma (Graves' disease being the most prevalent, responsible for 60%–90% of the cases of hyperthyroidism).
- Graves' thyroid disease is an autoimmune disease characterized by the triad of hyperthyroidism with diffuse goiter, ophthalmopathy, and dermopathy (occurring singly or in combination).
- Thyrotoxicosis refers to the clinical syndrome resulting from increased circulating levels of thyroid hormone.

RISK FACTORS

- Underlying heart disease
- Hypertension

ASSOCIATED CONDITIONS

- Atrial fibrillation
- CHF
- Hypertension
- Myocardial ischemia

Age-Related Factors

- Pediatric: rare
- Geriatric: apathetic thyrotoxicosis common; atrial fibrillation common presentation, as is weakness.
- Others: Young adults usually have Graves' disease

PREGNANCY

- Metabolic demands of pregnancy will exacerbate symptoms, and radioiodine is contraindicated in pregnancy.
- Careful management with an obstetrician and endocrinologist is desirable.

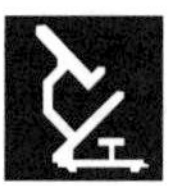

Diagnosis

DIFFERENTIAL DIAGNOSIS

- Emotional anxiety
- Pheochromocytoma
- Metastatic carcinoid
- Sprue
- Hyperparathyroidism

SIGNS AND SYMPTOMS

- History
  —Nervousness
  —Palpitations
  —Insomnia
  —Tremors
  —Diarrhea
  —Heat intolerance
  —Weight loss despite preserved or increased appetite
  —Fatigue
  —Increased perspiration
  —Weakness
  —Oligomenorrhea or amenorrhea
  —Stare, lid lag
  —Exertional dyspnea
- Cardiovascular findings
  —Sinus tachycardia
  —Atrial arrhythmias (especially atrial fibrillation)
  —Wide pulse pressure
  —Hypertension
  —Mid-systolic ejection murmur (left sternal boarder)
  —Active apical impulse
  —Loud S1
  —Loud P2
  —S3 (occasional)
  —Means-Lerman scratch (rare systolic scratch heard in the second left intercostal space during expiration)
  —Increased stroke volume, cardiac output, and cardiac work with decreased peripheral resistance

LABORATORY PROCEDURES

- Suppressed thyroid-stimulating hormone (sTSH) serum and increased free thyroxine index (FTI); normal levels exclude hyperthyroidism
- Serum T_3 only rarely needed (i.e., cases of T_3 toxicosis when both FTI and sTSH are low)
- High FTI and high sTSH indicate a TSH-producing tumor or peripheral hormone resistance.
- Thyroid-stimulating immunoglobulin assay if diagnosis is unclear

Drugs that May Alter Laboratory Results

Amiodarone is an iodine-rich benzofuran derivative that causes both hyperthyroidism and hypothyroidism. It also may affect thyroid function tests in the absence of clinical disease.

Pathologic Findings

Multinodular goiter, thyroiditis, opthalmopathy, dermopathy; no specific cardiovascular pathology

SPECIAL TESTS

- ECG (common but nonspecific)
  —Sinus tachycardia (40% of patients)
  —Atrial fibrillation (15%–25% of patients)
  —Shortening of atrio-ventricular conduction time along with functional refractory period transmits rapid atrial impulses
  —Intraatrial conduction disturbance causes prolongation or notched P wave and prolongation of the P-R interval (5%–15% of patients)
  —Second- or third-degree heart block (rare)
  —Interventricular conduction disturbances (right bundle branch block most common)

IMAGING STUDIES

- Echocardiography
  - —Measurement of cardiac chamber sizes, wall thickness, and ejection fraction
  - —Evaluation for associated mitral valve prolapse in Graves' disease
- Chest x-ray (nonspecific)
  - —Prominent left ventricle, aorta, and pulmonary artery
  - —Generalized cardiac enlargement
  - —Pulmonary edema (late)

DIAGNOSTIC PROCEDURES

Radioactive iodine uptake can be used in the differential diagnosis of hyperthyroidism with diffuse goiter, and in the diagnosis of ectopic struma ovarii, thyroiditis, and thyrotoxicosis factitia.

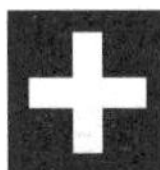

Treatment

GENERAL MEASURES

- Minor symptoms can be controlled medically as an outpatient.
- Unstable symptoms (i.e., thyroid storm or decompensated heart failure) require aggressive management and hospitalization.
- Prompt treatment of the hyperthyroid state is essential to the reduction of cardiovascular symptoms.
- Cardiovascular manifestations (CHF, atrial fibrillation) attributed solely to hyperthyroidism are reversible with treatment.
- Hyperthyroid patients with underlying cardiac disease may be resistant to therapy.

SURGICAL MEASURES

Thyroidectomy may be required in patients with a large, toxic, nodular goiter after medical stabilization or in medical therapeutic failures.

Medications

DRUG(S) OF CHOICE

- Beta-adrenergic blockade (e.g., propranolol 40–120 mg/day or atenolol 100 mg/day) appears to inhibit microsomal 5′-monodeiodinase which converts T_4 to T_3).
- Higher doses of atenolol can reduce symptoms of hyperthyroidism but do not change T_3 or rT_3 levels.
- Beta-blockers, verapamil, and diltiazem can rapidly rate control superventricular arrhythmias and reduce the hyperdynamic state (see Supraventricular Tachycardia chapter for dosing).
- Thyroid-suppressive drugs such as propylthiouracil (PTU; 100 mg every 2 hours during thyrotoxic crisis) or methimazole (20 mg/day) are the preferred drugs when heart failure complicates severe hyperthyroidism. Each blocks thyroid hormone and thyroid-stimulating immunoglobulin production. PTU also inhibits extrathyroidal conversion of T_4 to T_3.
- Digitalis glycosides can control ventricular rate in atrial fibrillation and are especially helpful in patients with heart failure. Higher doses may be required due to metabolic clearance. Target ventricular rate should be approximately 120 beats/min in order to avoid drug toxicity in the acute setting.
- Iodine (potassium iodine, sodium iodide, or an iodine-containing radiocontrast agent) suppresses the release of preexisting thyroid hormone.
- Diuretics reduce volume overload and pulmonary vascular congestion (see Congestive Heart Disease chapter for dosing).
- Warfarin therapy in atrial fibrillation for embolic prophylaxis
- Beta-blockers, calcium channel blockers, and nitrates for angina pectoris (see Angina chapter for dosing).

ALTERNATIVE DRUGS

- Radioiodine (^{131}I) is a safe alternative to PTU and methimazole.
- Contraindicated in pregnancy
- Usually avoided in the young

Contraindications

Refer to manufacturer's profile.

Precautions

Refer to manufacturer's profile.

Follow-up

PATIENT MONITORING

- Depends on frequency and severity of symptoms
- In Graves' disease, treat with PTU or methimazole for 6–12 months and follow up for recurrence.
- Treatment of arrhythmias and high-output failure can be weaned as symptoms resolve.
- Repeat tests as required (ECG, chest x-ray).
- Repeat thyroid levels to access for euthyroidism.
- CBC and liver functions to evaluate for complications of suppressive therapy (see Possible Complications below)

Possible Complications

- Agranulocytosis, vasculitis, hepatitis, and aplastic anemia are seen infrequently with suppressive therapy using PTU and methimazole.
- Hypothyroidism with ^{131}I
- Hypothyroidism or hypoparathyroidism after subtotal thyroidectomy

EXPECTED COURSE AND PROGNOSIS

- Overall clinical improvement in 1–2 weeks with euthyroidism by 2 months
- Cardiac manifestations usually take longer to resolve.
- Remission in approximately 50%
- Cyclics phases of exacerbation and remission
- Unpredictable
- May progress to thyroid failure with hypothyroidism
- General prognosis is good with gradual return of exercise tolerance and decrease in atrial irritability.

PATIENT EDUCATION

Organization

- American Heart Association, 7320 Greenville Ave., Dallas TX 75231; (214)373-6300

Activity

As tolerated after consulting with a physician

Diet

Low sodium and low fat (if underlying coronary artery disease)

Miscellaneous

SYNONYMS

- Graves' disease

ICD-9-CM

242.9 + 425.7 Hyperthyroid heart disease

BIBLIOGRAPHY

Braverman LE, Utiger RD. *The thyroid: a fundamental and clinical text,* 6th ed. Philadelphia: JB Lippincott, 1991.

Isselbacher KJ, Braunwald E, Wilson JD, et al. *Harrison's principles of internal medicine,* 13th ed. New York: McGraw-Hill, 1994.

Osborn LA. Thyroid hormone and the cardiovascular system. *Cardiol Clin* 1999;3:95–104.

Topol EJ, ed. *Textbook of cardiovascular medicine.* Philadelphia: Lippincott-Raven, 1998.

Author: Robert A. Taylor

Hypoplastic Left Heart Syndrome

Basics

DESCRIPTION

Hypoplastic left heart syndrome (HLHS) is described as underdevelopment of the left-sided cardiac structures, including the mitral valve, left ventricle, aortic valve, and aortic arch. Aortic and mitral valves may be either atretic or stenotic.

EPIDEMIOLOGY

- Incidence is 0.016%–0.036% of live births.
- 1.5% of infants with congenital heart disease
- Slight male predominance

Genetics

Recurrence risk for sibling of 0.05%; not associated with single specific chromosomal abnormality

RISK FACTORS

N/A

PREGNANCY

N/A

ASSOCIATED CONDITIONS

- Noncardiac
  —Associated with many different syndromes, including Turner's, Noonan's, and Holt-Oram; 28% of HLHS patients have a genetic disorder or extracardiac anomalies, including brain malformations.
- Cardiac
  —Associated with ventricular septal defects, small foramen ovale, anomalous pulmonary venous return
  —There is invariably a coarctation of the aorta.
  —HLHS may occur in the context of a double-outlet right ventricle or unbalanced atrioventricular canal defect.

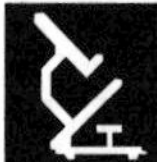

Diagnosis

SIGNS AND SYMPTOMS

- Typically presents in first week of life, may be diagnosed prenatally
- Early findings (days, prior to spontaneous closure of the ductus arteriosus) include tachypnea without retractions and mild cyanosis.
- Later findings (days to weeks, after spontaneous closure of the ductus arteriosus) include signs of low cardiac output, pallor, poor respiratory effort, decreased responsiveness, poor feeding, seizures, and oliguria.
- Physical findings following ductal closure include mild cyanosis, poorly palpable femoral pulses, and an active precordium with a single S2.
- There may be a nonspecific grade II/VI systolic murmur heard along the left sternal border.
- The murmur may be holosystolic and of a harsher quality in the presence of tricuspid regurgitation.
- The liver may be enlarged.

DIFFERENTIAL DIAGNOSIS

- Prior to ductal closure: persistent pulmonary hypertension of the newborn (PPHN, or persistence of the fetal circulation syndrome), sepsis
- Following ductal closure: sepsis, critical coarctation of the aorta, interrupted aortic arch

LABORATORY PROCEDURES

- Arterial blood gas reveals low pCO_2, slightly low pO_2.
- Following ductal closure, the infant develops a profound metabolic acidosis with elevation of liver enzymes and serum creatinine.

IMAGING STUDIES

- Chest x-ray findings are nonspecific and include:
  —Cardiomegaly with a globular appearance
  —Increased pulmonary vascular markings
- Echocardiography is the primary diagnostic study to be performed, and findings include the following:
  —Mitral and aortic atresia or stenosis
  —Markedly diminished left ventricular size, sometimes too small to be visualized
  —Hypoplasia of the ascending aorta and transverse arch
  —Prior to its closure, the ductus arteriosus is seen with flow from the pulmonary artery to the aorta.
  —Retrograde flow from the site of ductal entry up to the proximal aortic arch and coronary arteries
  —Flow across the foramen ovale from the left atrium to the right atrium.
- Clinicians must evaluate for tricuspid regurgitation, restriction to flow across the foramen ovale, pulmonary venous anatomy, right ventricular outflow tract obstruction, and right ventricular function.

SPECIAL TESTS

ECG findings include the following:

- Right superior axis deviation
- Right ventricular hypertrophy
- Right atrial enlargement
- Diminished R waves in leads V5 and V6
- Cardiac catheterization is not necessary for the diagnosis of HLHS.

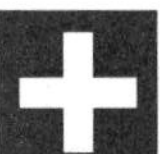

Treatment

GENERAL MEASURES

- Continuous i.v. infusion of prostaglandin E_1 at 0.05–0.1 μg/kg/min is necessary to maintain ductal patency and systemic output.
- Continuous positive airway pressure (CPAP) or intubation and mechanical ventilation may be required.
- Limitation of pulmonary blood flow may be achieved through hypoventilation and avoidance of supplemental oxygen.
- Diuresis and inotropic support are frequently required, especially for patients with a prolonged preoperative period.
- Balloon atrial septostomy may be required urgently if the atrial communication is restrictive.

SURGICAL MEASURES

- Surgical repair is delayed until liver, brain, and renal function recover.
- Surgical approach may consist of cardiac transplantation or the staged Norwood procedure.
- The Norwood procedure consists of three stages:
  - —Stage 1: Performed in the neonatal period. The right ventricle is used as the systemic ventricle. The proximal pulmonary artery is reconstructed to form the ascending aorta and is anastomosed to the descending aorta. Controlled pulmonary blood flow is supplied via a Blalock-Taussig shunt between the innominate artery and the pulmonary artery. The atrial septum is resected to allow unobstructed flow from the left atrium to the right atrium. The aortic coarctation is repaired.
  - —Stage 2: The bidirectional Glenn procedure usually is performed at 8–10 months of age. Cardiac catheterization is required prior to stages 2 and 3 to assess the hemodynamics and pulmonary artery anatomy. The shunt is taken down and the superior cava is connected directly into the pulmonary artery.
  - —Stage 3: The Fontan procedure is completed at approximately 2–3 years of age. The inferior vena caval flow is also directed into the pulmonary artery. Cyanosis is relieved.
- Combined approach entails planned transplantation with crossover to Norwood procedure if no donors are available. Alternatively, transplantation may follow stage 1 Norwood in the face of unfavorable hemodynamics.
- No intervention: This approach is occasionally used, but less commonly in recent years.

Follow-up

PATIENT MONITORING

- Frequent visits required
- Echocardiography, oxygen saturation, and hemoglobin measurements periodically obtained

EXPECTED COURSE AND PROGNOSIS

- 100% mortality without surgical intervention
- Cardiac transplantation
  - —Significant mortality awaiting transplantation due to shortage of neonatal donors
  - —If transplantation is performed, survival is approximately 85%.
  - —Significant morbidity present due to chronic immunosuppression and risks of infection and graft rejection
- Norwood procedure
  - —Greatest mortality in the immediately postoperative stage 1 period
  - —Prenatal diagnosis could affect probability of survival.
  - —Additional deaths may occur between stages 1 and 2.
  - —Low mortality following stages 2 and 3
  - —Morbidity due to recurrent coarctation of the aorta, restriction to flow across the atrial septum.
  - —Morbidity following stage 3 is similar to that in other Fontan patients, including pleural effusions, protein-losing enteropathy, poor cardiac output, and ventricular failure.
- Five-year survival is approximately 65%–70% in both groups when also considering deaths of infants awaiting transplantation.

PATIENT EDUCATION

- Parents of affected infants should be careful regarding maintaining adequate hydration because clotting of the shunt is a life-threatening event. Antibiotic prophylaxis against bacterial endocarditis is required prior to selected procedures.

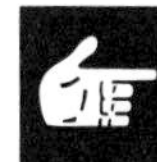

Miscellaneous

BIBLIOGRAPHY

Fyler C. *Nadas' pediatric cardiology.* Philadelphia: Hanley & Belfus, 1992.

Garson A, et al., eds. *The science and practice of pediatric cardiology,* 2nd ed. Baltimore: Williams & Wilkins, 1998.

Iannettoni MD, Bove EL, Crowley DC, et al. Improving results with first-stage palliation for hypoplastic left heart syndrome. *J Thorac Cardiovasc Surg* 1994;107:934–940.

Norwood WI, Kirklin JK, Sanders SP. Hypoplastic left heart syndrome: experience with palliative surgery. *Am J Cardiol* 1980;45:87–91.

Starnes VA, Griffin ML, Pitlick PT, et al. Current approach to hypoplastic left heart syndrome: palliation, transplantation, or both? *J Thorac Cardiovasc Surg* 1992;104:189–195.

Authors: Jeffrey H. Kern and Welton M. Gersony

Hypothyroid Heart Disease

Basics

DESCRIPTION

Cardiovascular manifestations of hypothyroidism include heart failure, pericardial effusion, arrhythmias, and premature atherosclerosis. Heart failure in hypothyroid patients usually occurs secondary to exacerbation of preexisting cardiac disease by the hemodynamic effects of hypothyroidism. Rarely, hypothyroidism alone may cause a cardiomyopathy with associated heart failure.

Incidence/Prevalence

Congenital hypothyroidism presents in 1/4,000 newborns worldwide. Hypothyroidism occurs in 2% of adult women and 0.1%–0.2% of adult men in North America.

Predominant Age

The peak incidence of hypothyroidism is between the ages of 30 and 60 years.

Predominant Sex

- Female

ETIOLOGY

Hypothyroidism results from decreased secretion of both thyroxine (T_4) and triiodothyronine (T_3), either due to thyroid gland destruction or secondary to pituitary or hypothalamic pathology.

RISK FACTORS

Preexisting heart disease increases the likelihood of cardiac involvement.

ASSOCIATED CONDITIONS

- Hypopituitarism
- Addison's disease

Age-Related Factors

- Pediatric: rare
- Geriatric: common

PREGNANCY

Heart disease due to hypothyroidism is unusual.

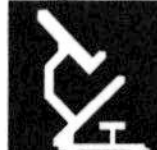

Diagnosis

DIFFERENTIAL DIAGNOSIS

The nephrotic syndrome may resemble myxedema (facial puffiness, pallor, anemia, and hypercholesterolemia).

SIGNS AND SYMPTOMS

- Symptoms
  —Exertional dyspnea
  —Fatigability
  —Rarely syncope
  —Angina during hormone replacement
- Signs
  —Bradycardia
  —Weak arterial pulses
  —Distant heart sounds
  —Nonpitting edema
  —Hypertension
  —Hypotension in severe myxedema
  —Rarely cardiac tamponade

LABORATORY PROCEDURES

- Thyroid-stimulating hormone (TSH)
  —Increased in thyroprivic or goitrous hypothyroidism
  —Normal or undetectable in pituitary or hypothalamic hypothyroidism; hyposecretion of other pituitary hormones
  —Decreased serum T_4 and free thyroxine index (FTI) are common to all types of hypothyroidism.
  —Serum T_3 in thyroid hypothyroidism may be reduced to a lesser degree than serum T_4.
  —Increased LDL and total cholesterol

Laboratory Results

- TSH elevated
- Free T_3 and free T_4 concentrations normal

Pathologic Findings

- Heart often pale, flabby, and grossly dilated in frank myxedema
- Microscopic examination in myxedema reveals myofibrillar swelling, loss of striations, and interstitial fibrosis.

SPECIAL TESTS

- ECG
  —Sinus bradycardia
  —Prolonged QTc interval
    - 450–519 msec in 14%–21% of hypothyroid patients
    - Rarely ≥520 msec (increased risk of malignant ventricular arrhythmias)
  —Atrioventricular and intraventricular conduction disturbances; incomplete or complete right bundle branch block
  —Reduced QRS voltage and flattening or inversion of T waves
  —Decreased P-wave amplitude

IMAGING STUDIES

- Chest x-ray
  —Cardiac enlargement due to chamber enlargement and/or pericardial effusion
  —Small heart with pituitary hypothyroidism and adrenal insufficiency

DIAGNOSTIC PROCEDURES

- Echocardiography (Doppler)
  —Pericardial effusion in approximately one-third of patients with myxedema
  —Rarely cardiac tamponade
    - Right atrial and/or right ventricular collapse in diastole
    - Respiratory cyclical variation tricuspid and mitral flow on Doppler echocardiography
  —Left ventricular dilatation with reduced contractility may occur.
- Coronary angiography in hypothyroid patients with angina often reveals severe coronary artery disease.

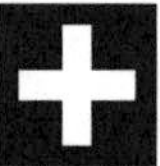

Treatment

GENERAL MEASURES

- Usually a normal metabolic state should be restored gradually in patients with heart disease. In adults, levothyroxine may be initiated at 25 μg/day and increased by 12.5- to 25-μg increments every 4–6 weeks until a euthyroid state is achieved.
- In known or suspected pituitary and hypothalamic hypothyroidism, treatment with hydrocortisone should precede thyroid replacement. Also, hydrocortisone should be given during rapid thyroid hormone treatment.
- Pericardiocentesis for rare cardiac tamponade

ADMISSION/DISCHARGE CRITERIA

- Moderate to severe heart failure
- QTc ≥520 msec, syncope, or ventricular tachycardia (monitored bed)
- Evidence of cardiac tamponade
- Severe angina

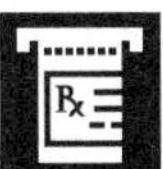

Medications

DRUG(S) OF CHOICE

- Unless contraindicated, beta-adrenergic blocking drugs can be added if thyroid hormone therapy exacerbates myocardial ischemia.
- Digitalis glycosides may be beneficial.
- When severe heart failure or cardiogenic shock results from hypothyroidism, intravenous T_3 is recommended.
- Subclinical hypothyroidism
  —L-T_4 25 μg/day decreases lipoprotein (a) levels
- Hypothyroidism
  —Titration to daily L-T_4 doses of 150 μg or higher prevents atherosclerosis progression.
- Severe angina pectoris
  —Surgical or percutaneous revascularization may be performed with minimal thyroid replacement, followed by postoperative or post-procedural full thyroid replacement.
  —Beta-blockers may be tried cautiously if no contradiction, but may cause severe bradycardia.

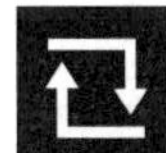

Follow-up

PATIENT MONITORING

- Thyroid tests (T_4, T_3, and TSH) should be measured every 4–6 weeks until a euthyroid state is attained. Optimum L-T_4 dose should be based on TSH and serum T_3.
- After patient euthyroid on appropriate L-T_4 dose, measure TSH and T_3 annually.

Possible Complications

- Unstable angina, heart failure, and pericardial tamponade

EXPECTED COURSE AND PROGNOSIS

Full recovery is expected, unless cardiac disease has developed.

PATIENT EDUCATION

Diet

- No-added-salt diet
- Reduced saturated fat and cholesterol diet

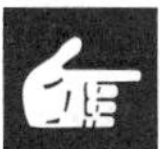

Miscellaneous

ICD-9-CM

244.9 + 429.9 Hypothyroid heart disease

BIBLIOGRAPHY

Braunwald E. *Heart disease: a textbook of cardiovascular medicine,* 5th ed. Philadelphia: WB Saunders, 1997.

Wilson J, Braunwald E, Isselbacher K, et al. *Harrison's principles of internal medicine,* 12th ed. New York: McGraw-Hill, 1991.

Osborn L. Thyroid hormone and the cardiovascular system. In: Crawford MH, ed. *The cardiology clinics annual of drug therapy.* Philadelphia: WB Saunders, 1999:97.

Author: Larry A. Osborn

Ischemia, Mesenteric

Basics

DESCRIPTION

- Primary mesenteric ischemia
  —Interruption of abdominal vascular circulation by arterial embolus, arterial or venous thrombosis, atherosclerotic stenosis, or nonocclusive vasospasm
  —Also known as mesenteric vasculopathy or mesenteric ischemic vasculopathy
- Secondary mesenteric ischemia
  —Compression of the vascular circulation from an extrinsic source

EPIDEMIOLOGY

- Accounts for 1/1,000 hospital admissions.
- Mean age for acute arterial embolus is 68 years, for acute arterial thrombosis 77 years, and for acute venous thrombosis 47–60 years.
- Men and women are affected equally.
- Chronic mesenteric ischemia may be present in 10%–20% of elderly patients by autopsy series, probably underreported because of multisystem disease; predilection for women in symptomatic patients, with mean age of 60.

RISK FACTORS

- Embolus
  —Cardiac thrombi from atrial fibrillation, recent myocardial infarction, valvular heart disease, dilated left atrium, dilated ventricle with mural thrombus (risk significantly reduced in patients who are chronically anticoagulated)
- Arterial thrombosis and chronic mesenteric ischemia
  —Atherosclerosis with associated risk factors (age, smoking, diabetes, hypertension, hyperlipidemia); also vasculitis (Behçet's, Buerger's, Churg-Strauss, Kawasaki, polyarteritis nodosa, Takayasu's, Wegener's, rheumatoid arthritis, lupus), hypercoagulable states (antiphospholipid antibodies; deficiency or mutations of protein C, protein S, and antithrombin III; sickle cell anemia; myeloproliferative disorders; oral contraceptives), trauma
- Venous thrombosis
  —Hypercoagulable states; also vasculitis, bowel obstruction, dehydration, pancreatitis, infections (appendicitis, diverticulitis), abdominal malignancy, abdominal trauma
- Nonocclusive intestinal mesenteric ischemia (NOMI)
  —Systemic hypotension (cardiogenic and cardiogenic shock), especially in elderly patients undergoing emergency cardiac or abdominal surgery; vasoconstricting drugs (e.g., cocaine, digoxin)
- Secondary mesenteric ischemia
  —Strangulated/ischemic bowel, abdominal malignancy, amyloidosis, neurofibromatosis, retroperitoneal fibrosis.

PREGNANCY

Pregnancy increases the risk of arterial and venous thrombosis in patients with preexisting hyper-coagulable states.

ASSOCIATED CONDITIONS

- Embolus
  —20% have synchronous emboli to upper or lower extremities. Prior emboli (cerebral, renal, lower extremity) are common.
- Arterial thrombosis and chronic mesenteric ischemia
  —Typically, diffuse and extensive atherosclerotic disease (coronary, cerebrovascular, peripheral vascular)
  —Less commonly systemic vasculitis
- Venous thrombosis: deep vein thromboses
- NOMI
  —Usually critically ill
  —With cardiogenic shock from aortic insufficiency
  —Myocardial infarction
  —Congestive heart failure
  —Renal failure
  —Hypovolemic shock from dehydration
  —Pancreatitis
  —Burns
  —Diarrhea
- Secondary mesenteric ischemia
  —Intraabdominal pathology (malignancy, infection, fibrosis, adhesions, trauma)

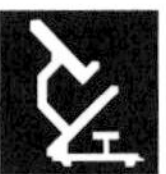

Diagnosis

DIFFERENTIAL DIAGNOSIS

- Bowel obstruction
- Perforated viscus
- Adhesions
- Appendicitis
- Cholecystitis
- Infectious colitis
- Pancreatitis
- Abdominal aortic aneurysm
- Abdominal abcess
- Abdominal malignancy
- Toxic megacolon
- Crohn's/ulcerative colitis
- Infectious colitis
- Pseudomembranous colitis

SIGNS AND SYMPTOMS

- Character, time course, and predominance of symptoms vary, depending on the cause and on the anatomic site of the ischemia.
- Abdominal pain, usually out of proportion to findings at physical examination, often poorly localized, precipitous with embolus, more insidious with thrombosis
- Urge to defecate (ischemic colitis)
- Classic triad (fear of eating, postprandial pain, weight loss) in chronic mesenteric ischemia
- Change in mental status (especially elderly patients)
- Abdominal distention (especially critically ill patients)
- Nausea and vomiting
- Diarrhea
- Lower gastrointestinal bleeding (common presenting sign in ischemic colitis)
- Fever
- Anorexia
- Upper gastrointestinal bleeding (in venous thrombosis, vague symptoms often delay diagnosis until esophageal variceal bleed)
- Physical signs minimal initially
- Later signs indicate bowel ischemia and necrosis
  —Fever
  —Tachycardia
  —Abdominal tympany
  —Peritoneal irritation
  —Abdominal distention from hypoperistalsis
  —Hypoactive bowel sounds from severe muscle ischemia
  —Fecal occult blood
  —In very late stages, hypotension, septicemia, and decreased mentation

LABORATORY PROCEDURES

- Routine blood tests show nonspecific markers of bowel injury
  —Hemoconcentration
  —Leukocytosis with left shift
  —Metabolic acidosis
  —Hyperamylasemia
  —Elevated serum lactate
  —Elevated serum alkaline phosphatase
  —Azotemia
  —Bacteremia
  —Specialized coagulation studies should be performed in cases of mesenteric vein thrombosis (antiphospholipid antibody, assays for protein C, protein S, Factor V Leiden, and antithrombin III).

IMAGING STUDIES

- Plain films (chest and abdominal x-ray) important to exclude other diagnoses
- Angiography should be performed immediately if acute mesenteric ischemia is suspected. It is diagnostic, differentiates embolus from thrombus, allows for planning surgical revascularization, and may provide means of therapy (papaverine infusion).
- CT or MRI diagnostic in 70%–100% of mesenteric venous thrombosis, and helpful in extrinsic vascular compression; unhelpful in arterial ischemia, delays diagnosis
- Ultrasonography not useful in acute ischemia, but excludes gallstones or appendicitis
- Avoid barium studies if angiography is planned; its utility is limited to acute ischemic colitis.

SPECIAL TESTS

- Abdominal paracentesis not widely used, may reveal blood-tinged fluid with high leukocytes and amylase
- Endoscopy useful only in acute and chronic ischemic colitis; preferred over barium studies in these entities because it allows mucosal brushings to exclude other diagnoses

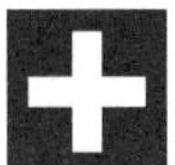

Treatment

GENERAL MEASURES

- Aggressive fluid resuscitation to replace losses from ischemic bowel
- Supplemental oxygen
- Optimize cardiac function; treat failure and arrhythmia (Swan-Ganz and Foley catheter monitoring)
- Discontinue vasoconstricting drugs (e.g., digoxin, vasopressin)
- Correct electrolyte and acid–base imbalances
- Broad-spectrum antibiotics
- Nasogastric tube to decompress ischemic bowel
- Rectal tube for ischemic colitis

SURGICAL MEASURES

- Embolism
  —Immediate vascular surgery for embolectomy and resection of nonviable bowel; second operation at 24–48 hours to evaluate areas of questionable viability
- Arterial thrombosis
  —Revascularization (bypass grafting) with resection of nonviable bowel; second operation at 24–48 hours to evaluate areas of questionable viability
- Venous thrombosis
  —General surgery only to resect nonviable bowel
- NOMI: general surgery only to resect nonviable bowel
- Secondary mesenteric ischemia: general surgery to resect extravascular disease
- Acute ischemic colitis: 20% require bowel resection
- Chronic ischemic colitis: only to relieve symptomatic stricture
- Chronic venous thrombosis: portosystemic shunting for intractable variceal bleeding
- Chronic mesenteric ischemia: arterial reconstruction for symptomatic patients

ADMISSION/DISCHARGE CRITERIA

- Admit for any indication of bowel ischemia requiring angiographic or surgical intervention.
- Discharge when vascular supply sufficient to prevent bowel ischemia and necrosis.

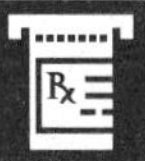

Medications

DRUG(S) OF CHOICE

- Heparin immediately if thromboembolism is suspected
- Warfarin long-term to prevent recurrent embolus or thrombosis
- Papaverine via affected artery (never systemic) for NOMI and preoperative arterial embolus or thrombosis
- Thrombolytics considered experimental for poor surgical candidates

Follow-up

PATIENT MONITORING

- Lifelong anticoagulation for most patients
- Monitor patients for extraintestinal emboli and thrombosis (coronary, cerebrovascular, peripheral vascular, deep vein thrombosis).

EXPECTED COURSE AND PROGNOSIS

- Acute arterial ischemia
  —Overall mortality rate 50%
  —If diagnosed before peritoneal signs, survival rate is 90%.
  —If bowel necrosis at time of diagnosis, mortality rate is 70%–90%.
  —Causes of death include extensive bowel necrosis, cardiopulmonary failure, hemorrhage, and recurrent emboli to other sites.
- Acute venous thrombosis
  —25%–30% mortality rate
  —Average hospital stay 26 days, with 55% incidence of major postoperative complications (infection, recurrent thrombosis)
- NOMI: very high mortality from underlying shock state and multiple organ failure
- Acute ischemic colitis
  —Most patients improve after 24 hours of expectant medical therapy (antibiotic, fluids, rectal tube).
  —60% mortality rate in surgical cases
  —Recurrence unusual
  —20% develop chronic colitis requiring elective surgery.
- Chronic arterial ischemia
  —80%–90% success following elective surgery
  —Myocardial disease and arterial reocclusion are important causes of death.

PATIENT EDUCATION

Because early intervention is key to survival, advise patients to seek immediate medical attention for symptoms of recurrent bowel ischemia.

Miscellaneous

ICD-9-CM

444.9 Embolism and thrombosis of unspecified artery or vein
557.9 Unspecified vascular insufficiency to intestine
557.1 Chronic vascular insufficiency of intestine

BIBLIOGRAPHY

Capell MS. Intestinal (mesenteric) vasculopathy I: acute superior mesenteric arteriopathy and venopathy. *Gastroenterol Clin North Am* 1998; 27:783–825.

Capell MS. Intestinal (mesenteric) vasculopathy II: ischemic colitis and chronic mesenteric ischemia. *Gastroenterol Clin North Am* 1998;27: 827–860.

Eldrup-Jorgenson J, Hawkins RE, Bredenberg CE. Abdominal vascular catastrophes. *Surg Clin North Am* 1997;77:1305–1320.

Author: Rosemary Mehl

Junctional Rhythm

Basics

DESCRIPTION

Normally the heartbeat is initiated by the sinus node (i.e., sinus rhythm).

- When it originates from the atrioventricular junction, it is called a junctional rhythm.
- A rhythm that is <100 beats/min is usually considered an escape rhythm, as during sinus bradycardia. If it is faster, it is called junctional tachycardia.

EPIDEMIOLOGY

- Depends on patient population, and can be seen in all ages

ETIOLOGY

- Idiopathic
- Junctional ectopic tachycardia (JET) is a rapid arrhythmia that can be life threatening seen in youth after congenital heart disease operations with beta-adrenergic stimulation.
- Seen in older individuals in concert with acute myocardial infarction (especially inferior with enhanced vagal tone) and as a manifestation of drug toxicity
- Catecholamine stimulation

RISK FACTORS

- None specific

PREGNANCY

N/A

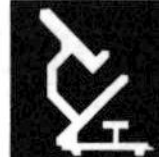

Diagnosis

DIFFERENTIAL DIAGNOSIS

- Atrioventricular (AV) nodal reentry
- AV reentry
- Permanent form of junctional reciprocating tachycardia, which virtually always has a deeply inverted P wave in ECG leads II, III, and aVF with the RP interval longer than the RR interval
- Ectopic atrial tachycardia
- Sinus tachycardia
- Atrial flutter

SIGNS AND SYMPTOMS

- Asymptomatic
- Palpitations
- Dyspnea
- Heart failure (if incessant, causing "tachycardia-associated cardiomyopathy")

LABORATORY PROCEDURES

- Only to assess drug levels if patient is thought to have toxicity

IMAGING STUDIES

N/A

SPECIAL TESTS

- ECG shows narrow QRS tachycardia without discernible P waves. If there is retrograde conduction to the atria, a P wave can be seen following the QRS.
- For the specific arrhythmia JET, there is often AV dissociation because the junctional rate is significantly greater than the atrial rate.

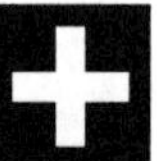

Treatment

GENERAL MEASURES

- Remove precipitating cause (toxic drug, catecholamine stimulation).

SURGICAL MEASURES

Usually a pacemaker is not needed.

ADMISSION/DISCHARGE CRITERIA

Usually arrhythmia is first recognized in inpatients. Discharge is determined by resolution of other medical problems.

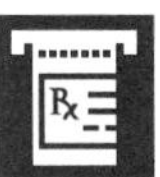

Medications

DRUG(S) OF CHOICE

- Drugs not often effective
- Sometimes substrate may be abatable, but risk for damage to normal AV conduction is significant (AV node or His bundle)
- For postoperative JET, beta-blockers, verapamil, procainamide (with hypothermia), and amiodarone have been used with varying success.
- For accelerated idioventricular rhythm in acute myocardial infarction, administration of antiarrhythmic drugs may suppress this escape pacemaker and lead to asystole.
  - —In this setting, observation is indicated because the junctional rhythm usually resolves.
  - —Especially common in inferior myocardial infarction. In the uncommon circumstance that it does not resolve, permanent pacemaker implantation may be indicated.

Follow-up

PATIENT MONITORING

Usually arrhythmia is transient and corrects during hospitalization for underlying cause.

EXPECTED COURSE AND PROGNOSIS

- Depends on underlying diseases

PATIENT EDUCATION

Depending on presentation and underlying disease:

- If observed in healthy athlete with high vagal tone, no intervention is necessary.
- Rarely, electrophysiologic study may be considered to identify substrate and perhaps cure with ablation (i.e., AV nodal reentry, AV reentry, ectopic atrial tachycardia).

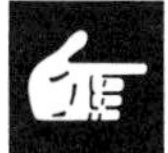

Miscellaneous

ICD-9-CM

427.89 Other, specified conduction disorders

BIBLIOGRAPHY

Hamdan MH, Scheinman MM. Role of invasive EP testing in the evaluation and management of junctional tachycardia. *Cardiol Electrophysiol Rev* 1997;4:439–442.

Walsh EP, Saul P, Sholler GF, et al. Evaluation of a staged treatment protocol for rapid automatic junctional tachycardia after operation for congenital heart disease. *J Am Coll Cardiol* 1997;29:1046–1053.

Author: Andrew E. Epstein

Left Ventricular Outflow Obstructive Lesions, Nonvalvular

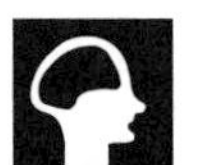

Basics

DESCRIPTION

Left ventricular outflow tract obstruction (LVOTO) may be valvar, subvalvar, or supravalvar. Combined lesions can occur. This chapter will discuss nonvalvular LVOTO.

- Subaortic obstructive defects include discrete fibromuscular ridges, hypertrophic cardiomyopathy idiopathic hypertrophic subaortic stenosis (HCM/IHSS) with systolic anterior motion of the mitral valve (SAM), accessory endocardial cushion tissue, and fibromuscular tunnel.
- Supravalvar aortic stenosis may occur as a discrete lesion immediately distal to the aortic valve, long segment narrowing of the transverse aortic arch, localized fibrous membrane, or discrete narrowing of the aorta, forming an aortic coarctation.

EPIDEMIOLOGY

- Subvalvar aortic stenosis constitutes 8%–20% of LV outflow tract obstruction. Supravalvar stenosis is the least common form.
- Discrete membranous subaortic obstruction: 2:1 male to female predominance
- Obstruction in HCM/IHSS occurs in 30/100,000 population
- Supravalvar obstruction is associated with William's syndrome in approximately 30% to 50% of cases; the remainder are non-William's and often familial.

ETIOLOGY

- HCM/IHSS is related to autosomal dominance in 50%; may occur with Friedreich's ataxia (autosomal recessive or dominant inheritance), LEOPARD syndrome, and Pompe's disease (glycogen storage disorder).
- Supravalvar aortic obstruction can occur as an autosomal-dominant trait; an elastin gene abnormality (7q11) has been determined to cause William's syndrome.
- No determined genetic etiology for other forms

PREGNANCY

- Potential poor tolerance of decreased systemic vascular resistance and increased blood volume, which accompanies pregnancy because of an inability to increase stroke volume; tachycardia may produce heart failure and myocardial ischemia
- HCM/IHSS may show improvement in symptomatology and reduction of outflow gradient and may be related to increased blood volume.

ASSOCIATED CONDITIONS

- Subvalvar outflow obstruction associated with valvar stenosis, aortic coarctation, ventricular septal defect, double outlet right ventricle, D-transposition of the great arteries, endocardial cushion defects.
- Supravalvular outflow obstruction is associated with peripheral pulmonic stenosis, ventricular septal defect, patent ductus arteriosus, pulmonary valve stenosis, and aortic coarctation. In William's syndrome, both supravalvar aortic stenosis and peripheral pulmonic stenosis are most often present. In adult life other arterial lesions may occur.

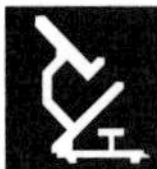

Diagnosis

DIFFERENTIAL DIAGNOSIS

- Valvar aortic stenosis

SIGNS AND SYMPTOMS

History

- Often asymptomatic; may be discovered only during referral for murmur evaluation
- Chest pain, dyspnea, and tachycardia are noted with severe HCM/IHSS, especially in adolescents and children. Chest pain is not anginal, although some studies have described evidence of ischemia.
- HCM/IHSS may present in infancy with congestive heart failure (CHF) with poor feeding/growth and respiratory distress.
- HCM/IHSS may be associated with supraventricular and ventricular arrhythmias; most common is nonsustained ventricular tachycardia.
- HCM is the most common cause of sudden death in the adolescent population; family history of sudden early death often can be confirmed.

PHYSICAL EXAMINATION

- Discrete subvalvar obstruction
  —Soft murmur at left medial/left lateral sternal border radiating to upper sternal border and suprasternal notch
  —No systolic ejection click
  —Early diastolic murmur of aortic insufficiency may be audible.
  —Pulses are usually symmetric.
- HCM/IHSS
  —Variable
  —Often healthy appearing, may have normal examination results
  —Often increased apical impulse
  —S1 normal; S2 may be paradoxically split with delayed closure of aortic valve
  —Systolic ejection murmur at left lower sternal border and apex; increases with decreased preload (i.e., Valsalva maneuver)
  —May be holosystolic murmur at apex and axilla with associated mitral regurgitation; often difficult to discern from outflow murmur
- Supravalvar obstruction
  —Features of William's syndrome may be present, including elfin facies.
  —Thrill often palpable at suprasternal notch and carotid vessels
  —No systolic click
  —Blood pressure differential between right and left arms may be present.
  —Systolic ejection murmur at base of heart radiating to neck
  —Murmur of aortic insufficiency may be present.
  —Coexistent murmur of peripheral pulmonic stenosis may be present.

LABORATORY PROCEDURES

- ECG
  —LV hypertrophy in proportion to degree of obstruction: may be normal to severe
  —Prominent hypertrophy accompanied by ST- and T-wave changes
- Holter
  —Holter monitor important to revealing possible arrhythmias, especially with HCM
  —Supraventricular arrhythmias and ventricular arrhythmias can be documented, especially runs of nonsustained ventricular tachycardia
- Chest x-ray
  —Usually normal cardiac silhouette and pulmonary vascular markings, although a congestive heart may cause pulmonary vascular congestion
  —Cardiomegaly may be present late, and enlargement of the LV downward, leftward, and posterior gives the appearance of an elongated heart in the frontal view extending down to the left hemidiaphragm, whereas the lateral view reveals a convex and globular posterior shadow.
  —Aortic root may appear dilated with fixed subaortic obstruction and may appear smaller with supravalvar obstruction.
  —Calcification generally only seen with valvar stenosis

IMAGING STUDIES

- Echocardiogram
  —Excellent modality for diagnosis and examining 2-D anatomy of obstruction
  —Allows for evaluation of degree/location of hypertrophy
  —Gradient across obstruction may be estimated by Doppler.
  —Identification of aortic root dilatation, which can be associated with fixed subaortic obstruction
  —Visualization of supravalvar stenosis, degree of narrowing
  —Evaluation of LV size, septal and free wall thickness
  —Identifies associated lesions
- Cardiac catheterization/angiography
  —Mean left atrial pressure and left ventricular end-diastolic pressure may be elevated
  —Accurate measurement of gradient across obstruction
  —Ventriculogram shows location and dimensions of obstruction and quality of ventricular function
  —Identifies associated lesions, especially peripheral pulmonic stenosis

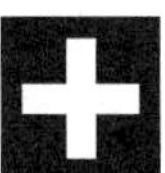

Treatment

GENERAL MEASURES

- Dependent on nature/degree of obstruction
- Discrete membranous subaortic obstruction tends to be progressive; will usually be referred for surgical resection at time of identification if >30 mm Hg; some patients remain stable with mild gradients
- No vigorous physical activity (e.g., weight lifting, competitive sports)
- Dual-chamber pacing in HCM/IHSS may improve symptomatology and reduce outflow gradient.
- Increased degree of gradient in HCM/IHSS is not correlated directly to increased risk of sudden death.
- Gradient in HCM may be variable.

SURGICAL MEASURES

- Fibromuscular ridge with discrete membranous obstruction is resected surgically and may recur or require reoperation. Obstruction is generally removed circumferentially during cardiopulmonary bypass and accessed through the aortic valve; septal myotomy also may be performed.
- HCM/IHSS referred for myectomy; at times mitral valve repair dependent on degree of obstruction
- Tunnel-type obstruction may have a history of repeated resections; use of Ross procedure (pulmonary autograft) is recommended.
- Removal of accessory endocardial cushion tissue to relieve LVOTO; may need mitral valve replacement.

ADMISSION/DISCHARGE CRITERIA

Admission

- Signs/symptoms of LV outflow compromise: poor perfusion, hypotension, CHF, myocardial infarction, arrhythmia
- Progressive increase in degree of obstruction

Discharge

- Resolution of above status after supportive care or surgical intervention

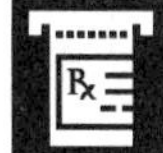

Medications

DRUG(S) OF CHOICE

- Antiarrhythmic therapy not required in most cases
- Calcium channel blockers may improve diastolic function in HCM/IHSS
- Atrial fibrillation prominent in HCM/IHSS, especially following surgery
- High-dose beta-adrenergic blockade thought to improve survival in childhood HCM/IHSS; may be only means of control for ventricular arrhythmias in HCM/IHSS
- Anticongestive measures for late LV dilatation and CHF

Follow-up

PATIENT MONITORING

- Dependent upon degree of obstruction, symptomatology, surgical history

EXPECTED COURSE AND PROGNOSIS

- Surgery for a discrete membranous obstruction usually yields a good result but can recur; gradient may persist despite surgical resection; aortic insufficiency and heart block are potential complications of surgery.
- HCM/IHSS courses are age dependent. Symptomatic infants have a poor prognosis, with high mortality. The usual course is slow progression of symptoms with risk of sudden death. Some patients remain stable for many years.
- Risk factors for death in HCM/IHSS include family history of sudden death, higher LV end-diastolic pressure, syncope, history of CHF.
- Supravalvar aortic stenosis may remain stable for years with mild obstruction, and surgical results are usually excellent. Peripheral pulmonary stenosis rarely leads to right ventricular dysfunction and may regress during childhood. Other arterial stenoses may emerge.

PATIENT EDUCATION

- No vigorous activity/competitive sports
- Higher incidence of sudden death with HCM/IHSS than general population, especially during or following exercise
- Endocarditis prophylaxis

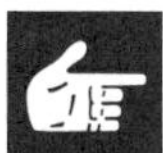

Miscellaneous

BIBLIOGRAPHY

Kuck KH. Arrhythmias in hypertrophic cardiomyopathy. *Pacing Clin Electrophysiol* 1997;20(Part 2):2706–2713.

Ostman-Smith I, Wettrell G, Risenfeld T. A cohort study of childhood hypertrophic cardiomyopathy. *J Am Coll Cardiol* 1999;34:1813–1822.

Rayburn ST, Netherland DE, Heath BJ. Discrete membranous subaortic stenosis: improved results after resection and myectomy. *Ann Thorac Surg* 1997;64:105–109.

Takeuchi M, Abe H, Kuroiwa A. Effect of dual chamber pacing on coronary flow velocity in a patient with hypertrophic obstructive cardiomyopathy. *Pacing Clin Electrophysiol* 1996;19(Part 1):2153–2155.

Emmanouildes, et al. *Moss & Adams,* 5th ed. 1995.

Bruce CJ, et al. Fixed left ventricular outflow tract obstruction presumed hypertrophic obstructive cardiomyopathy: implications for therapy. *Ann Thorac Surg* 1999;68:100–104.

Fyler D. *Nadas pediatric cardiology.* Copyright 1992, Donald Fyler, MD.

Garson, et al. *The science and practice of pediatric cardiology,* 2nd ed. 1997.

Morris CA. Genetic aspects of supravalvular aortic stenosis. *Curr Opin Cardiol* 1998;13: 214–219.

Fedderly RT. Left ventricular outflow obstruction. *Pediatr Clin North Am April* 1999.

Kim YM, et al. Natural course of supravalvar aortic stenosis and peripheral pulmonary arterial stenosis in William's syndrome. *Cardiol Young* 1999;9:37–41.

Perloff JK. The clinical recognition of congenital heart disease, 4th ed. 1994.

Oakley CM. Pregnancy and congenital heart disease. *Heart* 1997;78:12–14.

Kitchiner D, et al. Prognosis of supravalve aortic stenosis in 81 patients in Liverpool (1960–1993). *Heart* 1996;75:396–402.

Kizilbash AM, et al. Spontaneous variability of left ventricular outflow tract gradient in hypertrophic obstructive cardiomyopathy. *Circulation* 1998;97:461–466.

Berger S, Dhala A, Friedberg, DZ. Sudden cardiac death in infants, children, and adolescents. *Pediatr Clin North Am* 1999;46: 221–234.

Authors: David Crowe and Welton M. Gerson

Long QT Syndrome

Basics

DESCRIPTION

- The QT interval is prolonged on the ECG.
- Patients may be identified fortuitously, after an episode of syncope or palpitations, or during family screening.

EPIDEMIOLOGY

The prevalence is estimated to be 1/5,000 individuals, but this estimate is uncertain. Any age can be affected.

ETIOLOGY

The long QT syndrome (LQTS) is a genetic disorder.

- Multiple genes have been identified causing the syndrome.
- Abnormalities affect the sodium and potassium channels.
  - —LQT1 mediated by potassium channel gene on chromosome 11
  - —LQT2 mediated by potassium channel gene on chromosome 7
  - —LQT3 mediated by sodium channel gene on chromosome 3
  - —LQT4 mediated by gene with uncertain function on chromosome 4
  - —LQT5 mediated by potassium channel gene on chromosome 21
  - —LQT6 mediated by potassium channel gene on chromosome 21

RISK FACTORS

- Female gender
- Absolute length of QT interval
- History of syncope
- Family history of unexpected, premature sudden death

PREGNANCY

There is not a firm contraindication for pregnancy. Arrhythmias are sometimes exacerbated by pregnancy, and the risk of genetic transmission to the offspring has to be considered and discussed.

ASSOCIATED CONDITIONS

- None

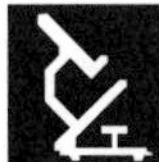

Diagnosis

DIFFERENTIAL DIAGNOSIS

- Ischemia
- Electrolyte disturbances (hypokalemia, hypocalcemia)
- Brugada syndrome
- Central nervous system injury
- Any disease state that can alter cardiac repolarization and, therefore, the QT interval
- Drugs that prolong the QT interval (see the Appendix for the table Drugs that Can Prolong the QT Interval).

SIGNS AND SYMPTOMS

- Syncope and presyncope
- Cardiac arrest

LABORATORY PROCEDURES

- None

IMAGING STUDIES

Although there are reports of abnormal sympathetic innervation identified by positron emission tomography (PET) scanning and ^{123}I metaiodobenzylguanidine, these are for research purposes only.

SPECIAL TESTS

Measurement of the QT interval on the ECG is the foundation of the diagnosis. Although genetic testing is available in research settings, genotyping is not clinically available.

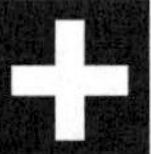

Treatment

GENERAL MEASURES

Beta-blockers are mainstays of therapy.

- Pacing to prevent bradycardia and left sympathectomy are time-honored treatments.
- Because of the efficacy of implantable defibrillators (ICDs) to prevent sudden, arrhythmic death, they are being used more frequently.

SURGICAL MEASURES

Two surgical interventions are used to manage LQTS:

- Left cervicothoracic sympathectomy is a time-honored approach to decrease the risk of torsades de pointes ventricular tachycardia. Permanent pacing, either atrial- or ventricular-based, shortens the QT interval and also decreases the risk of torsades de pointes ventricular tachycardia.
- The ICD is used for secondary prevention of death in patients resuscitated from cardiac arrest, and for "high-risk" individuals, such as those from families with a high rate of premature death from LQTS.

ADMISSION/DISCHARGE CRITERIA

- If the presentation of LQTS is cardiac arrest, ICD implantation is recommenced.
- If the syndrome is diagnosed incidentally, discussion about risk of disease (cardiac arrest) must be discussed. If an ICD is desired, admission is then planned.
- If the patient presents with syncope and the ECG pattern of LQTS is recognized, he or she should be hospitalized because recurrence may not spontaneously terminate.

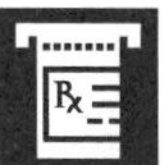

Medications

DRUG(S) OF CHOICE

- Beta-blockers are mainstay of therapy.
- They are thought to be most beneficial for patients with LQT1 and LQT2 syndromes.
- Because the sodium channel is the basis of LQT3, recent data suggest a possible benefit from mexiletine for these patients. The use of this drug, however, is not generally considered a mainstay of therapy.
- A large number of drugs can cause QT interval prolongation and precipitate torsades de pointes ventricular tachycardia in these patients.

Follow-up

PATIENT MONITORING

Family screening is indicated with ECGs recorded in first-degree relatives at the least. The disease cannot be prevented, but interventions can decrease the risk of syncope, cardiac arrest, and death.

EXPECTED COURSE AND PROGNOSIS

- Guarded, but depends on the gene involved, symptoms (prior syncope increases risk of death), and family history

PATIENT EDUCATION

- Learn contraindicated drugs.
- Prevent hypokalemia and hypomagnesemia.
- Genetic counseling is indicated for patients with LQTS who are considering having children.

Diet

- No special diet

Activity

Try to avoid situations that induce startle reflexes.

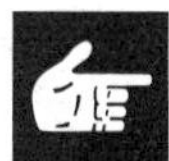

Miscellaneous

ICD-9-CM

427.1 Paroxysmal ventricular tachycardia

See also: Ventricular fibrillation; Ventricular tachycardia; Brugada syndrome; Sudden death.

ORGANIZATIONS

Sudden Arrhythmia Death (SADS) Foundation, 508 E. South Temple, Suite 20, P.O. Box 58767, Salt Lake City, UT 84102; http:www.sads@sads.org.

BIBLIOGRAPHY

Moss AJ. Management of patients with the hereditary long QT syndrome. *J Cardiovasc Electrophysiol* 1998;9:668–674.

Roden DM, Lazzara R, Rosen M, et al. Multiple mechanisms in the long-QT syndrome: current knowledge, gaps, and future directions. *Circulation* 1996;94:1196–2012.

Author: Andrew E. Epstein

Lyme Disease and the Heart

Basics

DESCRIPTION

Lyme disease is a multisystem infection caused by *Borrelia burgdorferi*, a spirochetal organism transmitted by the Ixodes tick (deer tick).

- Stage 1. Early localized (3–32 days after tick bite) erythema chronicum migrans (90%) and flulike illness
- Stage 2. Early disseminated (weeks to months) multiorgan involvement, most commonly neurologic (10%) and carditis (1%–8%)
- Stage 3. Late disseminated (months to years) arthritis (up to 50%), and neurologic syndromes
  - —Cardiac manifestations typically occur 1–2 months after onset of infection.
  - —Conduction system disease: first-, second-, or third-degree atrioventricular (AV) block, bundle brunch block, fascicular block
  - —Tachyarrhythmias
    - Myocarditis and pericarditis
    - Cardiomyopathy and congestive heart failure rare in the United States

EPIDEMIOLOGY

- Lyme disease is the leading tickborne disease in the United States.
- Overall incidence 4.4/100,000

Incidence

- Between May and August
- Highest prevalence in northeastern coastal states, the upper Midwest, and Northern California
- Can occur at any age, most common in children and young adults
- Males affected as often as females
- Myocarditis was reported in 8% of U.S. patients before widespread use of antibiotic for erythema migrans most recent data <1%.

ETIOLOGY

- Causal microorganism *B. burgdorferi*, transmitted by the bite of Ixodes ticks
- Chronic arthritis related to HLA DR-4

RISK FACTORS

- Exposure to tick-infested area

PREGNANCY

N/A

ASSOCIATED CONDITIONS

N/A

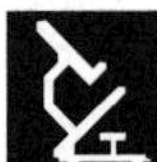

Diagnosis

DIFFERENTIAL DIAGNOSIS

- Rheumatic myocarditis, viral myocarditis
- Juvenile rheumatoid arthritis
- Babesiosis, ehrlichiosis

SIGNS AND SYMPTOMS

- Cardiac symptoms
  - —Asymptomatic
  - —Light-headedness
  - —Dizziness
  - —Syncope
  - —Dyspnea
  - —Palpitations
  - —Chest pain

LABORATORY PROCEDURES

- IgG–IgM burgdorferi antibodies (positive ELISA or immunofluorescent assay result should be confirmed by Western blot). Poor sensitivity early, as antibodies develop slowly: 30%–40% seropositive patients early, 60%–70% 2–4 weeks after infection
- Culture of skin lesions and polymerase chain reaction of skin biopsy and blood

IMAGING STUDIES

- Echocardiogram: Dilated cardiomyopathy is rare.

SPECIAL TESTS

- ECG
  - —Atrioventricular conduction system disease in up to 90% of patients with Lyme disease: first-, second-, or third-degree AV block, bundle brunch block, fascicular block, tachyarrhythmias, nonspecific ST segment or T-wave changes

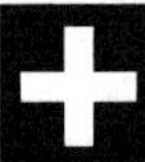

Treatment

GENERAL MEASURES

- Preventive measures when in grassy or wooded areas, including wearing light-colored clothing, long pants tucked into socks or boots, and long-sleeved shirts, and using tick repellent
- Prophylactic antibiotic therapy is not necessary.

SURGICAL MEASURES

N/A

ADMISSION/DISCHARGE CRITERIA

- Hospitalize patients with significant PR prolongation or second-degree or complete AV block until antibiotics have been initiated and the heart block has responded.
- Temporary pacing may be necessary.

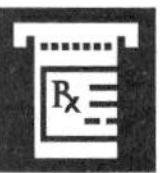

Medications

DRUG(S) OF CHOICE

- Most manifestations of Lyme disease resolve spontaneously without treatment.
- Antibiotics may hasten resolution and prevent disease progression.
- Myocarditis
  —Oral treatment for first-degree heart block: doxycycline (100 mg b.i.d. for 14 days), amoxicillin (500 mg t.i.d. for 14 days), cefuroxime axetil 500 mg b.i.d. for 14 days
  —For advanced (second- or third-degree) heart block, no proof that i.v. treatment is more effective than oral treatment: ceftriaxone (2 g i.v. daily for 14 days)
  —Vaccine LYMERIX: recommended for individuals over 15 years of age who live or work in grassy or wooded areas and whose exposure is frequent or prolonged

Follow-up

PATIENT MONITORING

Patients with severe Lyme disease should be monitored with ECG during weeks and months after tick bite to detect conduct abnormalities.

EXPECTED COURSE AND PROGNOSIS

- Prognosis of cardiac manifestations of Lyme disease is usually good.
- Temporary pacemaker may be required in up to one-third of cases.
- Complete recovery occurs in most (up to 90%).
- Late complications such as dilated cardiomyopathy occur rarely.

PATIENT EDUCATION

Protection against tick exposure should be emphasized in endemic areas.

Organization

- American Lyme Disease Foundation, One Financial Plaza, Hartford, CT 66103; (860)525-2000; hotline (800)886-LYME; lymefnd@aol.com

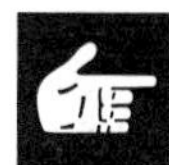

Miscellaneous

ICD-9-CM

088-8 Other specific arthropod-borne disease
088-81 Lyme disease

BIBLIOGRAPHY

Cox J, et al. Cardiovascular manifestations of Lyme disease. *Am Heart J* 1991;122:1449–1455.

Nadelman RB, Wormser GP. Lyme borreliosis. *Lancet* 1998;352:557–565.

Nagi K, et al. Cardiac manifestations of Lyme disease: a review. *Can J Cardiol* 1996;12:503–506.

Sigal L. Early disseminated Lyme disease: cardiac manifestations. *Am J Med* 1995;89(suppl 4A):25–29.

Author: Maria Cecilia Bahit

Marfan's Syndrome

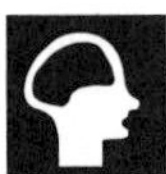

Basics

DESCRIPTION

Marfan's syndrome describes a clinical constellation reflecting connective tissue disease of varying severity.

- The clinical presentation ranges from severe congestive heart failure in the fetus/neonate, to the relatively asymptomatic adult.
- Genetic expression and penetrance determine the clinical manifestations.
- Mitral valve prolapse (MVP) with or without mitral regurgitation and aortic root dilatation are the most common cardiac findings.
- The ultimate complication of the disease is aortic dissection with or without aortic valve insufficiency.
- The aim of management is to closely monitor or even retard aortic root growth and, if possible, replace the aorta prophylactically, before dissection occurs.
- Spontaneous pneumothorax, lens dislocation, and scoliosis/lordosis can all be among the presenting findings in Marfan's syndrome.
- Patients are unusually tall with long, slender fingers and toes.
- They may report being "double-jointed" (abnormal appendicular joint mobility).
- The trunk is short compared with leg length, and there can be anterior chest deformity (pectus excavatum or carinatum), giving the patient with Marfan's syndrome a characteristic appearance.
- Hernias and lumbosacral spine widening of the neural canal (dural ectasia) also may be present.

EPIDEMIOLOGY

- Marfan's syndrome is relatively common.
- There is no predilection for race or sex.
- Age at presentation is usually dependent on the severity of the disease:
  —Mild scoliosis in a tall child may result in a screening echocardiogram, which shows MVP and a dilated aortic root.
  —Opthalmologic examination may result in the diagnosis of lens dislocation (50%).
  —In some cases, other members of the family with "familial tall stature" are then diagnosed with Marfan's disease.
  —A hydropic fetus may have severe MVP/mitral regurgitation on fetal echocardiographic evaluation, and at birth be found to have long digits and heart failure syndrome.
  —Myriad presentations reflect Marfan's as a multisystem disease with protean manifestations.

Prevalence

- About 1/10,000 population in the United States

ETIOLOGY

- Marfan's syndrome is autosomal dominant.
  —25%–30% are sporadic, new, dominant mutations. There is full penetrance, but considerable clinical variability.
  —Sporadic cases demonstrate a paternal age effect: in a small series, the fathers were older than fathers in the general population (37 years vs. 30 years).
  —Linkage to chromosome 15 has been established. The gene product, fibrillin, is abnormal in Marfan's syndrome.

RISK FACTORS

The cardiovascular complications of Marfan's syndrome are often more severe in young children (infantile type) with new mutations.

PREGNANCY

- Many women with Marfan's syndrome have had multiple successful pregnancies.
- Marfan's syndrome patients with prominent cardiac manifestations are often discouraged from pursuing pregnancy because of increased risk of aortic dissection.

ASSOCIATED CONDITIONS

- Marfan's syndrome is a multisystem disease.
- In addition to the above characteristics, dolichocephaly, high arched palate, arachnodactyly, striae atrophicae, hernias, and pes planus may all be seen.

Diagnosis

DIFFERENTIAL DIAGNOSIS

- Homocystinuria
- Klinefelter's syndrome
- Fragile-X syndrome
- Ehlers-Danlos syndrome
- Erdheim's cystic medial necrosis
- Congenital contractural arachnodactyly
- Stickler's syndrome may present with similar connective tissue findings.
- Diagnosis of Marfan's syndrome requires the presence of two major criteria plus several minor criteria in another system:
  —Positive family history fulfills one major criterion.
  —Other major criteria are ectopia lentis, dilatation or dissection of the ascending aorta, and lumbosacral dural ectasias.
  —At least four of the following should be present:
    - Pectus carinatum
    - Pectus excavatum
    - Positive wrist sign
    - Positive thumb sign
    - Reduced upper to lower segment ratio
    - Arm span to height ratio of >1.05
    - Scoliosis or spondylolisthesis
    - Medial displacement of the medial malleolus
    - Protrusio acetabulae
    - Spontaneous pneumothoraces, striae atrophicae, and recurrent hernias are also useful signs for diagnosis.

SIGNS AND SYMPTOMS

- Near-sightedness (myopia) in a patient with subluxation of the lenses, particularly if the patient is tall, should provoke concern for Marfan's syndrome.
- Acute chest pain in a tall person, or, relentless "tearing" chest pain in an adolescent or adult with few risk factors for angina, should stimulate concern for ascending aortic or thoracoabdominal aortic dissection.
- Spontaneous pneumothorax in a person of tall stature, with prominent digits, and/or pes planus may be the first presentation of Marfan's syndrome.
- Tall patients with scoliosis or lordosis should be evaluated carefully to see if any other criteria for Marfan's syndrome are satisfied.
- Patients presenting with a new apical murmur, a mid-systolic click at the left lower sternal border, or a diastolic murmur at the left middle to right upper sternal border should be assessed for other Marfan's criteria.
- The positive wrist sign indicates joint hyperextensibility in that the little finger covers the nail of the thumb when one hand is wrapped around the other, at the wrist.
- The positive thumb sign indicates joint hyperextensibility in that the thumb extends beyond the ulnar surface of the hand when the patient is asked to stretch the thumb across the palm.
- The upper-to-lower segment ratio averages 0.85 in patients with Marfan's syndrome (normal ratio 0.93). The upper segment of height is the distance from the top of the head to the pubic bone; the lower segment is the length from the pubic bone to the bottom of the foot. This abnormally low ratio in patients with Marfan's syndrome reflects their abnormally long limbs.
- The arm span is frequently longer than the height in patients with Marfan's syndrome. In the general population, arm span is usually less than or equal to length.

LABORATORY PROCEDURES

- Urine amino acid analysis in the absence of pyridoxine supplementation should be obtained to rule out homocystinuria.
- Blood should be obtained to search for deletions/alterations on the fibrillin gene.

IMAGING STUDIES

- Transthoracic echocardiography looks for and quantifies aortic root dilatation, compared with normal values for age and body surface area. MVP with or without regurgitation and aortic insufficiency as well as heart function are also assessed. In patients who image well, false lumina in the ascending aorta may be seen.
- Magnetic resonance angiography delineates false lumina in patients presenting with possible aortic dissection.

- Arteriography is used to confirm aortic dissection.
- Lumbosacral MRI confirms the presence of dural ectasias.

SPECIAL TESTS

- ECG to evaluate left atrial and left ventricular enlargement complements echocardiography.
- Genetic sequencing may become routine in the future to identify and confirm the abnormality on chromosome 15, and the resultant deficit within fibrillin.

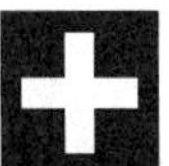

Treatment

GENERAL MEASURES

- Adults and children are routinely followed by the cardiologist or pediatric cardiologist in addition to the primary caregiver. Depending on the level of aortic root dilatation, and the rate of the dilatation, follow-up intervals should be between 3 and 12 months.
- Because Marfan's syndrome is the most common etiology of aortic dissection in youth, rough competitive sports are discouraged. Moderately strenuous or nonstrenuous recreational activities are permissible (e.g., badminton, baseball, curling, golf, table tennis, archery, bowling and riflery).
- All patients with valvar involvement should receive endocarditis prophylaxis prior to dental work or invasive procedures.
- Chest pain, back pain, and abdominal pain in a Marfan's syndrome patient should provoke a prompt evaluation for aortic dissection.

SURGICAL MEASURES

- Emergency surgery during dissection or rupture is mandatory.
- Prophylactic aortic root replacement should be performed when the aortic root diameter reaches or exceeds 5 cm, because the risk of dissection increases substantially at greater diameters.
- Mitral valve replacement may be necessary for severe regurgitation.

ADMISSION/DISCHARGE CRITERIA

Management is on an outpatient basis, unless aortic dissection or elective aortic/mitral surgery is undertaken.

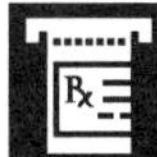

Medications

DRUG(S) OF CHOICE

- Use of beta-blockade or calcium channel blockers has been advocated in adults.
- Although wall stress is increased in the acute intravenous administration of these drugs in the catheterization laboratory, long-term use may decrease the rate of aortic root dilatation.
- Advantages of long-term beta-blockade have not been proven in growing children, whose aortic root size is predicated on their age and body surface area.
- Bacterial endocarditis prophylaxis for dental and invasive procedures

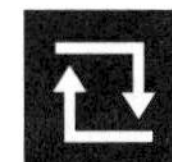

Follow-up

PATIENT MONITORING

- Close regular visits for assessment of possible signs and symptoms.
- Serial echocardiography is mandatory, because aortic root dilatation can occur without symptoms.

EXPECTED COURSE AND PROGNOSIS

- Prognosis is predicated on which major manifestations of Marfan's syndrome are present.
  - —Even with aggressive medical therapy and appropriate vigilance, aortic dissection and death have occurred.
  - —Replace the root prophylactically at 5–5.5 cm.
  - —Clinical course is dependent on the rate of aortic root dilatation, and on mitral valve status.
  - —Heart failure symptoms from mitral regurgitation can usually be medically managed.
  - —If accompanied by cardiomyopathy, the prognosis is more guarded; heart transplantation may be considered.
  - —Operative mortality rate for aortic root replacement is less than 2%, if myocardial function is good preoperatively.

PATIENT EDUCATION

- Activities are limited, as discussed previously.
- Diet should be the AHA diet for both children and adults.
- The National Marfan Foundation of the United States can supply information and support, although treatment must be individualized by the cardiologist/pediatric cardiologist.

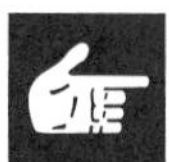

Miscellaneous

ICD-9-CM

759.82

BIBLIOGRAPHY

Beighton P, et al., eds. *McKusick's heritable disorders of connective tissue,* 5th ed. St. Louis: Mosby-Year Book, 1993.

Gott VL, et al. Replacement of the aortic root in patients with Marfan's syndrome. *N Engl J Med* 1999;340:1307–1313.

Haouzi A, et al. Heterogeneous aortic response to acute beta-adrenergic blockade in Marfan syndrome. *Am Heart J* 1997;133:60–63.

Rios AS, et al. Effect of long-term beta-blockade on aortic root compliance in patients with Marfan syndrome. *Am Heart J* 1999;137: 1057–1061.

Authors: Donna M. Timchak and Welton M. Gersony

Mitral Regurgitation, Adult

Basics

DESCRIPTION

Mitral regurgitation (MT) is the backflow of blood from the left ventricle (LV) to the left atrium during systole.

EPIDEMIOLOGY

Prevalence

Estimates of the disease prevalence are confounded by the observation that a small degree of physiologic MT can be detected on careful Doppler echocardiography in as many as 80% of normal healthy people.

CAUSES

- Myxomatous degeneration of the mitral valve is the most common cause of mitral regurgitation in United States. It accounts for about 65% of causes of pure mitral regurgitation.
- Mitral annular calcification
- Rheumatic heart disease
- Congenital malformation
- Ruptured chordae tendineae
- Ruptured papillary muscle
- Infective endocarditis
- Marfan's syndrome
- Ehlers-Danlos syndrome
- Pseudoxanthoma elasticum
- Systemic illness/drug effects (e.g., lupus vasculitis)
- Functional:
  - —Ischemic
  - —Dilated cardiomyopathy
  - —Infiltrative/restrictive cardiomyopathy
  - —Hypertrophic cardiomyopathy

RISK FACTORS

N/A

PREGNANCY

Patients with mitral regurgitation tolerate pregnancy well, but it might precipitate congestive heart failure in case of severe mitral regurgitation with LV systolic dysfunction.

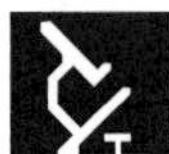

Diagnosis

DIFFERENTIAL DIAGNOSIS

- The murmur of mitral regurgitation has to be differentiated from that of aortic stenosis and hypertrophic cardiomyopathy.
- Dynamic auscultation is helpful in that situation; mitral regurgitation murmur increases with squatting and during the strain phase of Valsalva due to decrease in preload, but that of aortic stenosis is diminished.
- Handgrip increases the murmur of mitral regurgitation due to increase in the afterload with an opposite effect on aortic stenosis and hypertrophic obstructive cardiomyopathy murmurs.

SIGNS AND SYMPTOMS

Signs

- Brisk carotid upstroke with early peak and rapid decline secondary to backward flow into the left atrium instead of forward flow across the aortic valve.
- Precordial palpation usually reveals a normal apical impulse early in the disease with a displaced diffuse apex late in the course of the disease due to LV dilatation.
- Left parasternal pulsations can be appreciated with the onset of right ventricular failure or with systolic expansion of the left atrium with anterior displacement of the right heart when severe mitral regurgitation is present.
- On cardiac auscultation, the patient with mitral regurgitation typically has a soft S1 with a holosystolic murmur that is loudest at the apex and radiates to the axilla. The intensity of the murmur correlates with the severity of mitral regurgitation of organic etiology, contrary to functional mitral regurgitation, when it is grade 4 or above or grade 2 or below.
- S2 is normal early in the disease. An accentuated pulmonary component of S2 can be appreciated with the onset of pulmonary hypertension. S3 can be heard over the apex secondary to the increased rate and velocity of early diastolic filling.

Symptoms

- Mitral regurgitation secondary to ischemic disease or dilated cardiomyopathy will have symptoms typical of the underlying disease. However, patients with mitral regurgitation secondary to leaflet disease will remain symptomatic for many years.
- The typical initial presentation will be exercise intolerance in the form of exertional dyspnea. This is followed by symptoms of pulmonary congestion and congestive heart failure.
- The onset of symptoms may coincide with a period of increased hemodynamic burden (e.g., pregnancy, infection, etc.) or with the onset of atrial fibrillation.

LABORATORY PROCEDURES

N/A

IMAGING STUDIES

Electrocardiography

Findings in patients with mitral regurgitation are nonspecific and include left atrial enlargement, atrial fibrillation, and LV hypertrophy in patients with severe mitral regurgitation.

Chest X-ray

- Chest radiography may be normal early in the disease with left atrial enlargement later on. During the decompensated stage, evidence of pulmonary involvement becomes apparent.
- Pulmonary hypertension is manifested as increased size of central pulmonary arteries with peripheral attenuation of pulmonary vessels.

Echocardiography

- An initial 2-D Doppler study is indispensable in the management of mitral regurgitation.
- It estimates the LV and left atrial volumes, LV ejection fraction (EF), and the severity of mitral regurgitation.
- It helps in disclosure of the anatomic cause of mitral regurgitation.
- Serial echocardiograms help in the decision making regarding timing of surgery.
- It should be performed after mitral valve surgery to establish a baseline status.

Transesophageal Echocardiography

- It is useful for evaluation of patients in whom transthoracic echocardiography is inconclusive.
- It should be performed intraoperatively to establish the anatomic basis of mitral regurgitation and guide repair.

SPECIAL TESTS

Cardiac catheterization can be performed to assess the severity of mitral regurgitation as well as to delineate coronary anatomy.

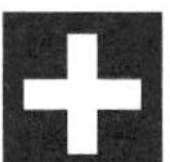

Treatment

GENERAL MEASURES

- Recommendations for left ventriculography and hemodynamic measurement in mitral regurgitation:
  —When noninvasive tests are inconclusive regarding the severity of mitral regurgitation, LV function, or need for surgery
  —When there is discrepancy between clinical and noninvasive findings regarding severity of mitral regurgitation

SURGICAL MEASURES

- Mitral valve replacement or repair
  —Acute symptomatic mitral regurgitation
  —Patients with severe mitral regurgitation and NYHA class II–IV symptoms with EF >60% and end-systolic dimension <45 mm.
  —Patients with severe mitral regurgitation with EF 50%–60% and end-systolic dimension 45–50 mm regardless of the symptoms
  —Patients with severe mitral regurgitation with EF 30%–50% and/or end-systolic dimension 50–55 mm regardless of the symptoms
  —Asymptomatic patients with severe mitral regurgitation and atrial fibrillation in the presence of preserved LV function.
  —Asymptomatic patients with severe mitral regurgitation and severe pulmonary hypertension with preserved LV function.
  —Asymptomatic patients with severe mitral regurgitation with EF 50%–60% or end-systolic dimension 45–50 mm
  —Patients with severe LV dysfunction (EF <30% and/or end-systolic dimension >55 mm) in whom chordal preservation is likely
  —Asymptomatic patients with severe mitral regurgitation and preserved LV function in whom mitral valve repair is highly likely
  —Patients with mitral valve prolapse and severe mitral regurgitation in the presence of preserved LV function who have recurrent ventricular arrhythmias despite medical therapy
- Recommendations for coronary angiography in mitral regurgitation:
  —When mitral valve surgery is contemplated in patients with angina or history of myocardial infarction
  —When mitral valve surgery is contemplated in patients with one or more risk factors for coronary artery disease
  —When ischemia is suspected as a causal factor in mitral regurgitation

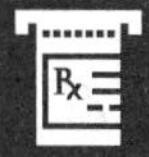

Medications

DRUG(S) OF CHOICE

- Vasodilators
  —There are no long-term studies to indicate that they are beneficial in asymptomatic patients with normal LV function.
  —Symptomatic patients should be referred for surgery.
- Atrial fibrillation
  —Rate control can be achieved with beta-blockers, calcium channel blockers, digitalis, or, rarely, amiodarone if cardioversion is a factor.
  —Anticoagulation using warfarin is indicated in patients with mitral regurgitation and atrial fibrillation with a target INR of 2–3.

Follow-up

PATIENT MONITORING

- Asymptomatic patients with normal LV function should be evaluated clinically on a yearly basis. Echocardiography is recommended every 6–12 months if mitral regurgitation is severe.
- Patients should be followed postoperatively because some might worsen after surgery, and in case of mitral valve replacement they should be anticoagulated.

Prevention

Prophylaxis against infective endocarditis and recurrent rheumatic fever, if applicable, is indicated.

Complications

- Atrial arrhythmias
- Congestive heart failure
- Sudden cardiac death
- Pulmonary hypertension with right-sided heart failure
- Recurrent rheumatic fever
- Systemic embolization
- Prosthetic valve-related complications

EXPECTED COURSE AND PROGNOSIS

- For the patients with symptoms from severe mitral regurgitation, surgical intervention improves long-term outcome and relieves symptoms.
- Surgical treatment of mitral regurgitation secondary to LV dilation and systolic dysfunction, dilated cardiomyopathy, or ischemic heart disease remains controversial with the possibility of worsening of LV function after surgery as a result of increased afterload.

PATIENT EDUCATION

Asymptomatic patients should be educated to report any symptoms, which can be confirmed objectively using an exercise test.

Activity

There is no limitation for asymptomatic patients with mild to moderate mitral regurgitation with normal LV function. There is no evidence that vigorous exercise accelerates the progression of mitral regurgitation.

Diet

- Low-salt diet for congestive heart failure

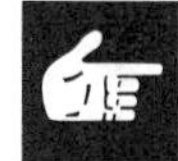

Miscellaneous

ICD-9-CM

424.0

BIBLIOGRAPHY

Bonow RO, Carabello B, de Leon AC Jr, et al. ACC/AHA guidelines for the management of patients with valvular heart disease: a report of the American College of Cardiology/American Heart Association Task Force on Practice Guidelines (Committee on Management of Patients with Valvular Heart Disease). *J Am Coll Cardiol* 1998;32:1486–1588.

Otto C. *Valvular heart disease,* 1st ed. Philadelphia: WB Saunders, 1999.

Quinones MA. Management of mitral regurgitation: optimal timing for surgery. *Cardiol Clin* 1998;16:421–436.

Rahimtoola SH, et al. *Hurst's the heart,* 9th ed. New York: McGraw-Hill, 1998.

Authors: Amr El-Shafei, Steven Herrmann, Madhukar Gupta, and Bernard R. Chaitman

Mitral Regurgitation, Pediatric

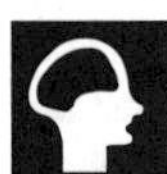

Basics

DESCRIPTION

Congenital abnormalities of the mitral valve result in incompetence during systole (ventricular contraction), causing regurgitation of blood into the left atrium with each left ventricular (LV) contraction.

Systems Affected

- Cardiovascular

ETIOLOGY

Genetics

Isolated congenital mitral insufficiency is a rare congenital anomaly in pediatric patients.

CAUSES

- Most often seen in association with other congenital heart defects, connective tissue disease, or metabolic/storage disease
- Secondary/acquired mitral regurgitation is seen following acute rheumatic fever, Kawasaki disease, cardiomyopathy, and endocarditis in children.

RISK FACTORS

- History of rheumatic fever
- Endocardial cushion defect
- Mitral valve prolapse
- Connective tissue disease

Diagnosis

DIFFERENTIAL DIAGNOSIS

The main considerations for differential diagnosis of mitral regurgitation include:

- Acquired heart disease such as acute rheumatic fever or chronic rheumatic heart disease
- Congenital mitral regurgitation alone or in association with endocardial cushion defects or mitral valve prolapse
- Connective tissue disease
- Acute trauma, infarcted papillary muscle
- On physical examination, the murmur should be distinguished from a ventricular septal defect murmur

SIGNS AND SYMPTOMS

- General
  —Symptoms usually depend on the severity and acuity of mitral regurgitation, although patients may be asymptomatic even with severe mitral regurgitation
  —Chronic mitral regurgitation is usually well-tolerated in children
- History
  —History of murmur
  —History of rheumatic fever
  —History of connective tissue disease
  —History of mitral valve prolapse
- Most common signs and symptoms
  —Shortness of breath
  —Tachypnea
  —Increased frequency of respiratory tract infections
  —Cough
  —Fatigue
  —Poor feeding
  —Exercise intolerance
- Other signs and symptoms
  —Growth failure, if advanced
- Physical examination (cardiovascular)
  —Increased precordial activity
  —Right ventricular heave if associated with increased pulmonary arterial pressure
  —Laterally displaced LV impulse
  —Increased intensity of second heart sound if pulmonary arterial pressure is elevated
  —S3 may be loud
  —Murmur of mitral regurgitation is a high-frequency, pansystolic, blowing sound heard best at the apex with radiation to the axilla (appreciated best when patient is supine and leaning leftward).
  —If the mitral regurgitation is moderate to severe, a low-frequency diastolic rumble may be appreciated at the apex, which represents increased diastolic flow across the mitral valve.

SPECIAL TESTS

- ECG
  —May remain normal until mitral regurgitation is severe
  —Left atrial enlargement (manifested by broad, notched P waves prominent in lead II)
  —Prominent LV forces
  —Right ventricular hypertrophy may eventually be present in severe cases with pulmonary hypertension.
  —If left atrial enlargement is severe, atrial arrhythmias may be observed.

IMAGING STUDIES

- Chest x-ray
  —Cardiomegaly (enlarged left atrium and LV)
  —Pulmonary venous congestion
  —Pulmonary edema (if severe mitral regurgitation)
- Echocardiography
  —Detailed visualization of the mitral valve and valve apparatus
  —LV systolic function is normal to increased because the ventricle is unloaded. If "normal," it must be compared with previous echocardiogram to ensure that function has not deteriorated.
  —Left atrium may appear dilated.
  —Color Doppler can be used to qualitatively assess mitral regurgitation.
  —If severe, pulmonary venous flow reversal may be observed (i.e., reflux into the pulmonary veins).
- Cardiac catheterization
  —May be indicated if echocardiogram is not conclusive regarding the cause of mitral regurgitation, cardiac function, associated lesions, or degree of pulmonary hypertension.
  —Mitral valve anatomy, cardiac output, pulmonary vascular resistance, and associated lesions should be assessed.
  —Pressure tracings demonstrate an elevated pulmonary capillary wedge pressure *a* wave or an elevated left atrial *a* wave if the left atrium is entered.

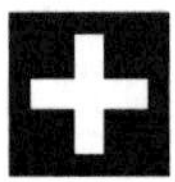

Treatment

GENERAL MEASURES

- Outpatient except for complications or surgery
- Treatment options are medical or surgical.
- For children, the size/age of the patient is an important factor in selecting a treatment plan because the smaller the patients are more likely they will need serial valve replacements as they outgrow an initial prosthetic valve.
- Medically manage if possible. If medical therapy fails, consider valvuloplasty if technically feasible and use mitral valve replacement as a final option.
- Timing of surgery is controversial, although recent literature indicates that in children, unlike adults, ventricular function appears to be preserved and improves postoperatively.

SURGICAL MEASURES

- Mitral valve repair and mitral valve replacement (MVR) are the surgical options and are indicated if medical therapy fails.
- Mitral valve repair is preferred if technically feasible to avoid complications related to size and growth, as well as anticoagulation.
- The type of mitral valve repair depends on the type of mitral valve defect. For a regurgitant valve, annuloplasty or valvuloplasty is performed. In the larger child, the annulus may be supported by a DeVega or Carpentier ring (this will not grow with the child).
- Mitral valve leaflet cleft or chordae tendineae abnormalities usually can be repaired surgically.
- MVR is reserved for patients with moderate to severe mitral regurgitation who failed medical management and who are not candidates for valve repair.
- Most common type of prosthetic valve is the St. Jude bileaflet tilting disk valve for children.
- Current operative mortality rate is $<5\%$.

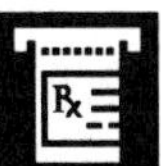

Medications

DRUG(S) OF CHOICE

- Mild to moderate chronic mitral regurgitation often can be managed medically with digoxin and diuretics.
- Angiotensin-converting enzyme inhibitors may be used for afterload reduction, although they are usually reserved for moderate to severe mitral regurgitation (the long-term use in children has not been well studied).
- If mitral regurgitation is acute, patients are usually more symptomatic because the uncompensated left atrium has a sudden increase in volume overload. These patients usually require i.v. afterload reduction with nitroprusside or hydralazine in addition to digoxin or i.v. inotrope and diuretics.
- If atrial arrhythmias are present, antiarrhythmic medications should be administered as needed.
- If mitral regurgitation is secondary to rheumatic fever, following initial treatment, long-term prophylaxis is necessary: 1.2 million units penicillin G benzathine i.m. every 4 weeks or penicillin V 250 mg orally b.i.d.
- Bacterial endocarditis prophylaxis is necessary per AHA guidelines.
- For patients who undergo MVR, anticoagulation (heparin) should be started within 8–12 hours of surgery at a dose that achieves a partial thromboplastin time of 1.7–2.0 times normal. Oral anticoagulation may also be started once there are no active surgical issues such as chest tubes or pacing wires, requiring removal.
- Warfarin should be dosed to achieve an INR of 2.0–3.0. Discontinue heparin once warfarin is in the therapeutic range.

Contraindications

- Penicillin allergy

Precautions

Refer to manufacturer's profile of each drug.

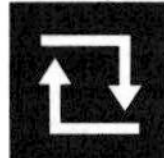

Follow-up

PATIENT MONITORING

- Close, regular follow-up is essential to monitor for progression of symptoms or change in physical status.
- For patients who underwent MVR, close attention should be directed to the crisp mechanical sound of the prosthetic valve at the apex on examination. Absence of this finding may indicate thrombus of the valve or valve malfunction.
- Recommendations for unoperated patients regarding frequency of visits, serial echocardiograms, and ECGs depend on the severity of mitral regurgitation.
- Close monitoring of the INR following MVR
- Children are at particular risk for bleeding because of their activity level.
- Children have up to a 2% risk of thromboembolic events, even with appropriate anticoagulation.

Prevention/Avoidance

- Bacterial endocarditis prophylaxis for dental and invasive procedures is continued for life.
- Rheumatic fever prophylaxis when indicated

Possible Complications

- Complications of anticoagulation may arise in patients with prosthetic mitral valves (i.e., bleeding or thrombosis).
- Recurrent rheumatic fever
- Bacterial endocarditis
- Pulmonary edema
- Atrial arrhythmias

EXPECTED COURSE AND PROGNOSIS

- Preoperatively, most patients with mild to moderate mitral insufficiency can be medically managed; however, patients who demonstrate LV dysfunction or atrial arrhythmia may be at increased risk for surgery and for long-term postoperative arrhythmias.
- Although LV function may worsen in the immediate postoperative period, children generally appear to have recovery of LV function with time.
- After MVR in children, eventual re-replacement will be required.

PATIENT EDUCATION

- Patients should be educated about signs of worsening symptoms or the presence of palpitations, which may indicate new onset of an atrial arrhythmia.
- Bacterial endocarditis prophylaxis as per AHA guidelines.
- Patients receiving anticoagulation with prolonged bleeding or easy bruisability should contact their physician. Children receiving anticoagulation need to be restricted from rough physical activities.

Activity

- Adequate rest and reasonable physical activity
- Patients on oral anticoagulation are restricted from contact sports.

Diet

- No restrictions

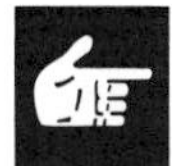

Miscellaneous

BIBLIOGRAPHY

Bradley LM, et al. Anticoagulation therapy in children with mechanical prosthetic cardiac valves. *Am J Cardiol* 1985;56:533–535.

Carpentier A, Branchini B, Cour C, et al. Congenital malformation of the mitral valve. Pathology and surgical treatment. *J Thorac Cardiovasc Surg* 1976;7:854–857.

Garson A Jr, Bricker JT, Fisher DJ, et al. *The science and practice of pediatric cardiology,* 2nd ed. New York: Williams & Wilkins, 1998.

Krishnan US, Gersony WM, Berman Rosenzweig E, et al. Late left ventricular function after surgery for children with chronic symptomatic mitral regurgitation. *Circulation* 1997;96:4280–4285.

Emmanaulides GC, Allen HD, Riemenschneider TA, Gutgesell HP, eds. *Moss and Adams' heart disease in infants, children, and adolescents including the fetus and young adult,* 5th ed. New York: Williams & Wilkins, 1995.

Skoularigis J, Sinovich V, Houbert G, et al. Evaluation of long-term results of mitral valve repair in 254 young patients with rheumatic mitral regurgitation. *Circulation* 1994;90:167–174.

Authors: Erika Berman Rosenzweig and Welton M. Gersony

Mitral Stenosis

Basics

DESCRIPTION

Mitral stenosis causes obstruction to left ventricular (LV) inflow at the level of the mitral valve and results from structural abnormalities that prevents proper opening during diastolic LV filling.

EPIDEMIOLOGY

Prevalence

- During the past 40 years, the prevalence and incidence of rheumatic fever has decreased dramatically.
- In 1960, mitral stenosis accounted for 43% of all valve disease at European centers compared with 9% in 1985.

ETIOLOGY

N/A

CAUSES

- Rheumatic heart disease is by far the most common cause of mitral stenosis.
- Degenerative
  - —Carcinoid syndrome
  - —Fabry's disease
  - —Mucopolysaccharidosis
  - —Whipple's disease
  - —Gout
  - —Rheumatoid arthritis
  - —Obstruction by large vegetation
  - —Congenital mitral stenosis accounts for $<$1% of cases.

RISK FACTORS

N/A

PREGNANCY

N/A

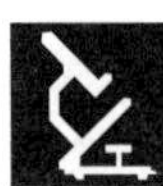

Diagnosis

DIFFERENTIAL DIAGNOSIS

- Causes of mid-diastolic murmur (MDM)
  - —Austin-Flint: MDM in patients with aortic insufficiency secondary to decreased opening of mitral valve in diastole due to the eccentrically directed jet of aortic regurgitation
- MDM with patent ductus arteriosus and ventricular septal defect: occurs due to increased flow across the mitral valve
- MDM in constrictive pericarditis secondary to constriction ring at the AV groove level
- Cor triatriatum
- Tricuspid stenosis: Its murmur increases during inspiration as well as during the release phase of Valsalva.
- Atrial septal defect: MDM over the tricuspid secondary to increased flow across the tricuspid valve

SIGNS AND SYMPTOMS

Signs

- Mitral facies (malar flush), secondary to decrease in cardiac output in patients with severe mitral stenosis, is rarely seen in the Western world.
- Palpable tapping first heart sound (S1)
- Accentuated S1 because of the prolonged mitral inflow prevents the leaflets from returning to the normal resting position before LV pressure increases abruptly at the onset of systole.
- Accentuated pulmonary component of the second heart sound with the development of pulmonary hypertension.
- Diastolic mid-diastolic rumbling murmur heard strictly at the apex with presystolic accentuation coinciding with atrial contraction
- Signs of pulmonary hypertension and right-sided heart failure occur later in mitral stenosis.

Symptoms

- Some patients are asymptomatic.
- The chief complaint in patients with mitral stenosis is dyspnea.
- Exertional dyspnea, orthopnea, paroxysmal nocturnal dyspnea, and even acute pulmonary edema
- Symptoms may be precipitated by factors that increase blood flow across the mitral valve or shorten the diastolic time, such as emotional or physical stress, infection, fever, pregnancy, or atrial fibrillation with rapid ventricular response.
- Patients with severe mitral stenosis eventually develop pulmonary hypertension with secondary right-sided heart failure manifested by elevated jugular venous pressure, hepatomegaly, ascites, and lower limb edema.
- Atrial arrhythmias: about 30%–40% of patients with mitral stenosis develop atrial fibrillation.
- Hemoptysis is a rare manifestation of end-stage mitral stenosis.

LABORATORY PROCEDURES

N/A

IMAGING STUDIES

ECG

- It is a relatively insensitive technique for detection of mitral stenosis.
- P mitrale is defined as a broad and bifid P wave in lead II or broad and/or deep negative component of the biphasic P wave in lead V1. It is a sign of left atrial enlargement.
- Atrial fibrillation or flutter may be seen.

Chest X-ray

- The classic features are left atrial enlargement with normal LV contour and enlarged pulmonary artery.
- Pulmonary congestion: Interstitial edema might show itself as Kerly B lines initially.
- Other features include hemosiderosis and mitral valve calcification.

Echocardiography

- 2-D and Doppler echocardiography is now considered the diagnostic modality of choice for diagnosis and assessment of the severity of mitral stenosis.
- Echocardiography demonstrates restricted mobility of the anterior leaflet with diastolic doming as well as fixed posterior leaflet.
- Mitral valve area can be estimated using 2-D echocardiography by planimetry or Doppler using pressure half-time.

SPECIAL TESTS

- Cardiac catheterization
  - —To perform percutaneous mitral balloon valvotomy
  - —To assess the severity of mitral regurgitation in patients considered for the percutaneous procedure when the echocardiogram is not adequate to assess the mitral valve

PATHOLOGY

- The most characteristic pathologic finding is fusion of the leaflet edges along the commissures between the anterior and posterior leaflets.
- Additional features include fusion, thickening, and shortening of the mitral valve chordae; fibrosis and thickening of the valve leaflets; and superimposed calcification.

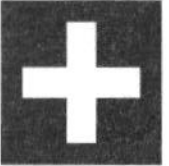

Treatment

GENERAL MEASURES

Prophylaxis against infective endocarditis and recurrent rheumatic fever, if applicable, is indicated.

SURGICAL MEASURES

Percutaneous Mitral Balloon Valvotomy

- Patients with mitral stenosis (mitral valve area <1.5 cm^2) and NYHA class II or more symptoms and valve morphology suitable for balloon valvotomy in the absence of atrial thrombus and moderate to severe mitral regurgitation
- Patients with mitral stenosis (mitral valve area <1.5 cm^2) and pulmonary hypertension (pulmonary artery systolic pressure $>$50 mm Hg at rest and 60 mm Hg during exertion) and valve morphology suitable for balloon valvotomy in the absence of atrial thrombus and moderate to severe mitral regurgitation

• Patients with mitral stenosis (mitral valve area <1.5 cm²) and NYHA class III or more symptoms and a nonpliable calcified valve who are at high risk for surgery in the absence of atrial thrombus and moderate to severe mitral regurgitation
• Patients with mitral stenosis (mitral valve area <1.5 cm²) and valve morphology suitable for balloon valvotomy who have new-onset atrial fibrillation in the absence of atrial thrombus and moderate to severe mitral regurgitation

Mitral Valve Replacement

• Patients with mitral stenosis (mitral valve area <1.5 cm²) and NYHA class II or more symptoms who are not candidates for balloon valvotomy and mitral valve repair
• Patients with mitral stenosis (mitral valve area <1.0 cm²) and severe pulmonary hypertension with NYHA class I–II symptoms who are not candidate for balloon valvotomy and mitral valve repair

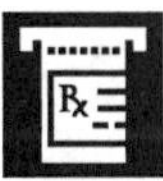

Medications

DRUG(S) OF CHOICE

• Mitral stenosis is a mechanical problem and medical therapy cannot be expected to cause regression or delay progression of disease.
• Beta-blockers and calcium channel blockers can be used to manage exertional symptoms related to rapid heart rate.
• Intermittent diuretics can be used to if there is evidence of pulmonary vascular congestion.
• Digitalis does not benefit patients with mitral stenosis and normal sinus rate unless there is atrial fibrillation or right or left ventricular dysfunction.

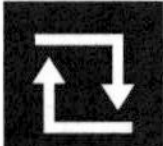

Follow-up

PATIENT MONITORING

N/A

Prevention

• Prophylaxis against infective endocarditis and rheumatic fever

Complications

• Atrial arrhythmias
• Pulmonary hypertension with right-sided heart failure
• Hemoptysis
• Recurrent rheumatic fever
• Systemic embolization may occur in 10%–20% of patients with mitral stenosis (cerebral 75%; peripheral 33%; visceral 66%).

EXPECTED COURSE AND PROGNOSIS

• In studies conducted before the surgical era, the 10-year mortality rate ranged from 33% to 70%, with a 20-year mortality rate of 80%–87%.
• In these historical studies the incidence of heart failure was about 60%, and about 20% of the patients had embolic events.

Diet

• Low-sodium diet with the development of congestive heart failure

Activity

Patients should counsel to avoid unusual physical stresses.

PATIENT EDUCATION

N/A

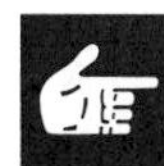

Miscellaneous

ICD-9-CM

394.0

BIBLIOGRAPHY

Bonow RO, Carabello B, de Leon AC Jr, et al. ACC/AHA guidelines for the management of patients with valvular heart disease: a report of the American College of Cardiology/American Heart Association Task Force on Practice Guidelines (Committee on Management of Patients with Valvular Heart Disease). *J Am Coll Cardiol* 1998;32:1486–1588.

Bruce CJ, Nishimura R. Clinical assessment and management of mitral stenosis. *Cardiol Clin* 1998;16:375–404.

Otto C. *Valvular heart disease,* 1st ed. Philadelphia: WB Saunders, 1999.

Rahimtoola SH, et al. *Hurst's the heart,* 9th ed. New York: McGraw-Hill, 1998.

Authors: Steven Herrmann, Amr El-Shafei, Madhukar Gupta, and Bernard R. Chaitman

Mitral Valve Prolapse

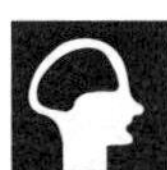

Basics

DESCRIPTION

Mitral valve prolapse is exaggerated billowing of the mitral valve leaflets into the left atrium during systole without valve coaptation, resulting in mitral regurgitation.

ETIOLOGY

Genetics

The mitral valve prolapse syndrome is thought to be at least partly heritable, with an autosomal-dominant mode of transmission with variable penetrance.

Prevalence

- One of the most prevalent cardiovascular abnormalities, affecting 3%–5% of the general population
- Females are affected twice as often as males.

Age

Mitral valve prolapse has been described in all groups, but is most common in young women.

CAUSES

- Myxomatous degeneration of the mitral valve apparatus

RISK FACTORS

- Mitral valve prolapse generally is a primary cardiovascular disorder. Several conditions are associated with it, although none definitely causal. These include the following:
    —Marfan's syndrome
    —Ehlers-Danlos syndrome
    —Pseudoxanthoma elasticum
    —Periarteritis nodosa
    —Osteogenesis imperfecta
    —Myotonic dystrophy
    —Von Willebrand's disease
    —Hyperthyroidism
- Mitral valve prolapse tends to be seen in patients with asthenic body habitus, straight backs, shallow chest wall, and pectus excavatum.

PREGNANCY

- No contraindications to pregnancy

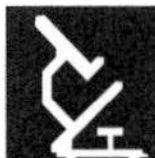

Diagnosis

DIFFERENTIAL DIAGNOSIS

- Mitral regurgitation
- Tricuspid regurgitation
- Tricuspid valve prolapse
- Papillary muscle dysfunction
- Hypertrophic obstructive cardiomyopathy

SIGNS AND SYMPTOMS

- The majority of patients with mitral valve prolapse are asymptomatic.
- However, many patients have increased anxiety, fatigue, palpitations, orthostatic hypotension, and evidence of autonomic dysfunction.
- Chest pain is a frequent complaint, although it is generally atypical with regard to angina.
- The chest pain with mitral valve prolapse usually occurs at rest and is sharp in character.

LABORATORY PROCEDURES

- Auscultatory examination shows a systolic click at least 0.14 seconds after the first heart sound, occurring just after the carotid upstroke.
- The ejection click is best heard with the stethoscope diaphragm at the left sternal border and is followed by a middle to late crescendo systolic murmur lasting until the second heart sound.
- Occasionally only the ejection click or the murmur alone will be present.
- The duration of the murmur corresponds with the severity of the mitral regurgitation.
- Arterial vasodilation, augmented contractility, and decreased venous return cause the click and murmur to move toward S1.
- Thus, dynamic auscultation with amyl nitrate, early Valsalva, or upright posture causes the click and murmur to move toward S1.
- Squatting, leg raise, and isometric exercise delays the click and murmur toward S2.

IMAGING STUDIES

- The ECG is usually normal in asymptomatic patients. However, biphasic T waves and nonspecific ST segment abnormalities, perhaps secondary to papillary muscle ischemia, may be noted in leads II, III, and aVF.
- Paroxysmal supraventricular tachycardia is the most frequent arrhythmia noted with mitral valve prolapse, although premature atrial beats, ventricular beats, and sinus node dysfunction with bradyarrhythmias are also common.
- M-mode echocardiography shows posterior movement of the mitral valve leaflets in mid-systole.
- On 2-D echocardiography, the valve leaflets are thickened and redundant and prolapse back into the atrium during systole.
- The parasternal view is the most specific for the diagnosis of mitral valve prolapse using the prolapse criteria.
- Color flow Doppler usually shows a mitral regurgitant jet.

PATHOLOGY

- Myxomatous proliferation of the middle layer (spongiosa) of the valve, resulting in increased mucopolysaccharide deposition and myxomatous degeneration
- By electron microscopy, the collagen fibers in the valve leaflets are disorganized and fragmented.
- With increased stroma deposition, the valve leaflets enlarge and become redundant.
- The endothelium is usually noncontiguous and a frequent site for thrombus or infective vegetation.

SPECIAL TESTS

Cardiac catheterization also can visualize the mitral valve leaflets prolapsing into the atium as well as a scalloped appearance of the leaflets consistent with redundant tissue.

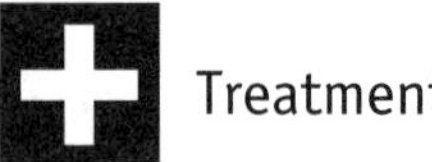

Treatment

GENERAL MEASURES

- Reassurance is necessary with the asymptomatic patient.
- Patients with neurologic symptoms should be considered for aspirin or anticoagulation therapy.
- Patients with mitral regurgitation should be treated with afterload reduction or considered for mitral valve repair or replacement.
- Patients with arrhythmias or long QT syndromes should have 24-hour ECG monitoring.
- Electrophysiologic studies may be considered in symptomatic patients because of the rare association of mitral valve prolapse and sudden cardiac death.

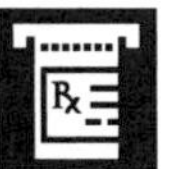

Medications

DRUG(S) OF CHOICE

- Beta-blockers are the drug of choice for patients with mitral valve prolapse and palpitations.
- Chest pain syndromes are also best treated with beta-blockers.
- Angiotensin-converting enzyme inhibitors if mitral regurgitation is moderate to severe

ALTERNATIVE DRUGS

- Hydralazine and nitrates in combination for afterload reduction

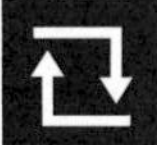

Follow-up

PATIENT MONITORING

- Asymptomatic patients should be followed with transthoracic echocardiogram every 3–5 years.
- Patients with more severe mitral regurgitation should be followed more frequently.

Prevention

- Endocarditis prophylaxis is recommended for patients with both the mid-systolic click and mitral regurgitant murmur.
- Women under the age of 45 with the systolic click only may not require prophylaxis unless undergoing upper respiratory or genitourinary procedures.

Complications

- Sudden cardiac death (very rare)
- Chordae rupture
- Endocarditis
- Fibrin emboli
- Heart failure with progressive mitral regurgitation

EXPECTED COURSE AND PROGNOSIS

For most patients, prognosis is excellent.

PATIENT EDUCATION

Patient education as to avoidance of alcohol, caffeine, stimulants, and nicotine may be sufficient to control symptoms in some instances.

Activity

No limitations unless heart failure or anginal symptoms predominate

Diet

Sodium and water restriction should be encouraged if the mitral regurgitation is severe enough to affect left ventricular function.

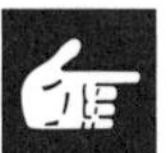

Miscellaneous

SYNONYMS

- Systolic click-murmur syndrome
- Barlow's syndrome
- Billowing mitral cusp syndrome
- Myxomatous mitral valve
- Floppy valve syndrome
- Redundant cusp syndrome

ICD-9-CM

354.9

See also: Mitral regurgitation

BIBLIOGRAPHY

Alexander RW, ed. *Hurst's the heart.* New York: McGraw-Hill, 1998.

Braunwald E, ed. *Heart disease: a textbook of cardiovascular medicine,* 5th ed. Philadelphia: WB Saunders, 1997.

Topol EJ, ed. *Textbook of cardiovascular medicine.* Philadelphia: Lippincott-Raven, 1998.

Authors: Steven Herrmann, Amr El-Shafei, Madhukar Gupta, and Bernard R. Chaitman

Multifocal Atrial Tachycardia

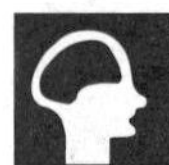

Basics

DESCRIPTION

Multifocal atrial tachycardia (MAT) is characterized by a rate greater than 100 beats/min and the following:

- Discrete P waves of varying morphology from at least three different foci
- Irregular variation in PP, PR, and RR intervals reflecting absence of dominant pacemaker
- Isoelectric baseline between P waves

EPIDEMIOLOGY

Prevalence depends on level of sickness of population and location where assessment is performed.

- May occur at any age, but usually in older individuals
- Rarely seen in children and then occurs in the absence of structural heart disease and is usually self-limited (months)
- Although MAT occurs primarily in patients with lung disease in intensive care units, it can occur in critically ill patients in any setting.

ETIOLOGY

MAT usually occurs during critical illness, especially in the setting of chronic lung disease. Beta-agonists and methylxanthine derivatives (theophylline) may be contributory.

RISK FACTORS

- Chronic lung disease
- Recent surgery
- Diabetes

PREGNANCY

N/A

ASSOCIATED CONDITIONS

See above regarding Etiology.

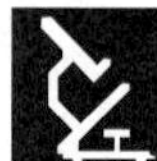

Diagnosis

DIFFERENTIAL DIAGNOSIS

- Wandering atrial pacemaker (multiple P-wave morphologies, but average atrial rate <100 beats/min; common in elderly patients who are otherwise well)
- Multiple premature atrial contractions (can identify dominant, e.g., sinus, P waves)
- Atrial fibrillation (no clear P waves)
- Atrial tachycardia (regular with only one morphology P wave)

SIGNS AND SYMPTOMS

- None
- Palpitations
- Dyspnea
- Hypotension

LABORATORY PROCEDURES

N/A

IMAGING STUDIES

N/A

SPECIAL TESTS

ECG is the only diagnostic test.

- Discrete P waves of varying morphology from at least three different foci
- Atrial rate greater than 100 beats/min
- Isoelectric baseline between P waves
- Irregular variation in PP, PR, and RR intervals reflecting absence of dominant pacemaker

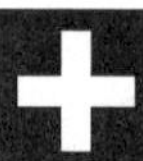

Treatment

GENERAL MEASURES

- Optimize pulmonary and general care.
- Reverse causes of illness and debility.
- Avoid theophylline.

SURGICAL MEASURES

N/A

ADMISSION/DISCHARGE CRITERIA

Usually arrhythmia is first recognized in inpatients. Discharge is determined by resolution of other medical problems.

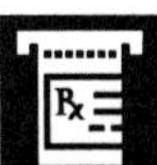

Medications

DRUG(S) OF CHOICE

- Verapamil usual drug of choice
- Amiodarone reported to be useful in children with MAT in need of therapy

Precautions

- Beta-blockers are controversial and may be difficult if not impossible to use in patients with serious lung disease.
- Digoxin is not helpful.
- Classic antiarrhythmics are not useful (procainamide, quinidine).

ALTERNATIVE DRUGS

Intravenous magnesium may be helpful.

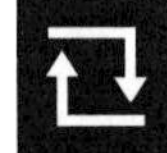

Follow-up

PATIENT MONITORING

MAT is usually an acute problem and does not require long-term monitoring following hospital release.

- During the acute phase, there must be vigilance for hypotension, hypoxia, and excessive myocardial demand.
- Caregivers should maintain nutrition, especially in intensive care units.

EXPECTED COURSE AND PROGNOSIS

- Depends on underlying disease

PATIENT EDUCATION

N/A

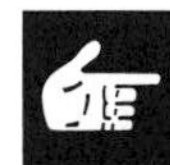

Miscellaneous

SYNONYMS

- Chaotic atrial rhythm
- Chaotic atrial tachycardia

ICD-9-CM

427.89 Other, specified cardiac dysrhythmias

See also: Atrial premature beats; Atrial fibrillation.

BIBLIOGRAPHY

Kastor JA. Multifocal atrial tachycardia. *N Engl J Med* 1990;1713–1717.

Scher DL, Arsura EL. Multifocal atrial tachycardia: mechanisms, clinical correlates, and treatment. *Am Heart J* 1989;118:574–580.

Shine KI, Kastor JA, Yurchak PM. Multifocal atrial tachycardia: clinical and electrocardiographic features in 32 patients. *N Engl J Med* 1968;279:344–349.

Author: Andrew E. Epstein

Muscular Dystrophy and the Heart

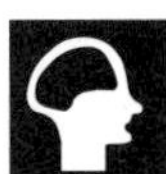

Basics

DESCRIPTION

The muscular dystrophies are progressive hereditary degenerative diseases of skeletal muscles.

- Primary manifestations include progressive muscle wasting secondary to intrinsic defects of the muscle fiber.
- Myopathies and polymyopathies not included.
- Cardiac involvement is variable, but frequent, and includes dilated cardiomyopathy and conduction defects.
- The dystrophies can be classified according to pattern of inheritance, clinical types, and the defective gene product:
- X-linked, dystrophinopathies
  - —Classic Duchenne's dystrophy and Becker's muscular dystrophy
  - —X-linked, nondystrophinopathies: Emery-Dreifuss muscular dystrophy
  - —Autosomal: myotonic muscular dystrophy (Steinert's disease), limb-girdle dystrophies of Erb, and facioscapulohumeral dystrophy of Landouzy-Dejerine

Systems Affected

- Cardiac and musculoskeletal

ETIOLOGY

Genetics

- Duchenne's/Becker's
  - —X-linked recessive
  - —One-third of cases sporadic
  - —The genetic mutations affect the protein dystrophin, which is absent (Duchenne's) or altered (Becker's).
  - —Gene locus is located on the short arm of the X chromosome. Females are carriers.
- Others
  - —Variable inheritance
  - —Gene located

Predominant Age

- Mean age 12 years, range 5–45

Predominant Sex

- Male

PREGNANCY

- Prenatal diagnosis possible
- Females with cardiomyopathy due to muscular dystrophy at risk for deterioration during pregnancy
- Female carriers rarely have cardiomyopathy.

ASSOCIATED CONDITIONS

- Respiratory insufficiency, pneumonias, and mild retardation (Duchenne's and myotonic dystrophy)
- Chronic bronchitis, bronchiectasis, cataract, baldness, gonadal atrophy, and megacolon (myotonic dystrophy)
- Transient ischemic attack and stroke

Age-Related Factors

- Pediatric: usual age of onset
- Others: some present in middle age

ETIOLOGY

Incidence/Prevalence

- Duchenne's
  - —Incidence 1/3,300 male, live births (13–33/100,000)
  - —Prevalence 3/100,000 population
  - —Most common lethal X-linked disease
  - —Found in every part of the world with little ethnic variation
  - —The disease is present at birth.
  - —Overt clinical symptoms usually do not manifest before age 2–5.
  - —The heart is commonly involved, with ECG abnormalities and DCM being most typical.
- Becker's
  - —Rarer than Duchenne's
  - —Incidence 3–6/100,000 male births
  - —Presents clinically at mean age of 12 years, range 5–45 years
  - —The degree of cardiac involvement is more variable and less frequent than for Duchenne's, but may eventually affect 80% of patients.
- Others
  - —Males and females
  - —Onset childhood to adolescence or adulthood
  - —Myotonic dystrophy most common adult form of muscular dystrophy
  - —Variable cardiac involvement includes cardiomyopathy and conduction defects.

SIGNS AND SYMPTOMS

- Clumsy, waddling gait, frequent falls, difficulties rising from floor; wheelchair bound; pseudohypertrophy of calves, lumbar lordosis and kyphoscoliosis
- Mild mental retardation (nonprogressive)
- Impaired breathing and coughing leading to frequent pneumonias
- Systolic impulse at the left sternal border; short, impure grade I–III/VI mid-systolic murmur at the left second interspace and loud P2
- Mid-systolic click and late systolic murmur of mitral valve prolapse or holosystolic murmur of mitral regurgitation
- S3 or S4 gallop
- Dilated cardiomyopathy with heart failure (enlarged heart and increased pulmonary markings) involving predominantly the left ventricle (LV; late sign)
- Inappropriate sinus tachycardia (persistent or labile, gradual or abrupt onset)
- Atrial flutter (often preterminal)
- PACs, junctional rhythm, sustained supraventricular tachycardia, premature ventricular contractions (uniform/multiform), couplets, nonsustained ventricular tachycardia
- Becker's
  - —Cardiac involvement may occur at an early age and is unrelated to the extent of the musculoskeletal disorder.
  - —Appreciable cardiac involvement can occur in patients without significant muscular disability, whereas others with progressive muscular atrophy and weakness may have little cardiac involvement.
  - —Findings include:
    - Muscular weakness and atrophy similar to Duchenne's but later onset and less rapid progression
    - Dilated cardiomyopathy involving both ventricles
    - Fascicular block, bundle branch block, third-degree atrioventricular (AV) block
    - Malignant ventricular arrhythmias
- Others
  - —Atrophy and weakness specific for type
  - —Atrial fibrillation/atrial flutter and atrial standstill. Bradycardia and first degree AV block.
  - —Varying degree of AV block, including third-degree block and slow junctional rhythms leading to syncope and sudden death.
  - —Dilated cardiomyopathy and malignant ventricular arrhythmias possible
  - —Mental retardation

ETIOLOGY

- Hereditary

RISK FACTORS

- Family history

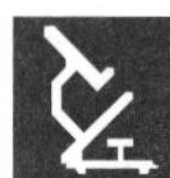

Diagnosis

DIFFERENTIAL DIAGNOSIS

- The major differential diagnoses to consider in young adults with muscular dystrophy presenting with heart failure is idiopathic and postviral dilated cardiomyopathy.
- In individuals with Duchenne's, abnormal ECG findings can resemble pulmonary hypertension and right ventricular hypertrophy.
- For all dystrophies, conduction disturbances due to other causes should be considered.

LABORATORY PROCEDURES

- Elevated creatinine kinase (CK) and CK and MB fraction (CK-MB); not useful for diagnosis of cardiac involvement
- Increased CO_2 with profound worsening with O_2 supplementation (Duchenne's, myotonic dystrophy)

Pathologic Findings

- Duchenne's
  - —Predilection for specific regions of the myocardium: the posterobasal and posterolateral LV walls (fibrous replacement) with relative sparing of IVS, right ventricle, and atria

—Often there is a small vessel coronary arteriopathy characterized by hypertrophy of media with luminal narrowing.
—Occult cardiac disease is present at an early age, evident by abnormal ECG, but overt cardiac disease usually follows severe muscular dysfunction in the terminal stages.

SPECIAL TESTS

- Duchenne's
  —ECG
    - Simplest and most reliable tool for detecting cardiac involvement
    - Tall right precordial R waves and increased R/S amplitude
    - Deep Q waves on leads I, aVL, V5–6
    - Abnormal terminal force of P waves, especially in V1 with negative deflection >20 msec and 0.1 mV, or broad and notched P waves in V2
    - Short P-R interval, or in late stage prolonged P-R interval
    - Minor RVCD, LPFB, LAFB, RBBB or rarely bifascicular block

IMAGING STUDIES

- Duchenne's
  —Chest x-ray
    - Thoracic deformities
    - High diaphragms
    - Reduction in anteroposterior dimensions, causing increased transverse heart size
    - Evidence of left heart failure in terminal stages
  —Echocardiogram
    - Hyperechoic regions in the posterobasal LV wall
    - Segmental or global LV hypokinesis and dilatation
    - Mitral regurgitation
    - Mitral valve prolapse
    - In some patients, systolic function appears normal, but diastolic dysfunction is present.
  —Thallium scintigraphy/SPECT
    - Regional perfusion defects (posterobasal and lateral LV wall) in metabolic abnormal but viable myocardium
- Becker's, Emery-Dreifuss, myotonic dystrophy
  —Chest x-ray
    - May show evidence of heart failure with enlarged heart and prominent pulmonary vasculature
  —Echocardiogram
    - May show dilated cardiomyopathy
    - For myotonic dystrophy, normal systolic function is common, with evidence of diastolic dysfunction.

DIAGNOSTIC PROCEDURES

- Duchenne's
  —Endomyocardial biopsy
  —Electron microscopy
    - Abnormalities of mitochondria, C bands, sarcoplasmic reticulum, and nuclei
- Becker's
  —ECG
    - Conduction defects as for Duchenne's, but also left bundle branch block, complete heart block, and malignant ventricular arrhythmias
- Others
  —ECG
  —Atrial fibrillation/flutter/standstill, junctional rhythms, third degree AV block
  —IVCD, H-V interval prolongation, RBBB, increased P-R interval, LAFB, increased QRS duration, third-degree AV block, ventricular tachycardia (rare)

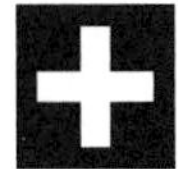

Treatment

GENERAL MEASURES

- Hospitalization only for those with heart failure, arrhythmias, or other serious illness
- Supportive, prevention of contractures, bipap at night (Duchenne's)
- Symptomatic, treatment of heart failure and serious arrhythmias
- Treatment follows guidelines used for cardiomyopathy and conduction abnormalities due to any cause.

SURGICAL MEASURES

- Pacemaker if high-degree AV block present (Becker's, Emery-Dreifuss, myotonic dystrophy, occasional Limb-Girdle dystrophies)

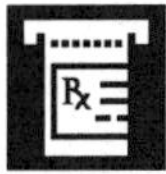

Medications

DRUG(S) OF CHOICE

- There are no specific medications for muscular dystrophy, but in the treatment of complications some should be avoided:
  —Procainamide/phenytoin: may worsen muscle weakness
  —Verapamil i.v.: may cause fatal respiratory arrest
  —Halothane, suxamethonium, isoflurane, succinylcholine: can cause malignant hyperthermia and cardiac arrest during anesthesia

ALTERNATIVE DRUGS

N/A

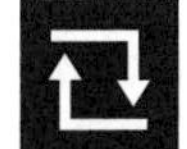

Follow-up

PATIENT MONITORING

- Depends on severity/character of symptoms
- Severe heart failure, malignant arrhythmias, and symptomatic conduction disturbances require hospitalization.

Prevention/Avoidance

- Genetic counseling

Possible Complications

- Heart failure, cardiac arrest, death

EXPECTED COURSE AND PROGNOSIS

- Duchenne's
  —Relentless, progressive course
  —Most wheelchair bound at the end of first decade
  —Death likely from pulmonary infections and respiratory failure in the second decade
  —Cardiac involvement may cause the death.
  —Rapid progressive preterminal heart failure may follow years of circulatory stability.
  —Systemic emboli may be caused by a dilated, hypokinetic LV.
  —Only 20%–25% survive beyond 25 years.
- Becker's
  —Slower progression than Duchenne's
  —Usually unable to walk by age 25–30 years
  —Adult patients generally have cardiomyopathy
  —Heart failure often the cause of death
  —Serious ventricular arrhythmias may occur and cause sudden death
  —Pacemaker often required for high-degree AV block
  —Death usually occurs in fifth decade.
- Others
  —Slowly progressive
  —Benign course compared with Duchenne's
  —Pacemaker placement may be required
  —Sudden death may occur due to high degree AV block.

PATIENT EDUCATION

Organization

Muscular Dystrophy Association USA, National Headquarters, 3300 E. Sunrise Dr., Tucson, AZ 85718; 1-800-572-1717

Activity

- As tolerated

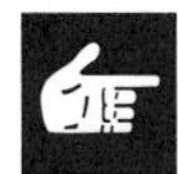

Miscellaneous

ICD-9-CM

359.1 + 425.8 Cardiomyopathy due to progressive muscular dystrophy

BIBLIOGRAPHY

Adams RD. *Principles of neurology,* 6th ed. New York: McGraw-Hill, 1997.

Braunwald E. *Heart disease: a textbook of cardiovascular medicine,* 5th ed. Philadelphia: WB Saunders, 1997.

Hearst A. *The heart.* 1998.

Author: Kirsten Tolstrup

Myocardial Infarction

Basics

DESCRIPTION

- Prolonged myocardial ischemia resulting in myocardial injury and necrosis
- Subdivided into Q-wave infarction (usually presenting as ST elevation) and non-Q-wave infarction (usually presenting as ST segment depression/nondiagnostic ECG/normal ECG). The distinction is important because the initial therapeutic strategy and clinical course differ.

EPIDEMIOLOGY

Incidence

- 900,000 cases per year; 30% die

Age

- Incidence increases with age

Sex

- More men affected than women

ETIOLOGY

- Coronary atherosclerotic disease (>90%): acute plaque rupture with thrombus formation
- Coronary vasospasm: variant/Prinzmetal's angina, cocaine
- Coronary emboli: endocarditis, mural thrombi
- Congenital coronary anomalies
- Thrombotic disease: hypercoagulable states, sickle cell disease, oral contraceptive use
- Coronary vasculitis: Takayasu, Kawasaki, polyarteritis nodosa, lupus, scleroderma, rheumatoid arthritis, allograft rejection
- Aortic dissection: proximal type with coronary ostial involvement
- Trauma: coronary dissection/laceration
- States with oxygen demand exceeding supply: hypotension, severe left ventricular hypertrophy (LVH), aortic stenosis

RISK FACTORS

Major Risk Factors

- Advancing age
- Sex: males, postmenopausal females not on estrogen
- Family history of premature coronary atherosclerotic heart disease
- Dyslipidemia: elevated LDL, low HDL
- Diabetes mellitus
- Smoking
- Hypertension
- Obesity: particularly central/truncal obesity
- Sedentary life-style

Other Risk Factors

- Elevated lipoprotein(a)
- Elevated plasma homocysteine
- Hypertriglyceridemia
- Psychosocial factors: stress, social isolation, depression
- Inflammatory markers: elevated C-reactive protein
- Prothrombic factors: elevated fibrinogen

PREGNANCY

- Rare, estimated incidence 0.01%
- Causes include coronary spasm, dissection, atherosclerosis, thrombosis

ASSOCIATED CONDITIONS

- Peripheral vascular disease

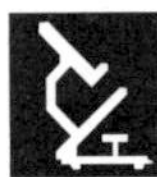

Diagnosis

DIFFERENTIAL DIAGNOSIS

- Cardiovascular: unstable angina, pericarditis, aortic dissection
- Pulmonary: pulmonary embolus, pleurisy/pneumonia, pneumothorax
- GI: esophageal disorders (spasm, reflux), peptic ulcer disease, biliary disease, pancreatitis
- Muscular: costochondritis, chest wall pain
- Psychiatric

SIGNS AND SYMPTOMS

Signs

- Anxiousness
- Diaphoresis, skin pallor
- JVP elevated with right ventricular (RV) infarction, severe LV failure
- Basilar rales with LV dysfunction
- Soft S1 and S2 with decreased contractility; S3; S4 very common
- Pericardial friction rub
- Systolic murmur at apex; mitral regurgitation from papillary muscle dysfunction/rupture, VSD

Symptoms

- Chest pain
- Dyspnea
- Pain in abdomen, neck, jaw, arm, back
- Nausea/vomiting
- Diaphoresis
- Palpitations, syncope
- Sudden death
- Cerebrovascular accident (CVA)
- Sudden confusion, weakness
- Severe apprehension

LABORATORY PROCEDURES

ECG

ECG provides the most important initial information to guide management.

- Acute ST elevation: ST segment elevation localizes area of myocardial injury and usually results in Q-wave myocardial infarction (MI)
  - —Exception: posterior: ST depression in leads V1–V2, up to V4; large R wave in V1
- ST depression/nondiagnostic ECG changes/normal ECG
  - —Usually results in non-Q-wave MI (if cardiac enzymes positive)

Serum Markers

- Creatinine kinase (CK) and MB fraction
  - —CK nonspecific; in MM, BB, MB fractions
  - —CK-MB sensitive and specific; traditional cardiac enzyme to detect myocardial damage/diagnose MI
  - —Elevation onset at 4–6 hours, peak at 14–36 hours (depending on reperfusion therapy), returns to normal at 48–72 hours
- Troponin T and I
  - —Elevation onset at 4–6 hours, peak at 24–36 hours (depending on reperfusion therapy), returns to normal in 10–14 days
  - —Very sensitive, highly specific
  - —Replaced LDH as test of choice to diagnose MI >48 hours from onset
- Myoglobin
  - —Elevation onset at 2 hours, returns to normal at 7–12 hours
  - —Nonspecific; limited clinical utility lies in early peak

IMAGING STUDIES

Echocardiogram

- Useful to assess wall motion abnormalities; unable to distinguish reliably severe ischemia versus acute infarction versus old infarction
- Information about ejection fraction (EF), mechanical complications

Nuclear Medicine Studies

- Limited use in acute MI
- Rarely used to diagnose RV infarction or when MI cannot be diagnosed by standard means

Cardiac Catheterization

Coronary angiography used in conjunction with primary percutaneous transluminal coronary angioplasty in acute MI setting

SPECIAL TESTS

N/A

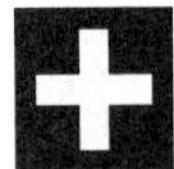

Treatment

GENERAL MEASURES

- Oxygen
- Alleviate pain: nitrates, morphine
- Alleviate anxiety: anxiolytics
- Telemetry/cardiac care unit (CCU) monitoring
- Bed rest first 12 hours
- NPO/clear liquid diet first 12 hours
- Stool softener
- Keep plasma K and Mg optimal.

SURGICAL MEASURES

- PTCA: as above
- Coronary artery bypass grafting (CABG): in acute setting, reserved for hemodynamic insta-

bility or refractory angina not amenable to PTCA or with failed PTCA and coronary anatomy amenable to CABG

ADMISSION/DISCHARGE CRITERIA

- CCU monitoring
  - —Monitor in CCU 1–3 days depending on course; discharge 4–7 days depending on course (variable clinical practice).
  - —Monitor for complications
- Mechanical/hemodynamic disturbances
  - —Heart failure/cardiogenic shock
  - —RV infarction
    - Usually in setting of inferior infarction
    - Suspect with hypotension, elevated JVP (Kussmaul's sign), clear lungs
    - Maintain RV preload, inotropic support
  - —New systolic murmur: papillary muscle dysfunction, papillary muscle rupture, VSD
  - —Cardiac rupture (free wall)
  - —Ventricular aneurysm
- Arrhythmias
  - —PVCs: usually require no treatment
  - —Accelerated idioventricular rhythm occurs with reperfusion, usually requires no treatment
  - —Ventricular tachycardia: lidocaine/direct current (DC) cardioversion
  - —Ventricular fibrillation: DC cardioversion
  - —Atrioventricular (AV) block: pacing more often needed with anterior MI than inferior MI
  - —Bundle branch blocks
- Recurrent chest pain
  - —Recurrent ischemia/infarction
  - —Early pericarditis
- LV thrombus with possible embolization
- Dressler's syndrome: late autoimmune pericarditis

Medications

DRUG(S) OF CHOICE

Acute ST Elevation MI

The goal is early reperfusion with thrombolytic therapy or primary PTCA.

- Thrombolytics
  - —Indications
    - ST elevation >1 mm in two or more contiguous leads
    - New left bundle branch block with history suggesting acute MI
    - Benefit if given <12 hours after symptom onset, greatest benefit 6 hours
  - —Contraindications
    - Absolute contraindications: active internal bleeding (not menses), intracranial neoplasm or recent head trauma, prolonged CPR, suspected aortic dissection, pregnancy, history of hemorrhagic CVA or recent nonhemorrhagic CVA, blood pressure >200/120 mm Hg, recent trauma or surgery in preceding 2 weeks, allergy to chosen thrombolytic
    - Relative contraindications: distant nonhemorrhagic CVA, recent trauma or surgery beyond 2 weeks, active PUD, hemorrhagic retinopathy, bleeding diathesis, prior recent streptokinase or APSAQ (for these agents)
- Agents available
  - —Tissue plasminogen activator (tPA): 90 mg i.v. in accelerated regimen; 15 mg i.v. bolus then 0.75 mg/kg (50 mg maximum) over 30 minutes then 0.5 mg/kg (35 mg maximum) over 60 minutes; concomitant i.v. heparin required
  - —Streptokinase: 1.5 million units i.v. over 30–60 minutes
  - —APSAC: 30 units i.v. over 5–10 minutes
  - —Recombinant plasminogen activator: 15 megaunits i.v. bolus, and repeat in 15–30 minutes
- Catheterization/PTCA: Alternative to thrombolytic therapy if performed at experienced center in timely fashion (primary PTCA), if thrombolytics contraindicated, with failed thrombolytics (rescue PTCA), or in cardiogenic shock
- Aspirin
- Beta-blocker
- Intravenous unfractionated heparin or low-molecular-weight heparin (LMWH)
- Nitrates
- Angiotensin-converting enzyme (ACE) inhibitor: acutely in <24 hours with anterior MI, CHF
- Lidocaine: prophylactic lidocaine not routinely indicated

Acute ST Depression or No ECG Change MI

- Aspirin
- Intravenous unfractionated heparin or LMWH
- Beta-blocker
- Nitrates
- ACE inhibitor
- Consider IIb/IIIa glycoprotein inhibitor.

Follow-up

EXPECTED COURSE AND PROGNOSIS

- 50% of MI-related deaths within 1 hour of symptom onset, before patient reaches hospital, primarily from ventricular arrhythmias
- Current hospital mortality rate 5%–10%
- In-hospital mortality and complication rates higher with Q-wave infarction compared with non–Q-wave infarction; 2-year mortality rates the same in the two groups (up to 30%)
- Main risk factors for serious cardiac events, death: increased age, EF <40%, recurrent ischemia at rest or with minimal exertion, CHF, VT/VF episode

Risk Stratification

- Estimate EF (echo, multigated acquisition)
- Stress testing (exercise or pharmacologic with echocardiography, nuclear imaging) versus catheterization prior to discharge (clinical practice varies)
- Electrophysiologic study with VT/VF >48–72 hours into MI for possible AICD

PATIENT EDUCATION

Secondary Prevention

- Smoking cessation
- Control blood pressure.
- Control diabetes mellitus.
- Aspirin
- Beta-blocker
- HMG-CoA reductase inhibitor: LDL goal <100 mg/dl
- ACE inhibitor
- Consider anticoagulation in selected cases (controversial).

Diet

- AHA step I diet (<30% total calories from fat with less than one-third being saturated fat, low cholesterol)

Activity

- Cardiac rehab, exercise prescription

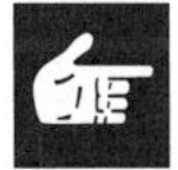

Miscellaneous

ICD-9-CM

410.9 Acute myocardial infarction, unspecified site
410.7 Subendocardial myocardial infarction
410.0 Acute myocardial infarction of anterolateral wall

INTERNET RESOURCES

- www.acc.org/clinical/guidelines
- www.americanheart.org

BIBLIOGRAPHY

Alexander RW, et al. Diagnosis and management of patients with acute myocardial infarction In: *Hurst's the heart,* 9th ed. New York: McGraw Hill, 1998, 1345–1416.

Antman EM, Braunwald E. Acute myocardial infarction. In: *Heart disease: a textbook of cardiovascular medicine,* 5th ed. 1184–1288.

Ryan TJ, et al. Guidelines for the management of patients with acute myocardial infarction. A report of the American College of Cardiology/ American Heart Association Task Force on Practice Guidelines. *J Am Coll Cardiol.* Philadelphia: W.B. Saunders, 1997;28:1328–1428 and 1999;34:890–911.

Authors: Vineet Kaushik and Nanette K. Wenger

Myocarditis

Basics

DESCRIPTION

Myocarditis is an inflammatory condition involving the heart that can be due to a variety of causes, including a direct viral infection.

- There are many kinds of inflammatory myocarditis including giant cell myocarditis, hypersensitivity myocarditis, viral myocarditis, and eosinophilic myocarditis.
- All are quite unique and have various responses to treatment and natural histories.
- In general, physicians tend to equate viral myocarditis with myocarditis in general.
- The treatment of viral inflammatory myocarditis is highly variable because of inconsistent responses to immunosuppressive therapy.

EPIDEMIOLOGY

- The epidemiology of viral inflammatory myocarditis is poorly understood.
- It apparently follows cyclical patterns that change over the years.
- The incidence may vary from decade to decade.

ETIOLOGY

- Infectious agents (viruses, bacteria, fungi, parasites, rickettsia, spirochetes)
- Toxins (cocaine)
- Hypersensitivity due to medications (e.g., clozapine)
- Chemotherapy (daunorubicin, doxorubicin)
- Radiation
- Giant cell

RISK FACTORS

- There are no obvious factors for the development of acute myocarditis.
- It is believed that some patients will develop viral myocarditis following a self-limited viral illness, but the nature of this association is poorly understood.

PREGNANCY

Inflammatory myocarditis can occur during pregnancy, in which case the stress of pregnancy can potentially aggravate the development of heart failure.

ASSOCIATED CONDITIONS

- None

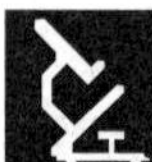

Diagnosis

DIFFERENTIAL DIAGNOSIS

- The differential diagnosis of inflammatory myocarditis includes idiopathic dilated cardiomyopathy and acute myocardial infarction.
- The onset of myocarditis can clearly mimic acute myocardial infarction with regional wall motion abnormalities on echocardiography, an increase in serum enzymes, and chest pain.
- Myocarditis can only be diagnosed definitively by tissue analysis.
- When there is suspicion of myocarditis, a myocardial biopsy may be indicated.
- This is somewhat controversial, because the treatment of acute inflammatory viral myocarditis is currently poorly defined, and basically consists of treatment for heart failure.
- Nevertheless, some patients will respond to immunosuppressive therapy, including corticosteroids.

SIGNS AND SYMPTOMS

- Shortness of breath
- Fatigue
- Chest pain
- All of the manifestations of acute and chronic heart failure

LABORATORY PROCEDURES

There are no specific laboratory procedures, although acute and convalescent titers for viral antibodies may be of some value.

IMAGING STUDIES

Imaging studies such as echocardiography are nonspecific and show either regional or global ventricular dysfunction.

SPECIAL TESTS

- Myocardial biopsy of the right ventricle is the most helpful special test.
  - —Because of possible sampling error, at least four biopsy samples should be obtained during the procedure.
  - —Histopathologic diagnosis of inflammatory myocarditis can be difficult, even by an experienced pathologist.

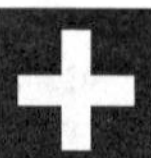

Treatment

GENERAL MEASURES

Management of inflammatory myocarditis is basically the management of heart failure and therefore includes loop diuretics, angiotensin-converting enzyme inhibitors, β-adrenergic blockers, and in some cases left ventricular assist devices and heart transplantation.

SURGICAL MEASURES

- Heart transplantation

ADMISSION/DISCHARGE CRITERIA

- Admission and discharge criteria are similar to those for heart failure.
- Patients are usually admitted to the hospital when there is acute severe hemodynamic compromise that requires intravenous diuretics and support with drugs such as nitroprusside and positive inotropic agents.

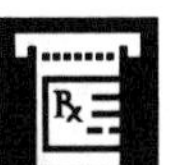

Medications

DRUG(S) OF CHOICE

Corticosteroids have been shown to be of no benefit.

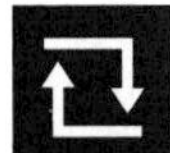

Follow-up

PATIENT MONITORING

- As for other etiologies of heart failure

EXPECTED COURSE AND PROGNOSIS

- Many patients spontaneously improve following the onset of viral inflammatory myocarditis.
- Patients with giant cell myocarditis may have a somewhat worse prognosis than patients with lymphocytic inflammatory myocarditis. Careful follow-up is always indicated.
- Some patients may demonstrate a rapid downhill course and require mechanical support and even heart transplantation.
- Although heart transplantation can be performed in these patients, there can be an exaggerated tendency toward rejection, particularly in the early posttransplantation follow-up phase.

PATIENT EDUCATION

- Patients need to be educated with information about myocarditis, just as they would be for any heart illness culminating in heart failure.
- Patients should be told that there is a higher likelihood of the spontaneous resolution with viral myocarditis compared with other forms of acute heart failure.
- Giant cell myocarditis has a poor prognosis, and affected patients may require transplantation.
- When heart failure is present, patients must be informed about the treatment and expected course of the syndrome.

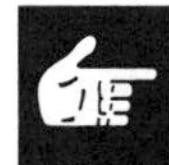

Miscellaneous

ICD-9-CM

428.0 Failure, heart, congestive

BIBLIOGRAPHY

Kilian J, et al. Myocarditis and cardiomyopathy associated with clozapine. *Lancet* 1999;354: 1841–1845.

Rodkey SM, Ratliff NB, Young JB. Cardiomyopathy and myocardial failure. In: Topol EJ, ed. *Comprehensive cardiovascular medicine.* Philadelphia: Lippincott-Raven, 1998:2593–2594.

Wynne J, Braunwald E. The cardiomyopathies and myocarditides. In: Braunwald E, ed. *Heart disease: a textbook of cardiovascular medicine,* 5th ed. Philadelphia: WB Saunders, 1997:1414–1426.

Authors: Gary S. Francis and Deepak L. Bhatt

Noonan's Syndrome

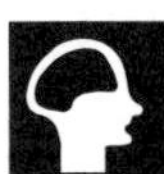

Basics

DESCRIPTION

Noonan's syndrome is a mendelian inherited syndrome characterized by a characteristic phenotypic stigmata.

Systems Affected

- Cardiovascular, endocrine, urologic, otologic, neurologic, and hematologic

Genetics

- An autosomal-dominant pattern of inheritance has been established. Many cases may be new stigmata. Normal karyotype. To date, familial pedigree studies have isolated the locus of Noonan's syndrome to several chromosomes, including 12 and 18.
- A large proportion (20%–30%) of first-generation family members of individuals with Noonan's syndrome are also affected with Noonan's syndrome.

Prevalence

The overall prevalence is not well established, but is approximately 1/2,000 newborns, males affected as often as females.

Age at Presentation

Fetal to adult; the mean age at diagnosis is approximately 9 years.

ASSOCIATED CONDITIONS

- Cardiovascular (50% of cases)
  - —Pulmonary valve dysplasia and stenosis: most common lesion (50%–75% of cases)
  - —Hypertrophic cardiomyopathy: typically asymmetric and can be associated with subaortic or subpulmonic stenosis (25%–33% of affected individuals)
  - —Atrial septal defect (ASD): (27% of cases)
  - —Tetralogy of Fallot
  - —Conduction abnormalities
  - —Rarely aortic stenosis and coarctation
- Endocrine/urologic
  - —Gonadal dysfunction: hypofunction of testes in males
  - —Cryptorchidism
  - —Short stature
  - —Renal abnormalities
- Otologic
  - —Progressive sensorineural hearing deficits (50% of cases)
- Neuropsychological
  - —Mental retardation (25% of cases)
  - —Developmental delay
- Hematologic/oncologic
  - —Coagulopathies
  - —Chronic myelomonocytic leukemia or "benign" monoclonal gammopathy
  - —Malignant schwannoma
- Neurologic
  - —Cerebrovascular disease such as moyamoya

Sex

- Male and female

PREGNANCY

- Pregnancy is possible, but may be high risk in women with severe manifestations; 50% of offspring of affected mothers will have Noonan's syndrome.

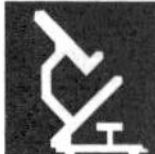

Diagnosis

DIFFERENTIAL DIAGNOSIS

- Turner's syndrome
- Cardio-facial-cutaneous syndrome
- LEOPARD syndrome
- Costello syndrome
- Neurofibromatosis: Noonan's syndrome. In the context of isolated pulmonary stenosis or peripheral artery stenosis, may see right-axis deviation and right ventricular hypertrophy.

SIGNS AND SYMPTOMS

The phenotype varies with the age at presentation.

Fetal

- Increased nuchal fluid
- Possible hydrops
- Pleural effusions
- Normal karyotype on amniocentesis
- Brachycephaly or growth retardation
- Shortened femora
- Renal abnormalities

Infant

- Cardiac abnormalities
  - —Systolic ejection murmur of pulmonary stenosis
  - —Possible ejection click
  - —If left ventricular hypertrophy with outflow obstruction is present, the patient may have typical symptoms of exertional dyspnea, chest pain, palpitations, postural hypotension, or syncope.
- Edema of hands and feet
- High arched palate
- Short or webbed neck
- Pectus carinatum or excavatum
- Cubitus valgus
- Typical facies: malformed posteriorly rotated ears, antimongoloid palpebral slant, ptosis, broad flat nose
- Undescended testes with possible hypogonadism
- Cardiovascular malformations: predominantly ASD, pulmonary stenosis, and hypertrophic cardiomyopathy

Childhood and Adolescence

- Short stature
- Developmental delay
- Characteristic cardiac malformations
- Sexual maturation delay of approximately 2 years

LABORATORY PROCEDURES

N/A

SPECIAL TESTS

ECG

- Isolated pulmonary stenosis or peripheral pulmonary artery stenosis may be seen.
- Right axis deviation and right ventricular hypertrophy
- If associated with asymmetric left ventricular hypertrophy, left axis deviation with left ventricular hypertrophy may be seen.
- Conduction abnormalities: typically first degree atrioventricular block

Audiometry

- Sensorineural or conductive hearing losses
- Developmental/psychosocial testing
  - —May reveal varying degrees of cognitive, behavioral, and psychosocial deficits

IMAGING STUDIES

- Fetal ultrasonography
  - —Subcutaneous edema of nuchal skin folds
  - —Generalized fetal edema
  - —Renal abnormalities
  - —Short femora
  - —Cardiac abnormalities
- Transthoracic or fetal echocardiography
  - —Pulmonary stenosis, ASD, asymmetric hypertrophic cardiomyopathy, tetralogy of Fallot, rarely aortic stenosis
- X-ray
  - —Chest: enlarged cardiac silhouette secondary to left or right ventricular hypertrophy
  - —Extremity: bone age studies in association with growth hormone therapy for growth retardation
- Cardiac catheterization
  - —Diagnostic catheterization rarely required
  - —Pulmonary stenosis with doming or dysplastic pulmonary valve
  - —Hypertrophic cardiomyopathy with possible ventricular outflow tract obstruction

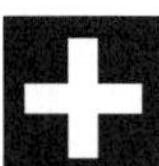

Treatment

GENERAL MEASURES

Treatment depends on age of diagnosis and presentation to medical attention. All individuals with heart lesions associated with an increased risk for endocarditis should receive appropriate prophylaxis prior to dental or invasive procedures. Regarding hypertrophic cardiomyopathy, see Hypertrophic Cardiomyopathy chapter.

- Prenatal
  —Parental counseling is advised regarding potentially affected systems, especially cardiac and renal. Timing and mode of delivery should be organized through the efforts of a high-risk perinatal team.
- Newborn
  —Patients with fetal hydrops should receive supportive, nutritional, and respiratory care in an experienced center where neonatal, renal, and cardiac care can be provided.
- Infancy and childhood
  —Early recognition of and intervention for cognitive or developmental delays
  —Identification and management of hearing deficits
- Adolescence and adulthood
  —Early evaluation and recognition of growth delay
  —Appropriate referral for management of pubertal delay

SURGICAL MEASURES

- Cardiac
  —Interventional cardiac catheterization with balloon dilation of pulmonary valvar stenosis or peripheral pulmonary artery stenosis; often poor results for dysplastic pulmonary valve stenosis
  —Myotomy or myomectomy for severe left ventricular outflow tract obstruction due to hypertrophic cardiomyopathy
  —Surgical or transcatheter device ASD closure
  —Surgical repair of pulmonary stenosis, tetralogy of Fallot, or other lesions
- Orthopedic
  —Leg-lengthening procedures for short stature
- Otologic
  —Placement of hearing aid devices for sensorineural deficits or myringotomy tubes for conductive hearing loss

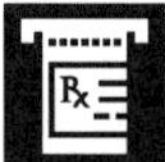

Medications

DRUG(S) OF CHOICE

- In symptomatic patients with hypertrophic cardiomyopathy, results may be achieved with:
  —Beta-adrenergic receptor-blocking agents such as propranolol
  —Calcium channel blockers such as verapamil or diltiazem
  —Disopyramide
- Growth hormone therapy beginning as early as 8 years of age for children with growth retardation/short stature

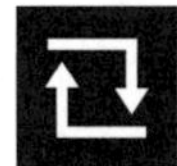

Follow-up

PATIENT MONITORING

- Routine lifelong outpatient visits with attention to systems discussed above, especially cardiovascular, renal, endocrine, and otologic
- A well-coordinated multidisciplinary approach is required.

Prevention/Avoidance

If cardiac defects are present, administer bacterial endocarditis prophylaxis for dental and invasive procedures as per the AHA guidelines.

EXPECTED COURSE AND PROGNOSIS

Overall, the prognosis and outcomes have improved significantly. This is due to early recognition and treatment of associated cardiac malformations and short stature.

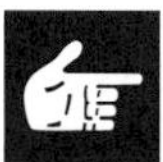

Miscellaneous

SYNONYMS

- Female pseudo-Turner's syndrome
- Male Turner's syndrome
- Ullrich's syndrome

BIBLIOGRAPHY

Emmanouilides GC, et al. *Moss and Adams' heart disease in infants, children and adolescents,* 5th ed. Baltimore: Williams & Wilkins, 1995.

Grange CS, Heid R, Lucas SB, et al. Anesthesia in a parturient with Noonan syndrome. *Can J Anaesth* 1998;45:332–336.

Harland M, Burch M, McKenna WM, et al. A clinical study of Noonan syndrome. *Arch Dis Child* 1992;67:178–183.

Ishizawa A, Oho S, Dodo H, et al. Cardiovascular abnormalities in Noonan syndrome; the clinical findings and treatments. *Acta Pediatr Jpn* 1996;38:84–90.

Nisbet DL, et al. Prenatal features of Noonan syndrome. *Prenatal Diagnosis* 1999;19:642–647.

Rudolph AM. *Rudolph's pediatrics,* 19th ed. East Norwalk, CT: Appleton & Lange, 1991.

Authors: Eric D. Fethke and Welton M. Gersony

Obesity and the Heart

Basics

DESCRIPTION

Heart failure can occur owing to a marked increase in the workload of the heart secondary to density.

EPIDEMIOLOGY

- The prevalence of obesity is increasing in the United States.
- Development of heart failure is more likely in the morbidly obese, those with a body mass index greater than 40 kg/m^2.
- The same level of obesity is more likely to lead to cardiac hypertrophy in women compared with men.

ETIOLOGY

- Obesity leads to ventricular hypertrophy, independent of the effects of blood pressure.
- The effects of obesity and hypertension in causing hypertrophy appear synergistic.
- The longer obesity has been present, the more likely it is that heart failure will develop.

RISK FACTORS

- Sedentary life-style, television viewing, family history of obesity

PREGNANCY

- Contraindicated with severe, symptomatic heart failure

ASSOCIATED CONDITIONS

- Sleep apnea, pulmonary hypertension
- Osteoarthritis
- Acanthosis nigricans
- Gallbladder disease
- Depression
- Hypertension
- Diabetes
- Hyperlipidemia
- Coronary artery disease

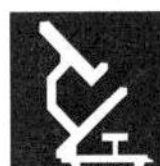

Diagnosis

DIFFERENTIAL DIAGNOSIS

- Other causes of left ventricular hypertrophy and dilatation

SIGNS AND SYMPTOMS

- Obesity
- Hypertension
- Dyspnea
- Loud P2
- Jugular venous distension
- Edema
- Hepatomegaly
- S3

LABORATORY PROCEDURES

ECG may show a prolonged QT interval

IMAGING STUDIES

- Chest x-ray may show cardiomegaly.
- Transthoracic echocardiography may provide suboptimal images due to body habitus.
- Left ventricular hypertrophy may be seen on echocardiography, as may right and left ventricular dilatation.

SPECIAL TESTS

- If endomyocardial biopsy is performed, myocyte hypertrophy is seen.
- Right heart catheterization shows elevated pressures.

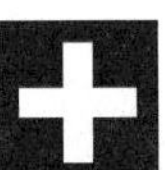

Treatment

GENERAL MEASURES

- Weight loss is paramount.
- Dieting, such as with a supervised very low calorie diet, and exercise can be very useful.
- Behavioral modification, encouraging a more active life-style, is of benefit.
- Diet should also be low sodium.
- Consultation with a nutritionist can be useful.

SURGICAL MEASURES

Gastric bypass can lead to effective weight loss.

ADMISSION/DISCHARGE CRITERIA

- As for heart failure of any etiology
- Patients may require prolonged inpatient dieting.

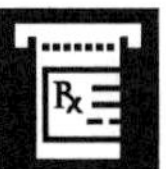

Medications

DRUG(S) OF CHOICE

- The combination of fenfluramine and phentermine (Phen-Fen) was effective in establishing a modest amount of weight loss, but is definitely associated with an increased rate of pulmonary hypertension, and very likely can lead to valvular regurgitation, usually minor and reversible. This latter observation led to the withdrawal of this medication.
- Control of concomitant high blood pressure is important.

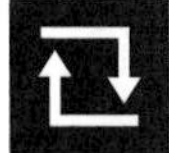

Follow-up

PATIENT MONITORING

Follow the patient's weight.

EXPECTED COURSE AND PROGNOSIS

- Sudden death is more common in the morbidly obese.
- Significant weight loss can reverse cardiomyopathy due to obesity.

PATIENT EDUCATION

- Engage in at least 30 minutes of moderate exercise daily.
- Restrict caloric intake.
- Limit sedentary activities such as watching television.

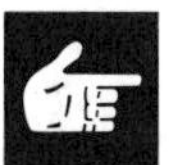

Miscellaneous

ICD-9-CM

428.0 Failure, heart, congestive

BIBLIOGRAPHY

Alpert MA, Hashimi MW. Obesity and the heart. *Am J Med Sci* 1993;306:117–123.

Alpert MA, Terry BE, Mulekar M, et al. Cardiac morphology and left ventricular function in normotensive morbidly obese patients with and without congestive heart failure, and effect of weight loss. *Am J Cardiol* 1997;80:736–740.

Carson JL, Ruddy ME, Duff AE, et al. The effect of gastric bypass surgery on hypertension in morbidly obese patients. *Arch Intern Med* 1994;154:193–200.

De Simone G, Devereux RB, Roman MJ, et al. Relation of obesity and gender to left ventricular hypertrophy in normotensive and hypertensive adults. *Hypertension* 1994;23:600–606.

Duflou J, Virmani R, Rabin I, et al. Sudden death as a result of heart disease in morbid obesity. *Am Heart J* 1995;130:306–313.

Kasper EK, Hruban RH, Baughman KL. Cardiomyopathy of obesity: a clinicopathologic evaluation of 43 obese patients with heart failure. *Am J Cardiol* 1992;70:921–924.

Stone NJ. Diet, nutritional issues, and obesity. In: Topol EJ, ed. *Comprehensive cardiovascular medicine.* Philadelphia: Lippincott-Raven, 1998:63–66.

Authors: Deepak L. Bhatt and Gary S. Francis

Orthostatic Hypotension

Basics

DESCRIPTION

Orthostatic hypotension is defined as a decrease in blood pressure of over 20 mm Hg systolic, or 10 mm Hg diastolic, upon standing or during head-up tilt. It is also known as postural hypotension.

EPIDEMIOLOGY

- Occurs in 14%–30% of individuals over 65 years of age
- Increases with age

ETIOLOGY

Genetics

Most cases are not caused by hereditary illness. Exceptions are rare and include autosomal-dominant familial amyloid neuropathy and porphyria; as well as autosomal-recessive familial dysautonomia-Riley-Day syndrome; beta-hydroxylase deficiency; and aromatic L-amino acid decarboxylase deficiency.

RISK FACTORS

- Age over 65
- Hypertension

PREGNANCY

N/A

ASSOCIATED CONDITIONS

Refer to Differential Diagnosis below.

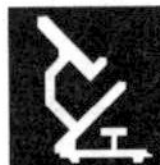

Diagnosis

DIFFERENTIAL DIAGNOSIS

Non-neurogenic Causes

- Hypovolemia (blood loss or dehydration)
- Vasodilation (vigorous exercise or excessive heat)

Neurogenic Causes

- Drugs
  - —Central nervous system–mediated (methyldopa, reserpine, clonidine, barbiturates, amphetamine, anesthetics, minoxidil)
  - —Peripheral nervous system–mediated (alpha-blockers, beta-blockers)
  - —Combination central and peripheral (tricyclic antidepressants, phenothiazines, levodopa)
  - —Autonomic neuropathy (alcohol, vincas)
  - —Vascular dilatation (nitrates, hydralazine, angiotensin-converting enzyme inhibitors, angiotensin-II antagonists, potassium channel blockers, calcium antagonists, endothelin antagonists).
- Metabolic diseases (diabetes mellitus, chronic renal failure, chronic liver disease, vitamin B_{12} deficiency, alcohol-induced, Fabry's, Tangier's, porphyria)
- Inflammatory (Guillaine-Barré, transverse myelitis)
- Infections (syphilis, HIV, Chagas, botulism, tetanus, herpes zoster)
- Neoplasia (brain tumors, especially third ventricle or posterior fossa, paraneoplastic)
- Connective tissue disease (rheumatoid arthritis, lupus)
- Surgery/trauma (sympathectomy, spinal cord transection)
- Neurally mediated (vasovagal, carotid sinus hypersensitivity, micturition syncope, cough syncope, swallow syncope)
- Primary chronic autonomic failure syndromes (Shy-Drager, Parkinson's)
- Secondary neuropathies (congenital growth factor deficiency, familial amyloid neuropathy, Riley-Day syndrome, dopamine beta-hydroxylase deficiency, aromatic L-amino acid decarboxylase deficiency)
- Primary acute and subacute dysautonomias

SIGNS AND SYMPTOMS

- May be asymptomatic, especially if long-standing
- Classically associated with head-up positional change
- Dizziness, visual disturbances, loss of consciousness/syncope, impaired cognition, seizures (cerebral hypoperfusion)
- Lower back/buttock pain or suboccipital/paracervical "coathanger" pain (muscle hypoperfusion)
- Angina pectoris
- Oliguria
- Falls (especially in elderly)
- Fatigue, lethargy
- Blood pressure decreases after 3 minutes in the upright position (usually standing, but sitting is acceptable in severely orthostatic individuals)
  - —Non-neurogenic causes produce tachycardia and sometimes sweating.
  - —Neurogenic causes include a decrease in blood pressure without tachycardia.

LABORATORY PROCEDURES

- Tilt-table measurement of blood pressure in supine and upright position
- Testing after liquid meal challenge, exercise testing, or carotid massage is helpful in determining cause.
- Plasma catecholamine measurements in supine and upright positions may help in differentiating certain neurologic conditions.

IMAGING STUDIES

N/A

SPECIAL TESTS

- May be used to determine suspected cause: MRI (for brain or spinal cord lesions), genetic testing (for familial amyloid neuropathy), sural nerve biopsy

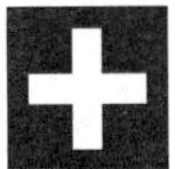

Treatment

GENERAL MEASURES

- Correction of non-neurogenic causes (e.g., hypovolemia) is curative.
- For neurogenic orthostatic hypotension, discontinue medications that may be causative.
- Avoid sudden head-up position changes, prolonged recumbency, straining during micturition/defecation, and vasodilatory stimuli (e.g., alcohol, large meals, overheating, vigorous exercise).
- Head-up tilt at night may increase blood pressure by activation of renin–angiotensin–aldosterone system.
- Ensure adequate fluid and salt intake.
- Identify body positions (leg-crossing, stooping) that may attenuate hypotension.
- Elastic stockings and abdominal binders may help, but often are not acceptable to patients.

SURGICAL MEASURES

Cardiac pacemakers are rarely indicated, except in some forms of neurally mediated syncope, such as carotid hypersensitivity.

ADMISSION/DISCHARGE CRITERIA

- Admit if hypotension is severe enough to cause ischemic end-organ damage (heart, brain, abdominal viscera).
- Discharge when blood pressure is sufficient to perfuse major organs.

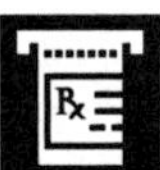

Medications

DRUG(S) OF CHOICE

- Mineralocorticoids (fludrocortisone) reduce salt loss and expand volume.
- Sympathomimetics (ephedrine, midodrine) cause vasoconstriction. Use with caution in patients with ischemic heart disease, peripheral vascular disease, or urinary retention.
- Desmopressin reduces nocturnal polyuria.
- Caffeine and octeotride are beneficial in postprandial hypotension.
- Erythropoietin expands red cell mass and blood volume in patients with renal failure.
- Prostaglandin synthetase inhibitors (indomethacin), dopamine blockers (metoclopramide), and beta 2-blockers prevent vasodilation.
- Dopamine agonists and beta-blockers with intrinsic sympathetic activity (pindolol) increase cardiac output.

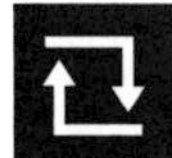

Follow-up

PATIENT MONITORING

Ambulatory blood pressure monitoring may be helpful for evaluation of therapeutic measures. At times, however, dissociation between blood pressure and symptoms may occur.

EXPECTED COURSE AND PROGNOSIS

- Prognosis is determined by underlying cause rather than the postural hypotension itself.
- In non-neurogenic orthostatic hypotension, treatment of cause and/or reversal of the underlying deficit may be curative.
- Goals of therapy for chronic orthostatic hypotension are to ensure mobility and prevent falls that can cause substantial morbidity and mortality.

PATIENT EDUCATION

Education and cooperation are essential for nonpharmacologic preventative measures, as detailed in General Measures.

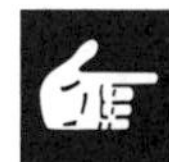

Miscellaneous

ICD-9-CM

458.0

BIBLIOGRAPHY

Mathias CJ, Kimber JR. Postural hypotension: causes, clinical features, investigation, and management. *Annu Rev Med* 1999;50:317–336.

Topol E, ed. *Textbook of cardiovascular medicine.* Philadelphia: Lippincott-Raven, 1998: 1807–1831.

Author: Rosemary Mehl

Osteogenesis Imperfecta and the Heart

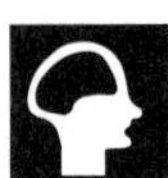

Basics

DESCRIPTION

Osteogenesis imperfecta (OI) is a genetic disorder characterized by bones that break easily, often from little or no apparent cause.

- The basic defect is abnormal synthesis of type I collagen molecules.
- Valvular dysfunction and aortic root dilation are associated with this disorder. There are four types of this disease:
    - —Type I: mild bone fragility, blue sclera, abnormal dentition (IB), hearing loss in most, and autosomal-dominant inheritance
    - —Type II (lethal): extreme bone fragility, blue sclera, abnormal dentition, autosomal-recessive inheritance, or sporadic
    - —Type III: severe bone fragility, bluish sclera at birth, abnormal dentition, hearing loss, and autosomal-recessive or autosomal dominant inheritance
    - —Type IV: variable bone fragility, normal sclera, abnormal dentition (IVB), hearing loss, and autosomal-dominant inheritance

EPIDEMIOLOGY

Prevalence

- 1/30,000 births
- Best estimate suggests a minimum of 20,000 and possibly as many as 50,000 cases of OI in the United States.
- Aortic root dilation occurs in 12% of affected individuals.
- Valvular heart disease is seen in approximately 2%–4% of cases, predominately aortic regurgitation.

Age

- Several forms of the disease lead to premature death during early childhood.
- Cardiac manifestations noted in patients 5–64 years of age

Sex

No apparent association with gender noted

ETIOLOGY

Most forms of OI are caused by imperfectly formed collagen as a result of a genetic defect.

- Collagen is the major protein of the body's connective tissue.
- In OI, a person has either less collagen or a poorer quality of collagen.
- The dysfunctional collagen results in weakening of the aortic annulus and dilation of the aorta.
- There is no clear association between aortic root dilation and aortic insufficiency.
- The valvular abnormalities appear to be secondary to structural defect of the valve tissue rather than a secondary effect from root dilation.

Genetics

- OI can be dominantly or recessively inherited.
- Sporadic forms also may occur.
- The aortic root dilation appears to segregate in families affected by OI.

RISK FACTORS

- Family history of this disorder
- Blood pressure is not related to degree of aortic root dilation in this population, although hypertension should be treated appropriately in affected individuals.

PREGNANCY

Genetic counseling is recommended for prospective parents if one or both are affected by this disorder.

ASSOCIATED CONDITIONS

Mitral valve prolapse (MVP) has been noted in some surveys of OI, but the inconsistent association with this common disorder probably reflects coinheritance of OI and MVP, rather than MVP secondary to the collagen defect of OI.

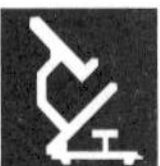

Diagnosis

DIFFERENTIAL DIAGNOSIS

- The cardiac disorders are not the presenting manifestations of OI. These are detected in patients in whom the diagnosis of OI is already known.
- Dyspnea may be related to mechanical difficulties of respiration (rib fractures, kyphoscoliosis, etc.).
- Other connective tissue diseases cause similar cardiac involvement:
    - —Marfan's disease
    - —Cystic medial necrosis
    - —Ehlers-Danlos syndrome

SIGNS AND SYMPTOMS

- History of bone fractures without significant trauma
- Family history of osteogenesis imperfecta
- Most are asymptomatic from cardiac disease (see chapters on Aortic Regurgitation and Mitral Regurgitation for further discussion).

LABORATORY PROCEDURES

N/A

IMAGING STUDIES

- Echocardiography is used to diagnose the valvular abnormalities seen with OI.
- Aortic root abnormalities also can be detected by CT scan or MRI of the thorax.

SPECIAL TESTS

Collagen testing from a skin biopsy is used to determine the amount of collagen present and its structure.

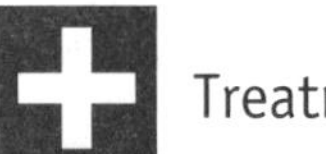

Treatment

GENERAL MEASURES

- There is no cure for the underlying defect in OI.
- Activity is restricted due to the risk of fractures.
- Hypertension should be treated.
- No specific pharmacologic therapy for patients with aortic root dilation without hypertension

SURGICAL MEASURES

- Aortic valve replacement may be undertaken when appropriate (see chapter on Aortic Regurgitation)
- May be complicated by bleeding problems secondary to platelet dysfunction and capillary fragility

ADMISSION/DISCHARGE CRITERIA

- Admission for aortic valve replacement in appropriate individuals is on an elective basis, with discharge based on standard postoperative protocols.

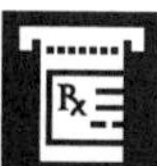

Medications

DRUG(S) OF CHOICE

N/A

ALTERNATIVE DRUGS

Beta-blockade has not been advocated to slow progression of aortic root dilation (as is done in Marfan's).

Follow-up

PATIENT MONITORING

With cardiac valve involvement, serial echocardiograms and symptoms are followed to determine timing of surgery.

EXPECTED COURSE AND PROGNOSIS

The prognosis for an individual with OI varies greatly depending on the type of OI, and the number and severity of symptoms.

- Type I: good life expectancy
- Type II: lethal
- Type III: decreased life expectancy, where few reach adulthood
- Type IV: good life expectancy

Expected Complications (Noncardiac)

- Numerous fractures
- Restricted activity
- Short stature
- Brain damage
- The majority of OI patients that have cardiac involvement are asymptomatic, and the cardiac conditions are rarely the cause of morbidity and mortality in this disorder.

PATIENT EDUCATION

Organization

- Osteogenesis Imperfecta Foundation, 804 W. Diamond Avenue, Suite 210, Gaithersburg, MD 20878; phone (301)947-0083 or (800)981-2663; Fax (301)947-0456; Internet site: www.oif.org

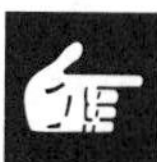

Miscellaneous

ICD-9-CM

765.51 Osteogenesis imperfecta

BIBLIOGRAPHY

Hortop J, et al. Cardiovascular involvement in osteogenesis imperfecta. *Circulation* 1986; 73:54–61.

Wheeler VR, et al. Cardiovascular pathology in osteogenesis imperfecta type IIA with a review of the literature. *Pediatr Pathol* 1988;8:55–64.

Wong RS, et al. Osteogenesis imperfecta and cardiovascular diseases. *Ann Thorac Surg* 1995;60:1439–1443.

Author: Daniel T. Price

Pacemakers

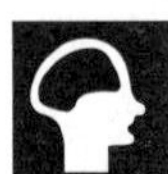

Basics

DESCRIPTION

A pacemaker is an implantable device designed to treat bradycardia. On occasion, pacemakers can be used to prevent and treat tachycardias. The indications for pacemaker implantation are detailed in the ACC/AHA Guideline referenced below. The general indications include:

- Bradycardia
- Atrioventricular (AV) block
- Conduction disturbances with acute myocardial infarction
- Tachycardia prevention
- Possibly for dyspnea and angina in hypertrophic cardiomyopathy and congestive heart failure in dilated cardiomyopathy

EPIDEMIOLOGY

Over 1 million people in the United States have pacemakers, and there are about 435 new implantations per 1,000,000 people each year. Pacemakers are implanted in appropriate candidates irrespective of age.

ETIOLOGY

N/A

RISK FACTORS

- Related to underlying diseases leading to arrhythmia problem
- The most common cause of heart disease in the United States is atherosclerosis. Thus, the majority of patients with pacemakers have coronary artery disease.

PREGNANCY

- No contraindication from pacemaker per se, although underlying heart disease may be a contraindication (e.g., valve disease with anticoagulation, cardiomyopathy).

ASSOCIATED CONDITIONS

- See Risk Factors above.

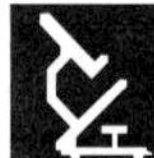

Diagnosis

DIFFERENTIAL DIAGNOSIS

N/A

SIGNS AND SYMPTOMS

- Related to the indication for pacemaker implantation, not the device itself

LABORATORY PROCEDURES

N/A

IMAGING STUDIES

- Related only to evaluation of cardiac disease leading to electrical disease
- Possible tests include echocardiography, exercise testing, and cardiac catheterization with coronary and ventricular angiography.

SPECIAL TESTS

Ambulatory monitoring, telemetry, Holter monitoring, and electrophysiologic study can all be used to establish arrhythmia disturbance to provide indication for pacemaker implantation.

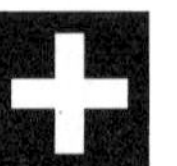

Treatment

GENERAL MEASURES

Follow-up is discussed below.

SURGICAL MEASURES

Pacemakers are now generally implanted by cardiologists and electrophysiologists, often in a catheterization laboratory or dedicated electrophysiology laboratory.

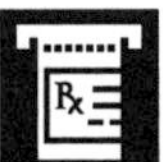

Medications

DRUG(S) OF CHOICE

Drugs are often used with pacemakers to:

- Decrease the frequency of arrhythmia occurrence
- Treat concomitant diseases, such as atrial fibrillation and coronary artery disease (e.g., beta-blockers, nitrates, aspirin, angiotensin-converting enzyme inhibitors, etc.)

Follow-up

PATIENT MONITORING

- Cardiologist generally performs follow-up.
- Pacemakers are usually checked over the telephone with intermittent office visits.

EXPECTED COURSE AND PROGNOSIS

- Variable and depends on underlying heart disease
- Patients with AV block have a worse prognosis than those with sinus node dysfunction, probably because the former have greater degrees of structural heart disease.

PATIENT EDUCATION

- Compliance with telephone and office follow-up should be emphasized.
- Patients should be taught to be vigilant for pacemaker complications, including infection, bleeding, lead fracture, and device failure.
- Avoidance of electromagnetic interference, including MRI scans, some tanning booths, and arc welder generators, is important. Note that microwave use is not contraindicated with modern pacemakers. Cell phones may be used contralateral to the site of the pacemaker.

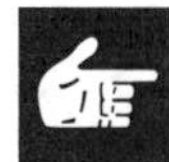

Miscellaneous

ICD-9-CM

Not applicable because pacemakers are not diseases, but rather a treatment.

See also: AV block; Sick sinus syndrome

BIBLIOGRAPHY

Goldschlager N. Recognition and management of patients with bradyarrhythmias. In: Goldman L, Braunwald E, eds. *Primary cardiology.* Philadelphia: WB Saunders, 1998:353–370.

Goldschlager N. Bradycardias and pacemakers. In: Wachter RM, Goldman L, Hollander H, eds. *Hospital medicine.* Baltimore: Williams & Wilkins (in press).

Gregoratos G, Cheitlin MD, Conill A, et al. ACC/AHA guidelines for implantation of cardiac pacemakers and antiarrhythmia devices: a report of the American College of Cardiology/American Heart Association Task Force on Practice Guidelines (Committee on Pacemaker Implantation). *J Am Coll Cardiol* 1998;31:1175–1206.

Author: Andrew E. Epstein

Paget's Disease and the Heart

Basics

DESCRIPTION

Paget's disease is a disorder manifested by rapid bone growth.

- There is increased vascularity of bone and increased blood flow through the cutaneous tissue overlying the involved bone, possibly secondary to local heat production by metabolically hyperactive affected bone.
- For an increased cardiac output to occur in Paget's disease, there must be at least a 15% increase in involvement of the skeleton with an increase in alkaline phosphatase.
- The increased cardiac output may precipate heart failure if underlying heart disease is present.
- Augmentation of cardiac output obligated by the increased flow may not be manageable by the diseased heart, leading to heart failure.
- For example, if there is underlying severe aortic stenosis, the added demands placed on the heart by the need for increase flow through new vasculature may lead to clinical deterioration and heart failure.

EPIDEMIOLOGY

- Paget's disease is not uncommon, occurring in 3%–4% of subjects over age 40 years.
- White individuals over age 55 are the group predominantly affected.
- There is an increased incidence of Paget's in first-degree relatives.
- Autosomal-dominant transmission has been described in certain cases.
- Heart failure due to Paget's disease is unusual, but could easily go unrecognized.

ETIOLOGY

The etiology of Paget's disease is unknown.

RISK FACTORS

There are no known risk factors.

PREGNANCY

N/A

ASSOCIATED CONDITIONS

- Metastatic calcification
- Headache
- Hearing loss

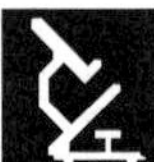

Diagnosis

DIFFERENTIAL DIAGNOSIS

- There must be a high index of suspicion to diagnose Paget's disease.
- Patients may notice that their hat size is increasing.
- The enlarged bones may be painful, deformed, and warm.
- Deafness and nerve compression can occur when it involves the skull.

SIGNS AND SYMPTOMS

- Increase in hat size
- Skin warmth (over the skull, tibia)

LABORATORY PROCEDURES

- There is a marked increase in plasma alkaline phosphatase, derived from overactive osteoblasts.
- Urinary hydroxyproline

IMAGING STUDIES

The sizes of the affected bones are increased radiographically.

SPECIAL TESTS

Occasionally bone biopsy is undertaken to exclude other bone disease such as osteomalacia.

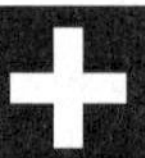

Treatment

GENERAL MEASURES

Treatment for pain may consist of simple analgesics.

SURGICAL MEASURES

Fractures of pagetic bone require the usual surgical treatment.

ADMISSION/DISCHARGE CRITERIA

- As for heart failure of any etiology

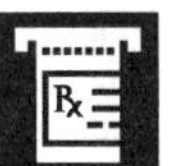

Medications

DRUG(S) OF CHOICE

- Bisphosphonates may be given to reduce excess bone turnover.
- Calcitonin is also widely used to treat Paget's disease.

Follow-up

PATIENT MONITORING

- As for heart failure of any etiology

EXPECTED COURSE AND PROGNOSIS

- As for heart failure of any etiology

PATIENT EDUCATION

- As for heart failure of any etiology

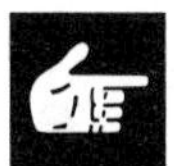

Miscellaneous

ICD-9-CM

428.0 Failure, heart, congestive

BIBLIOGRAPHY

Heistad DD, Abboud FM, Schnid PG, et al. Regulation of blood flow in Paget's disease of bone. *J Clin Invest* 1975;55:69.

Authors: Gary S. Francis and Deepak L. Bhatt

Paradoxical Embolism

Basics

DESCRIPTION

A paradoxical embolism is caused by emboli that originate in the venous system and reach the arterial system via a right-to-left cardiac or extracardiac shunt. The presumptive diagnosis requires four clinical criteria:

- Venous thrombosis
- Communication between right and left circulations
- Right-to-left atrial pressure gradient during the entire or a portion of the cardiac cycle
- Systemic embolism in the absence of common cardioembolic substrates
  - —The diagnosis is definite when a thrombus lodged across an intracardiac shunt is demonstrated.
  - —About 50% embolize predominantly to the lower extremities, 35%–40% to the brain, and 10%–15% to the coronary, renal, splenic, or mesenteric arteries.
  - —Two or more sites of embolism occur in 25% of patients.
  - —Pulmonary embolism is demonstrated in two-thirds of patients and deep vein thrombosis in 40%.
  - —Patent foramen ovale is present in 72% of patients, atrial septal defect in 12%, pulmonary arteriovenous fistula in 12%, and ventricular septal defect in 4%.

Systems Affected

- Cardiovascular

ETIOLOGY

Genetics

Atrial or ventricular septal defects and other congenital shunts have a genetic etiology.

Incidence/Prevalence

- Paradoxical embolism is an uncommon clinical syndrome described in all races, different age groups, and both sexes.
- Its true incidence and prevalence are unknown.

Predominant Age

- The fourth decade of life

Predominant Sex

- 2:1 female to male ratio

RISK FACTORS

- High risk: those with an intra- or extracardiac communication and deep vein thrombosis or pulmonary embolism.
- Moderate risk: those with right atrial hypertension due to chronic obstructive pulmonary disease, ischemic or myopathic right ventricular dysfunction, or atrial fibrillation
- Low risk: those with normal right atrial pressure who exhibit transient spontaneous or induced (respiration, Valsalva, or coughing) right-to-left atrial pressure gradient

ASSOCIATED CONDITIONS

- Intra- or extracardiac communication, peripheral vein thrombosis, pulmonary embolism, and right atrial hypertension
- In autopsy studies the prevalence of patent foramen ovale ranges from 22% to 34%, but most (85%) are 2–5 mm and the minority (15%) are 6–10 mm in diameter.
  - —The latter are more likely to be associated with embolism.
  - —By saline contrast echocardiography in patients <55 years of age with systemic embolism, but no cardiac disease, the prevalence of patent foramen ovale ranges from 25% to 50%.
  - —This contrasts with a 3%–15% prevalence in subjects undergoing echocardiography for reasons other than cardioembolism.
- The prevalence of secundum-type atrial septal defect in adults is probably <1%.
- Thus, paradoxical embolism occurs mostly in association with a patent foramen ovale.
- Risk factors for deep vein thrombosis and pulmonary embolism include postoperative status, inactivity due to obesity, myocardial infarction, congestive heart failure, venous insufficiency, primary or secondary hypercoagulable states, and *in situ* right atrial thrombosis.
  - —*In situ* right atrial thrombosis occurs in patients with atrial fibrillation, those undergoing right atrial cannulation during cardiopulmonary bypass, or in those with right atrial catheters.

Age-Related Factors

- Pediatric: rare
- Geriatric: less common
- Others: middle age peak incidence

PREGNANCY

Hypercoagulable state increases the incidence of venous thromboembolism.

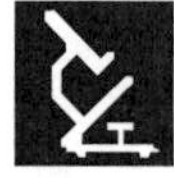

Diagnosis

DIFFERENTIAL DIAGNOSIS

- Most common causes of cerebral or peripheral arterial embolism are atheroemboli from carotid arteries or aortic atheromatous disease or cardioembolism due to atrial fibrillation, mitral stenosis, prosthetic heart valves, anterior myocardial infarction, dilated cardiomyopathy, and infective or noninfective endocarditis.
- Less commonly, systemic and venous thrombosis or pulmonary embolism can be seen in patients with cardiomyopathy and left ventricular thrombus and congestive heart failure leading to vein thrombosis.
- Rarely, dilated cardiomyopathy with right and left heart thrombi and embolism or right and left heart valves endocarditis and embolism are seen.

SIGNS AND SYMPTOMS

- The signs and symptoms of deep vein thrombosis and pulmonary embolism that usually precede those of systemic embolism are described in other sections of this book.
- Paradoxical embolism implies recurrent pulmonary embolism because right atrial hypertension is usually preexistent for a recurrent and migrating venous thrombi to traverse a left-to-right shunt.
- The vascular distributions, signs, and symptoms of paradoxical embolism are those of transient ischemic attack, stroke, or peripheral embolism described in the chapter on Arterial Embolism.

LABORATORY PROCEDURES

No specific laboratory abnormalities are reported.

Pathologic Findings

- Cardiac shunt defect and evidence of peripheral vascular embolism

SPECIAL TESTS

Transesophageal echocardiography with or without saline contrast study may be needed in patients with technically limited or equivocal transthoracic echocardiograms, in those with suspected right atrial or ventricular thrombi, or in those with embolism of undefined etiology.

IMAGING STUDIES

- Imaging studies in patients with suspected paradoxical embolism should include those described in the chapter on Arterial Embolism.
  - Brain CT, MRI/magnetic resonance angiography (MRA), carotid duplex ultrasonography/MRA, and angiography
  - Transthoracic echocardiography with saline contrast and during Valsalva or coughing
    - —Bubbles seen in the left atrium within the first three cardiac cycles suggest an interatrial septal defect.
    - —Bubbles seen after three cardiac cycles suggest a pulmonary arteriovenous communication.
  - If systemic embolism has occurred and an interatrial septal defect is demonstrated, studies for detection of deep venous thrombosis and pulmonary embolism should be performed.

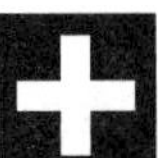

Treatment

GENERAL MEASURES

- Those related to deep venous thrombosis, pulmonary embolism, and arterial embolism that are described elsewhere in this book

SURGICAL MEASURES

- In patients with hemodynamically compromising main or proximal pulmonary artery thrombosis not candidates for thrombolytic therapy, pulmonary thromboembolectomy, interatrial septal defect closure, and inferior vena cava interruption via insertion of a filter or surgical plication should be considered.
- In patients with peripheral embolism, surgical or percutaneous thromboembolectomy is indicated when limb ischemia persists despite adequate anticoagulation.
- Recurrent paradoxical embolism despite adequate anticoagulation requires interruption of the inferior vena cava via filter or surgical plication and closure of the interatrial septal defect or patent foramen ovale.

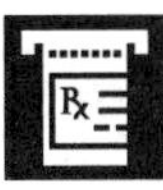

Medications

DRUG(S) OF CHOICE

- If deep vein thrombosis or pulmonary embolism is diagnosed, the patient is hemodynamically stable, and the risk for cerebral hemorrhagic infarction is low, heparin i.v. bolus and continuous infusion to a partial thromboplastin time 1.5–2.5 times control is indicated.
- Warfarin is started on days 2–3 and heparin discontinued on day 7–10 or when INR therapeutic (INR 2–3).
- If no contraindications, thrombolytic therapy should be considered in patients with
  - —Peripheral embolism and a large pulmonary embolism with hemodynamic compromise
  - —Peripheral embolism with jeopardized limb viability
- In patients with suspected paradoxical embolism, but no evidence of vein thrombosis or pulmonary embolism, the use of heparin and long-term anticoagulation lacks supportive data.

Contraindications

Refer to manufacturer's literature.

Precautions

Refer to manufacturer's literature.

Significant Possible Interactions

Warfarin interacts with many drugs.

ALTERNATIVE DRUGS

N/A

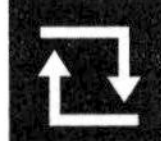

Follow-up

PATIENT MONITORING

- Monitoring of warfarin therapy

Prevention/Avoidance

Avoid activities, situations, or drugs that increase risk of venous thromboembolism.

Possible Complications

Limb or organ injury or loss due to embolism

EXPECTED COURSE AND PROGNOSIS

- Limited prospective and longitudinal data are available.
- These patients' clinical course is related to the severity of pulmonary and arterial embolism.
- Paradoxical embolism suggests recurrent pulmonary embolism that in combination with a stroke portends a poor prognosis.
- Patients with peripheral embolism have better prognosis.
- Most (70%) patients demonstrate full recovery of neurologic or peripheral pulse deficits, whereas 10% have persistent deficits. The remaining 20% die, and pulmonary embolism is the main cause.

PATIENT EDUCATION

- As described in the corresponding sections of pulmonary and arterial embolism

Activity

- As tolerated

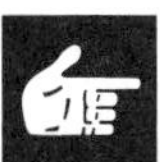

Miscellaneous

ICD-9-CM

444.9 Paradoxical embolism
434.1 Cerebral embolism
444.22 Peripheral artery embolism
415.1 Pulmonary embolism
451.9 Thrombophlebitis

BIBLIOGRAPHY

De Belder MA, Tourikis L, Leech G, et al. Risk of patent foramen ovale for thromboembolic events in all age groups. *Am J Cardiol* 1992; 69:1316–1320.

Gill TJ, Campbell CC. Radial artery occlusion by paradoxical embolism: a case report. *J Hand Surg* 1995;20:406–407.

Loscalzo J. Paradoxical embolism: clinical presentation, diagnostic strategies, and therapeutic options. *Am Heart J* 1986;July:141–145.

Nagelhout DA, Pearson AC, Labovitz AJ. Diagnosis of paradoxic embolism by transesophageal echocardiography. *Am Heart J* 1991;121:1552–1554.

Nelson C, Snow F, Barnett M, et al. Impending paradoxical embolism: echocardiographic diagnosis of an intracardiac thrombus crossing a patent foramen ovale. *Am Heart J* 1991;122: 859–862.

Ofori CS, Moore LC, Hepler G. Massive cerebral infarction caused by paradoxical embolism: detection by transesophageal echocardiography. *J Am Soc Echocardiogr* 1995;8:563–566.

Ranoux D, Cohen A, Cabanes L, et al. Patent foramen ovale: is stroke due to paradoxical embolism? *Stroke* 1993;24:31–34.

Schreiter SW, Phillips JH. Thromboembolus traversing a patent foramen ovale: resolution with anticoagulation. *J Am Soc Echocardiogr* 1994; 7:659–662.

Speechly-Dick ME, Middleton SJ, Foale RA. Impending paradoxical embolism: a rare but important diagnosis. *Br Heart J* 1991;65:163–165.

Author: Carlos A. Roldan

Patent Ductus Arteriosus

Basics

DESCRIPTION

Functional closure of the ductus arteriosus usually occurs within the first 24 hours of life. Complete obliteration of the lumen is usually completed in the first weeks of life.

Systems Affected

- Cardiovascular

ETIOLOGY

Genetics

A genetic factor may be present in some cases. Siblings of patients with a patent ductus arteriousus (PDA) have as high as a 2%–4% incidence of having a PDA themselves.

Incidence/Prevalence

In the United States, as an isolated lesion, a persistent PDA has been estimated to occur in 1/2,000 to 1/5,000 live births and represents 9%–12% of all congenital heart lesions.

- There is an increased incidence in premature infants and those with hypoxemia.
- A rubella infection early in pregnancy has a high association with persistent patency of the ductus arteriosus.

Predominant Sex

- Female more than male

RISK FACTORS

- Prematurity and hypoxemia contribute to persistent patency of the ductus arteriosus.
- Rubella infection early in pregnancy has a high association with persistent patency of the ductus arteriosus.

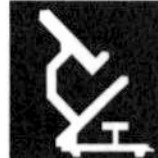

Diagnosis

DIFFERENTIAL DIAGNOSIS

The following lesions also cause continuous or to-and-fro murmurs. Usually these lesions can be ruled out by the physical examination, and almost always by echocardiography.

- Aortopulmonary window
- Venous hum
- Arteriovenous fistula
- Ruptured sinus of Valsalva
- Truncus arteriosus
- Absent pulmonary valve

SIGNS AND SYMPTOMS

- Most common signs and symptoms: The clinical findings depend on the magnitude of left-to-right shunt through the PDA and the ability of the heart to manage the extra volume load.
- Two major factors control the degree of shunting:
  —Diameter and length of the ductus arteriosus
  —Systemic and pulmonary vascular resistance
- Premature infants
  —Diagnosis often made in first week of life, because left-to-right shunt begins early; premature infants usually have low pulmonary vascular resistance from birth.
  —Classical machinery murmur is usually not present.
  —Systolic murmur which may extend into early diastole is heard best at the left sternal border in the second and third intercostal spaces.
  —Hyperactive precordium
  —Widened pulse pressure
  —Prominent pulses
  —If a large shunt is present, patients will have signs of congestive heart failure.
- Term infants, older children
  —Small PDA
    - Usually not symptomatic
    - Normal first and second heart sounds
    - Murmur usually systolic in infancy and then continuous murmur heard best at second left intercostal space in older child
    - Prominent peripheral pulses
    - Slightly increased arterial pulse pressure

  —Moderate PDA
    - Patients may have signs of congestive heart failure in infancy.
    - Loud continuous murmur with machinery quality at left upper sternal border
    - Increased heart rate
    - Bounding pulses
    - Widened pulse pressure
    - Hyperdynamic precordium

  —Large PDA
    - Usually have signs of congestive heart failure in first few months of life
    - Murmur usually is continuous.
    - Increased heart rate
    - Bounding pulses
    - Widened pulse pressure
    - Hyperdynamic precordium
    - May have mid-diastolic rumble at apex
    - May eventually progress to pulmonary vascular disease and right-to-left shunt if untreated

LABORATORY PROCEDURES

N/A

IMAGING STUDIES

- Chest x-ray
  —The x-ray findings vary in proportion to the degree of left-to-right shunting.
  —With a larger shunt, there is cardiomegaly with enlargement of the left ventricle, left atrium, and prominent pulmonary vasculature.

SPECIAL TESTS

- ECG
  —Small ductus: ECG is normal.
  —Larger ductus: increased left ventricular forces, occasionally left atrial enlargement
  —Larger ductus with pulmonary hypertension: increased biventricular forces

DIAGNOSTIC PROCEDURES

- Echocardiography
  —The ductus is best imaged in a high left parasternal view.
  —Color flow mapping is essential to demonstrate flow through the ductus.
  —Continuous wave Doppler is useful for estimating the pulmonary artery pressure.
  —If there is a significant shunt, left atrial and left ventricular dilatation (and possible left ventricular hypertrophy) may be seen.
  —Echocardiography has an important role in excluding other significant intracardiac lesions, especially ductal-dependent lesions.
- Cardiac catheterization
  —Catheterization is rarely needed to make the diagnosis.

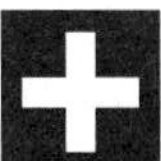

Treatment

GENERAL MEASURES

- General supportive measures in premature infants include maintaining an adequate hematocrit and fluid restriction.
- Indomethacin has been used successfully to close a patent ductus arteriosus in a large proportion of premature infants. It has not been shown to be effective in term infants.
- The classic small or large ductus arteriosus should be eliminated, the timing of which is determined by the presence or absence of symptoms.
- The term *silent ductus* refers to echocardiographic findings of a minimal color Doppler shunt diagnostic or suggestive of a tiny PDA in a patient with no other physical or laboratory evidence of a PDA. In most cases the echocardiographic study was done for a nonspecific systolic murmur that might well have been classified by a cardiologist as functional without an ultrasonographic study. These patients can be followed without intervention. Although endocarditis with silent ductus specifically is virtually unreported, it may be prudent to nevertheless recommend appropriate antibiotic prophylaxis.

SURGICAL MEASURES

- With modern surgical techniques, surgical closure has achieved nearly a 100% success rate with almost no mortality risk and low morbidity.
- Neither the size of the patient nor that of the ductus arteriosus are limiting factors. Although there have been reports of recanalization after ligation alone, and other rare complications (injury to the recurrent laryngeal nerve, injury to the thoracic duct with chylothorax, or accidental ligation of the left pulmonary artery, descending aorta, or carotid artery), surgical ligation or division of the ductus arteriosus has been the standard for more than 60 years.
- Recently, some institutions have begun video-assisted thoracoscopic ligation of the PDA. This approach may reduce the postoperative convalescence period and may be associated with less chest wall deformity.
  —A potential drawback is greater difficulty controlling intraoperative bleeding. More experience with this procedure will determine the future role it may play in ductal closure.

Catheter Closure

—Catheter closure of a PDA was first introduced over 20 years ago and is now accepted as the preferred therapy at most institutions.
—Size of the patient and of the ductus arteriosus are factors that currently limit its use, but new techniques are expanding its applicability.
—Studies report high success rates with few complications, which include coil embolization, left pulmonary artery stenosis, and femoral vessel occlusion.

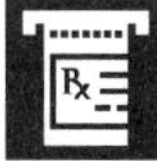

Medications

DRUG(S) OF CHOICE

- Infants with signs of congestive heart failure can be managed briefly with anticongestive medications; standard treatment for symptomatic patients is elimination of the ductus arteriosus on an urgent basis.
- A patient with a PDA should receive bacterial endocarditis prophylaxis according to the recommended AHA guidelines.

Possible Complications

- Congestive heart failure, usually in young infants with a large ductus arteriosus
- Bacterial endocarditis
- Aneurysm of the ductus arteriosus
- Pulmonary vascular disease

Follow-up

EXPECTED COURSE AND PROGNOSIS

- In premature infants, persistent patency of the PDA is common. The great majority will close as the patient matures, but in the context of respiratory distress syndrome, early pharmacologic or surgical intervention is often required.
- Term infants with PDA rarely have spontaneous closure.
- Patients with untreated PDA are at risk for the possible complications listed above.

ASSOCIATED CONDITIONS

PDA can be an isolated lesion or can be associated with virtually all other congenital heart defects.

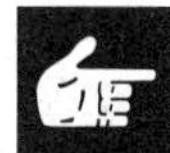

Miscellaneous

BIBLIOGRAPHY

Balzer DT, Spray TL, McMullin D, et al. Endarteritis associated with a clinically silent patent ductus arteriosus. *Am Heart J* 1993;125:1192.

Brook MM, Heymann MA. Patent ductus arteriosus. In: *Moss and Adams' heart disease in infants, children, and adolescents,* 5th ed. Baltimore: Williams & Wilkins, 1995:746.

Gersony WM, Peckham GJ, Ellison RC, et al. Effects of indomethacin in premature infants with patent ductus arteriosus: results of a national collaborative study. *J Pediatr* 1983; 102:895.

Goyal VS, Fulwani MC, Ramakantan R, et al. Follow-up after coil closure of patent ductus arteriosus. *Am J Cardiol* 1999;83:463.

Hines MH, Bensky AS, Hammon JW Jr., et al. Video-assisted thorascopic ligation of patent ductus arteriosus: safe and outpatient. *Ann Thorac Surg* 1998;66:853.

Ing FF, Sommer RJ. The snare-assisted technique for transcatheter coil occlusion of moderate to large patent ductus arteriosus: immediate and intermediate results. *J Am Coll Cardiol* 1999;33:1710.

Kirklin JW, Barratt-Boyles BG. Patent ductus arteriosus. In: *Cardiac surgery,* 2nd ed. New York: Churchill Livingstone, 1993:851.

Lloyd TR, Beekman RH, Moore JW, et al. The PDA Coil Registry: 250 patient-years of follow-up [Abstract]. *J Am Coll Cardiol* 1996;27(suppl 2):34.

Shim D, Fedderllly RT, Beekman RH, et al. Follow-up of coil occlusion of patent ductus arteriosus. *J Am Coll Cardiol* 1996;28:207.

Authors: Karen Altmann and Welton M. Gersony

Pectus Excavatum

Basics

DESCRIPTION

Pectus excavatum is also known as funnel chest.

- Depression of the sternum so that the ribs on each side protrude farther anteriorly than the sternum
- This condition is associated with connective tissue disorders such as Marfan's syndrome, Poland's syndrome, Pierre Robin syndrome, and scoliosis.
- There is an increased incidence of mitral valve prolapse, Wolf-Parkinson-White syndrome, and atrial septal defect.

Systems Affected

- Musculoskeletal, cardiovascular, and pulmonary

EPIDEMIOLOGY

Incidence/Prevalence

- 0.4%–2% of the general population.
- Increased incidence in people with a family history

Predominant Sex

More males affected than females

ASSOCIATED CONDITIONS

- Marfan's syndrome
- Poland's syndrome
- Scoliosis
- Pierre Robin syndrome

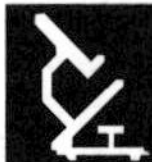

Diagnosis

SIGNS AND SYMPTOMS

- Diagnosis by physical examination: depression of the sternum so that the ribs on each side protrude farther anteriorly than the sternum
- Most patients are asymptomatic. Cardiopulmonary symptoms such as fatigue and decreased exercise tolerance have been reported.
- Heart murmur is evident in 40%–50% of cases, most commonly a systolic murmur that mimics pulmonic stenosis. This may be secondary to kinking of the pulmonary artery or changes in the diameter of the right ventricular outflow tract.
- Splitting of the second heart sound is also commonly found.

IMAGING STUDIES

Chest X-ray

The degree of sternal depression can be appreciated.

- The heart is displaced to the left and rotated.
- Parasternal soft tissues may be seen as an increased density over the inferomedial portion of the left hemithorax.
- Occasionally an unusual mediastinal configuration can mimic a mediastinal mass.

Echocardiogram

- Compression of the right atrium or right ventricle may be seen.
- Morphologic changes in the right ventricle have been reported.
- These include right ventricle dilatation, rounded apex, sacculations in the free wall, and hypertrophy of the moderator band.

SPECIAL TESTS

ECG

Increased left sided potentials related to leftward displacement of the heart may be seen, as may right ventricular conduction delay.

Pulmonary Function Tests

A slightly decreased vital capacity is commonly found, as is an occasional restrictive lung pattern.

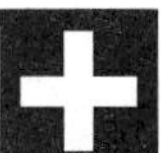

Treatment

GENERAL MEASURES

Physicians should be aware of associated conditions and cardiac abnormalities. ECG and echocardiogram should be considered.

SURGICAL MEASURES

This chest wall deformity can be surgically repaired.

- The majority of people will not have a functional benefit.
- There are case reports suggesting symptomatic and hemodynamic improvements.
- Sometimes the defect is repaired for cosmetic reasons.

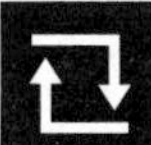

Follow-up

PATIENT MONITORING

Determined by symptoms and associated conditions

EXPECTED COURSE AND PROGNOSIS

Dependent on any other related conditions (e.g., Marfan's syndrome)

PATIENT EDUCATION

Activity

- No restrictions

Diet

- No restrictions

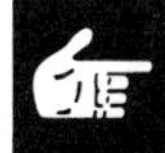

Miscellaneous

SYNONYMS

- Funnel chest

BIBLIOGRAPHY

Fraser RG, Pare JA, Pare PD, et al. *Diagnosis of diseases of the chest.* Philadelphia: WB Saunders, 1991.

Guller B, Hable K. Cardiac findings in pectus excavatum in children: review and differential diagnosis. *Chest* 1974;66:165–171.

Mocchegiani R, Bandano L, Lestuzzi C, et al. Relation of right ventricular morphology and function in pectus excavatum to the severity of the chest wall deformity. *Am J Cardiol* 1995;76:941–946.

Shamberger RC, Welch KJ. Cardiopulmonary function in pectus excavatum. *Surg Gynecol Obstet* 1988;166:383–391.

Authors: Richard Mascolo and Gerard P. Aurigemma

Pericardial Tamponade

Basics

DESCRIPTION

Pericardial tamponade is defined as fluid accumulation of any nature in the pericardial space resulting in an increase in intrapericardial pressures.

- Tamponade encompasses a spectrum of conditions, from asymptomatic elevation of intrapericardial pressure to hemodynamic compromise with hypotension and electromechanical dissociation (EMD).
- In some instances, tamponade affects only discrete regions of the heart, from loculated effusion or clot.
- The rate of fluid accumulation has important implications for the developing tamponade.
- Acute tamponade develops after rapid accumulation of pericardial fluid. Only 100–200 mL of fluid is required to increase intrapericardial pressures acutely, owing to the limited distensibility of the pericardium.
- Conversely, the more common chronic tamponade develops after gradual accumulation of pericardial fluid. As much as 1–1.5 L of fluid may accumulate in the slowly distending pericardium before tamponade occurs.
- Gradual accumulation allows the pericardium to stretch and compensate for the increasing volume without increasing pressure.
- Physical examination findings may be less reliable in cases of chronic tamponade.

Systems Affected

- Cardiovascular

ETIOLOGY

Incidence/Prevalence

- Unknown

CAUSES

- When intrapericardial pressure exceeds right ventricular (RV) pressure, RV dysfunction ensues.
- With decreased RV output, left ventricular (LV) output decreases, resulting in systemic hypotension.
- The most common causes of tamponade include trauma, malignancy, uremia, postcardiac surgery, and idiopathic causes.
- Other less common causes include viral syndrome, lupus, rheumatoid arthritis, radiation injury, myocardial infarction, iatrogenic causes (e.g., cardiac catheterization, pacemaker placement), aortic dissection, and infection (e.g., sepsis, tuberculosis, fungus).
- Rarely, tamponade from pneumopericardium may occur after barotrauma from mechanical ventilation.

RISK FACTORS

- Conditions that would predispose to the above, including renal failure, a history of chest/mediastinal radiotherapy, coagulopathy, etc.

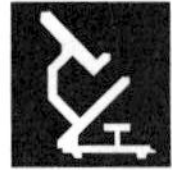

Diagnosis

DIFFERENTIAL DIAGNOSIS

- Pericardial tamponade should be considered when hypotension is present and accompanied by the above risk factors.
- Other more common causes of hypotension must be considered: hypovolemia/hemorrhage, sepsis, tension pneumothorax, massive pulmonary embolus, arrhythmia, myocardial infarction, congestive heart failure or cardiomyopathy, aortic dissection, constrictive pericarditis, etc.

SIGNS AND SYMPTOMS

- Presentation varies, usually with nonspecific symptoms including dyspnea, fatigue, chest pain, syncope, hypotension, and shock.
- In severe cases, EMD can occur. On physical examination:
  - —Tachycardia
  - —Tachypnea
  - —Clear lungs on auscultation
  - —Pulsus paradoxus is a greater than normal decrease in systolic blood pressure with inspiration. It is measured as the difference between the first Korotkoff sound heard intermittently (only at end expiration) and the first Korotkoff sound heard regularly (throughout the respiratory cycle). A difference of >10 mm Hg is abnormal. This finding is nonspecific for tamponade.
  - —Beck's triad consists of (a) decreased arterial pressure, (b) increased central venous pressure, and (c) quiet heart on examination. It is a rare finding, especially in the medical patient with insidious onset of tamponade.
  - —Kussmaul's sign is the absence of the normally expected decrease, or even a paradoxical increase, in central venous pressure with inspiration.
  - —Pericardial friction rub, fever, etc., accompanying the underlying condition leading to tamponade

LABORATORY PROCEDURES

N/A

SPECIAL TESTS

- ECG findings may include:
  - —Diffuse low voltage, most helpful when a decrease in voltage is observed on serial tracings
  - —PR or ST-segment changes consistent with pericarditis
  - —Nonspecific ST-segment or T-wave changes
  - —Electrical alternans is periodic variation of the amplitude of the P-QRS complex—rare, but highly specific. Involvement of the QRS complex alone is less specific.

IMAGING STUDIES

- Chest x-ray: a globular heart or rapid changes in the cardiac silhouette on serial radiographs may be seen. However, findings are nonspecific, and usually not helpful.
- Transthoracic echocardiography is the most sensitive and specific noninvasive diagnostic test. Characteristic findings by two-dimensional and Doppler studies include:
  - —RV collapse in early diastole
  - —Right atrial collapse in late diastole
  - —Reciprocal respiratory variation in RV and LV diastolic dimension
  - —Inferior vena cava plethora with a decrease in the usually observed inspiratory collapse
  - —Swinging heart (in the pericardial fluid)
  - —Decreased LV filling with inspiration, with increased filling with expiration; reciprocal changes observed for the RV
- Echocardiographic changes may appear before symptoms.
- Transesophageal echocardiography may be helpful in locating loculated effusions or clots that are difficult to visualize by transthoracic examination.

DIAGNOSTIC PROCEDURES

Pulmonary artery catheter monitoring: Equalization of pressures may be observed between the pulmonary arterial diastolic pressure and central venous pressure.

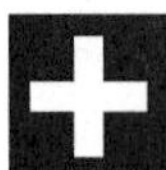

Treatment

GENERAL MEASURES

- Rapid infusion of intravenous fluid may be used for temporary hemodynamic support in preparation for pericardiocentesis.
- Acute tamponade is more likely to respond to intravenous fluid therapy than chronic tamponade.
- Vasoactive agents are of unproven benefit and should be considered only as a bridge to definitive treatment by drainage.

SURGICAL MEASURES

Percutaneous Techniques

- Needle pericardiocentesis
  —Emergent percutaneous drainage of pericardial fluid to relieve intrapericardial pressure
  —Pericardiocentesis should be performed by a skilled and experienced physician.
  —After administration of local anesthesia, a large-bore needle is inserted in the skin via a fifth intercostal or subxiphoid approach and advanced into the pericardial space.
  —ECG monitoring and full resuscitative equipment are essential, and single-lead ECG monitoring of the advancing needle may be helpful in avoiding the myocardium.
  —If possible, pericardial fluid may be located echocardiographically prior to needle insertion.
  —Care must be taken not to injure the myocardium or epicardial coronary arteries.
  —Pericardiocentesis may be followed by placement of an indwelling catheter and closed drainage.
  —Continuous drainage is preferred because pericardial effusions may reaccumulate after initial needle drainage.
- Balloon pericardiotomy
  —A balloon is advanced into the pericardium.
  —Dilation of the balloon creates a potential pathway for drainage of pericardial fluid into the pleural space, without the use of catheter drainage.
  —Complications include pneumothorax and the need for thoracentesis or chest tube.

Invasive Techniques

- Pericardiotomy (pericardial window)
  —The preferred method of drainage if circumstances allow and wider pericardial excision is not required
  —The pericardium is approached via a xiphisternal or subxiphoid incision. The pericardium is opened and allowed to drain via a small chest tube.
  —This method has the advantage of pericardial biopsy for diagnosis, as well as improved clearance of thicker pericardial fluids (e.g., fibrinous debris or clot).
  —Drainage into the peritoneum is an alternative to tube drainage.
- Pericardiectomy
  —Indicated when more extensive removal of the pericardium is required
  —Under these circumstances, thoracotomy or median sternotomy approaches are used.

ADMISSION/DISCHARGE CRITERIA

- Asymptomatic pericardial effusion requires semiurgent evaluation.
- Hemodynamic instability necessitates immediate treatment by evacuation of the pericardial fluid.

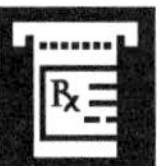

Medications

DRUG(S) OF CHOICE

Medical treatment is indicated only for the prevention of recurrent pericardial effusion and may preclude pericardiectomy. Appropriate consultation should be obtained before their use.

- Intrapericardial steroids: for hemodialysis patients and tamponade due to uremic pericarditis
- Intrapericardial tetracycline or chemotherapeutic agents: for malignant pericardial effusions
- Systemic chemotherapy
  —In small studies and meta-analyses, systemic chemotherapy for prevention of malignant effusions appears superior to pericardiocentesis alone.
  —It does not, however, approach the efficacy of intrapericardial or surgical treatment.

Precautions

Instillation of these agents may cause atrial arrhythmias and ventricular ectopy. Furthermore, tetracycline and chemotherapeutic agents act as sclerosing agents, which may cause pericardial constriction.

Follow-up

PATIENT MONITORING

Follow closely for signs or symptoms of reaccumulation of pericardial fluid.

Prevention/Avoidance

- Treatment and control of the underlying cause

Possible Complications

Inflammation of the pericardium, particularly in infection, may lead to scarring and ultimately pericardial constriction.

EXPECTED COURSE AND PROGNOSIS

- Variable, depending on the underlying cause and its reversibility
- Development of constrictive pericarditis may lead to impaired cardiac function.

PATIENT EDUCATION

Oranizations

- American Heart Association National Center, 7272 Greenville Avenue, Dallas, TX 75231; 1-800-AHA-USA1; http://www.americanheart.org/
- National Heart Lung and Blood Institute; http://www.nhlbi.nih.gov

Activity

- As clinically tolerated

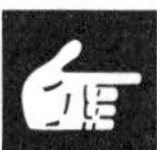

Miscellaneous

ICD-9-CM

423.9 Cardiac tamponade

See also: Pericarditis, constrictive; Pericardial effusion; Ventricular rupture; electromechanical dissociation

BIBLIOGRAPHY

Ameli S, Shah PK. Cardiac tamponade. Pathophysiology, diagnosis, and management. *Cardiol Clin* 1991;9:665–674.

Cummins RO, ed. *Advanced cardiac life support.* Dallas: American Heart Association, 1997.

Moores DWO, Dziuban SW Jr. Pericardial drainage procedures. *Chest Surg Clin North Am* 1995;5:359–373.

Tsang TSM, et al. Diagnosis and management of cardiac tamponade in the era of echocardiography. *Clin Cardiol* 1999;22:446–452.

Vaitkus PT, et al. Treatment of malignant pericardial effusion. *JAMA* 1994;272:59–64.

Author: James A. Kong

Pericarditis, Acute

Basics

DEFINITION

Acute pericarditis is inflammation of the pericardium lasting several days to 4–6 weeks. It is characterized by chest pain, pericardial friction rub, serial ECG changes, and pericardial effusion. It is the most common pathologic process involving the pericardium.

ETIOLOGY

- Idiopathic
- Viral infection (coxsackie A and B virus, echovirus, adenovirus, mumps, influenza, herpes simplex, HIV)
- Uremia
- Tuberculosis
- Postmyocardial infarction (acute fibrinous pericarditis, Dressler's syndrome)
- Postpericardiotomy associated with cardiac surgery
- Neoplasm (carcinoma of lung/breast, lymphoma, melanoma, or acute leukemia)
- Acute bacterial infection (*Streptococcus pneumoniae, Staphylococcus, Neisseria, Legionella, Mycoplasma,* Lyme disease)
- Fungal infection (histoplasmosis, coccidioidomycosis)
- Aortic dissection
- Collagen vascular disease (systemic lupus erythematosus, rheumatoid arthritis, scleroderma, polyarteritis nodosa)
- Drug-induced (procainamide, hydralyzine, isoniazid, minoxidil, methylsergide, phenytoin, anthracyclines, beta-lactam antibiotics)
- Radiation
- Hypothyroidism
- Pulmonary embolism
- Trauma

EPIDEMIOLOGY

Incidence

- 1/1000 hospital admissions and 2–5% autopsy series.
- Coincident chest pain and fever frequently occurring 1–2 weeks after a presumed viral respiratory illness.
- Acute pericarditis frequently occurs after injury to the myocardium or pericardium as seen following cardiac surgery (postpericardiotomy syndrome), trauma, or myocardial infarction (Dressler's syndrome).
- Chest pain typically 1-6 weeks following cardiac injury; some episodes may occur months/years later.

Predominant Age

- Occurs at all ages; most frequent in young adults

Predominant Sex

- Males affected more than females

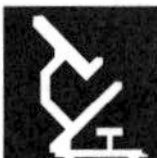

Diagnosis

DIFFERENTIAL DIAGNOSIS

- Acute myocardial infarction
- Myocarditis
- Early repolarization

SIGNS AND SYMPTOMS

- Chest pain/discomfort is typically sharp and localized to the retrosternal or left precordial region with radiation to the back, trapezius ridge, neck, or epigastrium. It is frequently aggravated by inspiration, movement, swallowing or lying supine, with pain relief or improvement upon sitting up or leaning forward. Pain is often absent in slowly developing tuberculous, postirradiation, and neoplastic or uremic pericarditis.
- Fever
- Dyspnea/orthopnea
- Fatigue/weakness
- Near syncope

PHYSICAL EXAMINATION

Pericardial Friction Rub

- High-pitched scratching or creaking sound pathognomonic of acute pericarditis
- Best heard at left sternal border with patient leaning forward using stethoscope diaphragm
- One to three components per cardiac cycle (ventricular systole, atrial systole, early ventricular filling)
- Frequently missed due to changing location and quality
- Most often confused with systolic murmurs of mitral or tricuspid regurgitation
- Correlates poorly with presence and size of pericardial effusion

Cardiac Tamponade

- Accompanies 10%–15% of patients with acute pericarditis
- Classic diagnostic quartet is tachycardia, hypotension, jugular vein distension, and pulsus paradoxus.
- Pulsus paradoxus is augmented decrease (>10–12 mm Hg) in systolic pressure with inspiration.

ECG Features

- Abnormal in ≥90% of cases of acute pericarditis
    - —Stage 1: Diffuse concave-upward ST-segment elevation involving multiple coronary artery territories with associated PR segment depression (80%), and absence of pathologic Q waves or reciprocal ST-segment depression
    - —Stage 2: ST junction returns to baseline accompanied by T-wave flattening
    - —Stage 3: Diffuse T-wave inversion observed during recovery period
    - —Stage 4: Return of T waves to normal
- Other ECG clues of acute pericarditis or large pericardial effusion
    - —Low QRS voltage
    - —Electrical alternans (<10% acute pericarditis) is regular alteration in the amplitude or configuration of ECG complexes seen with large effusions.
    - —Associated atrial arrhythmias or atrial premature beats

LABORATORY PROCEDURES

- Elevated erythrocyte sedimentation rate
- Moderate granulocytosis or lymphocytosis
- Moderate elevations of creatine phosphokinase (CK), creatine phosphokinase MB isoform (CK-MB), or cardiac troponin T or troponin I may occur and reflect accompanying epimyocarditis.
- Other helpful laboratory studies: tuberculin skin test, blood cultures, viral cultures, blood urea nitrogencreatinine, HIV test, viral cultures, thyroid studies, antinuclear antibody titer, rheumatoid factor, cold agglutinins, and fungal serologies

IMAGING STUDIES

- Little diagnostic value in uncomplicated acute pericarditis
- Enlargement of the cardiac silhouette with occasional "water-bottle" configuration seen with moderate/large effusions
- May demonstrate underlying cause or associated pleural effusion (usually left-sided)
- CT/MRI may confirm pericardial effusion or pericardial thickening and exclude aortic dissection

Echocardiography

- Absence of pericardial fluid does not exclude acute pericarditis.
- Capable of detecting, localizing, and estimating size of pericardial effusion and guiding pericardiocentesis
- Pericardial fluid depicted as echo-free space surrounding heart chambers
- May demonstrate right atrial/right ventricular diastolic collapse or exaggerated inspiratory tricuspid/pulmonic flow with reciprocal mitral flow supporting cardiac tamponade

Pericardiocentesis and Pericardial Biopsy

- Recommended in cases of cardiac tamponade or to exclude suspected purulent pericarditis

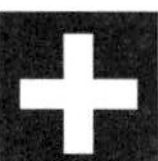

Treatment

GENERAL MEASURES

- Rest, avoidance of vigorous activity, and nonsteroidal antiinflammatory drugs are mainstays.
- Bed rest until chest pain and fever have diminished; frequent observation with vital sign monitoring and repeat echocardiography if a moderate-large effusion is present
- Avoidance of anticoagulation recommended to decrease risk of cardiac tamponade
- If anticoagulation is mandatory (mechanical heart valves), i.v. heparin preferred over oral anticoagulation
- Hospitalization recommended in following cases:
  —Rule out acute myocardial infarction
  —Exclude pyogenic process
  —Exclude and observe for cardiac tamponade and hemodynamic compromise
  —Parenteral analgesia for relief of refractory chest pain

SURGICAL MEASURES

- Pericardiocentesis
  —Increased jugular venous pressure, tachycardia, hypotension, and pulsus paradoxus generally signal cardiac tamponade and need for emergent pericardiocentesis.
  —Intravenous fluids and inotropic drugs may temporarily provide hemodynamic support prior to pericardiocentesis.
- Surgical subxiphoid pericardiotomy (pericardial window) or transthoracic endoscopic pericardiotomy
  —Limited palliative procedure for patients with poor prognosis
  —Operative mortality = 10%.
  —Procedure of choice for patients with expected long-term survival or loculated pericardial effusions
- Percutaneous balloon pericardiotomy
  —Palliative option for large pericardial effusions/tamponade
  —Echo or fluoroscopic guided insertion of dilating balloon into pericardial sac, creating tear in pericardium

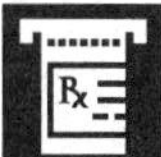

Medications

DRUG(S) OF CHOICE

- Aspirin (650 mg orally every 4 hours) or indomethacin (25–75 mg orally every 6–8 hours) for analgesia and antiinflammatory effect
- Morphine or meperidine (orally/i.v./i.m.) may be required for supplemental pain relief.
- Consider oral steroid (prednisone 40–80 mg/day) if chest pain persists beyond 48 hours. Steroid dose may be tapered after 5–7 days and discontinued after 3–6 weeks.

Chronic/Recurrent Pericarditis

- Reinsitute nonsteroidal antiinflammatory agents and/or steroids with more gradual tapering over several months.
- Chronic colchicine (1 mg orally daily) may improve symptoms and prevent recurrence.

Etiology-Specific Therapies

- Infectious (streptococcal/staphylococcal): i.v. beta-lactam with or without aminoglycoside or vancomycin; prompt drainage required if signs of tamponade or continued infection
- Neoplasm: pericardiocentesis as needed; balloon pericardiostomy, sclerotherapy, or limited subxiphoid surgical window performed for palliation
- Uremic: often responds to initiation or intensification of dialysis with surgery reserved for nonresponders or recurrent episodes

Follow-up

EXPECTED COURSE AND PROGNOSIS

- Most episodes are self-limited and resolve within 2–6 weeks.
- Notable complications include recurrent/chronic pericarditis (20%), cardiac tamponade (10%–15%), fibrosis or calcification of pericardium (constrictive pericarditis; 5%), effusive-constrictive pericarditis (5%), and arrhythmias, usually supraventricular tachycardias and premature atrial depolarizations.

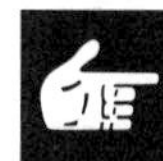

Miscellaneous

BIBLIOGRAPHY

Chou T. Pericarditis. In: *Electrocardiograpy in clinical practice,* 3rd ed. Philadelphia: WB Saunders, 1991:219–234.

Lorell BH. Pericardial diseases. In: Braunwald E, ed. *Heart disease: a textbook of cardiovascular medicine,* 5th ed. Philadelphia: WB Saunders, 1997:1478–1495.

Marriott HJ. Pericardial disease. In: *Bedside cardiac diagnosis.* Philadelphia: JB Lippincott, 1993:241–246.

Permanyer-Miralda G, Sagrista-Sauleda J, Soler-Soler J. Primary acute pericardial disease: a prospective series of 231 consecutive patients. *Am J Cardiol* 1985;56:623.

Spodick DH. The normal and diseased pericardium: current concepts of pericardial physiology, diagnosis, and treatment. *J Am Coll Cardiol* 1983;1:240–251.

Author: Michael P. Hudson

Pericarditis, Constrictive

Basics

DESCRIPTION

In constrictive pericarditis, a thick, inelastic pericardium encases the heart and restricts diastolic filling, leading to biventricular (RV > LV) diastolic dysfunction, venous engorgement, and diminished cardiac output. Ventricular filling is unimpeded during early diastole but is reduced abruptly by noncompliant pericardium at the end of the first third of diastole. It is typically an indolent, progressive process with symptoms appearing months to years after an acute pericarditis episode or pericardial trauma/surgery.

Effusive-Constrictive Pericarditis

- Accumulation of tense pericardial effusion plus thickened, fibrotic pericardium
- Hemodynamic features of tamponade before pericardiocentesis, and constriction afterward
- Diagnosis made by hemodynamic recordings before and after pericardiocentesis with continued elevation of right atrial/central venous pressures after removal of pericardial fluid
- Definitive treatment is complete pericardiectomy

EPIDEMIOLOGY

- 3:1 incidence men over women; wide age range (8–80 years)

ETIOLOGY

- Idiopathic/Unknown (40%)
- Tuberculosis (10%)
- Postcardiac surgery (5%–10%; incidence after coronary artery bypass grafting 0.3%)
- Postirradiation (5%)
- Other postinfectious pericarditis (postviral, bacterial/purulent, fungal/histoplasmosis)
- Collagen vascular disease (systemic lupus erythematosus, RA [rheumatoid arthritis])
- Drug-induced (procainamide, methylsergide, hydralyzine)
- Neoplasm
- Trauma (after pacemaker implantation)
- Uremic
- Asbestosis

CLINICAL MANIFESTATIONS

- Dyspnea/orthopnea/cough (78%)
- Abdominal distention/swelling (68%)
- Lower extremity edema (54%)
- Severe weakness and fatigue (25%)
- Weight loss/anorexia
- Chest pain (24%)
- Fever/nightsweats

Diagnosis

DIFFERENTIAL DIAGNOSIS

- Every patient with ascites, liver enlargement, and raised jugular venous pressure should be thoroughly investigated for constrictive pericarditis.
- Restrictive cardiomyopathy
- Biventricular congestive heart failure
- Hepatic cirrhosis
- Cor pulmonale
- Tricuspid valve stenosis or regurgitation
- Nephrotic syndrome

SIGNS AND SYMPTOMS

- Elevated jugular venous pressure with prominent X and Y venous descents (M- or W-shaped contour)
- Sinus tachycardia with normal or low-normal blood pressure
- Nonpalpable cardiac apical impulse
- Early diastolic pericardial knock with absence of S_3 and regurgitant murmurs
- Kussmaul's sign (jugular venous pressure fails to decrease with inspiration)
- Hepatosplenomegaly (>70%)
- Ascites: often more prominent than lower extremity edema
- Lower extremity edema
- Pulsus paradoxus (uncommon, fewer than one-third of cases)
- Peripheral cyanosis
- Muscle wasting/cachexia, particularly of upper extremities

LABORATORY PROCEDURES

- Generally nondiagnostic; erythrocyte sedimentation rate may be elevated; hypoalbuminemia and abnormal hepatocellular function tests

IMAGING STUDIES

Plain-film Chest Radiography

- Generally shows normal/small heart size and clear lung fields
- Calcification of pericardium in 40%–50% of cases
- Best seen on lateral view
- Calcification predominantly over right atrium/ventricle and in the atrioventricular grooves
- Prominent right superior mediastinum
- Left atrial enlargement

CT/MRI

- More accurate and useful than echocardiography or chest radiography for detecting thickened pericardium
- Abnormal pericardial thickness (>3 mm) on thoracic CT or MRI and characteristic hemodynamic changes usually confirm diagnosis.

Echocardiography

- Not reliable for detecting a thickened pericardium or excluding diagnosis
- Small ventricles, dilated atria, and thick pericardium
- Parallel motion of epicardium and parietal pericardium separated by 1-mm thick echo-free space strongly suggests thickened pericardium (M mode).
- Numerous suggestive echo findings may be present: dilated inferior vena cava/hepatic vein without respiratory variation, abrupt posterior motion of interventricular septum in early diastole (septal bounce), left ventricular (LV) posterior wall flattening, premature opening of pulmonary valve, and marked respiratory variation in diastolic atrioventricular flow velocities (>25% inspiratory decrease in mitral flow velocity)

SPECIAL TESTS

- Occult constrictive pericardial disease: diagnosed when the hemodynamic findings of constriction appear after rapid infusion of 1–2 L saline over 5–10 minutes
- Endomyocardial Biopsy: Rarely required; may be needed to exclude infiltrative/restrictive myocardial disease causing restrictive cardiomyopathy

ECG Findings

- Generally nonspecific: normal ECG rarely observed; low QRS voltage; notched P wave (P-mitrale); nondiagnostic ST-T wave abnormalities; atrial fibrillation or flutter

Catheterization Findings

- Elevation and equalization of pressures: <5 mm Hg difference between mean right atrial pressure, right ventricular diastolic pressure, and pulmonary capillary wedge pressure
- Prominent X and Y descents on the right atrial and pulmonary artery wedge pressure tracings (M or W configuration)
- Prominent early left/right ventricular diastolic filling pattern with "dip-and plateau" waveform ("square-root" sign)
- Lack of inspiratory decrease in right atrial pressure
- Modestly elevated right ventricular/pulmonary artery systolic pressure generally <60 mm Hg
- Right ventricular end-diastolic pressure >1/3 × right ventricular systolic pressure

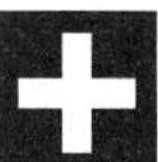

Treatment

GENERAL MEASURES

Progressive symptoms require confirmatory CT/MRI demonstrating pericardial thickening, right and left cardiac catheterization documenting constrictive physiology, and curative surgical pericardectomy.

SURGICAL MEASURES

- Surgical pericardial resection is definitive therapy with 5-year survival = 80%
- Most strongly indicated in NYHA functional class II–III
- Operative mortality = 3%–15%
- More extensive calcification, worse functional class (NYHA class IV), LV systolic dysfunction, history of neoplasm, renal insufficiency, and previous pericardial procedure predict poor postoperative survival
- Hemodynamic and symptomatic improvement usually rapid and progressive over several months, with 80%–90% survivors achieving NYHA I/II functional class

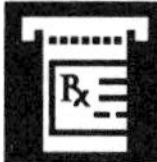

Medications

DRUG(S) OF CHOICE

- Mild symptoms are generally responsive to sodium restriction and diuretic therapy.
- Drugs that slow heart rate may be poorly tolerated.

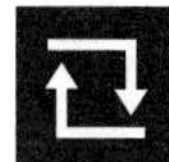

Follow-up

PATIENT MONITORING

- Progressive disease with minority of patients surviving 5 years without surgical repair

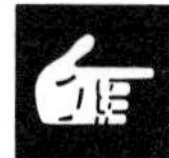

Miscellaneous

BIBLIOGRAPHY

Chou T. Pericarditis. In: *Electrocardiography in clinical practice,* 3rd ed. Philadelphia: WB Saunders, 1991:219–234.

Lorell BH. Pericardial diseases. In: Braunwald E, ed. *Heart disease: a textbook of cardiovascular medicine,* 5th ed. Philadelphia: WB Saunders, 1997:1496–1505.

Marriott HJ. Pericardial disease. In: *Bedside cardiac diagnosis.* Philadelphia: JB Lippincott, 1993:241–246.

Mehta A, Mehta M, Jain A. Constrictive pericarditis. *Clin Cardiol* 1999;22:334–344.

Vaitkus PT, Kussmaul WG. Constrictive versus restrictive cardiomyopathy: a reappraisal and update of diagnostic criteria. *Am Heart J* 1991; 122:1431.

Author: Michael P. Hudson

Pheochromocytoma

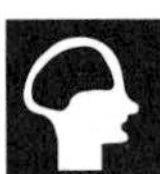

Basics

DESCRIPTION

Pheochromocytoma is a catecholamine-producing tumor that arises from chromaffin cells of neural crest origin.

- The majority occur in the adrenal glands.
- 10% are bilateral.
- 10% are extraadrenal.
- 10% are malignant.

EPIDEMIOLOGY

Incidence/Prevalence

- Occurs in approximately 0.1% of patients with hypertension in the United States

Predominant Age

- None

Predominant Sex

- Slightly more common in females than in males

Predominant Race

- None

ETIOLOGY

- Vast majority occur sporadically.
- Approximately 10% are inherited, usually in an autosomal-dominant pattern, often as part of a multiglandular neoplastic syndrome.
- When it occurs as part of multiple endocrine neoplasia (MEN) IIA, it is due to a genetic abnormality on chromosome 10.

RISK FACTORS

N/A

PREGNANCY

- Maternal and fetal mortality rates are high if maternal pheochromocytoma is not diagnosed antenatally.
- Once diagnosis has been made, the patient should be treated with phenoxybenzamine.
- First or second trimester: tumor should be excised as soon as patient has been adequately prepared with alpha-adrenergic blockers.
- Third trimester: patient should be treated with alpha-blockers until the fetus reaches viability, at which time the baby should be delivered by cesarian section. The tumor may be removed in the same operation.
- Vaginal delivery is extremely dangerous.
- Magnesium sulfate may be used to control hypertensive emergencies during labor and during resection of the tumor in a pregnant patient.

ASSOCIATED CONDITIONS

- MEN IIA (Sipple's syndrome): pheochromocytoma, medullary carcinoma of the thyroid, and hyperparathyroidism
- MEN IIB or MEN III syndromes: pheochromocytoma, medullary carcinoma of the thyroid, mucosal neuromas, ganglioneuromatosis, marfanoid habitus, and other connective tissue disorders
- Neurofibromatosis (von Recklinghausen's disease): Approximately 1% have pheochromocytoma; central or peripheral neurofibromas and café au lait spots are characteristic.
- Cerebelloretinal hemangioblastomatosis (von Hippel-Lindau syndrome): Pheochromocytoma occurs in 10%; retinal angiomas, cerebellar and spinal cord hemangioblastomas, renal cell carcinoma, and pancreatic or renal cysts also may occur.
- Carney's triad (rare): extraadrenal pheochromocytoma, gastric leiomyosarcoma, and pulmonary chondroma

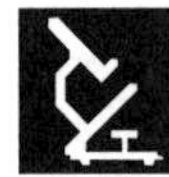

Diagnosis

DIFFERENTIAL DIAGNOSIS

- Hyperadrenergic essential hypertension
- Panic attacks
- Thyrotoxicosis
- Drug-induced states (e.g., amphetamines, cocaine)
- Migraine or cluster headaches
- Abrupt clonidine withdrawal
- Alcoholism
- Ingestion of tyramine-containing foods while taking monoamine oxidase inhibitors
- Hypoglycemia
- Paroxysmal tachycardias
- Acute myocardial infarction or angina pectoris
- Brain tumor or subarachnoid hemorrhage
- Aortic dissection
- Cardiovascular deconditioning
- Menopausal syndrome
- Neuroblastoma in a child
- Diencephalic or temporal lobe seizures
- Toxemia of pregnancy

SIGNS AND SYMPTOMS

Signs

- Hypertension: the major cardiovascular manifestation of pheochromocytoma.
  —Intermittent or sustained; spontaneous or provoked by acute physical stress
  —Classically labile, paroxysmal, and poorly responsive to standard antihypertensive drugs
  —May manifest itself as unusual blood pressure elevations after trauma or surgery
  —Episodes can be precipitated by exercise, palpation of the abdomen, smoking, contrast media, a variety of drugs and hormones, or contrast media.
- Tachycardia or reflex bradycardia
- Orthostatic hypotension
- Congestive heart failure: Up to 50% of patients have pathologic evidence of myocarditis or cardiomyopathy, which may be reversed when the tumor is removed.
- Myocardial ischemia/infarction
- ECG abnormalities/arrhythmias
- Weight loss
- Pallor
- Hypermetabolism
- Fasting hyperglycemia
- Tremor
- Increased respiratory rate
- Decreased gastrointestinal motility
- Psychosis (rare)
- Flushing (rare)

Symptoms

- Sudden "spells" with headache, palpitations, sweating, nervousness, tremulousness, nausea, and vomiting
- Pain in chest/abdomen
- Weakness/fatigue
- Dizziness
- Heat intolerance
- Paresthesias
- Constipation
- Dyspnea
- Visual disturbances
- Seizures

LABORATORY PROCEDURES

- Twenty-four hour urine collection for measurement of unconjugated catecholamines (epinephrine and norephinephrine) or their metabolites [metanephrines and vanillylmandelic acid (VMA)]
  —Must be collected when the patient is obviously hypertensive
  —Many drugs alter urinary levels of catecholamines, metanephrines, and VMA, so the patient should be off all medications if possible (including antihypertensive medications).
  —Measurement of plasma catecholamines

IMAGING STUDIES

- Once the diagnosis of pheochromocytoma has been made with biochemical tests, an imaging study should be performed to localize the tumor.
- CT of the adrenals
  —Provides precise anatomic information and can detect tumors larger than 0.5 cm in diameter.
  —Safe, easy, widely available, relatively inexpensive
- MRI of the adrenals
  —Provides anatomic information
  —Provides some histologically specific information about the tumor
- ^{131}I-metaiodobenzylguanidine scan
  —Uses a radioisotope that localize in chromaffin tissue
  —Useful in localizing extraadrenal or other difficult-to-find pheochromocytomas
- Arteriography
  —Rarely indicated
  —May precipitate a hypertensive crisis

SPECIAL TESTS

- Clonidine suppression test
  —Clonidine administration normally results in lower levels of plasma cataecholamines. In

patients with pheochromocytoma, plasma catecholamine levels are not under normal physiologic control and remain the same or increase after administration of clonidine.
—Test is useful only if basal plasma catecholamine levels are abnormally elevated.

- Provocative test with glucagon
  —Blood is drawn for plasma catecholamines before and 2 minutes after the intravenous administration of glucagon (1.0 mg as a bolus).
  —Blood pressure and heart rate should be closely monitored, and phentolamine must always be readily available for the treatment of any episodes of severe hypertension.
- Measurement of plasma concentration of chromogranin A
  —Elevated in patients with pheochromocytoma
- Vena caval sampling for catecholamines
  —Rarely indicated
  —Occasionally used when tumors cannot be located with other techniques
- Measurement of plasma concentration of neuron-specific enolase: may be useful in differentiating benign from malignant pheochromocytoma
- ECG
  —Abnormal in up to 75% of patients
  —Abnormalities include T-wave inversion, left ventricular hypertrophy, short P-R interval with narrow QRS complex, supraventricular arrhythmias, ST segment elevation or depression
- Echocardiogram
  —Left ventricular hypertrophy
  —During a hypertensive crisis, may show systolic anterior motion of anterior mitral valve leaflet, paradoxical septal motion, and proximal excursion of the posterior wall

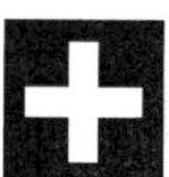

Treatment

GENERAL MEASURES

- A team consisting of an internist, anesthesiologist, and surgeon should work together to adequately prepare and follow the patient.
- Because the patients are hypovolemic, sodium intake must be adequate to prevent profound postural hypotension upon initiation of medical therapy and postoperatively; this may require intravenous infusion of saline.
- A beta-blocker should never be used prior to adequate alpha-receptor blockade, because severe hypertension may occur secondary to unopposed alpha-adrenergic receptor stimulation by circulating catecholamines.

SURGICAL MEASURES

- Treatment of choice is surgical removal.
- Preparation of the patient should begin at least 7–10 days prior to surgery (see Medications below).
- The operating room should be as calm and quiet as possible.
- An intraarterial line should be placed for continuous blood pressure monitoring.
- Anesthesia should be obtained with halogenated hydrocarbon agents (enflurane or isoflurane), which are unlikely to produce sensitization of the myocardium to catecholamine-induced arrhythmias.
- Management of hypertensive emergencies during surgery may be managed with infusions of either phentolamine or sodium nitroprusside.
- For most abdominal tumors, either a subcostal or a midline incision is adequate.

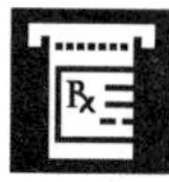

Medications

DRUG(S) OF CHOICE

- Phenoxybenzamine
  —A nonspecific alpha-adrenergic antagonist
  —Should be administered orally beginning at least 7–10 days prior to surgery
  —Initial dose is 10 mg twice daily. Dosage should be increased to an average of 0.5–1.0 mg/kg daily, administered in two divided doses.
- Prazosin, terazosin, doxazosin
  —Specific alpha 1-adrenergic antagonists
  —All have the potential to cause severe postural hypotension, so should be given at bedtime.
- Labetalol
  —alpha- and beta-antagonist
  —Both oral and intravenous formulations are available.
  —Disadvantage is that it has four times more beta-antagonistic activity than alpha-antagonistic activity, so often there is more slowing of the heart rate than control of hypertension.
- Metyrosine
  —Competitive inhibitor of tyrosine hydroxylase, the rate-limiting step in catecholamine biosynthesis.
  —When used in conjunction with alpha-antagonists, it may provide more stable blood pressure control.
  —Inhibits catecholamine synthesis in the brain (as well as in the periphery), often causes sedation, and can cause extrapyramidal signs (rare). Central nervous system toxicity may manifest as vivid or frightening dreams and is reversible.
  —Calcium antagonists
- Various chemotherapeutic combinations with or without radiation therapy have been used to treat malignant pheochromocytoma (after aggressive surgical resection).

ADMISSION/DISCHARGE CRITERIA

- Outpatient management except for complications or surgery

Follow-up

PATIENT MONITORING

- Repeat urine collection for catecholamines, metanephrines, and/or VMA once at least 5–7 days after surgery
- Urine collection and measurements should be made if symptoms reappear, or yearly, if the patient remains asymptomatic, for a total of 5 years.

EXPECTED COURSE AND PROGNOSIS

- Persistence or recurrence after surgery can occur if the tumor was disrupted or incompletely resected, if a second primary was present and not resected, or if metastatic disease was not appreciated.
- Long-term survival of patients after the successful removal of a benign pheochromoctyoma is essentially the same as for age-matched controls.
- Approximately 25% of patients remain hypertensive, but this is usually easily controlled with medication.

PATIENT EDUCATION

Patients should be made aware of symptoms/signs of pheochromocytoma and counseled to notify a physician if these recur after surgical resection.

Organizations

- National Adrenal Diseases Foundation (NADF), 505 Northern Boulevard, Great Neck, NY 11021; (516)487–4992
- American Cancer Society, 1599 Clifton Road NE, Atlanta, GA 30329; (404)320–3333

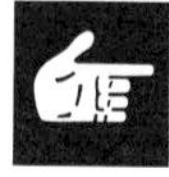

Miscellaneous

ICD-9-CM

255.6

BIBLIOGRAPHY

Kaplan NM. Systemic hypertension: mechanisms and diagnosis. In: Braunwald E, ed. *Heart disease,* 5th ed. Philadelphia: WB Saunders, 1997:829–830.

Keiser HR. Pheochromocytoma and related tumors. In: Degroot LJ, ed. *Endocrinology,* 3rd ed. Philadelphia: WB Saunders, 1995:1853–1877.

Radtke WE, Kazmier FJ, Rutherford BD, et al. Cardiovascular complications of pheochromocytoma crisis. *Am J Cardiol* 1975;35:701–705.

Williams GH, Lilly LS, Seely EW. The heart in endocrine and nutritional disorders. In: Braunwald E, ed. *Heart disease,* 5th ed. Philadelphia: WB Saunders, 1997:1897–1899.

Author: Deborah L. Ekery

Pickwickian Syndrome

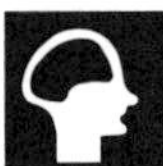

Basics

DESCRIPTION

Pickwickian syndrome is characterized by temporary, recurrent interruptions of respiration during sleep. Typical features include nocturnal wakefulness, daytime sleepiness, and obesity.

Systems Affected

- Cardiovascular and pulmonary

EPIDEMIOLOGY

Incidence/Prevalence

- Approximately 2.5 million people in the United States suffer from sleep apnea.
- The majority of sleep apnea sufferers are at least 20% over ideal body weight.

Predominant Age

- Middle-aged adults

Predominant Sex

Males outnumber premenopausal females 30:1.

ETIOLOGY

- Obesity
- Pharyngeal obstruction

RISK FACTORS

- Moderate to severe obesity
- Male gender
- Narrowed upper airway/short, thick neck
- Enlarged adenoids or tonsils
- Decreased muscle tone of the soft palate, uvula, and pharynx
- Use of sedative or hypnotic agents
- Alcohol consumption

PREGNANCY

Pregnancy is contraindicated in women with severe pulmonary hypertension.

ASSOCIATED CONDITIONS

- Coronary artery disease
- Hyperlipidemia
- Diabetes mellitus
- Hypothyroidism
- Obstructive sleep apnea
- Chronic obstructive pulmonary disease
- Degenerative joint disease

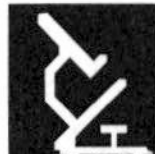

Diagnosis

DIFFERENTIAL DIAGNOSIS

- Chronic mountain sickness
- Central sleep apnea
- Narcolepsy
- Ondine's curse
- Infantile apnea

SIGNS AND SYMPTOMS

- Daytime sleepiness/somnolence
- Loud nocturnal snoring
- Morning headaches
- Extreme obesity
- Hypoventilation
- Muscle twitching
- Cyanosis
- Periodic respiration
- In advanced cases: right ventricular heave, prominent P2 component of the second heart sound, right ventricular failure (elevated jugular venous pressure, hepatomegaly, lower extremity edema)

LABORATORY PROCEDURES

- Arterial blood gas: hypoxia and hypercapnia are common; widened A-a gradient
- Serum bicarbonate: usually elevated
- Complete blood count: polycythemia common

Pathologic Findings

- Extreme obesity primarily involving the trunk and pharyngeal area
- Small pharyngeal cavity due to redundant palatal tissue, fat deposition in the soft tissues of the pharynx, or superficial fat masses in the neck that compress the pharynx
- Palatal soft tissue edema

SPECIAL TESTS

- ECG: may reveal right ventricular hypertrophy denoted by tall, peaked P waves in leads II, aVF, V_1 through V_3, clockwise rotation, right axis deviation, R/S ratio in lead V_1 greater than 1, qR pattern in aVr, inverted T waves in leads V_1 through V_4 and the inferior leads.

IMAGING STUDIES

- Chest x-ray: may demonstrate dilatation of the main pulmonary artery and its branches, underperfusion of the peripheral pulmonary artery branches, and decreased prominence of the aortic knob due to counterclockwise rotation of the heart on a posteroanterior film; filling of the retrosternal space on a lateral film of the chest
- Echocardiography: can confirm cor pumonale and assess pulmonary artery pressures

Diagnostic Procedures

- Polysomnography

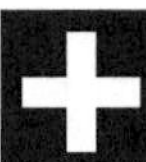

Treatment

GENERAL MEASURES

- Patients with severe hypoxemia, severe hypercapnia, heart failure, syncope, or marked arrhythmias should be hospitalized.
- Weight reduction
- Elevation of the head with pillows or elevation of the head of the bed by 6–8 inches
- Avoid alcohol.
- Avoid sedative and hypnotic agents.

SURGICAL MEASURES

- Uvulo-palato-pharyngoplasty
- Tracheotomy

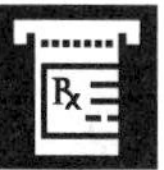

Medications

DRUG(S) OF CHOICE

- Theophylline: in low doses and moderate doses causes mild cortical arousal with increased alertness; lowers vascular resistance
- Protriptyline: mild alerting and improved attention likely due to enhancement of dopamine-mediated processes
- Clomipramine: dimilar to protriptyline
- Pemoline: amphetamine variant that is a central nervous system stimulant; mild alerting, improved attention
- Nicotine: mild alerting action with stimulation of the nicotinic receptors in the brain; large concentrations stimulate the respiratory center
- Progesterone: enhances respiratory drive

Contraindications

Refer to manufacturer's literature.

Precautions

Refer to manufacturer's literature.

Significant Possible Interactions

- Theophylline interacts with a wide variety of medications; refer to manufacturer's literature for specific details.
- Tricyclic agents, when taken in combination with other antidepressants can lead to excessive sedation.
  —There are several documented drug interactions with tricyclic agents; refer to manufacturer's literature for further details.
- Progesterone may increase blood pressure and lower HDL in some patients.
- Drugs that may alter laboratory results
  —Diuretics may lead to contraction alkalosis and elevation of bicarbonate levels; excessive intake of antacids may lead elevated bicarbonate
- Disorders that may alter laboratory results
  —A diffusion defect, a right-to-left shunt (intracardiac or intrapulmonary), or V/Q mismatch can produces a widened A-a gradient.
  —Renal disorders, disorders producing metabolic or respiratory alkalosis, mineralocorticoid excess, and congenital chloridorrhea can lead to elevations in the bicarbonate level.
  —Hemoconcentration, extreme physical exercise, and polycythemia vera lead to an elevated hematocrit.

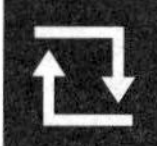

Follow-up

PATIENT MONITORING

- Depends on the frequency and severity of the patient's complaints
- Hospitalization for oxygen therapy, heart failure management, and arrhythmia management may be necessary in extreme cases.

Prevention/Avoidance

- Adherence to a low-fat/low-calorie diet
- Regular aerobic/fat-burning exercise
- Tobacco cessation
- Avoid alcohol consumption.
- Avoid sedatives.

Possible Complications

- Cardiac
  —Systemic hypertension, sinus arrhythmias, extreme bradycardia, sinus arrest, asystole, atrial flutter, atrial fibrillation, ventricular tachycardia, syncope, right ventricular hypertrophy, right heart failure (cor pulmonale), left heart failure
- Respiratory
  —Hypoxemia, hypercarbia, pulmonary hypertension
- Neurologic
  —Morning headaches, excessive daytime sleepiness, slowed mentation, sleepwalking, blackouts, automatic robotlike behavior, bedwetting
- Psychiatric
  —Hallucinations, anxiety, irritability, aggressiveness, jealousy, suspiciousness, irrational behavior, loss of interest in sex
- Hematologic
  —Polycythemia

EXPECTED COURSE AND PROGNOSIS

- Variable, dependent on the degree of obesity, pharyngeal obstruction, pulmonary hypertension, and right ventricular dysfunction
- In cases of overt right ventricular failure with severe pulmonary hypertension, a patient's life expectancy is 6 months to 1 year.

PATIENT EDUCATION

Organizations

- National Organization for Rare Disorders
- American Narcolepsy Association, Inc.
- Narcolepsy and Cataplexy Foundation of America
- Narcolepsy Network
- NIH/National Institute of Neurological Disorders and Stroke

Activity

- As tolerated
- Exercise program after physician's approval

Diet

- Low fat
- Low sodium

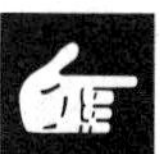

Miscellaneous

ICD-9-CM

278.8

BIBLIOGRAPHY

Braunwald E. *Heart disease: a textbook of cardiovascular medicine,* 5th ed. Philadelphia: WB Saunders, 1997.

Fauci AS, Braunwald E, Isselbacher KJ, et al. *Harrison's principles of internal medicine,* 14th ed. New York: McGraw-Hill, 1998.

Thoene JG. *Physicians guide to rare diseases.* New Jersey: Dowden Publishing, 1992.

Author: Phoebe A. Ashley

Pregnancy and the Heart

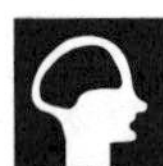

Basics

DESCRIPTION

Maternal blood volume and cardiac output increase up to 50% by 32 weeks of pregnancy and continue at that level until delivery.

- These changes put unique stress on the patient with underlying heart disease and may contribute to the development of certain heart diseases (peripartum cardiomyopathy).
- There are three general patient presentations
  - —Uncorrected congenital heart disease, which can be divided into:
    - Predominant volume loads such as atrial septal defects, patent ductus arteriosus
    - Pressure loads such as pulmonic valve stenosis, coarctation of the aorta, aortic valve disease
    - Complex often cyanotic congenital heart disease such as tetralogy of Fallot
  - —Acquired heart disease
    - Most common are rheumatic heart disease, coronary heart disease, and peripartum cardiomyopathy.
  - —Corrected congenital or acquired heart disease
    - Common issues here are the patient with a prosthetic valve or partially corrected defects.

Systems Affected

Cardiovascular, pulmonary

ETIOLOGY

Genetics

Women with congenital heart disease have an increased risk of having children with congenital heart disease.

Incidence/Prevalence

Maternal heart disease occurs in 1%–4% of pregnancies.

Predominant Age

- Young adults

Predominant Sex

- Female
- Prognosis worsens with heart disease and advancing age of the mother.

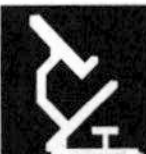

Diagnosis

DIFFERENTIAL DIAGNOSIS

- Heart disease versus normal hemodynamic changes of pregnancy

SIGNS AND SYMPTOMS

- Clinical presentation of pregnancy complicated by heart disease depends on the underlying disease, its severity, and the stage of pregnancy.
- Fatigue and dyspnea, common symptoms of heart disease, are common with normal pregnancies.
- Chest pain from gastroesophageal reflux must be distinguished from angina.
- Palpitations are common during pregnancy (often sinus tachycardia).
- Fever and night sweats are common during normal pregnancy.
- Alterations in the cardiovascular physical examination due to the normal hemodynamic changes of pregnancy must be distinguished from pathologic changes due to heart disease.
- Normal pregnancy may be associated with:
  - —Heart rate in the upper range of normal
  - —Systolic blood pressure increases as pregnancy progresses to levels largely determined by the patient's age and parity (increases with both).
  - —Higher values for blood pressure are recorded upright or in the left lateral position and the lowest levels in the supine position when the gravid uterus compresses the inferior vena cava and reduces venous return to the heart.
  - —An enlarged apical impulse and third heart sound are often present.
  - —The first and second heart sounds are often loud and exhibit increased splitting. Fourth heart sounds are rare and suggest the presence of heart disease.
  - —Systolic heart murmurs are common in pregnancy and result from the increased stroke volume and hyperkinetic state of pregnancy.
  - —A continuous murmur may be heard due to increased blood flow to the breasts (mammary souffle), and venous hums heard in the aortic area may mimic aortic regurgitation.
  - —True diastolic murmurs are rare in pregnancy and suggest heart disease.

Pathologic Findings

- Depend on specific heart disease

IMAGING STUDIES

- Use of chest x-rays is of limited value in pregnancy because of the potential hazards of exposing the fetus to radiation.
- Cardiac silhouette is altered by the elevation of the diaphragm, making specific chamber enlargement difficult to diagnose accurately.
- Echocardiography is the diagnostic test of choice.

Diagnostic Procedures

- ECG can be very useful, but a leftward shift in the axis and ST-T wave changes can occur normally in pregnancy.
- Pulmonary artery catheterization can be performed with a flow-directed catheter without the use of fluoroscopy
- Left heart catheterization can be performed with abdominal shielding and use of a brachial approach to minimize exposure of the fetus to radiation, but should only be performed if the diagnostic information cannot be obtained by other less invasive methods.

SPECIAL TESTS

Confirmation of pregnancy

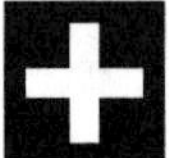

Treatment

GENERAL MEASURES

- Outpatient evaluation and treatment unless the fetus or the mother's life is threatened
- Prompt treatment of infections
- Prevention and treatment of anemia with iron supplements
- Vaginal delivery is generally preferred with pain control to avoid tachycardia and hemodynamic monitoring in selected patients to guide therapy during delivery

SURGICAL MEASURES

- When decompensation threatens the mother's life and aggressive pharmacologic therapy is insufficient, surgical correction of any correctable lesions should be considered.
- Risk to the mother is not particularly higher when pregnant, but fetal loss is not uncommon.
- In the case of mitral stenosis, percutaneous balloon valvotomy may be accomplished with less risk to the fetus.
- Cesarian section should be reserved for obstetrical reasons because it puts more stress on the heart.

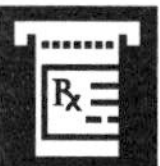

Medications

DRUG(S) OF CHOICE

- For heart failure
  —Digoxin is safe, but blood levels need to be monitored.
  —Furosemide or other diuretics are safe, but potassium levels need to be monitored.
  —Hydralazine is safe in those patients who do not respond to digoxin and diuretics.
- For arrhythmias
  —Digoxin is useful for controlling the heart rate in supraventricular arrhythmias.
  —Beta-blockers can be added if digoxin does not control the heart rate.
  —Verapamil is relatively safe unless heart failure is present.
  —Quinidine is safe in therapeutic doses but can cause abortion at toxic doses.
  —Procainamide is relatively safe.
  —Lidocaine for ventricular tachyarrhythmias is relatively safe.
- For anticoagulation
  —Heparin is preferred because it is not teratogenic but there is risk of hemorrhage.

Contraindications

Angiotensin-converting enzyme inhibitors increase the incidence of stillbirths and should be avoided. Amiodarone causes fetal hypothyroidism and premature births. Warfarin causes birth defects and fetal death, especially if used in the first trimester.

Precautions

See manufacturer's literature on each product.

Significant Possible Interactions

Digoxin levels can be increased by concomitant use of calcium channel blockers or quinidine. Many drugs increase warfarin levels.

ALTERNATIVE DRUGS

Newer drugs such as angiotensin receptor blockers, type I-C and III antiarrhythmic drugs, and low-molecular-weight heparin have not been used extensively in pregnancy, but may be of use in selected patients.

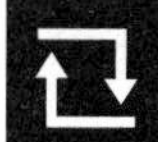

Follow-up

PATIENT MONITORING

Pregnant patients with heart disease need frequent visits with the obstetrician and cardiologist, and coordination of delivery plans with an anesthesiologist.

Prevention/Avoidance

- Fluid retention, excessive weight gain, and infections should be avoided if possible.
- Antibiotic prophylaxis to prevent bacterial endocarditis is controversial for normal labor and delivery, but should be considered in those at the highest cardiac risk (prosthetic valve, conduits) or with the greatest risk of bacteremia (infected uterus).

Possible Complications

- Fetal abnormalities, fetal death, maternal death, worsening of heart disease (bacterial endocarditis)

EXPECTED COURSE AND PROGNOSIS

Maternal mortality rates depend on the underlying cardiac condition.

- Less than 1%
  —Left-to-right shunts at the atrial, ventricular, and ductal levels
  —Pulmonary valve disease
  —Corrected congenital heart disease
  —Bioprosthetic valves
  —Mild to moderate mitral stenosis
- 5%–10%
  —Moderate to severe mitral stenosis
  —Mechanical prosthetic valves
  —Aortic stenosis
  —Coarctation of the aorta
  —Uncorrected congenital heart disease
  —Marfan's syndrome with normal aorta
- 25%–50%
  —Pulmonary hypertension
  —Complicated coarctation of the aorta (aortic stenosis or severe hypertension)
  —Marfan's syndrome with dilated aorta

PATIENT EDUCATION

Prenatal care is critical for patients with heart disease.

Activity

Restrict activity to decrease the burden on the heart.

Diet

Dietary sodium restriction to reduce fluid accumulation; dietary restriction of calories to keep weight gain appropriate

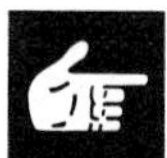

Miscellaneous

ICD-9-CM

674.82 Post-partum cardiomyopathy

BIBLIOGRAPHY

Clark SL. Cardiac disease in pregnancy. *Obstet Gynecol Clin North Am* 1991;18:237.

Elkayam U, Gleicher N, eds. The evaluation of the cardiac patient. In: *Principles and practice of medical therapy in pregnancy*, 2nd ed. E. Norwalk, CT: Appleton & Lange, 1991.

Author: Michael H. Crawford

Premature Ventricular Contractions

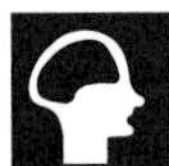

Basics

DESCRIPTION

Premature ventricular contractions (PVCs) involve depolarization of the ventricle with inscription of QRS earlier than expected.

- The depolarization is initiated in the ventricles, causing the QRS morphology to be bizarre and not typical of depolarization via the normal conducting system.
- The term *premature ventricular contraction* is in one respect a misnomer because there can be depolarization without contraction. However, the term is so ingrained in the medical lexicon that its continued use is reasonable.

EPIDEMIOLOGY

- Frequent after myocardial infarction, and ubiquitous as age increases and in setting of cardiomyopathy
- May occur at any age, but prevalence increases with age, and PVCs are ubiquitous in the elderly

ETIOLOGY

- Reentry, automaticity, and triggered mechanisms
- Most frequently seen in structural heart disease, especially during acute and after myocardial infarction, and cardiomyopathy
- Drug toxicity (digitalis, QT-prolonging agents)
- Sympathetic stimulation (e.g., beta-agonists used to treat bronchospasm, caffeine)
- Slow heart rates during which ventricular beats may represent escape rhythms

RISK FACTORS

- Increasing age
- Structural heart disease

PREGNANCY

- Contraindications related to underlying heart disease
- No contraindication if structurally normal heart; symptoms may increase during pregnancy

ASSOCIATED CONDITIONS

Because the frequency of ischemic heart disease and cardiomyopathy increases with age, PVCs are seen in association with these diseases.

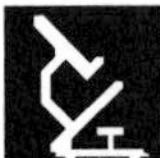

Diagnosis

DIFFERENTIAL DIAGNOSIS

Atrial premature contractions (APCs) with aberrancy.

SIGNS AND SYMPTOMS

- Symptoms may be absent.
- Palpitations
- Dyspnea
- On physical examination, PVCs are associated with early beats followed by a pause that may either be compensatory (depolarization does not change timing of intrinsic rhythm) or not.
  - —Giant *a* waves are seen in the neck veins because with the PVC there is atrial contraction against a closed tricuspid valve.
  - —There may be an absent peripheral pulse with the early beat because the heart has not had time to fill in diastole, and the contraction pattern of the ventricles is abnormal.

LABORATORY PROCEDURES

- None

IMAGING PROCEDURES

Depends on age and suspicion for heart disease

- Echocardiogram
- Perfusion imaging to evaluate ischemia (e.g., thallium) and ejection fraction
- MRI (also called nuclear magnetic resonance, or NMR)

SPECIAL TESTS

- ECG
- Ambulatory (Holter) monitor
- Event recorder
- Evaluate for underlying heart disease
  - —Ischemia (exercise test)
  - —Myocardium (echocardiogram, MRI)
- Pathology: Depends on substrate, but usually scar/fibrosis. Sometimes in a structurally normal heart, PVCs arise from triggered activity or automatic focus in normal tissue

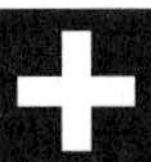

Treatment

GENERAL MEASURES

- Treat underlying heart disease.
- Beta-blockers if ischemic heart disease
- Because there is no evidence that treatment of PVCs extends life and that treatment may even increase mortality (Cardiac Arrhythmia Suppression Trial), first therapy should be reassurance and avoidance of therapy if possible.
- The Canadian Amiodarone Myocardial Infarction Arrhythmia Trial and the European Myocardial Infarction Amiodarone Trial showed that prophylactic amiodarone following myocardial infarction does not improve overall survival.
- See chapter on Ventricular Tachycardia for management of nonsustained ventricular tachycardia (PVCs occur in runs of three or more).
  - —For patients with ischemic heart disease and low left ventricular ejection fractions, electrophysiologic study can be justified, and if sustained ventricular tachycardia is induced, an implantable defibrillator can be offered (refer to Buxton et al. and Mess et al. in Bibliography).
- The best prevention of PVCs is the prevention of heart disease.

SURGICAL MEASURES

Not applicable; however, some PVCs may be "cured" by ablation of arrhythmia focus in right ventricular outflow tract and in fascicles of His-Purkinje system.

ADMISSION/DISCHARGE CRITERIA

All attempts should be made to avoid treating PVCs per se. Beta-blockers and anxiolytics can be started on an outpatient basis. For patients with structural heart disease, admission is indicated for loading of drugs with proarrhythmic potential (class I drugs, e.g., quinidine, procainamide, disopyramide, sotalol).

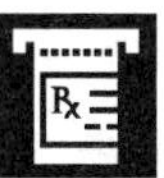

Medications

DRUG(S) OF CHOICE

- No therapy is ideal.
- Beta-blocker if ischemic heart disease
  —Even though beta-blockers may not suppress PVCs, they will increase survival.
  —In symptomatic patients beta-blockers may decrease symptoms by decreasing vigor of post-PVC beat that is usually responsible for the palpitation (increased contraction after pause via Starling principle).
- Lidocaine is usually used in acute settings, such as myocardial infarction.
  —Lidocaine should not be used prophylactically because meta-analyses suggest an increase in mortality due to bradycardic deaths when the drug is used in this manner.
  —If the patient has had ventricular tachycardia or ventricular fibrillation, lidocaine is the usual first antiarrhythmic drug chosen.
- Primary antiarrhythmic drug should be chosen for long-term use if reassurance not satisfactory.
- Amiodarone or sotalol if structural heart disease
- Anxiolytic sometimes helpful if patient worried about palpitations

Contraindications

Class IC drugs are contraindicated, and all class I drugs are probably inadvisable in ischemic heart disease.

- Proarrhythmia
  —May manifest as increased mortality from class I drugs in ischemic heart disease
  —Torsades de pointes ventricular tachycardia with class IA and class III drugs
  —Avoid class I and III drugs if corrected QT interval prolonged at baseline.

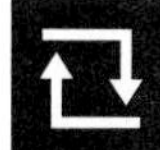

Follow-up

PATIENT MONITORING

- Monitor on-line with telemetry and record ECGs at least daily in acute setting.
- Outpatients may have repeat Holter monitors or event recorders to correlate symptoms with the rhythm if empiric therapy does not decrease symptoms.

EXPECTED COURSE AND PROGNOSIS

- Normal if structurally normal heart
- Decreased survival if ischemic heart disease
- Controversial if cardiomyopathy

PATIENT EDUCATION

- Teach patients that PVCs per se are not a cause for mortality by themselves, and that antiarrhythmic drug treatment may worsen prognosis.
- In setting of structurally normal heart, prognosis is normal. There is no indication for treatment in the absence of symptoms.
- No specific diet is indicated, although in some individuals caffeine may increase frequency of PVCs.
- Teach that antiarrhythmic drugs may be proarrhythmic.

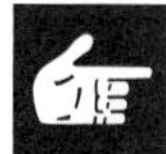

Miscellaneous

SYNONYMS

- Premature ventricular beats
- Premature ventricular depolarizations
- Ventricular premature contractions
- Ventricular premature beats
- Ventricular premature depolarizations

ICD-9-CM

427.69 Ventricular premature beats, contractions, or systoles

BIBLIOGRAPHY

Buxton AE, Lec KL, Fisher JD, et al. A randomized study of the prevention of sudden death in patients with coronary artery disease. *N Engl J Med* 1999;341:1882–1890.

Cairns JA, Connolly SJ, Roberts R, et al., for the Canadian Amiodarone Myocardial Infarction Arrhythmia Trial Investigators. Randomised trial of outcome after myocardial infarction in patients with frequent or repetitive ventricular premature depolarisations: CAMIAT. *Lancet* 1997;349:675–682.

The Cardiac Arrhythmia Suppression Trial II Investigators. Effect of the antiarrhythmic agent moricizine on survival after myocardial infarction. *N Engl J Med* 1992;327:227–233.

Echt DS, Liebson PR, Mitchell LB, et al. Mortality and morbidity in patients receiving encainide, flecainide, or placebo: The Cardiac Arrhythmia Suppression Trial. *N Engl J Med* 1991;324:781–788.

Epstein AE, Bigger JT, Wyse DG, et al. Events in the Cardiac Arrhythmia Suppression Trial (CAST): mortality in the entire population enrolled. *J Am Coll Cardiol* 1991;18:14–19.

Julian DG, Camm AJ, Frangin G, et al. Randomised trial of effect of amiodarone on mortality in patients with left-ventricular dysfunction after recent myocardial infarction: EMIAT. *Lancet* 1997;349:667–674.

Moss AJ, Hall WJ, Cannom DS, et al. Improved survival with an implanted defibrillator in patients with coronary disease at high risk for ventricular arrhythmia. *N Engl J Med* 1996; 335:1933–1940.

Author: Andrew E. Epstein

Prostheti
c Valves

Basics

DESCRIPTION

There are two classes of heart valves: mechanical prostheses, with rigid manufactured occluders, and biological or tissue valves, with flexible leaflet occluders of animal or human origin.

Mechanical Valves

These are three different types by design:

- Ball valve: Starr-Edwards
- Disk valve
  - —Bjork-Shiley tilting disk valve
  - —Medtronic Hall
- Bileaflet
  - —St. Jude
  - —Duromedics
  - —CarboMedics

Biological Valves

- Porcine
  - —Hancock
  - —Carpentier-Edwards
  - —Toronto stentless
- Pericardial
  - —Carpentier-Edwards
- Homograft
  - —Noncommercial
  - —Cryolife
- Autologous
  - —Pulmonary autograft

Complications

- Structural valvular deterioration
- Nonstructural dysfunction
- Valve thrombosis
- Embolism
- Bleeding events
- Operated valvular endocarditis

RISK FACTORS

- Atrial fibrillation
- Left ventricular (LV) systolic dysfunction
- Previous thromboembolism
- Hypercoagulable states

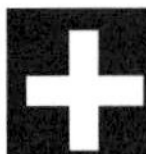

Treatment

GENERAL MEASURES

Embolic Event During Adequate Antithrombotic Therapy

In such patients, antithrombotic therapy should be adjusted as follows:

- Warfarin, INR 2–3: Warfarin dose should be increased to achieve INR of 2.5–3.5.
- Warfarin, INR 2.5–3.5: Warfarin dose may need to be increased to achieve INR of 3.5–4.5.
- Not already on aspirin: Aspirin 80–100 mg/day should be initiated.
- Warfarin plus aspirin 80–100 mg/day: Aspirin dose may be increased to 325 mg/day if higher dose of warfarin in not achieving the desired clinical results.
- Aspirin alone: Aspirin dose may need to be increased to 325 mg/day and/or warfarin added to achieve INR of 2.0–3.0.

Antithrombotic Therapy in Patients Requiring Noncardiac Surgery

- The risk of increased bleeding during the procedure performed with a patient receiving antithrombotic therapy has to be weighed against the risk of thromboembolism caused by stopping antithrombotic therapy.
- In general, patients on warfarin should stop warfarin 72 hours before the procedure and restart in the afternoon on the day of the procedure or after control of active bleeding.
- Patients taking aspirin should stop taking aspirin 1 week before the procedure and restart the day after the procedure or after the control of active bleeding.
- Therapy should be individualized in unusual circumstances.

SURGICAL MEASURES

Thrombosis of Prosthetic Heart Valves

- Patients who have a large clot, those with evidence of valve obstruction, and those in NYHA classes III or IV because of prosthetic thrombosis should undergo early/immediate operation.
- Thrombolytic therapy for a prosthetic valve obstructed by thrombus is associated with significant risks and is often ineffective and is reserved for those patients in whom surgical intervention carries high risk and those with contraindications to surgery.
- Patients with a small clot who are in NYHA functional class I or II and those with LV systolic dysfunction should have in-hospital, short-term i.v. heparin therapy. If this is unsuccessful, they may receive a trial of continous infusion thrombolytic therapy over several days.

Reoperation to Replace a Prosthetic Heart Valve

- Reoperation to replace a prosthetic heart valve is a serious clinical event.
- It is usually required for moderate to severe prosthetic dysfunction (structural and nonstructural), dehiscence, and prosthetic endocarditis.
- Reoperation also may be indicated for recurrent thromboembolism, severe intravascular hemolysis, severe recurrent bleeding from anticoagulant therapy, thrombosed prosthetic valve, and valve prosthesis–patient mismatch.

Major Criteria for Valve Selection

- In general mitral valve repair is preferable to MVR, provided it is feasible and the appropriate skill and experience are available to perform the procedure successfully.
- Carefully selected patients with aortic regurgitation (AR) or aortic stenosis (AS) in whom the valve is not calcified are also candidates for valve repair, with the same provisos as mitral valve repair and with the recognition that information regarding the early and late results of aortic valve repair for AR is quite limited at this time.
- The major advantages of a mechanical valve are an extremely low rate of structural deterioration and a better survival rate in younger patients.
- The major disadvantages are the increased incidence of bleeding due to the need for antithrombotic therapy and the cost and disadvantages of antithrombotic therapy.
- The major advantages of a bioprosthesis (whether porcine or pericardial) are a lower bleeding rate and lack of need for antithrombotic therapy.
- The major disadvantage is the increased rate of structural valve deterioration and hence the need for reoperation in younger patients.
- Pericardial bioprostheses may have a lower rate of structural valve deterioration than porcine bioprostheses in patients ≥65 years of age.
- The following are general recommendation for valve replacement:
  - —Patients with expected long life spans
  - —Patients with a mechanical prosthetic valve already in place in a different position than the valve to be replaced
  - —Patients in renal failure, on hemodialysis, or with hypercalcemia
  - —Patients requiring warfarin therapy because of risk factors for thromboembolism
- Recommendations for valve replacement with a bioprosthesis:
  - —Patients who cannot or will not take warfarin therapy
  - —Patients ≥65 years of age needing AVR who do not have risk factors for thromboembolism
  - —Patients considered to have possible compliance problems with warfarin therapy
  - —Patients ≥70 years of age needing MVR who do not have risk factors for thromboembolism

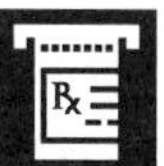

Medications

DRUG(S) OF CHOICE

- Antibiotic prophylaxis
  —Infective endocarditis: All patients with prosthetic heart valves need appropriate antibiotic prophylaxis against infective endocarditis.
  —Rheumatic carditis: Patients with rheumatic heart disease continue to need antibiotic as prophylaxis against recurrence of rheumatic carditis.
- Antithrombotic therapy
  —All patients with mechanical valves require warfarin therapy.
  —Even with the use of warfarin, the risk of thromboemboli is 1%–2% per year, but the risk is considerably higher without treatment with warfarin.
  —The risk of a clinical thromboembolism is ~0.7% per year in patients with biological valves in sinus rhythm.
  —The risk of embolism is greater with a valve in the mitral position (mechanical or biological) than with one in the aortic position.
  —With either type of prosthesis or valve location, the risk of emboli is probably higher in the first few days and months after valve insertion before the valve is fully endothelialized.
  —First 3 months after valve replacement:
    - Warfarin, INR 2.5–3.5

  —≥3 months after valve replacement:
    - Mechanical valve
    - Aortic valve replacement (AVR) with no risk factor
    - Bileaflet valve or Medtronic Hall valve: warfarin, INR 2.0–3.0
    - Other disk valves or Starr-Edwards valve: warfarin, INR 2.5–3.5
    - AVR with risk factor: warfarin, INR 2.5–3.5
    - Mitral valve replacement (MVR): warfarin, INR 2.5–3.5
- Bioprosthesis
  —AVR and no risk factor: aspirin, 80–100 mg/day
  —AVR with risk factor: warfarin, INR 2.0–3.0
  —MVR and no risk factor: aspirin, 80–100 mg/day
  —MVR and risk factor: warfarin, INR 2.5–3.5
- The following recommendations should also be considered in some subset of patients:
  —Addition of aspirin 80–100 mg once daily if not already on aspirin in patients with risk factor
  —Warfarin, INR 3.5–4.5, in high risk patients when aspirin cannot be used

Follow-up

PATIENT MONITORING

- The first outpatient evaluation after valve surgery usually occurs 3–4 weeks after discharge.
- The workup on this visit should include complete or interval history and physical examination, ECG, chest x-ray, 2-D and Doppler echocardiography, complete blood count, blood urea nitrogen/creatinine electrolytes, lactic dehydrogenase (LDH), and INR, if indicated.
- The asymptomatic uncomplicated patients thereafter need to be followed only at 1-year intervals, at which time a complete history and thorough examination should be performed. ECGs and chest x-ray are not routinely indicated but are valuable in individual patients. The frequency with which 2-D and Doppler echocardiography should be performed in uncomplicated patients is uncertain.
- Once regurgitation is detected, close follow-up with 2-D and Doppler echocardiography every 3–6 months is indicated.
- Any patient with a prosthetic heart valve who does not improve after surgery or who later shows deterioration of functional capacity should undergo appropriate testing, including 2-D and Doppler echocardiography and, if necessary, transesophageal echocardiography and cardiac catheterization with angiography to determine the cause.

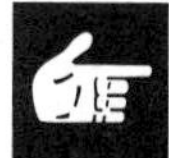

Miscellaneous

BIBLIOGRAPHY

Alexander RW, ed. *Hurst's the heart.* New York: McGraw-Hill, 1998.

Bonow et al. ACC/AHA Guidelines for the management of patients with valvular heart disease. *J Am Coll Cardiol* 1998;32:1486–1588.

Braunwald E, ed. *Heart disease: a Textbook of cardiovascular medicine,* 5th ed. Philadelphia: WB Saunders, 1997.

Feigenbaum H, ed. *Echocardiography,* 5th ed. Baltimore: Williams & Wilkins, 1993.

Author: Madhukar Gupta

Pulmonary Atresia with Intact Ventricular Septum

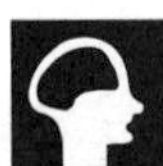

Basics

DESCRIPTION

This type of atresia of the pulmonary valve has no ventricular septal defect.

- The main and branch pulmonary arteries are almost always normal.
  - —Forward flow may be present in early fetal life.
  - —The ductus arteriosus is usually patent in the neonate for a few days, but when closure occurs, there are no alternate sources of pulmonary blood flow.
  - —Pulmonary collateral vessels are not prominent.
- A broad spectrum of coronary artery abnormalities are common, varying from coronary atresia (observed in stillborns) to mild stenoses. Myocardial blood flow may be dependent on right ventricular (RV) sinusoids in some cases.

EPIDEMIOLOGY

Incidence/Prevalence

- 0.07/1,000 births, 1% of congenital heart disease, 3% of critically ill children

Predominant Age

- Newborn

Predominant Sex or Race

- None

ETIOLOGY

- Unknown

PREGNANCY

- Patients who undergo surgery with four-chamber anatomy, normal coronary arteries, and mild to moderate pulmonary valve stenosis are at low maternal and fetal risk during pregnancy.
- Pregnancy is not recommended for women who have undergone the Fontan procedure, and those with coronary artery disease or ventricular dysfunction.

ASSOCIATED CONDITIONS

- Rare

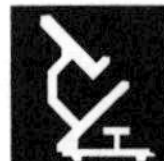

Diagnosis

DIFFERENTIAL DIAGNOSIS

The differential diagnosis of a newborn with cardiac cyanosis also includes critical pulmonary stenosis with intact ventricular septum, transposition of the great arteries, total anomalous venous return, tricuspid atresia, Ebstein's anomaly, tetralogy of Fallot, and pulmonary atresia with ventricular septal defect (extreme tetralogy variant).

SIGNS AND SYMPTOMS

- Severe cyanosis
- Tachypnea
- Normal S1
- Single S2
- May have regurgitant murmur at left lower sternal border due to tricuspid insufficiency
- As ductus arteriosus closes, severity of symptoms progress
- May have low cardiac output, with myocardial ischemia

History

- Severe cyanosis within 3 days of birth
- Persistent tachypnea, may develop respiratory distress
- Murmur may be audible

LABORATORY PROCEDURES

Arterial saturation <70%; less severe hypoxia in patients receiving prostaglandins to keep ductus patent

Pathologic Findings

- Usually slightly small to normal valve annulus with fused leaflets
- Small or miniscule RV chamber with severe myocardial hypertrophy; 20% have large, usually dysfunctional RV; tricuspid valve annulus size correlates with RV size
- Slightly small but confluent pulmonary arteries; few pulmonary arterial collaterals
- Coronary artery abnormalities are frequent.
- Myocardial function is often abnormal.
- Restrictive atrial communication is rare; foramen ovale is dilated.
- Tricuspid annulus may be large in 5%–10% of cases and tricuspid insufficiency may be present. A few patients with large chambers may have Ebstein's deformity.
- Mitral valve abnormalities are rare.

IMAGING STUDIES

- Heart size is most often normal; large right atrium if tricuspid regurgitation is significant. Decreased pulmonary vascular markings are usual, unless ductus is widely patent.
- Echocardiography
  - —Documents small to miniscule RV chamber and tricuspid valve and no ventricular septal defect
  - —Some cases have large RV chamber.
  - —Slightly small to normal pulmonary valve annulus and pulmonary arteries
- Echocardiography (Doppler)
  - —Absence of flow across right ventricular outflow tract
  - —Assesses severity of tricuspid regurgitation qualitatively, and may allow prediction of RV pressure
  - —Right-to-left flow across atrial septum

SPECIAL TESTS

- ECG
  - —Normal sinus rhythm
  - —Axis 0–120 degrees
  - —Most often normal axis
  - —May have right axis if a large RV chamber is present
  - —Usually decreased RV voltage, V1 and V3R.
- Cardiac catheterization
  - —Documents atresia of the RV outflow tract
  - —Demonstrates size of pulmonary arteries and status of the ductus arteriosus
  - —Evaluates for RV dependent coronary circulation
  - —RV angiogram can demonstrate filling of coronary arteries retrograde via myocardial sinusoids. Coronary angiogram also is required to observe for stenoses in the coronary circulation.

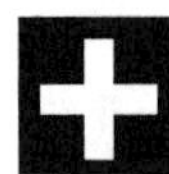

Treatment

GENERAL MEASURES

- Without treatment, prognosis is extremely poor; most neonates die within days.
- Prostaglandin is administered to maintain ductal-dependent pulmonary blood flow. Cardiac catheterization is performed to assess for coronary abnormalities or RV-dependent coronary circulation.

SURGICAL MEASURES

The size of the right ventricular chamber and tricuspid valve will determine if a four-chamber repair can be achieved. There are several approaches to repair depending on the PA with IVs anatomic findings.

- If the tricuspid valve annulus and RV are miniscule, a Blalock-Taussig shunt procedure alone is performed urgently in the neonatal period. These patients will likely undergo multiple operations in childhood, eventually leading to a Fontan type of circulation. (All superior vena cava and inferior vena cava blood flows passively to the lungs, and the left ventricle pumps oxygenated blood to the body.)
- Patients with small but not tiny tricuspid valves may undergo most often with an associated Blalock-Taussig shunt relief of right ventricular outflow tract (RVOT) obstruction.
- Patients with RV-dependent coronary circulation eventually may undergo a Fontan procedure that will incorporate an RV with systemic pressure into the systemic circulation so that the distal coronary arteries will be perfused. The prognosis often is poor with this type of anatomy.
- Late surgery
  —Reopen RVOT later in childhood.
  —Eliminate shunts in patients with good four-chamber anatomy.
  —Perform Fontan procedure for patients without functional right ventricle.

ADMISSION/DISCHARGE CRITERIA

The anatomy and surgical requirements for the individual patient determine admission, length of stay, and discharge criteria. Relief of cyanosis and satisfactory feeding are necessary before discharge in the neonatal period

Medications

DRUG(S) OF CHOICE

- At birth virtually all patients require prostaglandin to maintain ductal patency.
- Pressors (e.g., dopamine) and diuretics may be needed in the newborn period
- Endocarditis prophylaxis

Contraindications

- Allergies to any medicine

Precautions

- Refer to manufacturer's profile of each drug.

Significant Reactions

Refer to manufacturer's profile of each drug.

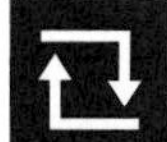

Follow-up

PATIENT MONITORING

- Follow-up should be tailored to the type of repair the patient has undergone.
- Specific issues include:
  —Arterial oxygen saturation and hemoglobin concentration to assess the adequacy of pulmonary blood flow
  —Pulmonary outflow gradients in patients with RVOT repairs
  —Growth of the RV chamber
  —Follow for sign or symptoms of ventricular ischemia

EXPECTED COURSE AND PROGNOSIS

- With no intervention, most patients die in the neonatal period. The remainder will die in infancy. Death is due to profound hypoxia and ventricular failure. A few patients with persistent patency of the ductus arteriosus will survive into childhood.
- There is an increased incidence of sudden death among surgically palliated infants, most likely due to left ventricular ischemia or dysfunction and a fatal arrhythmia.
- With intervention, the clinical course will depend on the adequacy of the RV. Overall, the 4-year survival rate is 64%. It must be noted that patients with adequate RVs and only one surgical procedure do better than patients who have multiple operations and ultimately undergo a Fontan operation. A child with a two-ventricle repair without coronary disease may have a relatively normal childhood, although exercise tolerance may be decreased. As the patient grows, the need for additional surgeries to enlarge the RVOT may be needed. 50% of patients will undergo an additional procedure, but ultimate prognosis may be favorable.

PATIENT EDUCATION

- Parents must be informed about the benefits of surgery and possible outcomes with the variations of this lesion.
- Patient's activity should be self-limited, based on cardiac status.

Diet

No restrictions are necessary.

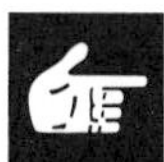

Miscellaneous

ICD-9-CM

746.01

BIBLIOGRAPHY

Bonow RO, Carabello B, de Leon AC Jr, et al. ACC/AHA guidelines for the management of patients with valvular heart disease: a report of the American College of Cardiology/American Heart Association Task Force on Practice Guidelines (Committee on Management of Patients with Valvular Heart Disease). *J Am Coll Cardiol* 1998;32:1486–1588.

Fyler DC. *Nadas' pediatric cardiology.* St. Louis: Mosby-Year Book, 1992.

Garson A, Bricker JT, Fisher DJ, et al. *The science and practice of pediatric cardiology,* 2nd ed. Baltimore: Lippincott Williams & Wilkins, 1997.

Hanley FL, Sade RM, Blackstone EH, et al. Outcomes in neonatal pulmonary atresia with intact ventricular septum. A multiinstitutional study. *J Thorac Cardiovasc Surg* 1993;105: 406–427.

Authors: David Brick and Welton M. Gersony

Pulmonary Edema, High-Altitude

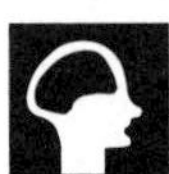

Basics

DESCRIPTION

High-altitude pulmonary edema (HAPE) is a form of noncardiogenic pulmonary edema that occurs after ascending to altitudes above 8,000 feet.

- Usually occurs in young, healthy persons who have quickly ascended to altitude and then engaged in physical exertion before they have become acclimated
- Can also occur in persons who reside at high altitude and return home after a few days at lower altitude

Systems Affected

- Pulmonary

ETIOLOGY

Genetics

- Unknown

Incidence/Prevalence

- In the United States, occurs in 0.2%–15% of the population, depending on factors such as age, sex, and rate of ascent
- Incidence ranges from 1/10,000 Colorado skiers to 1/50 climbers on Mt. McKinley.

Predominant Age

- Young adults

Predominant Sex

- Males affected more than females

Age-Related Factors

- Pediatric: Children more susceptible
- Geriatric: Recovery may be slower

ETIOLOGY

- Decreased PO_2 plays a central role.
- Pulmonary edema is thought to be secondary to increased capillary permeability and increased pulmonary artery pressure without increased pulmonary capillary wedge pressure.
- Pronounced hypoxia-induced pulmonary vasoconstriction may lead to overperfusion of the less obstructed portions of the vascular bed, leading to endothelial injury and pulmonary edema.

RISK FACTORS

- Altitude achieved (increased incidence with higher altitude)
- Rate of ascent (increased incidence associated with more rapid ascents)
- Cold exposure
- Prior history of HAPE

PREGNANCY

- Women with low-risk pregnancies should experience no difficulties up to approximately 10,000 feet.
- Women with high-risk or late-term pregnancies should avoid high altitudes.

ASSOCIATED CONDITIONS

- Hypothermia
- Acute mountain sickness (AMS)
- High-altitude cerebral edema

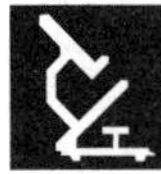

Diagnosis

DIFFERENTIAL DIAGNOSIS

- Viral or bacterial upper respiratory infection
- Pneumonia
- Congestive heart failure
- Laboratory procedures
- No characteristic findings in common laboratory tests
- Complete blood count: frequent leukocytosis
- Arterial blood gas: respiratory alkalosis and low oxygen saturation

SIGNS AND SYMPTOMS

- Symptoms begin within 2–5 days of a rapid ascent.
- Most cases are preceded by symptoms of AMS.
  - —Early symptoms
    - Dyspnea on exertion
    - Fatigue, decreased exercise tolerance
    - Weakness
    - Dry cough
  - —Late signs and symptoms
    - Tachycardia
    - Tachypnea
    - Rales
    - Pink-tinged frothy sputum
    - Cyanosis
    - Fever (usually $<38.5°C$)
    - Confusion

LABORATORY PROCEDURES

- No characteristic findings in common laboratory tests
- Complete blood count: frequent leukocytosis
- Arterial blood gas: respiratory alkalosis and low oxygen saturation

Pathologic Findings

- Lung edema

IMAGING STUDIES

- Chest x-ray
  - —Diffuse, peripheral patchy infiltrates, may be unilateral or bilateral
  - —Becomes more homogeneous in advanced cases and during recovery

SPECIAL TESTS

N/A

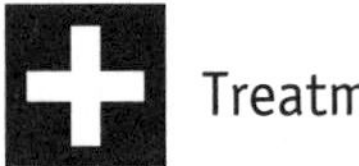

Treatment

GENERAL MEASURES

- If patient can maintain oxygen saturation above 90%, can be discharged on home oxygen with next day follow-up
- Must have reliable person with them to observe for worsening condition
- Admission required for patients unable to maintain saturations above 90%, who can be discharged when clinically improved and maintaining oxygenation
- Immediate improvement in oxygenation is the treatment of choice:
  - —Descent is critical, at least 3,000 feet as soon as possible
  - —Supplemental oxygen at 2–6 L/min to keep oxygen saturation above 90%
  - —If descent not feasible, use a hyperbaric bag to simulate descent
  - —May benefit from continuous positive airway pressure mask if available

SURGICAL MEASURES

N/A

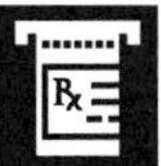

Medications

DRUG(S) OF CHOICE

- Prevention
  —Nifedipine 20 mg every 8 hours or 30–60 mg of sustained release daily in patients with history of HAPE
  —Diazoxide treatment
  —Nifedipine 20 mg every 6 hours
  —High-flow oxygen to maintain oxygen saturation above 90%

Contraindications

Refer to manufacturer's literature.

Precautions

Refer to manufacturer's literature.

ALTERNATIVE DRUGS

N/A

Follow-up

PATIENT MONITORING

N/A

Prevention/Avoidance

- Slow rate of ascent
- Average increase in sleeping altitude 1,000–1,200 ft/day above 8,000 feet
- No ascent to higher altitude with symptoms of AMS
- Descent when symptoms of AMS do not improve after a day of rest.
- Diet high in carbohydrates may be beneficial.
- Avoidance of alcohol
- Limit activity for first 1–2 days.
- Drink plenty of fluids.

Possible Complications

- Death, arrhythmias, cardiac arrest

EXPECTED COURSE AND PROGNOSIS

- Untreated and unable to descend, mortality rate >50%
- Severe, advanced cases may require prolonged hospital course.
- Mild cases show improvement in symptoms within hours and complete recovery within 2–3 days.

PATIENT EDUCATION

- Persons with history of HAPE are at increased risk of recurrence.
- Rate of ascent and altitude achieved are critical in development of HAPE.

Activity

- As tolerated during recovery
- Vigorous exercise should be avoided until acclimatized to altitude.

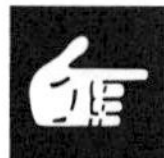

Miscellaneous

SYNONYMS

- Noncardiogenic pulmonary edema

ICD-9-CM

518.4 Acute edema of lung

BIBLIOGRAPHY

Auerbach P. *Wilderness medicine,* 3rd ed. St. Louis: CV Mosby, 1995.

Bartsch P. High altitude pulmonary edema. *Med Sci Sports Exerc* 1999;31(suppl):23–27.

Hultgren HN. High-altitude pulmonary edema: current concepts. *Annu Rev Med* 1996; 47:267–284.

Zafren K, Honigman B. High-altitude medicine. *Emerg Med Clin North Am* 1997;15:191–221.

Author: Gerald A. Charlton

Pulmonary Embolism

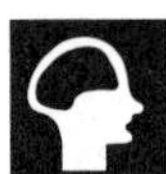

Basics

DESCRIPTION

Pulmonary embolism is defined as occlusion of a major pulmonary artery branch by a blood clot originating from the venous system of the body.

- Clinical presentation
  —Acute cor pulmonale: occlusion of more than two-thirds of the pulmonary circulation
  —Pulmonary infarction: complete occlusion of a distal branch of the pulmonary circulation.
  —Unexplained dyspnea: patients without acute cor pulmonale or pulmonary infarction

Systems Affected

- Pulmonary, cardiovascular.

ETIOLOGY

Genetics

- Hypercoagulable states (e.g., Factor V Leiden deficiency)

Incidence/Prevalence

- 250,000 cases/year; 50,000 deaths/year.

Predominant Age

- Increases with advancing age

Predominant Sex

- Males affected as often as females

CAUSES

- Propensity to venous thrombosis and pulmonary embolism increased by venous stasis, altered blood coagulability, and vascular injury (Virchow's triad)

RISK FACTORS

- Surgery, especially orthopedic, major abdominal, and thoracic
- Immobilization
- Occult cancer (hypercoagulable state)
- Oral contraceptive use
- Postpartum
- Obesity
- Advanced age
- Anticardiolipid antibodies (lupus erythematosus)
- Trauma to legs
- Advanced age
- Congestive heart failure

ASSOCIATED CONDITIONS

- Deep venous thrombosis
- Occult cancer
- Congestive heart failure
- Stroke
- Obesity

Age-Related Factors

- Pediatric: rare
- Geriatric: more common and often fatal
- Others: young women on oral contraceptives

PREGNANCY

- Increases the risk

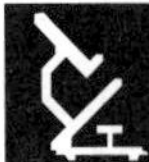

Diagnosis

DIFFERENTIAL DIAGNOSIS

- Acute myocardial infarction
- Pneumonia
- Congestive heart failure
- Pericarditis
- Pleurisy
- Anxiety neurosis/panic attacks

SIGNS AND SYMPTOMS

- Acute cor pulmonale
  —Dyspnea
  —Syncope
  —Cyanosis
  —Hypotension
  —Cardiopulmonary arrest
  —Anxiety
  —Tachypnea
  —Tachycardia
  —Jugular venous distention
  —Third heart sound
  —Right ventricular heave
  —Signs of deep venous thrombosis
  —ECG: new S1, Q3, T3 pattern, incomplete right bundle branch block or right ventricular ischemia.
  —Chest x-ray usually normal
  —Arterial blood gases: low PO_2, PCO_2
- Pulmonary infarction
  —Pleuritic chest pain
  —Dyspnea
  —Hemoptysis
  —Tachypnea
  —Lungs: rales, wheezes, or friction rub
  —Signs of deep venous thrombosis
  —ECG normal
  —Chest x-ray: elevated hemidiaphragm, peripheral infiltrate, or small pleural effusion
  —Arterial blood gases: normal or decreased PO_2, decreased PCO_2, alkalosis
- Unexplained dyspnea
  —Dyspnea
  —Anxiety
  —Tachycardia
  —Tachypnea
  —Signs of deep venous thrombosis
  —ECG usually normal
  —Chest x-ray normal
  —Arterial blood gases: normal or decreased PO_2, PCO_2

LABORATORY PROCEDURES

- Not helpful

Pathologic Findings

- Pulmonary infarction
- Pulmonary artery thrombi
- Deep venous thrombosis
- Cor pulmonale

SPECIAL TESTS

- None

IMAGING STUDIES

- V/Q scan: most useful if normal or highly suggestive of pulmonary embolism segmental perfusion defects
- Pulmonary angiography: intraluminal filling defects or arterial cut-offs
- Echocardiography: signs of cor pulmonale
- Ultrasonography of the leg veins to confirm deep venous thromboses
- Contrast venography to confirm deep venous thromboses

DIAGNOSTIC PROCEDURES

- Lung scan
- Pulmonary angiography
- Evidence of deep venous thrombosis and clinical features of one of the three presentations of pulmonary embolism

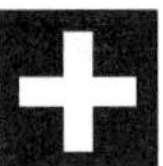

Treatment

GENERAL MEASURES

- Hospitalization, in the intensive care unit if unstable
- Oxygen as necessary
- Ventilatory assistance if needed
- Graduated leg compression stockings for deep venous thrombosis
- Emotional support (unexpected acute illness)

SURGICAL MEASURES

- Pulmonary thrombectomy for rare patient unresponsive to medical therapy or with chronic pulmonary hypertension from prior pulmonary embolism
- Inferior vena cava filter to prevent further thromboemboli in patients unresponsive to, refractory to, or contraindicated for medical therapy

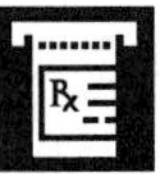

Medications

DRUG(S) OF CHOICE

- Intravenous heparin 5,000–10,000 units, followed by a continuous infusion to keep the partial thromboplastin time 1.5–2.5 times normal for at least 5 days
- Warfarin orally beginning 12–24 hours after heparin for at least 3 months
- Warfarin dose adjusted to increase the INR to 2.0–3.0 times normal (1.0)
- Thrombolytic therapy is indicated for patients with hemodynamic instability, right heart failure, massive pulmonary embolism, or extensive deep venous thrombosis: streptokinase 250,000 units over 30 minutes followed by 100,000 U/h for 24 hours or recombinant tissue plasminogen activator (rt-PA) 100 mg over 2 hours.

Contraindications

- The major contraindication to anticoagulation or thrombolytic therapy is active bleeding.
- Recent hemorrhagic stroke, intracranial disease or head trauma, a high risk of bleeding (recent surgery), and significant thrombocytopenia are contraindications to thrombolytic therapy.

Precautions

If the partial thromboplastin time and INR are adjusted appropriately, the risk of major hemorrhage can be minimized.

Significant Possible Interactions

Many drugs alter the metabolism of warfarin, making management by a specialized clinic desirable.

ALTERNATIVE DRUGS

Low-molecular-weight heparin given subcutaneously every 12 hours is an alternative to intravenous heparin and warfarin.

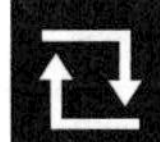

Follow-up

PATIENT MONITORING

The INR must be followed carefully in a patient on chronic warfarin.

Prevention/Avoidance

- Graduated compression stockings in susceptible patients (surgical patients)
- Periodic ambulation during long airplane or car trips
- Chronic warfarin or low-molecular-weight heparin therapy for high-risk patients
- Inferior vena cava interruption for high-risk patients

Possible Complications

- Pulmonary infarction
- Chronic pulmonary hypertension
- Right heart failure

EXPECTED COURSE AND PROGNOSIS

- With appropriate therapy hospital mortality rate is less than 10%.
- Long-term prognosis is determined by coexisting disease, residual pulmonary function, and level of pulmonary pressures.

PATIENT EDUCATION

- Avoidance of prolonged immobilization
- Weight loss

Activity

- Bed rest with leg movement exercises; ambulation as soon as possible

Diet

- Nothing special

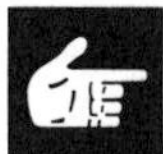

Miscellaneous

ICD-9-CM

415.1 Pulmonary embolism and infarction

See also: Thrombosis, deep vein

BIBLIOGRAPHY

Goldhaber SZ. Pulmonary embolic disease. In: Crawford MH, ed. *Current diagnosis and treatment in cardiology*. E. Norwalk, CT: Appleton & Lange, 1995.

Hyers TM, et al. Antithrombic therapy for venous thromboembolic disease. *Chest* 1998; 114:5615–5785.

Author: Michael H. Crawford

Pulmonary Hypertension, Primary and Secondary

Basics

DESCRIPTION

Pulmonary hypertension is defined as elevation of pulmonary arterial pressures to a mean of 25 mm Hg at rest or 30 mm Hg during exercise due to intrinsic abnormalities of pulmonary vasculature (primary pulmonary hypertension, PPH) or secondary causes including lung disease, chronic elevations of pulmonary venous pressures as a result of left heart disease (secondary pulmonary hypertension, SPH), and rare syndromes such as venoocclusive disease and pulmonary capillary hemangiomatosis.

EPIDEMIOLOGY

PPH

- Rare syndrome (incidence 2 per million)
- Female predominance (2.5:1); mean age 35 years
- Autosomal-dominant transmission in 6%, with one chromosomal locus mapped to 2q31-q32

ETIOLOGY

PPH

- Etiology unexplained by secondary causes
- Mechanisms: pulmonary arteriolar hypertrophy and remodeling due to sustained vasoconstriction, autoimmune mechanisms, *in situ* thrombosis
- Also see section on Associated Conditions.

SPH

- Heart disease
  - —Congenital heart disease with left-to-right shunting
  - —Acquired heart disease causing pulmonary venous hypertension (left ventricular failure or mitral or aortic valve disease)
- Pulmonary diseases
  - —Chronic obstructive lung disease (bronchitis, emphysema)
  - —Interstitial lung disease
  - —Pulmonary vascular disease: thromboembolism, collagen vascular disease, schistosomiasis/filariasis, Takayasu's arteritis, fibrosing mediastinitis
- Alveolar hypoventilation
  - —Abnormal chest bellows (e.g., poliomyelitis)
  - —Sleep apneas
  - —Disordered respiratory control (e.g., postencephalitis)

Other Etiologies

- Pulmonary venoocclusive disease: rare disease of unclear etiology
  - —Inflammatory and thrombotic obliterative process of pulmonary veins and venules
  - —Predominantly affects children and young adults
  - —Patients present with pulmonary edema and structurally normal left heart.
- Pulmonary capillary hemangiomatosis: very rare disease
  - —Infiltration of lung parenchyma and perivascular interstitium by proliferating microvessels, with a bleeding tendency
  - —Patients present with hemoptysis, and may behave like those with venoocclusive disease, but have abnormal perfusion scans and pulmonary angiograms.

RISK FACTORS

- Female sex

PREGNANCY

High risk to mother and fetus due to associated hemodynamic stresses, particularly in immediate postpartum period; oral contraceptives not recommended, because they may exacerbate pulmonary hypertension

ASSOCIATED CONDITIONS

- Anorectic agents (aminorex, dexfenfluramine, fenfluramine)
- Portal hypertension
- HIV infection
- Conditions associated with pulmonary hypertension; histopathologic findings of diffuse obliterative disease indiscernible from PPH

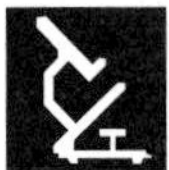

Diagnosis

DIFFERENTIAL DIAGNOSIS

- Heart disease: congenital heart disease with left to right shunting; cardiomyopathy and left ventricular failure; mitral or aortic valve disease
- Pulmonary diseases: chronic obstructive lung disease (bronchitis, emphysema); interstitial lung disease; pulmonary vascular disease (thromboembolism, collagen vascular disease, schistosomiasis/filariasis, Takayasu's arteritis, fibrosing mediastinitis)
- Alveolar hypoventilation: neuromuscular diseases (poliomyelitis); abnormal chest bellows (thoracic cage abnormality); sleep apneas; disordered respiratory control (e.g., postencephalitis)
- Pulmonary venoocclusive disease
- Pulmonary capillary hemangiomatosis

SIGNS AND SYMPTOMS

- Symptoms: dyspnea, fatigue, dizziness, chest pain, cough, hoarseness, orthopnea, effort syncope, edema, increased abdominal girth, palpitations
- Signs/physical examination findings: tachypnea, tachycardia, elevated jugular venous pressure with large *a* wave and large *v* wave if significant tricuspid regurgitation present, prominent right ventricular impulse, right ventricular S3 or S4 that increase with inspiration, loud pulmonic component (P2) of S2 or single S2, murmur of tricuspid regurgitation or pulmonic insufficiency, hepatomegaly, ascites, peripheral edema
- Findings or signs associated with underlying pulmonary disease (wheezes, rales, decreased excursion and air movement), and left heart disease, including those of mitral or aortic valve disease and dilated cardiomyopathy/left ventricular failure (murmur, S3)

LABORATORY PROCEDURES

See section on Special Tests.

IMAGING STUDIES

See sections on Investigations and Special Tests.

DIAGNOSTIC PROCEDURES

Investigations to confirm pulmonary hypertension and identify the causes include the following:

- ECG: right axis deviation, right atrial abnormality, right ventricular hypertrophy
- Chest x-ray: enlarged central pulmonary arteries, enlarged right atrium/ventricle, possible "pruning" of pulmonary vasculature, findings of left heart disease, including left atrial or ventricular enlargement
- Echocardiography with Doppler: right atrial/ventricular enlargement, right ventricular hypertrophy/dysfunction, elevated PA pressures, tricuspid/pulmonic insufficiency; may diagnose dilated cardiomyopathy, aortic and mitral valve disease, intracardiac shunts
- Right heart catheterization to assess right ventricular and pulmonary arterial pressures and pulmonary capillary wedge pressure (should be <15 mm Hg in PPH), and to rule out intracardiac shunts; consider pulmonary angiography if history and screening ventilation–perfusion (V/Q) scan suggest thromboembolic disease

SPECIAL TESTS

Special tests to consider to rule out secondary causes of pulmonary hypertension, depending on the history and physical examination findings, include the following:

- Echocardiography to rule out left heart disease
- V/Q scan to rule out chronic pulmonary embolism, with subsequent pulmonary angiography depending on result of V/Q scan; spiral CT scan to confirm pulmonary emboli
- Pulmonary function tests to rule out severe obstructive or restrictive patterns
- Sleep study to rule out sleep apnea
- Screen for collagen vascular diseases (scleroderma, systemic lupus erythematosus, polyarteritis nodosa)
- Screen for infectious etiologies: HIV, schistosomiasis, filariasis (highly recommended in excluding causes of SPH)

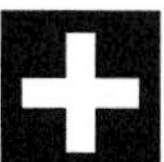

Treatment

GENERAL MEASURES

SPH

Three mechanisms contribute to development and worsening of SPH: (a) transmittance of high pulmonary venous pressures from left heart disease; (b) pulmonary endothelial dysfunction from elevated pressures, hypoxemia, and acidosis; and (c) remodeling/hypertrophy of pulmonary arterial tree over time due to elevated pressures and hypoxemia. Whereas the latter is irreversible, the first two have some reversibility. Treatment should aim to alter these factors:

- Treatment of left heart failure with diuretics, angiotensin-converting enzyme inhibitors, beta-blockers, digoxin, inotropes, and valve repair or replacement
- Treatment of hypoxemia and acidosis in hypoventilation syndromes with oxygen, continuous positive airway pressure, and mechanical ventilation
- Treatment of lung disease with bronchodilators, antibiotics, steroids, and smoking cessation
- Prevention of recurrent venous thromboembolic events with anticoagulants and/or vena caval filter
- Pulmonary thromboendarterectomy with chronic pulmonary emboli and proximal pulmonary arterial occlusion

PPH

Treatment includes:

- Supplemental oxygen to treat hypoxemia and vasoconstriction
- Vasodilators
  —Screen vasodilators include prostacyclin, adenosine, nifedipine, diltiazem, and inhaled nitric oxide (5–80 ppm).
  —Responders to vasodilators have improved survival, up to 95% at 5 years.
  —Initiate vasodilators under guidance of pulmonary artery catheter in catheterization laboratory or intensive care unit to assess tolerability and response.
  —Chronic therapy with prostacyclin (2–20 ng/kg/min), nifedipine (30–240 mg orally per day in increments), or diltiazem (120–900 mg orally per day in increments)
- Diuretics to treat right heart failure
  —Furosemide (40–500 mg/day) and spironolactone (25–100 mg/day) for ascites, edema, dyspnea
  —Closely monitor to avoid hypotension from overdiuresis (even in presence of edema, jugular venous distension) due to need for higher filling pressures in severely failing right ventricle.
- Inotropes such as dobutamine (2.5–7.5 μg/kg/min) or milrinone (0.35–0.75 μg/kg/min), either as temporary measure to improve right ventricular performance or chronically for patients with severe right ventricular failure refractory to above therapy.
- Chronic anticoagulation with warfarin (target INR 2.0–3.0) to prevent pulmonary emboli in presence of severe right heart failure appears to improve survival.
- Consider percutaneous atrial septostomy in normoxemic patients to improve left ventricular filling and cardiac output (at the expense of slightly worsening oxygenation from right-to-left shunt).
- Consider lung transplantation or heart–lung transplantation (in case of left-sided heart disease).

SURGICAL MEASURES

Consider percutaneous atrial septostomy, lung transplantation, heart–lung transplantation, inferior vena caval filter placement, and pulmonary thromboendarterectomy (see section on General Measures).

ADMISSION/DISCHARGE CRITERIA

Admission for patients with NYHA class IV symptoms or class II/III symptoms who require major dose adjustments of vasodilators, diuretics, inotropes under hemodynamic monitoring; discharge when stable on same medical, dietary, activity regimen as at home

Medications

DRUG(S) OF CHOICE

See PPH and SPH sections in General Measures.

Follow-up

PATIENT MONITORING

- Close frequent follow-up due to increased mortality rate
- Pneumococcal, influenza vaccines
- Monitor INR (2.0–3.0) on warfarin therapy.

EXPECTED COURSE AND PROGNOSIS

- PPH
  —Survival depends on clinical presentation; median survival 2.5 years.
  —Prognosis markedly improved if the patient responds to vasodilator therapy (up to 95% survival at 5 years)
  —Most deaths due to heart failure, sudden death (arrhythmia, pulmonary emboli), pneumonia, and other common causes of death
- SPH: depends on nature/reversibility of left heart disease

PATIENT EDUCATION

Diet

- Sodium, fluid restrictions to control heart failure

Activity

- As tolerated without symptoms
- Optimize exercise tolerance in cardiac rehabilitation program.
- Avoid high levels of activity (e.g., competitive sports).

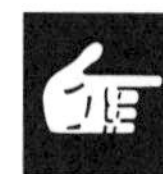

Miscellaneous

ICD-9-CM

416.0 Primary pulmonary hypertension
416.8 Other chronic pulmonary heart diseases: Pulmonary hypertension, secondary

INTERNET RESOURCES

- Pulmonary Hypertension Association website: volunteer support organization and source of information for patients with primary and secondary pulmonary hypertension. http://www.phassociation.org

BIBLIOGRAPHY

Fishman AP. Pulmonary hypertension. In: Alexander RW, Schlant RC, Fuster V, eds. *Hurst's the heart,* 9th ed. New York: McGraw-Hill, 1998: 1699–1717.

Higenbottam T, Stenmark K, Simonneau G. Treatments for severe pulmonary hypertension. *Lancet* 1999;353:338–340.

Newman JH, Ross JC. Chronic cor pulmonale. In: Alexander RW, Schlant RC, Fuster V, eds. *Hurst's the heart,* 9th ed. New York: McGraw-Hill, 1998:1739–1749.

Rubin LJ: Primary pulmonary hypertension. *N Engl J Med* 1997;336:111–117.

Authors: Pradyumna E. Tummala and Nanette K. Wenger

Pulmonic Regurgitation

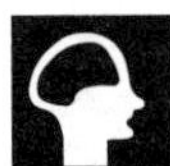

Basics

DESCRIPTION

Pulmonic regurgitation is incompetence of the pulmonary valve resulting in retrograde flow from the pulmonary artery to the right ventricle during diastole.

ETIOLOGY

Prevalence

- Uncommon

Age

Childhood cases are usually associated with other congenital heart defects; isolated cases are rare. Most cases occur during adulthood and are due to pulmonary causes.

CAUSES

- Dilation of pulmonary valve ring: pulmonary hypertension (PH) of any cause
- Dilation of pulmonary artery: idiopathic or secondary to connective tissue disorders such as Marfan's syndrome
- Pulmonic valve lesions: congenital malformation either alone or in association with other congenital anomalies, particularly tetralogy of Fallot, ventricular septal defect, and pulmonary valve stenosis
- Less common causes include trauma, iatrogenic causes (induced during surgical treatment of tetralogy of Fallot or congenital pulmonary stenosis), infective endocarditis, carcinoid syndrome, rheumatic involvement, syphilis, etc.

RISK FACTORS

N/A

PREGNANCY

Well tolerated in the absence of PH

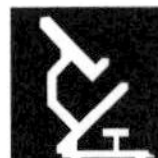

Diagnosis

DIFFERENTIAL DIAGNOSIS

- Aortic regurgitation

SIGNS AND SYMPTOMS

- Like tricuspid regurgitation, isolated pulmonary regurgitation (PR) is well tolerated for many years, until it complicates or is complicated by PH.
- Such patients usually present with signs and symptoms of right heart failure that includes swelling of feet, shortness of breath without much orthopnea, leg edema, ascites, hepatomegaly, venous distention (increased jugular venous pressure), and in long-standing cases splenomegaly.
- Physical examination may reveal palpable systolic pulsations in the left parasternal area (hyperdynamic right ventricle) and second left intercostal space (ICS; PH).
- A pulmonic tap due to pulmonary valve closure is usually easily heard at the second left ICS in patients with severe PH and PR.
- On auscultation there may be wide splitting of S2 due to a prolonged right ventricular ejection period, and P2 may be loud in the presence of PH.
- The diastolic murmur of PR is low pitched and is well heard at the left third and fourth ICS parasternally.
- A nonvalvular systolic ejection click and midsystolic ejection murmur, most prominent in the second left ICS also may be appreciated in severe PR.
- In the presence of right ventricular failure one may also hear S3 and S4 in the fourth ICS at the left parasternal area, which augments with inspiration.
- Graham Steell Murmur: This is the diastolic murmur of PR usually heard in the presence of severe PH. It is a high-pitched diastolic blowing decrescendo murmur that starts immediately after P2 and is most prominent at the left parasternal area in the second to fourth ICS.

LABORATORY PROCEDURES

- Nonspecific

PATHOLOGY

N/A

IMAGING STUDIES

- ECG
  - —In the absence of PH, ECG usually shows rSr (or rsR) configuration in the right precordial leads, indicative of right ventricular diastolic overload pattern.
  - —In patients with PH, ECG usually shows evidence of right ventricular hypertrophy.
  - —It usually shows right ventricular dilatation and in patients with PH right ventricular hypertrophy as well.
  - —Abnormal motion of the septum characteristic of volume overload of the right ventricle may be evident.
  - —The motion of the pulmonic valve may point to the cause of the PR. Pulsed Doppler detects PR extremely accurately.

SPECIAL TESTS

- Chest x-ray: Both pulmonary artery and right ventricle are usually enlarged, but these signs are nonspecific.
- Right heart catheterization may show elevated right ventricular end-diastolic pressure with or without PH.

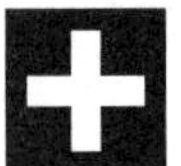

Treatment

GENERAL MEASURES

- PR per se is seldom severe enough to require specific treatment.
- Treatment of the primary condition responsible for PR usually ameliorates PR.

SURGICAL MEASURES

Surgical treatment of primary PR directed specifically toward the pulmonic valve (usually bioprosthesis) is rarely required for intractable right heart failure.

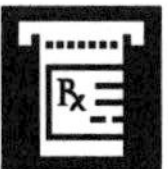

Medications

DRUG(S) OF CHOICE

- Diuretics when patient has volume overload
- Cardiac glycosides in the presence of right ventricular dilatation or failure

Precautions

Hypokalemia induced by loop diuretics may potentiate digoxin toxicity and arrhythmias.

ALTERNATIVE DRUGS

N/A

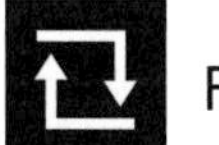

Follow-up

PATIENT MONITORING

- No recommendation for follow-up for isolated PR

Prevention

Routine use of antibiotics is not recommended in the absence of complex valvular lesions.

EXPECTED COURSE AND PROGNOSIS

- Usually very well tolerated for long time, also depends on treatment of the primary problem

PATIENT EDUCATION

Activity

No limitation until severe PH or reduced cardiac output due to right heart failure

Diet

- Low-sodium diet in the presence of right heart failure and fluid overload

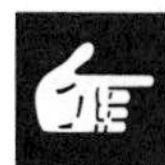

Miscellaneous

ICD-9-CM

424.3

BIBLIOGRAPHY

Alexander RW, ed. *Hurst's the heart.* New York: McGraw-Hill, 1998.

Bonow et al. ACC/AHA guidelines for the management of patients with valvular heart disease. *J Am Coll Cardiol* 1998;32:1486–1588.

Braunwald E, ed. *Heart disease: a textbook of cardiovascular medicine,* 5th ed. Philadelphia: WB Saunders, 1997.

Feigenbaum H, ed. *Echocardiography,* 5th edition. Baltimore: Williams & Wilkins, 1993.

Authors: Steven Herrmann, Amr El-Shafei, Madhukar Gupta, and Bernard R. Chaitman

Pulmonary Stenosis, Adult

Basics

DESCRIPTION

Pulmonic stenosis is obstruction to the right ventricular outflow tract leading to a hemodynamic pressure gradient across the right ventricle and pulmonary circulation.

ETIOLOGY

Prevalence

The congenital form is the most common form, but overall it is an uncommon finding.

Age

- Usually seen in children with associated congenital heart disease, may also be isolated
- Rare in adults due to acquired lesions, although patients with congenital pulmonary valvular lesion may present first during adulthood

CAUSES

- Peripheral pulmonary artery stenosis: localized or diffuse; commonly associated with supravalvular aortic stenosis, infantile hypercalcemia, and rubella syndrome (in association with patent ductus arteriosus)
- Pulmonary valve stenosis: commonly isolated lesion (7% of all congenital heart lesions); also occurs as part of Noonan's syndrome, tetralogy of Fallot, and rubella syndrome, and rarely acquired as part of carcinoid syndrome
- Pulmonary infundibular stenosis: rare as isolated lesion and usually associated with a ventricular septal defect (VSD) or tetralogy of Fallot, or in association with pulmonary valve stenosis
- Pulmonary subinfundibular stenosis: rarest form described and usually occurs as part of right-sided obstructive cardiomyopathy
- Compression from outside: cardiac tumors and aneurysm of sinus of Valsalva

RISK FACTORS

N/A

PREGNANCY

- Isolated mild or moderate pulmonary stenosis is rarely a significant impediment to successful pregnancy.
- Patients with cyanotic congenital heart disease generally tolerate the stresses of pregnancy worse than do patients with acyanotic lesions.

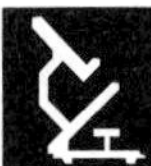

Diagnosis

DIFFERENTIAL DIAGNOSIS

- Aortic valve or subaortic stenosis
- VSD
- Ebstein's anomaly
- Atrial septal defect (ASD)

SIGNS AND SYMPTOMS

- The effect of pulmonary stenosis depends on severity, the structure and function of the rest of right ventricle, and the presence or absence of other associated lesions.
- Common symptoms are dyspnea and fatigue (low cardiac output), not orthopnea and paroxysmal nocturnal dyspnea.
- Other symptoms include the symptoms of right ventricle failure (leg edema, ascites, jaundice, etc.), cyanosis in patients with right-to-left shunt (associated ASD or patent foramen ovale), and retarded growth in children.
- Uncommon symptoms are dyspnea on exertion, angina, and symptoms due to endocarditis.
- Physical signs may include rounded plump face with isolated pulmonary stenosis, characteristic facies of Noonan's and William's syndrome, prominent or giant *a* waves in JVP, and left parasternal heave, suggestive of right ventricular hypertrophy.
- Auscultation reveals pulmonary ejection click in patients with valvular pulmonary stenosis and ejection systolic crescendo–decrescendo murmur usually best heard at the left second to fourth intercostal space (ICS).
- With mild stenosis A2 and P2 are well heard and widely split, but as stenosis becomes severe, P2 is delayed and softer and may be inaudible.
- With multiple peripheral pulmonary stenosis, P2 may be very loud.

IMAGING STUDIES

- ECG
  —May show right atrial abnormality, P pulmonale, incomplete or complete right bundle branch block, right axis deviation, and right ventricular hypertrophy
- Echocardiogram
  —The congenital pulmonary stenosis is usually characterized by fusion of the valve cusps and an incompletely formed raphe resulting in a domelike structure with a narrowed orifice.
  —Typically the valve annulus is normal in size.
  —In adults 2-D echo usually shows a thickened cusp with decreased excursion with doming during systole.
  —Poststenotic pulmonary dilatation is frequently evident, but its presence does not correlate with severity.
  —Doppler best assesses severity across the stenotic valve and assessment of peak instantaneous pressure gradient.

PATHOLOGY

Most patients with stenosis have a conical or dome-shaped pulmonary valve formed by fusion of valve leaflets.

SPECIAL TESTS

- Chest x-ray may show poststenotic dilatation of the pulmonary artery with oligemic lung fields, right ventricular hypertrophy, and right atrial enlargement.
- Cardiac catheterization confirms pressure gradient across stenotic pulmonary valve, and digital substraction or selective pulmonary angiography defines exact location, extent, and distribution of lesions in patients with peripheral pulmonary artery stenosis.

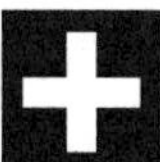

Treatment

GENERAL MEASURES

- Mild pulmonary stenosis is benign disease and usually does not require any treatment or intervention.
- Symptomatic patients with pulmonary stenosis and asymptomatic patients with moderate to severe stenosis (peak-to-peak gradient of >50 mm Hg) may be treated with balloon valvuloplasty, which is the procedure of choice for a typically domed, thickened valve.

SURGICAL MEASURES

Surgery is required for a dysplastic valve, as seen in Noonan's syndrome or patients with subinfundibular or peripheral pulmonary artery stenosis.

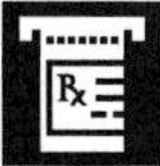

Medications

No medications shown to be effective.

DRUG(S) OF CHOICE

Precautions

- None

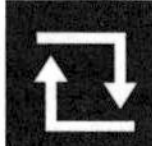

Follow-up

PATIENT MONITORING

- ECG and echocardiography in patients with moderate to severe pulmonary stenosis at interval of 3 years

EXPECTED COURSE AND PROGNOSIS

- Very good for patients with mild pulmonary stenosis
- Long-term data not available on balloon valvuloplasty but mid-term data (10 years) suggest results similar to surgical valvuloplasty

PATIENT EDUCATION

- Very low risk for infective endocarditis, except probably patients with severe pulmonary stenosis

Activity

- Applicable on patients with right ventricle failure.

Diet

- Low-sodium diet in patients with fluid overload

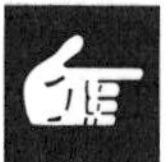

Miscellaneous

ICD-9-CM

424.3

BIBLIOGRAPHY

Alexander RW, ed. *Hurst's the heart.* New York: McGraw-Hill, 1998.

Bonow et al. ACC/AHA guidelines for the management of patients with valvular heart disease. *J Am Coll Cardiol* 1998;32:1486–1588.

Braunwald E, ed. *Heart disease: a textbook of cardiovascular medicine,* 5th ed. Philadelphia: WB Saunders, 1997.

Feigenbaum H, ed. *Echocardiography,* 5th ed. Baltimore: Williams & Wilkins, 1993.

Authors: Steven Herrmann, Amr El-Shafei, Madhukar Gupta, and Bernard R. Chaitman

Pulmonary Stenosis, Pediatric

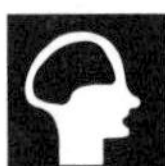

Basics

DESCRIPTION

Pulmonary stenosis (PS) is defined as obstruction to outflow from the right ventricle due to obstruction at the level of the pulmonary valve, the right ventricular outflow tract, or the branch pulmonary arteries.

System Affected

- Cardiovascular

Incidence

- Valvar PS is the second most common congenital heart lesion, occurring in 8%–12% of patients with congenital heart disease.
- Infundibular stenosis with an intact ventricular septum is rarely seen and accounts for only 5% of all cases of right ventricular outflow tract obstruction.
- Peripheral pulmonary artery stenosis (PPS), occurs in several forms, from a single obstructive lesion in the branch pulmonary arteries, to multiple lesions along the right and left pulmonary arteries, to branch pulmonary artery hypoplasia.
- Rarely an isolated lesion
- Neonatal PPS is transient, but has a reported incidence as high as 75%.

ETIOLOGY

Genetics

- Noonan's syndrome
  - —50% of patients have heart disease.
  - —75% of these have valvar PS with thickened dysplastic pulmonary valve leaflets.
- William's syndrome
  - —50% of the patients have cardiac defects; PPS is reported.
- Rubella syndrome
  - —50%–80% have heart disease, with PPS and patent ductus arteriosus being the most common lesions.

Predominant Age

- Congenital; murmur is heard shortly after birth

Sex

- Males and females are affected equally.

Diagnosis

DIFFERENTIAL DIAGNOSIS

- Valvar PS in the asymptomatic child must be differentiated from an atrial septal defect (ASD).
- The murmur is similar, but with an ASD there is a right ventricular impulse, a wide and fixed split of the second heart sound, and a mid-diastolic flow murmur over the tricuspid valve.
- There is mild cardiomegaly and the pulmonary vascular markings are increased on chest x-ray; the echocardiogram demonstrates the defect in the atrial septum.
- In the cyanotic infant with critical PS, tetralogy of Fallot reveals a similar picture.
- The echocardiogram demonstrates the large ventral septal defect that is part of tetralogy of Fallot.

SIGNS AND SYMPTOMS

- Valvar PS
  - —Children with valvar PS and an intact septum are asymptomatic and enjoy normal growth and development.
  - —The defect is discovered on auscultation soon after birth.
  - —There is no cyanosis.
  - —An ejection systolic murmur is heard at the left upper sternal border.
  - —The peak intensity of the systolic murmur is proportional to the severity of the obstruction.
  - —A systolic thrill may be palpated in the same area.
  - —The second heart sound is normal.
  - —An ejection click is often present early in systole.
  - —ECG reveals right axis deviation with right ventricular hypertrophy proportional to the amount of obstruction.
  - —The chest x-ray reveals normal heart size and pulmonary vascular markings.
  - —A prominent main pulmonary artery segment secondary to poststenotic dilatation of the pulmonary artery is common.
  - —Echocardiography reveals an abnormal pulmonary valve with a gradient estimated by Doppler echocardiography.
  - —Right ventricular hypertrophy may or may not be present depending on the severity of the obstruction.
- Critical valvar PS with intact ventricular septum presents in the neonatal period.
  - —The infant is cyanotic and right ventricular pressure is systemic or greater.
  - —Cyanosis results from right-to-left shunting across the foramen ovale.
  - —Long ejection systolic murmur with late peaking at left upper sternal border
  - —Second heart sound may be obscured by murmur.
  - —If cardiac output is compromised (in the most severe cases), murmur may be diminished.
  - —ECG reveals marked right axis deviation and right ventricular hypertrophy with strain.
  - —Chest x-ray reveals diminished pulmonary vascular markings and mild cardiomegaly.
  - —Echocardiography reveals thickened pulmonary valvar leaflets that dome in systole.
  - —A gradient across the valve can be estimated by Doppler echo. (See the Appendix for the table on Classification of Severity of PS.)
- PPS in the neonate
  - —Caused by flow acceleration at the acute angle of the bifurcation of the pulmonary artery into right and left branches
  - —This angle becomes less acute with growth and usually disappears by 2 months of age.
  - —Short grade 2/6 mid-systolic murmur at cardiac base
  - —Murmur radiates to axillae and back.
  - —No cardiac symptoms

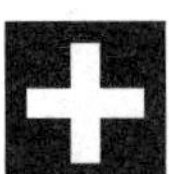

Treatment

GENERAL MEASURES

- Patients with mild PS do not require intervention.
- There is no need for cardiac catheterization, and the lesion does not tend to progress.
- When the PS is of moderate severity, patients undergo elective cardiac catheterization with anticipated balloon valvuloplasty.
- When the PS is severe, cardiac catheterization with interventional balloon valvuloplasty is recommended on an urgent basis.
- In the infant with critical PS, urgent balloon valvuloplasty is recommended. Prior to the procedure, the infant should be stabilized with a prostaglandin infusion, and any acidosis should be corrected.
- If valvuloplasty fails, emergent surgery to open the valve is necessary.

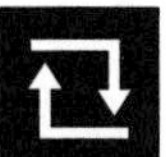

Follow-up

PATIENT MONITORING

- Children with mild pulmonary valve stenosis are followed as outpatients every 1–2 years with clinical examination, ECG, and periodic echocardiograms.
- There is no need for restriction in physical activity.

EXPECTED COURSE AND PROGNOSIS

- Patients with untreated moderate PS should be mildly restricted and followed as outpatients once or twice a year to assess progression of the stenosis.
- Following relief of the stenosis, unrestricted activity may be pursued.
- Patients with severe PS should be moderately restricted prior to valvuloplasty/surgery.
- Six months later, with evidence of relief of the obstruction, unrestricted activity is permitted.

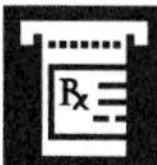

Medications

DRUG(S) OF CHOICE

- Bacterial endocarditis prophylaxis
- Prophylaxis is recommended by the AHA for all patients with PS. The incidence of BE is negligible (5.6/10,000 patient-years).

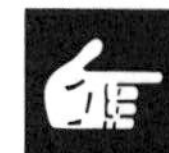

Miscellaneous

BIBLIOGRAPHY

Fyler DC, ed. *Nadas' pediatric cardiology*. Philadelphia: Hanley & Belfus, 1992:459–470.

Garson A Jr, Bricker JT, McNamara DG. Science and practice of pediatric cardiology. Vol. 2. Philadelphia: Lea & Fibiger, 1990:1382–1420.

Gersony WM, Hayes CJ, et al. Bacterial endocarditis in patients with aortic stenosis, pulmonary stenosis, or ventricular septal defect. In the report of the Second Natural History Study of Congenital Heart Defects (NHS-2). *Circulation* 87(suppl):121–126.

Hayes CJ, Gersony WM, et al. Results of treatment of patients with pulmonary stenosis. In the report of the Second Natural History Study of Congenital Heart Defects (NHS-2). *Circulation* 87(suppl):28–37.

Authors: Constance J. Hayes and Welton M. Gersony

Radiation Heart Disease

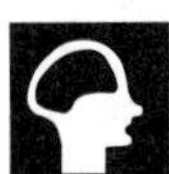

Basics

DESCRIPTION

- Radiation-induced heart disease may involve:
  - —Pericardium: effusion, scarring, constriction or tamponade; pericarditis is the most common cardiac manifestation of radiation injury
  - —Myocardium: myocardial infarction and left ventricular failure
  - —Coronary arteries: plaque formation, thrombosis, acute myocardial infarction and vessel rupture
  - —Conduction system: arrhythmias and conduction disorders
  - —Heart valves: mitral regurgitation
- Damage may present acutely or as long as 20 years after radiation exposure. It may be difficult to differentiate from clinical presentation of malignancy.

EPIDEMIOLOGY

- 10% of all patients requiring drainage of pericardial effusions have radiation-induced heart disease. Most are commonly associated with:
  - —Hodgkin's lymphoma: mantle field therapy associated with 5%–20% incidence of pericarditis
  - —Non-Hodgkin's lymphoma
  - —Breast carcinoma: <5% incidence of pericarditis
  - —Other thoracic tumors, including thymoma and tumors of the lung and esophagus (15% incidence of pericarditis)

ETIOLOGY

- Pericardial disease
  - —Direct damage (fibrosis of the parietal pericardium), hypersensitivity, vasculitis (fibrinous exudate results from damaged vessels)
- Myocardial disease
  - —Acute changes include inflammation and endothelial damage.
  - —Delayed changes include patches of fibrosis and scarring leading to interstitial myocardial fibrosis, usually of the anterior left ventricular and right ventricular walls.
- Coronary artery disease
  - —Endothelial damage
- Conduction system
  - —Secondary to ischemic fibrosis
- Heart valves
  - —Distortion secondary to fibrosis near valve rings

RISK FACTORS

- Radiation dose, volume of heart in radiation field, radiation fractionation, treatment duration, radiation source, anterior weighting of radiation
- Mediastinal radiation for Hodgkin's disease exposes a larger proportion of the heart than the treatment of breast carcinoma. Consequently, there are fewer cardiac complications in treatment of the latter, which can tolerate higher doses and longer duration of radiation.

PREGNANCY

N/A

ASSOCIATED CONDITIONS

- Pericardial disease
  - —Pericardial effusions, chronic constrictive pericarditis (effusion organizes and adheres)
- Myocardial disease
  - —Restrictive cardiomyopathy
- Coronary artery disease
  - —Premature atherosclerosis

Diagnosis

DIFFERENTIAL DIAGNOSIS

- Pericardial disease
  - —Effusion must be differentiated from that of malignancy. Effusions are usually larger, with tamponade more likely in malignant accumulations.
  - —Viral pericarditis
  - —Effusion secondary to radiation-induced hypothyroidism
- Myocardial disease
  - —Viral cardiomyopathy, drug-induced cardiomyopathy
- Coronary artery disease
  - —Ischemic heart disease

SIGNS AND SYMPTOMS

- Pericardial disease
  - —Acute pericarditis/effusion: usually not clinically evident. Symptoms include pain and malaise. Signs include fever, friction rub, and EKG abnormalities.
  - —Delayed pericarditis: may present as asymptomatic pericardial effusion with pleural effusions on chest x-ray; 50% of patients have dyspnea, jugular venous distension, and pulsus paradoxus
- Myocardial disease
  - —Results from constriction and severe heart failure
  - —May not be evident until after failed pericardiectomy
- Coronary artery disease
  - —Angina, acute myocardial infarction

LABORATORY PROCEDURES

- Pericardial fluid: routine infectious disease studies, and cytology to rule out malignant cells

IMAGING STUDIES

- Pericarditis/pericardial effusions
  - —ECG: ST-segment elevation throughout the precordium
  - —Chest x-ray: pleural effusions with delayed pericarditis
  - —Echocardiography: pericardial fluid accumulation

SPECIAL TESTS

- Pericardiocentesis: Effusion may be serous, serosanguineous, or hemorrhagic, with a high protein and lymphocyte content.
- Right heart catheterization

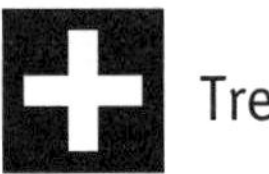

Treatment

GENERAL MEASURES

- According to presentation

SURGICAL MEASURES

- Pericardial effusions with hemodynamic compromise may require pericardial decompression/window, or pericardectomy for constrictive pericarditis.
- Operative mortality 21% versus 8% in idiopathic disease.
- Bypass surgery may be complicated by internal mammary artery damage or mediastinal fibrosis.

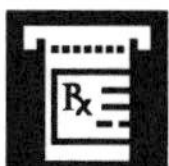

Medications

DRUG(S) OF CHOICE

- Nonsteroidal antiinflammatory drugs to control pain associated with early inflammation or effusion
- Corticosteroids reserved for use in severe pain

ADMISSION/DISCHARGE CRITERIA

Correlate with presentation.

Follow-up

PATIENT MONITORING

Asymptomatic pericardial effusions may be followed by physical examination and serial echo

EXPECTED COURSE AND PROGNOSIS

- Acute pericarditis usually terminates abruptly, is not treatment limiting and does not predict chronic changes.
- Pleural effusion treated surgically with a window has a late constriction rate near 75%.
- After pericardectomy, the 5-year survival rate is 51% (vs. 83% in nonradiation patients).
- Restrictive cardiomyopathy carries a poor prognosis.

PATIENT EDUCATION

Organizations

- American Heart Association National Center, 7272 Greenville Avenue, Dallas TX 75231; 1-800-AHA-USA1; www.americanheart.org

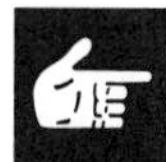

Miscellaneous

BIBLIOGRAPHY

Lorell BH. Pericardial diseases in heart disease. In: Braunwald E, ed. *A textbook of cardiovascular medicine,* 5th ed. Philadelphia: WB Saunders, 1997:1484–1534.

Selwyn AP. The cardiovascular system and radiation. *Lancet* 1983;2:152–154.

Stewart JR, Fajardo LF, Gillette SM, et al. Radiation injury to the heart. *Int J Radiat Oncol Biol Phys* 1995;31:1205–1211.

Author: Cheryl Russo

Renal Artery Stenosis

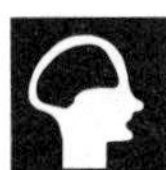

Basics

DESCRIPTION

Renal artery stenosis (RAS) is narrowing of the main renal artery and/or its major branches. Renovascular hypertension, the most common curable form of systemic hypertension, is composed of RAS and renal ischemia.

EPIDEMIOLOGY

- Occurs in up to 5% of the general population
- Accounts for 10%–45% of acute, severe, or refractory hypertension
- Age <20 years, usually female [fibromuscular dysplasia (FMD)]
- Age >45 years, men affected more than women

ETIOLOGY

- Atherosclerosis: usually involves the proximal one-third of the renal artery; also may be due to aortic atheroma encroaching on the renal artery ostium
- FMD: most common cause of renovascular hypertension in younger (primarily female) patients

Genetics

- Uncertain; may play a role in FMD

RISK FACTORS

- Age
- Coexisting atheromatous disease
- Tobacco use

PREGNANCY

N/A

ASSOCIATED CONDITIONS

- Atherosclerosis
- Malignant hypertension
- Ischemic nephropathy

Diagnosis

DIFFERENTIAL DIAGNOSIS

Intrinsic

- Renal segmental infarction
- Cholesterol embolus
- Takayasu's arteritis
- Polyarteritis nodosa
- Aneurysm of the renal artery
- Radiation-induced fibrosis
- Arterial embolus

Extrinsic

- Tumor (e.g., pheochromocytoma)
- Cysts
- Neurofibromatosis

SIGNS AND SYMPTOMS

- Hypertension in persons <20 or >50 years of age
- Acute-onset hypertension
- Hypertension resistant to drug therapy
- Azotemia with angiotensin-converting enzyme (ACE) inhibitors
- Abdominal bruit (40%); other bruits
- Hemorrhagic (grade III or IV) retinopathy
- Pulmonary edema

LABORATORY PROCEDURES

- Azotemia (if bilateral kidney involvement)
- Hypokalemia
- Proteinuria
- Elevated plasma renin activity

IMAGING STUDIES

- Renal scan: high false-negative rate (20%–25%)
- Captopril scan: sensitivity 92%, specificity 93%; positive and negative predictive values in high-risk populations approach 85%–90%; may miss bilateral disease
- Intravenous pyelogram: Findings include a decreased renal size and delayed caliceal appearance time when compared with the contralateral kidney (for unilateral stenosis); sensitivity 75%–80%, specificity 85%; may miss bilateral disease.
- Duplex ultrasonography: high positive and negative predictive values in a high-risk population (97%); however, it is time consuming and highly operator dependent
- Renal arteriography: currently the gold standard test
- Digital subtraction angiography: high dye load, injected centrally; sensitivity 88%, specificity 90%
- Magnetic resonance angiography: sensitivity of 90%–100% and specificity of 71%–96% for proximal artery stenoses of >50% stenosis (using renal arteriography as the reference standard).
- Spiral CT with contrast injection: sensitivity 98%, specificity 94%; accuracy may be lower in patients with creatinine >1.7 mg/dL due to reduced renal blood flow

SPECIAL TESTS

- Plasma renin activity
- Renal vein renin level
- Captopril test

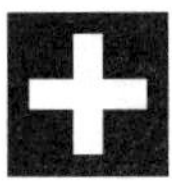

Treatment

GENERAL MEASURES

- Low suspicion for RAS: no further evaluation
- Moderate suspicion for RAS: noninvasive testing
- High suspicion for RAS: renal arteriogram or equivalent

MEDICAL MANAGEMENT

- Primary therapy for the patient with atherosclerotic disease who is considered not to be a candidate for renal artery revascularization
- Blood pressure control, lipid-lowering therapy, monitoring of renal function

SURGICAL MEASURES

- Surgery: primary indication for age <50–60 years (unilateral), age <60 years with renal insufficiency or diffuse or severe stenosis (bilateral)
  - —Aortorenal bypass (preferred)
  - —Endarterectomy
  - —Partial nephrectomy
- Renal angioplasty: primary therapy for FMD; also consider for nonsurgical candidate; increasing use as a general first approach prior to surgery
- Percutaneous angioplasty with or without stent

ADMISSION/DISCHARGE CRITERIA

N/A

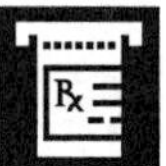

Medications

DRUG(S) OF CHOICE

- ACE inhibitors (with unilateral stenosis)
- Beta-antagonist
- Thiazide diuretic (with bilateral stenosis)
- Calcium channel antagonist
- Clonidine
- Lipid-lowering medications

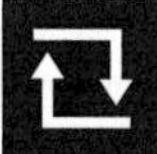

Follow-up

PATIENT MONITORING

Patients treated medically should be followed closely for continued or worsening hypertension, medication side effects, progressive atrophy of the kidney distal to the stenosis, and developing or worsening azotemia.

EXPECTED COURSE AND PROGNOSIS

- Surgical/angioplasty intervention
  —FMD: 58%–80% cured (diastolic blood pressure <90 mm Hg without medications); 35%–75% improved (15% decrease in diastolic blood pressure but still requiring medications); 7%–10% failed (<15% decrease in diastolic blood pressure)
  —Atheroma: 15%–22% cured, 57%–75% improved, and 10%–21% failed. Restenosis rate in atheromatous disease is 19%–25%, and 35% if the lesion is ostial.

PATIENT EDUCATION

- Cardiac and renal prudent diets.

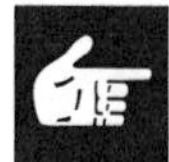

Miscellaneous

ICD-9-CM

440.1 Renal artery stenosis
401.9 Hypertension
402.01 Malignant hypertension

BIBLIOGRAPHY

Leier CV. Renal disorders and heart disease. In: Braunwald E, ed. *Heart disease: a textbook of cardiovascular medicine,* 5th ed. Philadelphia: WB Saunders, 1997:1914–1938.

Pickering TG. Renal artery disease. In: Topol EJ, ed. *Comprehensive cardiovascular medicine.* Philadelphia: Lippincott-Raven, 1998:3135–3150.

Pohl MA. Renal artery stenosis, renal vascular hypertension, and ischemic nephropathy. In: Schrier RW, Gottschalk CW, eds. *Diseases of the kidney,* 6th ed. Boston: Little, Brown, 1997: 1367–1423.

Author: David S. Bader

Renal Failure

Basics

DESCRIPTION

Renal failure is defined as progressive and irreversible destruction of the nephrons, regardless of cause, occurring over 3–6 months.

- Cardiac disease is the major cause (>40%) of mortality in patients with end-stage renal disease (ESRD). Cardiac arrest and acute myocardial infarction are the most common major cardiovascular events.
- Arrhythmia, left ventricular (LV) dysfunction, pericarditis, atherosclerotic and valvular heart disease are also prevalent.

EPIDEMIOLOGY

- In 1997, ESRD affected 2,947 per million U.S. population.
- The predominant age group is ≥65 years old.
- Males are affected more often than females.
- Blacks are affected more often than whites, who are affected more often than Asians.

ETIOLOGY

- Diabetes
- Hypertension
- Renovascular disease
- Glomerulonephritis
- Cystic kidney
- Other urologic causes

RISK FACTORS

Among patients with renal failure, there is a greater prevalence of the conventional cardiac risk factors.

- Diabetes
- Hypertension
- Tobacco
- Hyperlipidemia
- Male gender
- Family history of coronary artery disease (CAD)
- Obesity
- Metabolic abnormalities

PREGNANCY

N/A

ASSOCIATED CONDITIONS

- Anemia: diminished myocardial oxygen supply; increased cardiac workload
- Congestive heart failure (CHF)
  - —Approximately 35% of ESRD patients
  - —Both systolic and diastolic LV dysfunction
  - —Probability of developing pulmonary edema requiring hospitalization after the initiation of dialysis is 10% per year.
- Left ventricular hypertrophy (LVH): closely linked with hypertension, anemia, and pulmonary edema
- Dyslipidemia: elevated triglycerides and lipoprotein (a); lowered HDL cholesterol
- Hypertension: Either as a cause of renal failure or secondary to ESRD
- Pericarditis: approximately 10% of hemodialysis patients
- Valvular heart disease
  - —Aortic calcification 30%–55%
  - —Hemodynamically significant aortic stenosis 10%
  - —Mitral calcification 25%–50%
  - —Calcific mitral stenosis: rare
  - —Mitral regurgitation: common

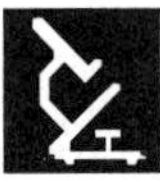

Diagnosis

DIFFERENTIAL DIAGNOSIS

N/A

SIGNS AND SYMPTOMS

The diagnosis of an acute coronary syndrome may be difficult in patients with renal failure

- Classical angina pectoris may not be present, as in the case of diabetic nephropathy.
- Silent ischemia may be present (15%–35%).
- Many patients have nonatherosclerotic ischemic heart disease with typical symptoms of angina pectoris, but with patent coronary arteries.
- Baseline ECG abnormalities secondary to LVH or electrolyte abnormalities are prevalent, limiting accurate assessment of myocardial ischemia.

LABORATORY PROCEDURES

- Cardiac troponin T and creatinine kinase and MB fraction often elevated in patients with renal failure, without evidence of myocardial ischemia/injury (false positive).
- Cardiac troponin I is a sensitive marker of myocardial ischemia/injury in renal failure.

IMAGING STUDIES

- Cardiac catheterization is the gold standard for defining coronary vasculature. This may lead to contrast-induced nephropathy (CIN), defined as an increase in creatinine of ≥1.0 mg/dL.
  - —Incidence ~10%
  - —Begins within 24–48 hours
  - —Peaks in 3–5 days
  - —Return to baseline creatinine in 7–10 days
  - —Need for temporary dialysis is uncommon
  - —Potential risks for developing CIN
    - Preexisting renal insufficiency
    - Diabetes
    - Volume depletion
    - Age
    - CHF
    - Hypertension
    - Dose of contrast (controversial)
    - High osmolarity contrast agent (controversial)
- Exercise ECG test: limited role due to high prevalence of abnormal baseline ECGs
- Exercise and dipyridamole nuclear imaging tests
  - —High incidence of abnormal resting nuclear images in patients with ESRD
  - —False-positive results with diffuse myocardial hypertrophy (may mimic a lateral wall myocardial infarction)
  - —Overall specificity 70%–75%, sensitivity 80%–88%, positive predictive value 70%–75%
  - —Exercise or dobutamine echocardiography: limited data available; promising for the evaluation of CAD in renal failure

SPECIAL TESTS

N/A

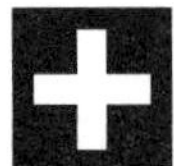

Treatment

GENERAL MEASURES

- Medical management of patients with renal failure and CAD follows the same general guidelines that have been established for patients with normal renal function.
- Specific attention is focused on the dosing of medications and careful monitoring of renal function.

Dialysis and the Cardiovascular System

- Advantages
  - —Normalizes intravascular volume
  - —Controls blood pressure
  - —Corrects metabolic abnormalities
  - —May improve LV systolic function
- Disadvantages
  - —Arteriovenous fistula increases cardiac output and may lead to high-output failure.
  - —Higher risk of infective endocarditis
  - —Dialysis-related hypotension
- ECG abnormalities and dysrhythmias during dialysis
  - —Decreased T-wave amplitude
  - —Increased QRS amplitude
  - —Prolonged or shortened QTc interval
  - —Ischemic-like ST segment and T-wave abnormalities
  - —Atrial fibrillation/flutter (28%)
  - —Ventricular ectopy (27%)
  - —Nonsustained ventricular tachycardia (20%)
- Peritoneal dialysis in CAD has the theoretical advantage of avoiding extremes in intravascular volume and electrolyte shifts, improved blood pressure control, avoidance of high-output states, and providing more constant acid–base equilibrium.

SURGICAL MEASURES

- Coronary artery bypass
  —Perioperative mortality rate of up to 10% in patients on dialysis
  —Dialysis can be performed on the day prior to surgery and immediately postoperatively or intraoperatively. Both approaches are safe and effective.
  —Risks for increased mortality and morbidity in patients with renal failure
    - Creatinine >2 mg/dL
    - Elevated blood urea nitrogen (linear relationship)
    - Acidosis
    - Electrolyte abnormalities
    - Fluid retention
    - Relative immunocompromise leading to infection
    - Bleeding secondary dysfunctional platelets
- Percutaneous transluminal coronary angioplasty and coronary stenting
  —Similar approach to the nonuremic patient
  —Initial technical results are as good, but re-stenosis rates may be higher

ADMISSION/DISCHARGE CRITERIA

N/A

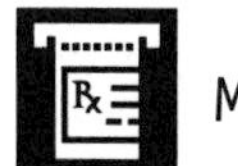

Medications

DRUG(S) OF CHOICE

Many cardiac medications are renally excreted. See standard references for a listing of renally excreted medications.

Follow-up

PATIENT MONITORING

Standard guidelines for patients with established CAD are followed. Serum creatinine should be checked 2–4 days after initiating or altering potentially nephrotoxic medications (e.g., angiotensin-converting enzyme inhibitors).

EXPECTED COURSE AND PROGNOSIS

- Patients with ischemic heart disease (IHD) and ESRD have up to 50% greater mortality than patients with ESRD alone.
- LVH, LV dilatation, and systolic dysfunction confer greater mortality independent of age, sex, diabetes, and IHD.
- Patients with CHF at baseline or at initiation of therapy for ESRD have a reported median survival of 36 months versus 62 months in those without CHF.
- Patients with recurrent CHF have a median survival of 29 months versus 45 months in those without recurrent CHF.

PATIENT EDUCATION

- Instructions regarding dietary regimen to optimize fluid and electrolyte status, particularly in those with CHF

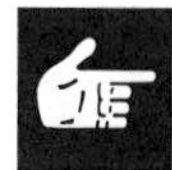

Miscellaneous

ICD-9-CM

586 Renal failure
593.9 Renal insufficiency
414.01 Coronary artery disease

BIBLIOGRAPHY

Foley RN, Harnett JD, Parfrey PS. Cardiovascular complications of end-stage renal disease. In: Schrier RW, Gottschalk CW, eds. *Diseases of the kidney,* 6th ed. Boston: Little, Brown, 1997: 2647–2660.

Hochrein J. The heart and the renal system. In: Topol EJ, ed. *Comprehensive cardiovascular medicine.* Philadelphia: Lippincott-Raven, 1998: 987–1000.

Leier CV. Renal disorders and heart disease. In: Braunwald E, ed. *Heart disease: a textbook of cardiovascular medicine,* 5th ed. Philadelphia: WB Saunders, 1997:1914–1938.

Author: David S. Bader

Rheumatic Fever

Basics

DESCRIPTION

Rheumatic fever (RF) is a systemic disease with multiorgan involvement. None of its manifestations, except for carditis, lead to permanent damage. In 1944, Jones criteria were introduced to guide the diagnosis of acute rheumatic fever (ARF). Those criteria were modified in 1956, revised in 1965 and 1984, and then updated in 1992. They are divided into major and minor criteria.

Major Criteria

- Carditis occurs in 40%–50% of the initial attacks of RF. The rheumatic process involves the endocardium, myocardium, and/or pericardium.
  —Carditis is more apt to recur if RF occurs in patients who have had carditis in the initial attack, thus increasing the risk of severe residual heart disease.
  —The term *mimetic carditis* was introduced to explain this phenomenon.
  —In the Utah outbreak of RF, 72% of the patients were diagnosed to have carditis by auscultation. Echocardiography/Doppler helped in the identification of additional 19%. The same group identified asymptomatic cardiac involvement in 47% of the patients with rheumatic polyarthritis.
- Arthritis mainly affects large joints. It moves from one joint to another, resulting in the typical picture of a migratory arthritis.
  —It occurs in about 75% of patients during the acute stage of the disease.
  —Joints are left without sequelae.
- Chorea (Sydenham's chorea or St. Vitus' dance) occurs without carditis or arthritis. It is usually associated with emotional instability. The latent period between streptococcal infection and chorea is 1–6 months. As a result, by the time the chorea is manifest, the antibodies and the acute-phase reactants are normal.
- Subcutaneous nodules
  —They range in diameter from 0.5 to 2 cm. They occur on the extensor surface of bony prominences.
  —They occur with severe carditis.
- Erythema marginatum
  —It is an area of erythema with an advancing edge and clearing center.
  —It is transient and found mainly over the trunk and inner aspects of the thighs and arms.
  —It is nonpruritic and blanches on pressure.

Minor Criteria

- Fever
- Arthralgia
- Prolonged PR interval

Laboratory Evidence Indicating Acute Infection

- Erythrocyte sedimentation rate (ESR) is almost always elevated (>60 mm/h). Congestive heart failure lowers ESR but not to normal levels.
- C-reactive protein
- Complete blood count usually demonstrates a moderate anemia. Leukocyte count is increased to moderate degree.

ETIOLOGY

Genetics

A familial clustering of RF was observed and is attributed to genetic factors that were not supported by studies of siblings and twins.

EPIDEMIOLOGY

Several epidemiologic studies over many years have demonstrated sequential relationship between the outbreaks of streptococcal pharyngitis and RF.

Prevalence

- RF is still the predominant cause of heart disease in children.
- In the United States, RF maintains its position as the leading cause of postnatally acquired heart disease in children.
- However, the United States is experiencing a dramatic decline in the incidence and prevalence of ARF.

Predominant Age

The school-age group had the highest attack rate.

CAUSES

Group A streptococci had been implicated as an initiative agent for ARF. Evidence of that is indirect and includes the following:

- Immunologic evidence: Initial as well as recurrent attacks of RF do not occur without a streptococcal antibody response.
- Clinical evidence: Septic sore throat preceding ARF and its recurrences has been recognized clinically for over 100 years.
- Prophylactic evidence: Convincing evidence is provided by the prevention of RF by penicillin therapy.

RISK FACTORS

- The school-age group had the highest attack rate.
- A familial clustering of RF was observed and is attributed to genetic factors that were not supported by studies of siblings and twins.
- However, two lymphocytes alloantigens have been identified in the sera of patients with well-documented RF in the past.

PREGNANCY

ARF tends to recur during pregnancy.

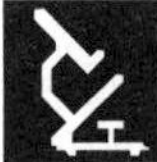

Diagnosis

DIFFERENTIAL DIAGNOSIS

- Fever and arthritis
  —Juvenile rheumatoid arthritis
  —Infective endocarditis
  —Sickle cell anemia
  —Polyarthritis
  —Immune complex disease
- Carditis
  —Functional murmurs
  —Myocarditis
  —Pericarditis
  —Mitral valve prolapse

SIGNS AND SYMPTOMS

- Requirement for diagnosis are two major criteria or one major plus one minor criteria. Evidence of recent streptococcal infection is an essential part of the diagnosis according to the updated criteria.
- Signs and symptoms of CHF in cases of carditis
- The unequivocal signs of carditis in a patient with RF are:
  —An organic heart murmur that was not previously present
  —Pericardial friction rub or effusion
  —Cardiac enlargement with or without heart failure.
- Arthralgia and arthritis
- Chorea
  —There is involuntary, uncoordinated, purposeless movement.
  —The tongue is affected with an inability to keep it protruded.
  —The handgrip is often unsustained (milkmaid hands).
  —Flexion of the wrist together with dorsiflexion of the interphalangeal joints gives "silver fork" deformity.
- Skin manifestations: subcutaneous nodules and erythema marginatum
- Fever

PATHOLOGY

Two main lesions characterize RF.

- Exudative-degenerative lesion
  —Consists of edema of the ground substance and fragmentation of collagen fibers as well as cellular infiltrate
  —Persists for 2–3 weeks and responds to antiinflammatory agents
- Proliferative lesion (Aschoff's nodule)
  —The myocardial nodule is usually oval in shape.
  —There is a paravascular aggregation of large multinucleated cells with basophilic cytoplasm.
  —Many of them have a characteristic owl-eye nucleus.
  —The origin of those nodules is controversial.

IMAGING STUDIES

Echocardiography might allow earlier diagnosis but ultimately may not prove to be superior.

SPECIAL TESTS

- Rapid detection of group A streptococci with specificity of ≥95% and more rapid identification of their presence in upper respiratory infection.
- Because the test has a low sensitivity, the negative test requires a throat culture confirmation.

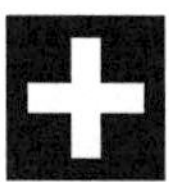

Treatment

GENERAL MEASURES

N/A

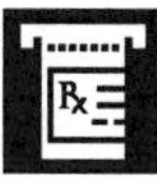

Medications

DRUG(S) OF CHOICE

- Benzathine: 600,000 units for patients weighing <60 pounds (i.m. once)
- Penicillin G: 1,200,000 units for patients weighing >60 pounds
- Aspirin
  - —Indicated in patients with arthritis, and usually results in rapid resolution of symptoms and signs
  - —The usual dosage is 90–120 mg/kg/day divided given at 4-hour intervals.
- Corticosteroids: Steroids result in rapid resolution of the inflammatory process, but there is no evidence that it terminates the disease or prevents residual damage.

ALTERNATE DRUGS

- Sulfadiazine
  - —0.5 g once daily for patients weighing <60 pounds
  - —1 g once daily for patients weighing >60 pounds
- Erythromycin: 250 mg twice daily (orally)
- For individuals allergic to penicillin:
  - —Erythromycin: 20–49 mg/kg/day (orally for 10 days)
  - —Azithromycin (orally, for 5 days)
    - 500 mg on first day
    - 250 mg/day for the next 4 days

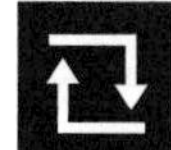

Follow-up

PATIENT MONITORING

- Patients should be monitored closely for evidence of heart failure.
- The sedimentation rate as well as C-reactive protein can be followed as a marker of activity.

Prevention

- Primary prevention: Prompt recognition and treatment represent primary RF prevention.
- Secondary prevention: For patients who have had a previous episode of RF, continuous antistreptococcal prophylaxis results in secondary prevention.
  - —Benzathine: 1,200,000 units for patients weighing <60 pounds i.m. every 4 weeks
  - —Penicillin G: 1,200,000 units for patients weighing >60 pounds every 3 weeks
- Duration
  - —RF with carditis or residual cardiac lesion: ≥10 years since the last episode at least till the age of 40 years
  - —RF with carditis but no residual cardiac lesion: 10 years or until adulthood, whichever is longer
  - —RF without carditis: 5 years or until the age of 21 years, whichever is longer

Complications

- Rheumatic valvular heart disease
- Congestive heart failure
- Recurrent ARF

EXPECTED COURSE AND PROGNOSIS

The presence or absence of carditis is an important determinant of the course and prognosis of ARF.

PATIENT EDUCATION

Diet

- No special diet unless heart failure is evident

Activity

- Patients must remain in bed during the acute febrile episode.
- Light activity can be allowed once the acute febrile episode is over.
- Patients with carditis should have rest until the signs of cardiac inflammation subside.

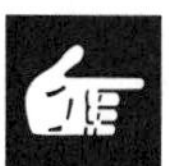

Miscellaneous

ICD-9-CM

391.0

See also: Individual valvular heart diseases

BIBLIOGRAPHY

Bonow RO, Carabello B, de Leon AC Jr, et al. ACC/AHA guidelines for the management of patients with valvular heart disease: a report of the American College of Cardiology/American Heart Association Task Force on Practice Guidelines (Committee on Management of Patients with Valvular Heart Disease). *J Am Coll Cardiol* 1998;32:1486–1588.

Kaplan EL. *Hurst's the heart,* 9th ed. New York: McGraw-Hill, 1998.

Otto C. *Valvular heart disease,* 1st ed. Philadelphia: WB Saunders, 1999.

Authors: Amr El-Shafei, Steven Herrmann, Madhukar Gupta, and Bernard R. Chaitman

Rheumatoid Arthritis

Basics

DESCRIPTION

Cardiac manifestations include the following:

- Pericarditis: a spectrum from asymptomatic disease to cardiac compression
- Valvular disease, usually regurgitation; in order of decreasing prevalence, mitral, aortic, tricuspid, and pulmonary
- Coronary arteritis (rarely causes significant dysfunction)
- Myocarditis
- Conduction pathway disease (most commonly first-degree heart block)
- Aortic arch disease
- Pulmonary hypertension

EPIDEMIOLOGY

- Pericarditis
  - —Most common cardiac lesion in rheumatoid arthritis (RA) patients
  - —11%–50% of patients have pericarditis.
  - —<1% develop cardiac compression
- Valvular
  - —At autopsy, rheumatoid granulomata involve valves in 3%–5% of patients.
  - —Echocardiography reveals 13% with mitral valve abnormalities.
- Coronary arteritis
  - —At autopsy, up to 20% of RA patients have coronary arteritis.
- Myocarditis
  - —Up to 20% of patients have nonspecific, focal myocarditis.
- Conduction disease
  - —Up to 10% of patients have various degrees of heart block.
- Aortic arch disease
  - —At autopsy, up to 5% of patients have involvement.
  - —Complicated by aneurysm formation

ETIOLOGY

In general, disease is fibrinous, granulomatous, and complement mediated.

- Pericarditis
  - —Fibrinous pericarditis
  - —Fibrous adhesions
  - —Rheumatoid granuloma/nodular type changes
- Valvular disease
  - —Nonspecific valvulitis with diffuse thickening and fibrosis
  - —Spares peripheral portions of the valve
  - —May be identical to rheumatoid nodule versus nongranulomatous valve inflammation
- Vascular disease
  - —Involvement usually limited to smaller intramyocardial arteries
  - —Pulmonary vasculitis
- Cardiomyopathy
  - —Drug-induced
  - —Myocarditis

RISK FACTORS

Pericarditis is associated with acute disease with other extraarticular involvement, usually in seropositive patients.

PREGNANCY

N/A

ASSOCIATED CONDITIONS

- Pleural effusion (found in half of patients with pericarditis and cardiac compression)
- Pericardial effusion
- Bacterial endocarditis (rarely, in association with valvular disease)

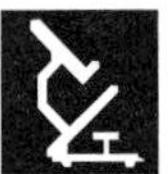

Diagnosis

DIFFERENTIAL DIAGNOSIS

- Pericardial disease
  - —Pericarditis (infectious, idiopathic)
  - —Pericardial effusion (infectious, inflammatory, idiopathic, neoplastic, radiation-induced)
- Valvular disease
  - —Endocarditis
  - —Liebman-Sachs
  - —Mitral valve prolapse
  - —Acute valvular incompetence
- Myocardial disease
  - —Ischemic
  - —Drug-induced
  - —Alcohol-related
  - —Infiltrative disorders

SIGNS AND SYMPTOMS

- Cardiac disease is often clinically inconspicuous and rarely life threatening.
- Often "silent heart disease" with three alterations typical of RA patients in absence of symptoms: posterior pericardial effusion, aortic root alterations, valvular thickening
- Pericarditis: chest pain, peripheral edema, orthopnea, friction rub, pericardial effusion (edema, dyspnea, tamponade, pulsus paradoxus)

LABORATORY PROCEDURES

- Tests for rheumatoid arthritis
- Rheumatoid factor, inflammatory indices (erythrocyte sedimentation rate, C-reactive protein)

IMAGING STUDIES

- ECG: first-degree atrioventricular block, precordial ST segment elevation with pericarditis
- Echocardiography: pericardial effusion, valvular disease, cardiomyopathy

SPECIAL TESTS

- Pericardiocentesis: Pericardial fluid reveals low glucose, low complement, variable white blood cell stain, culture, and sensitivities (acid fast bacillus, fungal)

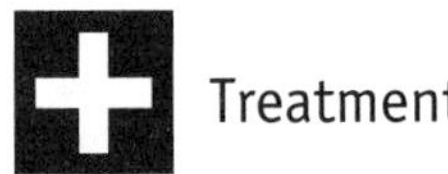

Treatment

GENERAL MEASURES

- Pericarditis: usually resolves with aggressive medical therapy for RA [steroids, nonsteroidal antiinflammatory drugs (NSAIDs), disease-modifying agents]
- Cardiomyopathy: appropriate heart failure medicines

SURGICAL MEASURES

- Pericardial effusion with compression: pericardiocentesis, surgical decompression/window
- Constrictive pericarditis: pericardiectomy
- Valvular: Rarely, involvement produces hemodynamic valve incompetence requiring valve replacement.

ADMISSION/DISCHARGE CRITERIA

- Follows clinical presentation

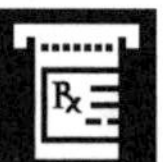

Medications

DRUG(S) OF CHOICE

- NSAIDs
- Corticosteroids
- Disease-modifying agents
- Immunosuppressives

Follow-up

PATIENT MONITORING

- Pericarditis: Watch for recurrence (15%) or pericardial effusion.

EXPECTED COURSE AND PROGNOSIS

- Pericarditis: favorable, although marker for decreased survival

PATIENT EDUCATION

Organization

- Arthritis Foundation, 1330 West Peachtree Street, Atlanta, GA 30309; www.arthritis.org

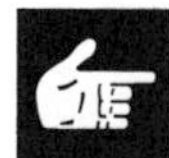

Miscellaneous

BIBLIOGRAPHY

Coblyn JS, Weinblatt ME. Rheumatic diseases and the heart. In: Braunwald E, ed. *A textbook of cardiovascular medicine,* 5th ed. Philadelphia: WB Saunders, 1997:1776–1778.

Corrao S, Sallí L, et al. Cardiac involvement in rheumatoid arthritis: evidence of silent heart disease. *Eur Heart J* 1995;16:253–256.

Mione S, Valentini G, Giunta A, et al. Cardiac involvement in RA: an echocardiographic study. *Cardiology* 1993;83:234–239.

Author: Cheryl Russo

Sarcoidosis and the Heart

Basics

DESCRIPTION

Cardiac involvement occurs in 25% of patients with systemic sarcoidosis and includes:

- Congestive heart failure (CHF): right-sided secondary to pulmonary disease; left-sided includes systolic and diastolic disease; global versus segmental abnormalities
- Chest pain: associated with abnormal functional study and normal angiogram
- Pericardial disease: rare, yet may be complicated by constriction or tamponade
- Valvular disease: secondary to papillary muscle involvement
- Conduction abnormality: Complete heart block is the most common clinical manifestation of cardiac involvement; right and left bundle branch block also may be seen.
- Ventricular arrhythmias: Ventricular tachycardia is the second most common presentation.
- Ventricular aneurysms: more common on the left than the right
- Coronary artery damage involving the intramural arteries

EPIDEMIOLOGY

Incidences include:

- CHF: 30%–40%
- Valvular involvement: <3%
- Complete heart block: 25%
- Ventricular tachycardia: 20% (11%–50%)
- Ventricular aneurysm: 8%–10%

ETIOLOGY

- No HLA type association
- Japanese disease with clinical variations: higher incidence of sudden death, and more infiltrative disease with associated high amount of replacement fibrosis
- Noncaseating granulomas involve the left ventricular free wall most often, followed by the ventricular septum, right ventricle, papillary muscle, right atrium, and left atrium.
- Surrounding involvement compresses/narrows the lumen of intramural arteries, producing chest pain. It serves as a focus for abnormal automaticity in ventricular arrhythmias. Replacement fibrosis narrows ventricular walls, increasing risk of aneurysm.

RISK FACTORS

Chronic steroid use may increase the rate of ventricular aneurysm. Ventricular aneurysms increase the risk of ventricular tachycardia.

PREGNANCY

N/A

ASSOCIATED CONDITIONS

- Hypercalcemia: secondary to sarcoidosis
- Hypokalemia: secondary to steroids

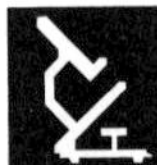

Diagnosis

DIFFERENTIAL DIAGNOSIS

- Heart failure: ischemic heart disease; other infiltrative disease (amyloid)
- Chest pain: acute myocardial infarction; pericarditis
- Conduction abnormalities: ischemic heart disease; medication-induced block

SIGNS AND SYMPTOMS

- Must have high clinical suspicion.
- Only 50% of patients with cardiac involvement of sarcoidosis are identified premortem.
- Physical examination for multiorgan involvement: skin involvement [lupus pernio (rash on nose, cheek, hands), erythema nodosum], hepatomegaly, lymphadenopathy, pulmonary involvement (dyspnea)
- Presentation ranges: asymptomatic with abnormal chest x-ray, fever, weight loss
- Cardiac presentations include complete heart block (syncope), ventricular tachycardia, heart failure, sudden death, and chest pain.

LABORATORY PROCEDURES

- Serum calcium
- Angiotensin-converting enzyme level: elevated in 80% patients with sarcoidosis

IMAGING STUDIES

- ECG: arrhythmia, conduction abnormalities
- Chest x-ray: right heart enlargement, pulmonary infiltrate, hilar adenopathy, pericardial effusion
- Echocardiography: septal thickening, pericardial effusion, ventricular dysfunction, valve regurgitation, ventricular aneurysm
- Gallium scan: active disease in lung and extrathoracic locations

SPECIAL TESTS

- Kveim-Siltzbach test, pulmonary function test, ophthalmologic examination to determine extent of sarcoid involvement
- Exercise stress test, Holter monitor for patients with cardiac involvement
- Endomyocardial biopsy: 20%–30% yield secondary to patchy disease or lower right ventricle involvement

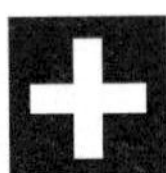

Treatment

GENERAL MEASURES

- Correlate with presentation.
- Pacemaker, defibrillator, heart failure medications, antiarrhythmic medications (caution with calcium and potassium abnormalities)

SURGICAL MEASURES

- Cardiac transplantation
- Valvular repair

ADMISSION/DISCHARGE CRITERIA

- Determined by clinical presentation
- Heart failure, arrhythmia, conduction abnormalities

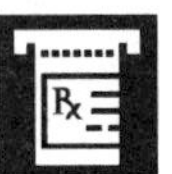

Medications

DRUG(S) OF CHOICE

Steroids are associated with aneurysm formation yet are known to change the course of the disease when started early.

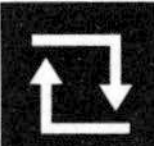

Follow-up

PATIENT MONITORING

- Physical examination
- ECG
- Holter monitor
- Echocardiography

EXPECTED COURSE AND PROGNOSIS

- In general, the mortality rate of sarcoidosis alone is low, but very high with cardiac involvement.
- Average survival with clinically significant disease is 1–2 years.
- Major causes of death are:
  —Sudden death (approaches 65% with significant disease)
- Heart failure
  —Pulmonary fibrosis
  —Pulmonary hemorrhage secondary to aspergilloma

PATIENT EDUCATION

Organization

- American Lung Association, 1740 Broadway, New York, NY 10019-4374; (212)315-8700, www.lungusa.org

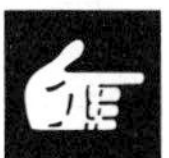

Miscellaneous

BIBLIOGRAPHY

Shammas RL, Movahed A. Sarcoidosis of the heart. *Clin Cardiol* 1993;16:462–472.

Sharma OP, Maheshwari A, Thaker K. Myocardial sarcoidosis. *Chest* 1993;103:253–258.

Author: Cheryl Russo

Scleroderma and the Heart

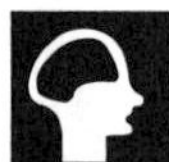

Basics

DESCRIPTION

Scleroderma is a multisystem disorder of unknown etiology characterized by cutaneous and visceral tissue fibrosis. There are two subsets:

- Diffuse or progressive systemic sclerosis (SSc) includes early and serious visceral involvement.
- Limited sclerosis (CREST; calcinosis, Raynaud's phenomenon, esophageal dysmotility, sclerodactyly, and telangiectasia) is associated with a long delay in visceral involvement. Survival is closely linked to the visceral involvement of the disease.

Conduction System Disease

- Common and often represents first manifestation of cardiac disease; may precede cutaneous lesions
- ECG abnormalities reported in up to 50% in some series (nonspecific ST-T wave, low voltage, right and left ventricular hypertrophy)
- Pseudoinfarction patterns have been observed on ECG in the posteroapical and anteroseptal regions
- Various degrees of heart block as well as rhythm disturbances (supraventricular tachycardia, ventricular tachycardia, bradyarrhythmias) common
- Fibrosis of sinoatrial node (most common), atrioventricular AV node, or His-Purkinje system seen at autopsy

Pericardium

- Pericarditis is common in systemic sclerosis (up to 70% of autopsy series)
- Effusion has been demonstrated on echocardiography in up to 40% of patients, whereas only one-third are symptomatic; reports of pericardial tamponade have been infrequent.
- No evidence of immune complexes or complement activation in pericardial fluid have been found.
- Found in limited scleroderma and mixed connective tissue disease, but not as frequent as diffuse SSc
- Constrictive pericarditis reported as a single case
- Pericardial disease does not appear to affect overall mortality in SSc

Myocardium

- Symptoms of myocardial involvement are usually those of CHF, although clinically evident myocardial disease is not common.
- Cardiomyopathy attributable to myocardial fibrosis is found in less than 10% of the diffuse variant.
- Myocarditis has been described but is considered rare.
- Postmortem lesions are seen in up to 80% and affect all chambers of the heart without coronary artery involvement.

Valvular Heart Disease

- Rarely produces lesions that affect only valvular tissue (other etiology should be sought if valvular disease present)

Coronary Artery Disease

- Involvement appears limited to the microvasculature due to changes in small arteries and arterioles leading to "intramyocardial Raynaud's phenomenon" as supported by catheterization studies demonstrating normal arteries with reduced perfusion and delayed runoff.
- Myocardial perfusion defects are common in diffuse scleroderma.
- Echocardiographic and reversible perfusion abnormalities have been demonstrated in up to 70% of patients when exposed to a cold stimulus, but the clinical significance remains unclear.
- Angina, myocardial infarction, and sudden death have been described.

Pulmonary Hypertension

- More common with limited disease variant
- In one report, 67% of patients with SSc who underwent cardiac catheterization had evidence of at least mild pulmonary hypertension.

EPIDEMIOLOGY

The incidence of scleroderma increases with age and peaks in the third to fifth decades of life.

- Women are affected three times as often as men.
- SSc is more frequent and severe in young black women.

Prevalence

- 13.4 to 75 per 100,000 persons
- Highest reported prevalence per ethnic group is found among the Choctaw Native Americans
- Rarity of disease and lack of a specific diagnostic test may contribute to an underestimation of incidence and prevalence.

ETIOLOGY

- Unknown

RISK FACTORS

Some studies have shown an association with HLA-DR1, -DR2, -DR3, and -DR5. Environmental factors associated with SSc and scleroderma-like illnesses include coal and gold mining (silica dust), polyvinyl chloride, benzine, toluene, and rapeseed oil.

ASSOCIATED CONDITIONS

- CREST, myopathy, symmetric polyarthritis, renal failure, sicca syndrome, hypothyroidism, trigeminal neuralgia, impotence

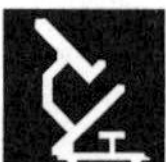

Diagnosis

DIFFERENTIAL DIAGNOSIS

- In early disease, SSc may initially be confused with other connective tissue diseases such as rheumatoid arthritis, systemic lupus erythematosus, polymyositis, or MCTD.
- Because SSc has numerous cardiac manifestations, the differential diagnosis includes the potential etiologies for each respective manifestation.

SIGNS AND SYMPTOMS

- Dyspnea, orthopnea, paroxysmal nocturnal dyspnea, palpitations, angina pectoris, distant heart sounds, elevated jugular venous pressure, pulsus paradoxus, precordial murmur, friction rub, pulmonary rales

LABORATORY PROCEDURES

- Antinuclear antibody is found in up to 95% of patients.
- Erythrocyte sedimentation rate may be elevated.
- Hypergammaglobulinemia (IgG) is found in approximately 50% of patients.
- Rheumatoid factor in low titer is present in 25% of patients.

PATHOLOGIC FINDINGS

- Range from focal myocardial involvement with contraction band necrosis to diffuse fibrotic replacement of both ventricles. These lesions occur in the absence of intraluminal coronary artery disease. An abnormal immune response has been indicated.
- It is suggested that contraction band necrosis in the myocardium is secondary to vascular spasm of the coronary arteries, which is similar to Raynaud's phenomenon occurring in the distal extremities.

IMAGING STUDIES

- Echocardiography is best for suspicion of pericarditis and pericardial effusion.
- Nuclear perfusion studies often demonstrate myocardial perfusion deficits of unknown clinical significance.

SPECIAL TESTS

- Primary evaluation of the cardiac status should be a 12-lead ECG and 24-hour ECG monitoring, followed by a thallium scan if indicated.
- Holter monitoring increases diagnostic yield of ECG abnormalities and is more sensitive compared with exercise or resting 12-lead ECG.

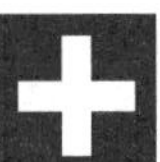

Treatment

GENERAL MEASURES

SSc cannot be cured, but treatment of involved organ system can relieve symptoms and improve function.

SURGICAL MEASURES

Heart–lung or single-lung transplantation may be a therapeutic option in those patients with severe symptomatic pulmonary hypertension without other significant systemic involvement.

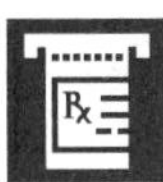

Medications

DRUG(S) OF CHOICE

- In uncontrolled studies, D-penicillamine reduced skin thickening and prevented the development of significant organ involvement.
- Glucocorticoids are indicated in those patients with inflammatory myositis or pericarditis, but high doses of steroids may play a role in precipitating renal crisis.
- Antiplatelet therapy may play a role in the treatment of SSc, but despite the therapeutic rationale, low doses of aspirin or dipyridamole did not show any benefit in a 2-year double blind study.
- If a Raynaud's-like phenomenon occurs in the heart, vasodilator or sympatholytic agents may have a role. Angiotensin-converting enzyme inhibitors are attractive not only as vasodilators, but may block angiotensin-induced myocardial fibrosis that has been shown in rabbits. These agents have experimental support demonstrating a decrease in perfusion abnormalities in patients with SSc.

Follow-up

PATIENT MONITORING

Routine history and physical examination will direct further diagnostic testing. Routine ECG may detect early cardiac involvement because conduction abnormalities often represent the first manifestation of SSc in the heart.

EXPECTED COURSE AND PROGNOSIS

The course of SSc is quite variable. Patients with limited scleroderma have a good prognosis. Prognosis is generally worse in patients with diffuse SSc, particularly when the onset occurs at an older age. In addition, males have a worse prognosis. Death occurs most often from cardiac, renal, or pulmonary involvement. The 10-year mortality rate has been estimated at 55% in patients with diffuse disease and 75% in those with limited disease. ECG evidence of heart involvement has been found to be associated with higher mortality.

PATIENT EDUCATION

Organizations

- Scleroderma Foundation: www.scleroderma.org
- Clinical Trials Listing Service: www.centerwatch.com

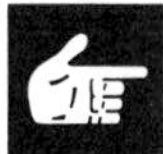

Miscellaneous

ICD-9-CM

Underlying Disease

710.1 Systemic sclerosis (includes CREST, progressive systemic sclerosis, and scleroderma)

Specific Manifestations

416.8 Pulmonary hypertension (secondary), unspecified
422.90 Acute myocarditis, unspecified
423.9 Pericardial disease, unspecified

BIBLIOGRAPHY

Anvari A, Graninger W, Schneider B, et al. Cardiac involvement in systemic sclerosis. *Arthritis Rheum* 1992;35:1356–1361.

Botstein GR, LeRoy EC. Primary heart disease in systemic sclerosis (scleroderma): advances in clinical and pathologic features, pathogenesis, and new therapeutic approaches. *Am Heart J* 1981;102:913–919.

Oram S, Stokes W. The heart in scleroderma. *Br J Med* 1961;23:243–259.

Sackner MA, Heinz ER, Steinberg AJ. The heart in scleroderma. *Am J Cardiol* 1966;17:542–559.

Topol EJ. *Cardiovascular medicine.* Philadelphia: Lippincott Williams & Wilkins, 1998:912–915.

Author: Christopher K. Dyke

Secundum Atrial Septal Defects

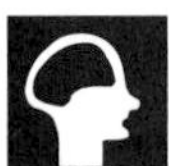

Basics

DESCRIPTION

A secundum atrial septal defect (ASD) is defined as the absence of septal tissue in the septum secundum, allowing for a free communication between the left and the right atrium at or near the level of the fossa ovalis.

- Defect size covers a wide spectrum, from a large fossa defect to multiple small perforations within the septum.
- The foramen ovale may or may not be included in the defect.
- A significant left-to-right shunt across the ASD causes enlargement of the right atrium and right ventricle, usually associated with normal pulmonary artery pressures.

EPIDEMIOLOGY

- Secundum ASDs are common, reported to occur in 7%–10% of children with congenital cardiac anomalies as the predominant cardiac lesion.
- The defect is more common in females (2:1).
- The condition is associated with a lack of early symptoms and the subtlety of the physical examination, which may delay the diagnosis into adult life. Thus, secundum ASDs are the most common form of congenital heart disease to present in the adult population.

ETIOLOGY

Isolated secundum ASDs are almost never associated with specific chromosomal abnormalities. However, there are certain skeletal malformations such as Holt-Oram syndrome with a reported incidence of ASDs as high as 50%.

PREGNANCY

- The presence of a large ASD does not adversely affect the outcome of pregnancy, but occasionally patients will have signs of mild congestive heart failure, and rarely severe decompensation.
- An infrequent complication associated with ASDs during pregnancy is paradoxical embolization across the ASD into the systemic circulation.

ASSOCIATED CONDITIONS

- ASDs may be associated with pulmonary valve stenosis, as well as with ventricular septal defects.
- The incidence of partial anomalous pulmonary venous return is 3% in patients with secundum defects as compared with 83% of those with a sinus venous ASD.
- Pulmonary vascular obstructive disease with right-to-left shunting may develop in patients with large ASDs that have been left unrepaired into middle age.

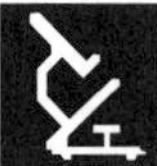

Diagnosis

DIFFERENTIAL DIAGNOSIS

The differential diagnosis for ASD includes mild pulmonary stenosis, because there are similarities in the physical examination.

- Partial anomalous pulmonary venous connections without an associated ASD, although unusual, can be confused with a secundum ASD because both result in a right heart volume load.
- The straight back syndrome with a systolic ejection murmur at the upper left sternal border and a prominent pulmonary artery on chest x-ray may superficially suggest the presence of an ASD.

SIGNS AND SYMPTOMS

- There are usually no symptoms related to an ASD in the pediatric age group. In the presence of a very large defect, mild dyspnea on exertion and easy fatigability may be seen, but such symptoms are often only appreciated in retrospect after repair of the ASD.
- Symptoms become more common in the fourth or fifth decade of life and include:
  - —Dyspnea on exertion
  - —Easy fatigability
  - —Congestive heart failure
  - —Atrial arrhythmias

Physical Examination

- An abnormal second heart sound that either is split widely and fixed or is persistently split, but varies somewhat with respirations
- A medium-pitched systolic ejection murmur is audible at the upper left sternal border related to increased blood flow across the pulmonary valve.
- The murmur may be prominent at the base and throughout the lung fields due to increased flow over the distal pulmonary vessels.
- A soft, early diastolic murmur may be heard at the lower left sternal border related to increased flow across the tricuspid valve.

LABORATORY PROCEDURES

- ECG usually shows right axis deviation and a right bundle branch block pattern over the right precordial leads. A left superior axis is consistent with a primum ASD.
- Chest x-ray may show mild to moderate cardiomegaly with a large right atrium, right ventricle, and pulmonary artery segment; pulmonary vascular markings are increased. Enlargement of the right ventricle is often only manifested on a lateral view. Many patients will have a relatively normal x-ray.
- Echocardiography is the optimal method for evaluating the anatomy of secundum ASDs. It is also essential to rule out associated abnormalities. The exact location and size of the ASD is visualized, and enlargement of the right atrium and right ventricle are defined.
- Cardiac catheterization is not necessary to establish a diagnosis of secundum ASD in any age group. It is only indicated to evaluate suspected pulmonary hypertension, or when interventional procedures are used as a form of therapy.

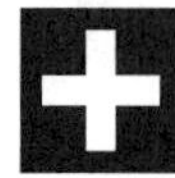

Treatment

GENERAL MEASURES

- Most children with a secundum ASD are asymptomatic.
- There is no indication for drug therapy for this condition.
- All patients with evidence of volume overload of the right ventricle on echocardiography should be referred for definitive closure.
- Some small to moderate ASDs may close spontaneously in the first 1–2 years of life, and for uncomplicated patients all approaches to closure should be delayed until the patients are at least 2 years of age.

SURGICAL MEASURES

- The most common form of repair of an ASD has been surgical closure of this defect using the standard technique of open heart surgery.
- More recently, methods of transcatheter closure of secundum ASDs have undergone investigation, and device repair has become an alternative to surgical closure of this defect. The recent results of transcatheter technique are excellent, with complete closure rates of 90%–95%. The complication rate is comparable with that of open heart surgery.

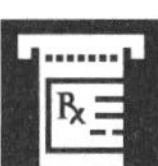

Medications

DRUG(S) OF CHOICE

- There are no medical therapies to treat a patient with an ASD.
- Associated arrhythmias may require treatment.

Follow-up

PATIENT MONITORING

- Patients repaired in the pediatric age group require minimal follow-up.
- Rarely, a patient will develop an atrial arrhythmia, but this is a very unusual event when ASD closure has been performed within the first two decades of life.
- In older patients who have congestive heart failure or pulmonary hypertension, the patient should be followed after surgery for evidence of progressive pulmonary hypertension or arrhythmia.
- The rare patient who develops pulmonary vascular obstruction later in life receives symptomatic therapy. ASD closure is not indicated in this group of patients and the prognosis is guarded.

EXPECTED COURSE AND PROGNOSIS

Long-term prognosis for children with a repaired ASD is excellent; a normal life span is expected. In the older patient who presents with symptoms, the life span may be shortened despite successful surgical closure.

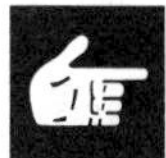

Miscellaneous

ICD-9-CM

745.5

BIBLIOGRAPHY

Beerman LB, Zuberbuhler JR. Atrial septal defect. *Paediatr Cardiol* 1987;22:541–562.

Kirklin JW, Barratt-Boyes BG. Atrial septal defect and partial anomalous pulmonary venous connection. In: *Cardiac surgery,* 2nd ed. Vol. I. New York: Churchill Livingstone, 1993.

Mandell V, Nimkin K, Hoffer FA, et al. Devices for transcatheter closure of intracardiac defects. *AJR* 1993;160:179–184.

Authors: William E. Hellenbrand and Welton M. Gersony

Sepsis and the Heart

Basics

DESCRIPTION

Sepsis is a systemic inflammatory response that is characterized by hypotension and multiorgan failure due to the release of inflammatory mediators.

- It is associated with considerable morbidity and mortality.
- Despite the traditionally recognized hyperdynamic myocardial response, the occurrence of myocardial dysfunction in septic shock is a well-documented phenomenon.

EPIDEMIOLOGY

Septic shock is the most common cause of death in intensive care units in the United States.

- Accounts for 400,000 cases and 100,000 deaths per year in the United States
- 25% develop cardiac dysfunction.
- Those with cardiac dysfunction have increased mortality rates from 20% up to 70%–90%.

ETIOLOGY

- The pathogenic mechanisms underlying the cardiac dysfunction in septic shock are very complex and are probably due to multiple factors.
- A number of humoral and intracellular mediators have been implicated in the cardiac dysfunction of sepsis, but the exact cause is not known.
- Possible causative agents and the data that exist to support their role in depressing cardiac function are listed as follows.

Endotoxin

Bacterial endotoxins are lipopolysaccharide molecules from the cell membrane of gram-negative bacteria released during infection.

- Contractile function is reduced when applied *in vitro* to adult myocytes.
- Infusion *in vivo* causes a classic septic hemodynamic response within 3–5 hours.
- Serum levels parallel the degree of myocardial depression.
- Causes induction of calcium-dependent nitric oxide synthase
- Stimulates the release of tumor necrosis factor-α (TNF-α)

TNF-α

TNF-α is expressed by macrophages within the myocardium and may act synergistically with interleukin-1β to depress myocardial function.

- Infusions of TNF-β result in myocardial depression within 1 hour.
- Pretreatment with monoclonal anti–TNF-α antibodies prevents septic shock in animals exposed to live bacteria or endotoxin.
- Induces negative inotropy by desensitizing the myofilament to the effects of calcium
- Disrupts excitation–contraction coupling
- Desensitizes the beta-receptor
- Induces nitric oxide synthase gene expression
- Induces cyclooxygenase enzyme-2 (COX-2)

COX-2

COX-2 is induced by endotoxin and other inflammatory mediators and produces prostaglandins.

- Higher prostacyclin and thromboxane levels are found in individuals with sepsis and are associated with increased mortality.
- May have indirect effects on coronary autoregulation and endothelial function

Free Radicals

Sepsis leads to increased oxidant stress.

- Causes increased left ventricular end diastolic diameter and decreased left ventricular contractility
- If leukocytes are removed from the perfusate in isolated rabbit hearts, myocardial depression is blocked.
- Reacts with nitric oxide to form peroxynitrate, which is implicated in cell membrane damage, enzyme dysfunction, and decreased mitochondrial function.

Platelet-Activating Factor (PAF)

PAF is produced by macrophages and endothelial cells after exposure to endotoxin.

- Plasma levels are increased in sepsis.
- Known to be a myocardial depressant in animals
- Receptor antagonists block the hemodynamic effects of endotoxin.

Catecholamines

Catecholamine levels are elevated in sepsis and are associated with the downregulation of cardiac beta-adrenoceptors.

- Dose of β-agonists often needs to be doubled with in the first 24 hours of treatment.
- Studies suggest that signal transduction in the β-adrenoceptor-adenylate cyclase system is disrupted in endotoxin models of sepsis.

Nitric Oxide (NO)

The role of NO in causing the systemic vasodilatation and hypotension of septic shock is well described; however, its effect on the myocardium has recently been investigated and may play a primary role in the myocardial dysfunction of sepsis. Many of the effects are mediated via cyclic guanosine monophosphate.

- NO is released in response to lipopolysaccharide and cytokines.
- Exposure of myocytes to cytokines and endotoxin leads to contractile dysfunction, which is temporally related to the synthesis of an inducible isoform of the NO synthase enzyme.
- Known to modulate both systolic and diastolic cardiac function
- Decreases contractility in isolated cardiac myocytes
- Causes alterations in protein kinase activity
- Decreases myofibril response to calcium
- Decreases cyclic adenosine monophosphate via phosphodiesterase.

Myocardial Ischemia

It was initially thought that myocardial ischemia played a major role in the cardiac dysfunction seen in sepsis; however, this does not appear to be a major mechanism.

RISK FACTORS

N/A

ASSOCIATED CONDITIONS

Other causes of a systemic inflammatory response syndrome are:

- Trauma
- Pancreatitis
- Burns

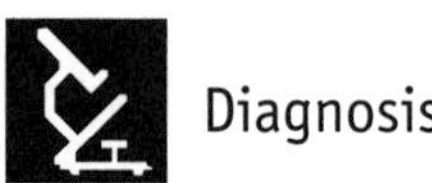

Diagnosis

DIFFERENTIAL DIAGNOSIS

Other causes of myocardial depression due to coexisting cardiac disease should always be considered.

SIGNS AND SYMPTOMS

Sepsis is a heterogeneous disease with varied clinical presentations and a hemodynamic picture that is complex and dynamic.

- The classic cardiovascular response to septic shock is profound peripheral vasodilatation (warm shock) leading to systemic hypotension. This causes an initial increase in cardiac index.
- Tachycardia and reduced afterload contribute to the increased cardiac output.
- Within 24 hours, most patients exhibit decreased systolic function (cold shock).
- The skin may rapidly change from warm and well perfused to cool and mottled over this short time.
- Assessment of intrinsic myocardial function is complicated by alterations in preload and heart rate.
- The myocardial dysfunction is usually reversible within 7–10 days among survivors.

LABORATORY PROCEDURES

The ECG demonstrates nonspecific findings (e.g., ST-T wave changes).

IMAGING STUDIES

Cardiac performance can be described and measured using several different noninvasive and invasive (see Special Tests) methods:

- Echocardiography may initially show hyperdynamic ventricular contractile function.
- Within 24 hours of onset, most patients exhibit globally decreased systolic function with a left ventricular (LV) ejection fraction of approximately 30% and an increase in LV end-diastolic diameter.
- This LV end-diastolic dilatation occurs without a corresponding increase in LV end-diastolic pressure, thus suggesting an increased left ventricular compliance.
- Those who die tend to have less profound myocardial depression and left ventricular dilatation, suggesting that these changes may be compensatory and protective.
- Several studies have demonstrated that the occurrence of LV end-diastolic dilatation is associated with a better prognosis.
- Radionuclide gated blood pool scanning demonstrates similar findings as noted above.

SPECIAL TESTS

Many clinical and experimental hemodynamic studies have attempted to characterize the myocardial dysfunction seen in sepsis independent of changes in heart rate and load:

- LVEF is usually depressed despite a normal stroke volume index (SVI).
- Stroke work index (SWI), which is the SVI multiplied by the mean arterial blood pressure, is depressed, and takes into account the reduced afterload.
- The preload-SWI relation (Frank-Starling relation) is shifted down and to the right. In a clinical setting, one can evaluate the pulmonary capillary wedge pressure in relation to the SWI during volume expansion to assess LV function.

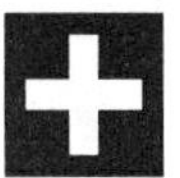

Treatment

GENERAL MEASURES

The mainstay of treatment for cardiac dysfunction during sepsis includes treatment of the underlying cause of the systemic inflammatory response, optimization of filling pressures, and possibly inotropic support.

- Correct hypotension to maintain end-organ perfusion
- Arterial and pulmonary artery monitoring catheters may be needed.
- Optimize oxygen delivery.
- Correct metabolic abnormalities.
- Inotropic agents include beta 1-adrenergic agents, cardiac glycosides, and possibly phosphodiesterase inhibitors.
- Immunomodulation: see Medications

SURGICAL MEASURES

N/A

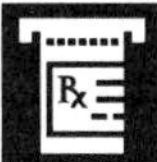

Medications

DRUG(S) OF CHOICE

- A number of immunomodulators have been developed to curb the cascade of inflammatory mediators.
- Although several trials have shown a favorable hemodynamic effect, no improvement in mortality has yet been demonstrated.
  —High-dose corticosteroids: Early animal studies have shown that dexamethasone blocks endotoxin-induced contractile dysfunction. More recent studies have failed to show any improvement in overall mortality.
  —Nonsteroidal antiinflammatory drugs: No hemodynamic or mortality benefit has ever been demonstrated.
  —Selective COX-2 inhibitors: not fully evaluated to date
  —Antilipopolysaccharide agents protect against the hemodynamic effects of sepsis, but no change in hypotension or mortality have been shown in human studies.
    - Anti-TNF-α antibodies improve LV function in patients with septic shock. Decreased mortality was demonstrated in early clinical trials, but no change in 28-day mortality rates was observed in recent larger studies.
    - NO synthase inhibitors increase systemic vascular resistance, mean arterial pressure, and LV SWI. The potential benefits may be limited by the increase in afterload and possible deleterious effect on cardiac output.

ADMISSION/DISCHARGE CRITERIA

N/A

Follow-up

PATIENT MONITORING

Patients with sepsis and any hemodynamic abnormalities, including hypotension and myocardial dysfunction, require intensive care and possibly invasive monitoring.

EXPECTED COURSE AND PROGNOSIS

Factors associated with a worse prognosis include:

- Lack of LV end-diastolic dilatation
- Persistent hyperdynamic profile
- Increased heart rate

PATIENT EDUCATION

N/A

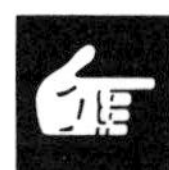

Miscellaneous

ICD-9-CM

785.59

BIBLIOGRAPHY

Grocott-Mason RM, Shah AM. Cardiac dysfunction in sepsis: new theories and clinical implications. *Intensive Care Med* 1998;24:286–295.

Piper RD. Myocardial dysfunction in sepsis. *Clin Exp Pharmacol Physiol* 1998;25:951–954.

Price S, et al. Myocardial dysfunction in sepsis: mechanisms and therapeutic implications. *Eur Heart J* 1999;20:715–724.

Author: Jarvis W. Lambert

Sick Sinus Syndrome

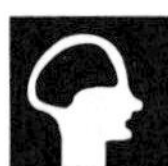

Basics

DESCRIPTION

The term *sick sinus syndrome* (SSS) incorporates a number of disorders involving impulse generation in the atria.

- Included are sinus bradycardia, sinus pauses or arrest, sinoatrial exit block, and the bradycardia–tachycardia syndrome (bradycardia alternating with atrial tachycardias, usually atrial fibrillation, but also atrial flutter and ectopic atrial tachycardia).
- Sinus pauses or arrest implies failure of normal intrinsic cardiac pacemaker function.
- Asymptomatic pauses of >2 seconds have been reported in >10% of patients undergoing ambulatory monitoring.
- Pauses of >3 seconds are uncommon, but frequent enough and asymptomatic such that pauses alone do not constitute evidence for pacemaker implantation.
- Patients may be symptomatic from paroxysmal tachycardia or bradycardia or both.

EPIDEMIOLOGY

Incidence increases with age.

ETIOLOGY

- Any structural heart disease
- Aging process
- Myocardial infarction leading to damage to the sinoatrial node or atria.

RISK FACTORS

- Structural heart disease
- Increasing age

PREGNANCY

- There is no specific contraindication to pregnancy.
- Extremely slow heart rates may compromise uterine blood flow, and atrial arrhythmias are more frequent during pregnancy.

ASSOCIATED CONDITIONS

- Structural heart disease

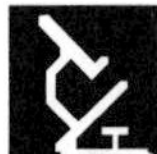

Diagnosis

DIFFERENTIAL DIAGNOSIS

Symptoms alone are not sufficient to assign a diagnosis of SSS. Symptoms must be correlated with the rhythm. This correlation is especially important when assessing the need and justification for permanent pacing. The differential diagnosis includes:

- Normal sinus arrhythmia
- Reversible causes of sinus node dysfunction such as drug toxicity
- Hypothyroidism

SIGNS AND SYMPTOMS

- None
- Lightheadedness
- Syncope
- Dyspnea, congestive heart failure
- Stroke if atrial fibrillation
- Fatigue
- In older persons, personality and memory changes, nausea, and nonspecific complaints
- Symptoms may be due to bradycardia itself, or to ventricular arrhythmias precipitated by bradycardia (e.g., torsades de pointes ventricular tachycardia).

LABORATORY PROCEDURES

- No laboratory test is needed to diagnose SSS.
- Thyroid function should be assessed because hypothyroidism may cause bradycardia.

IMAGING STUDIES

N/A

SPECIAL TESTS

- ECG
- Ambulatory monitor/event recorder
- Holter monitor/telemetry
- Rarely, invasive electrophysiologic study is needed to assess sinus node dysfunction.
- These studies are associated with a significant number of both false-positive and -negative test results.

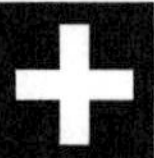

Treatment

GENERAL MEASURES

- If the SSS is due to nonessential drug therapy, those drugs should be stopped.
- When there is not a reversible cause of SSS, pacing is indicated to manage bradycardia and to allow drug therapy of tachycardia when it is present.
- Patients with SSS associated with atrial fibrillation (bradycardia–tachycardia syndrome) should be anticoagulated.
- There is no known way to prevent the development of intrinsic sinus node dysfunction.

SURGICAL MEASURES

The indications for pacemaker implantation are outlined in the American College of Cardiology/American Heart Association Guidelines referenced below and include:

- Sinus node dysfunction correlated with symptomatic bradycardia, including frequent sinus pauses that produce symptoms. In some patients, bradycardia is iatrogenic and will occur as a consequence of essential long-term drug therapy of a type and dose for which there are no acceptable alternatives.
- Symptomatic chronotropic incompetence
- Sinus node dysfunction occurring spontaneously or as a result of necessary drug therapy, with heart rate <40 beats/min when a clear association between significant symptoms consistent with bradycardia and the actual presence of bradycardia has not been documented
- In minimally symptomatic patients, chronic heart rate <30 beats/min while awake

ADMISSION/DISCHARGE CRITERIA

- When patients have extremely slow heart rates, severe symptoms, or ventricular arrhythmias as a result of bradycardia (torsades de pointes ventricular tachycardia), admission is warranted.
- Drug toxicity may be another indication for admission. Patients may be discharged after the arrhythmias have been treated.

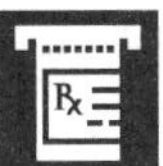

Medications

DRUG(S) OF CHOICE

There are no drugs to treat intrinsic sinus node dysfunction. Permanent pacing is usually required, and is very effective to relieve symptoms of sinus node dysfunction.

Follow-up

PATIENT MONITORING

- Pacemaker follow-up for those with permanent pacemakers
- For patients without pacemakers, systematic ECG and ambulatory monitoring are used to identify disease progression (e.g., longer pauses). This is especially true when new negatively chronotropic drugs are prescribed.

EXPECTED COURSE AND PROGNOSIS

Prognosis is governed by underlying heart disease and competing mortality. If SSS is associated with atrioventricular (AV) block, prognosis is worse than if AV block were absent.

PATIENT EDUCATION

- Mostly related to pacemaker follow-up in those with pacemakers
- If drug toxicity is the cause, counsel to take measures to avoid further toxicity.
- Recommendations regarding activity depend on hemodynamic consequences of bradycardias and tachycardias.

Diet

There is no specific diet.

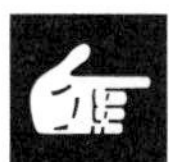

Miscellaneous

SYNONYMS

- Bradycardia–tachycardia syndrome
- Brady–tachy syndrome
- Sinus node dysfunction

ICD-9-CM

427.81 Sinoatrial node dysfunction

See also: Atrial premature beats; Atrial fibrillation; Atrial flutter; AV block; Pacemakers

BIBLIOGRAPHY

Gregoratos G, Cheitlin MD, Conill A, et al. ACC/AHA guidelines for implantation of cardiac pacemakers and antiarrhythmia devices: A report of the American College of Cardiology/American Heart Association Task Force on Practice Guidelines (Committee on Pacemaker Implantation). *J Am Coll Cardiol* 1998;31:1175–1206.

Author: Andrew E. Epstein

Sickle Cell Diseases and the Heart

Basics

DESCRIPTION

Sickle cell diseases are denoted by the presence of sickle- or crescent-shaped erythrocytes in the peripheral blood. Abnormally shaped red blood cells become rigid and lodge in capillaries, preventing the flow of oxygen to tissues and organs.

- Sickle cell diseases include sickle cell anemia, sickle cell-hemoglobin C disease, and sickle cell-thalassemia disease.
- The majority of the 50,000 persons in the United States with sickle cell disease are African Americans, although Asiatic Indians, Italians, Greeks, and other persons of Mediterranean ancestry are also afflicted.

Systems Affected

- Cardiovascular, respiratory, skeletal, hematologic, skin, immunologic, renal, gastrointestinal, genitourinary, and nervous

ETIOLOGY

Genetics

Sickle cell disease is inherited through a recessive gene.

Incidence/Prevalence

- Homozygotes (approximately 0.6% of blacks in the United States) have sickle cell anemia.
- Heterozygotes (8%–13% of blacks) carry the sickle cell trait and are not generally anemic; however, sickling has been demonstrated *in vitro*.
- Forty percent of the population in some areas of Africa carries the sickle cell trait.

Predominant Age

- Children and young adults

Predominant Sex

- Males and females affected equally

RISK FACTORS

Sickle cell crises are associated with the following:

- Hypoxia
- Infections
- Cold exposure
- Overexertion
- Dehydration
- Pregnancy
- General anesthesia

ASSOCIATED CONDITIONS

- Thalassemia
- Hemoglobin SC disease
- Hemoglobin C disease

Age-Related Factors

- Pediatric: common
- Geriatric: unusual in light of the high early mortality

PREGNANCY

- A relatively high rate of fetal loss occurs during pregnancy.
- Increases the risk of a sickle crisis
- May aggravate a patient's anemia
- On average, the maternal mortality rate is 1.6%.

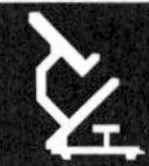

Diagnosis

DIFFERENTIAL DIAGNOSIS

- Hemoglobin SB thalassemia
- Hemoglobin SC disease
- Malaria and other parasitic blood dyscrasias
- Hemolytic uremic syndrome

SIGNS AND SYMPTOMS

Infants/Toddlers/Children

Onset of symptoms in most patients occurs in the first 3 years of life.

- Hemolytic anemia
- Acute attacks of pain: pain in the chest, abdomen, limbs, and joints
- Pallor of the tongue and lips
- Irritability
- Crying
- Poor eating habits
- Splenomegaly
- Hepatomegaly
- Jaundice
- Scleral icterus
- Cardiac murmurs

Adolescents/Young Adults

- Severe pain
- Delayed puberty
- Progressive anemia
- Leg ulcers
- Nosebleeds
- Dental disease
- Renal disease
- Aseptic necrosis of the femoral head
- Retinal lesions

Individuals 20 Years Old and Older

- Pain crises may become less frequent with advancing age
- Leg ulcers
- Retinitis
- Gallbladder disease
- Cardiac manifestations

Cardiomegaly Is the Rule

- Striking left atrial and biventricular enlargement often develop.
- In many cases left ventricular dilatation exceeds that expected by the degree of anemia.
  - —Left ventricular hypertrophy of the interventricular septum
  - —Decreased exercise capacity
  - —Increased resting cardiac output with a hemoglobin level below 7 g/dL of blood
  - —Increased cardiac contractility possibly secondary to a humoral, noncatecholamine positive inotropic factor
  - —Reduced maximum cardiac output at maximum exercise
  - —Hyperdynamic precordium
  - —Heart rate is generally normal to minimally increased; tachycardia should raise suspicion of congestive heart failure, myocardial dysfunction, or an acute decrease in hemoglobin
  - —Decreased peripheral vascular resistance secondary to peripheral vasodilatation, microvascular arteriovenous shunts, and decreased blood viscosity
  - —Right ventricular hypertrophy with eventual right heart failure
  - —Left ventricular enlargement secondary to chronic anemia and vascular occlusions
  - —Paradoxical splitting of the second heart sound
  - —Prominent third heart sound
  - —Ejection click due to pulmonary artery dilatation
  - —Valvular abnormalities: systolic murmurs (mitral and tricuspid regurgitation, systolic ejection murmur with wide radiation) and diastolic murmurs (mitral stenosis and aortic insufficiency)
  - —Patients with severe anemia may develop diastolic cardiac murmurs and dilatation of the aortic ring
  - —Myocardial infarction is relatively uncommon (patients with sickle cell disease may present with an acute myocardial infarction in the absence of atherosclerosis or coronary occlusion)
- Pulmonary manifestations
  - —Dyspnea
  - —Reduced vital capacity
  - —Pulmonary vascular congestion/pulmonary edema secondary to cardiac failure
  - —Pulmonary hypertension secondary to pulmonary infarction (from focal pulmonary sickling or thromboembolism) and venocclusive disease
  - —Cor pulmonale

LABORATORY PROCEDURES

- Normocytic red blood cells
- Red blood cell count of 2–3 million/μL
- Reticulocytosis of 10%–40%
- Leukocytosis with a left shift often develops during a crisis or bacterial infection. The white blood cell count may exceed 35,000/μL during an illness.
- Thrombocytosis is usually present.
- Bone marrow is hyperplastic, with a predominance of normoblasts. The bone marrow may become aplastic during "sickle crisis" or severe infection.
- Serum bilirubin is usually elevated.
- Fecal and urinary urobilinogen levels are also elevated.
- The erythrocyte sedimentation rate is generally low.

Pathologic Findings

- Arterial occlusions

SPECIAL TESTS

- The diagnosis of sickle cell anemia is made by the use of serum electrophoresis.
  —The homozygous state is denoted by the presence of only hemoglobin S with variable amounts of hemoglobin F.
  —The heterozygous state is denoted by the presence of both hemoglobin A and S (with more A than S present).
- Prenatal screening with recombinant DNA technology.

IMAGING STUDIES

- ECG may show right or left ventricular hypertrophy, myocardial infarction, or myocardial ischemia.
- Chest radiography may reveal cardiomegaly, pulmonary infiltrates, and enlarged pulmonary arteries.
- Exercise stress testing may be abnormal due to occlusive coronary artery disease.
- Echocardiography may confirm cor pulmonale, myocardial infarction, pulmonary hypertension, left ventricular hypertrophy, and valvular abnormalities.

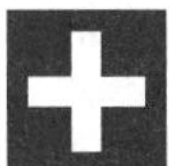

Treatment

GENERAL MEASURES

- Patients with sickle cell crisis are usually hospitalized and cared for in an ICU setting if hemodynamically unstable.
- Therapy is supportive.
- Blood transfusions should be administered only if the anemia is more severe than the patient's baseline anemia.
  —Goals of transfusion therapy should be to achieve a sickle cell concentration of <30% with a hematocrit of ≤46%.
  —Accepted indications for blood transfusion include the following:
    - Cardiopulmonary symptoms, particularly when the hemoglobin level is <5 g/dL.
    - High-output failure
    - Hypoxemia with PO_2 <65 mm Hg
    - Severe infection
    - Sepsis
    - Cerebral vascular accident
    - Organ failure
    - Prior to general anesthesia
    - Prior to surgery
    - Recalcitrant leg ulcers
    - Pregnancy
    - Crises should be managed with aggressive i.v. fluid hydration and analgesics.

SURGICAL MEASURES

- Allogenic bone marrow transplantation is the only currently available treatment that can cure sickle cell disease.
- Gene transfer therapy has the potential to provide marked improvement in or cure of patients with sickle cell disease.

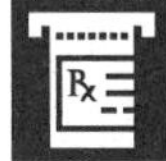

Medications

DRUG(S) OF CHOICE

- Hydroxyurea appears to decrease the incidence of pain crises and provide an increment in hemoglobin content.
- Folic acid 1 mg/day
- Erythropoietin may enhance erythropoiesis.
- Danazol is a drug currently being studied that may enable sickle cell erythrocytes to flow through very small capillaries.

Follow-up

PATIENT MONITORING

- Depends on the frequency and severity of the patient's symptoms

Prevention/Avoidance

- Antibiotics (prophylactic penicillin until the age of 6 years)
- Pneumococcal vaccine
- *Haemophilus influenzae* type b vaccine
- Regular check-ups
- Avoid becoming chilled.
- Dress warmly.
- Eat balanced meals.
- Ensure ample sleep.
- Practice deep breathing 5 minutes before going to sleep.

Possible Complications

- Organ failure
- Congestive heart failure
- Cardiac arrest
- Limb ischemia

EXPECTED COURSE AND PROGNOSIS

- The life span of patients with homozygous hemoglobin S (sickle cell disease) has increased to >40 years.
- Causes of death include intercurrent infections, multiple pulmonary emboli, thrombosis of a vital vascular bed, and renal failure.

PATIENT EDUCATION

Organizations

- National Organization for Rare Disorders (NORD)
- National Association for Sickle Cell Disease, Inc.
- NIH/National Heart, Lung and Blood Institute (NHLBI)
- Cooley's Anemia Foundation, Inc.
- The Canadian Sickle Cell Society
- March of Dimes Birth Defects Foundation
- National Center for Education in Maternal and Child Health (NCEMCH)

Activity

- As tolerated

Diet

- Ensure adequate nutrition and hydration.

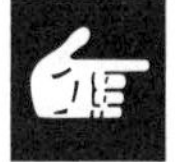

Miscellaneous

ICD-9-CM

282.60

BIBLIOGRAPHY

Berkow R. *The Merck manual of diagnosis and therapy.* New Jersey: Merck & Co., 1993.

Embury SH, Hebbel RP, Mohandas N, et al. *Sickle cell disease: basic principles and clinical practice.* Ch. 46. New York: Raven, 1994.

Fauci AS, Braunwald E, Isselbacher KJ, et al. *Harrison's principles of internal medicine.* New York: McGraw-Hill, 1998.

Thoene JG. *Physicians guide to rare diseases.* New Jersey: Dowden Publishing, 1992.

Author: Phoebe A. Ashley

Single Ventricle and Tricuspid Atresia

Basics

DESCRIPTION

This condition is characterized by a univentricular atrioventricular (AV) connection resulting in a single functioning ventricular chamber.

- The AV connections include a single-inlet ventricle associated with atresia of one of the AV valves (tricuspid atresia, mitral atresia), a double-inlet ventricle, and a common-inlet ventricle with an unbalanced AV connection. The latter is associated with AV septal defects (AV canal).
- The ventricular morphology is subdivided into dominant left ventricle, dominant right ventricle, and indeterminate ventricular morphology.
- The great vessel position may be normal, l transposed, d transposed, or doublet-outlet malposed.

System Affected

- Cardiovascular

ETIOLOGY

Genetics

- Most often multifactorial

EPIDEMIOLOGY

Incidence/Prevalence

- It has been reported that single-ventricle variants make up 1.1% of patients with congenital heart disease.
- Dominant left ventricular morphology makes up the majority, accounting for 74%–84%.
- A subset includes patients with asplenia and polysplenia associated with dextrocardia, abdominal heterotaxy, and a complex constellation of associated congenital heart lesions.
- Tricuspid atresia is the third most common form of cyanotic congenital heart disease, with a prevalence in clinical series of 0.3%–3.7%.
- The prevalence rate in autopsy series is 2.9%. Tricuspid atresia occurs in 1/15,000 live births.

Predominant Age

- Most patients present in early life in the neonatal or early infancy period.
- They present with cyanosis due to inadequate pulmonary blood flow (the majority) or congestive heart failure due to unobstructed pulmonary blood flow.

Predominant Sex

- Male predominance in tricuspid atresia with transposition of the great vessels

PREGNANCY

Pregnancy can cause marked deterioration in the status of a Fontan patient.

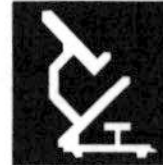

Diagnosis

DIFFERENTIAL DIAGNOSIS

The differential diagnosis is dependent on the associated anatomic lesions.

- Patients with obstruction to pulmonary blood flow
  —Tetralogy of Fallot
  —Pulmonary atresia with ventricular septal defect (VSD)
  —Transposition of the great arteries with VSD and pulmonary stenosis
  —Double-outlet right ventricle (RV) with VSD and pulmonary stenosis
- Patients with unobstructed pulmonary blood flow
  —Complete AV septal defect
  —Truncus arteriosus
  —Transposition of great arteries with large
  —Ventricular septal defect
  —Ventricular septal defect with coarctation of the aorta
  —Total anomalous pulmonary venous return
  —Double-outlet RV with VSD
  —Hypoplastic left heart syndrome
  —Interrupted aortic arch with large VSD

SIGNS AND SYMPTOMS

- Signs and symptoms are dependent on the associated anatomic lesions. The majority of patients with obstruction to pulmonary blood flow secondary to pulmonary atresia or severe pulmonary stenosis present in the newborn period or early infancy with severe cyanosis and hypoxemia secondary to restrictive pulmonary blood flow.
- Patients with unobstructed pulmonary blood flow present in early infancy with signs and symptoms of congestive heart failure:
  —Tachypnea
  —Tachycardia
  —Hepatomegaly
    - Poor feeding
    - Failure to thrive
    - Mild cyanosis

Physical Examination

- Systolic ejection murmur of pulmonary stenosis; or rarely, continuous murmur of ductus arteriosus or collateral blood flow
- Nonspecific systolic murmur at the left sternal border or systolic murmur of the AV valve; insufficiency diastolic flow murmur at the apex
  —Tachycardia
  —Gallop rhythm
  —Tachypnea
  —Hepatomegaly
  —Patients with associated coarctation of the aorta have diminished or absent pulses in the lower extremities and may present with low cardiac output syndrome and cardiogenic shock.

LABORATORY PROCEDURES

- Howell-Jolly bodies in asplenia syndrome and chromosome abnormalities in some patients (e.g., Down's syndrome)

PATHOLOGIC FINDINGS

- Ventricular morphology
  —Single left ventricle
  —Single right ventricle
    - Undifferentiated ventricle
- AV valves
  —Double-inlet ventricle
    - Single inlet ventricle with either tricuspid or mitral atresia or severe hypoplasia
  —Common AV valve with AV septal defect
- Pulmonary outflow tract: atretic or severely stenotic, unobstructed
- Aortic arch: normal coarctation of the aorta
  —Interrupted aortic arch

SPECIAL TESTS

- Oximetry: dependent on pulmonary blood flow; varies from 60% to 90%
- ECG
  —Tricuspid atresia with normal great arteries: short PR interval, left superior axis, and absent right ventricular forces
  —AV discordance with l transposition of the great arteries: AV conduction abnormalities, including complete AV block
  —Asplenia and polysplenia syndromes with abnormal situs; abnormal P-wave morphology
  —Other single ventricles: abnormal R-wave progression in precordial leads, although findings variable and nonspecific

IMAGING STUDIES

Chest X-ray

Findings are dependent on pulmonary blood flow:

- Pulmonary atresia or moderate to severe pulmonary stenosis: heart size normal with normal to decreased pulmonary vascular markings
- Unobstructed pulmonary blood flow, moderate to severe cardiomegaly with increased pulmonary vascular markings
- Additional abnormalities
  —Situs inversus or heterotaxy, dextrocardia or mesocardia, pulmonary venous obstruction; lungs have ground glass appearance with linear reticular pattern

Echocardiography

Echocardiography may diagnose and elucidate characteristics of the most complex single-ventricle variant. The segmental approach demonstrates:

- Abdominal and atrial situs
- Type and mode of AV connections
- Morphology and function of the main ventricular chamber
- Ventriculoarterial connections and relationships
- Systemic and pulmonary venous connections
- Status of the atrial septum

- Status of pulmonary valve and arteries
- Status of aortic arch AV valves and bulboventricular septum

Cardiac Catheterization

- Hemodynamic parameters
  —Systemic arterial saturation
  —Degree of intracardiac shunts
  —Pulmonary arterial pressure and resistance
  —Gradients between the main ventricle and pulmonary artery and ascending aorta
  —Gradient between ascending and descending aorta
  —Intraatrial gradients
  —Gradient between pulmonary capillary wedge pressure and ventricular end-diastolic pressure
- Angiography parameters
  —Pulmonary arterial architecture
  —Systemic and pulmonary venous return
  —Presence of aorticopulmonary collaterals
  —AV valve function
  —Ventricular function
  —Status of the bulboventricular foramen and aortic arch

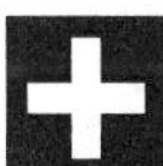

Treatment

GENERAL MEASURES

Treatment depends on associated cardiac defects and age of presentation.

- Severe pulmonary stenosis or pulmonary atresia: emergent establishment of an aorticopulmonary connection via pharmacologic (prostaglandin E_1) and subsequent surgical shunt
- Unobstructed pulmonary blood flow: medical treatment for congestive heart failure and subsequent surgical treatment to control pulmonary blood flow

SURGICAL MEASURES

Palliative Surgery

- Neonatal and early infancy
  —Systemic to pulmonary artery shunts (primarily modified Blalock-Taussig procedure) for patients with inadequate pulmonary blood flow
  —Atrial septectomy in patients with a restrictive atrial septal defect and stenosis or atresia of the left AV valve
  —Repair of coarctation of the aorta
  —Pulmonary artery banding for patients with unobstructed pulmonary blood flow and pulmonary artery hypertension to control pulmonary blood flow and pulmonary artery resistance
  —Repair of total anomalous pulmonary venous connection
- Late infancy and early childhood
  —Bidirectional Glenn shunt (superior vena cava to pulmonary artery anastomosis) increases effective pulmonary blood flow without increased volume load on ventricle.
  —Relief of subaortic stenosis

Definitive Surgery

The Fontan procedure with passive filling of the pulmonary arteries from the systemic venous system is the definitive surgical option.

- Interventional catheterization
  —Balloon atrial septostomy
  —Coil embolization of aorticopulmonary collaterals
  —Balloon dilatation and stenting of stenotic pulmonary arteries
  —Balloon dilation and stenting of coarctation of the aorta

Medications

DRUG(S) OF CHOICE

- Severe pulmonary stenosis or pulmonary atresia in the neonatal period treated with intravenous prostaglandin E_1 to establish patency of the ductus arteriosus
- Unobstructed pulmonary blood flow and congestive heart failure treated with digitalis and diuretics; may have associated coarctation of aorta requiring prostaglandin E_1 and pressors to maintain cardiac output

Follow-up

PATIENT MONITORING

Patients who have had a completed Fontan procedure must be considered as chronic cardiac patients for life.

EXPECTED COURSE AND PROGNOSIS

Physiology of the Fontan procedure predisposes patients to long-term complications:

- Progressive exercise intolerance
- Progressive ventricular dysfunction
- Chronic recurrent pleural effusions
- Chronic atrial arrhythmias, especially atrial flutter and intraatrial reentrant tachycardia
- Sinus and AV node dysfunction
- Thromboembolic events
- Protein-losing enteropathy
- Although the operative mortality rate is in the 5%–10% range and postoperative survival for 20 years is not uncommon, many of the survivors require chronic therapy for long-term complications, including anticongestive therapy, antiarrhythmic therapy, pacemakers, and anticoagulation.

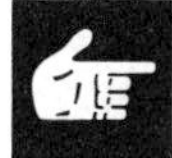

Miscellaneous

BIBLIOGRAPHY

Anderson RH, Becker AE. Historical review. In: Anderson RH, Crupi G, Parenzan L, eds. *Double inlet ventricle.* Tunbridge Wells, UK: Castle House, 1987 (Fontan operation in five hundred consecutive patients: factors influencing early and late outcome).

Béeri E, Maier SE, Landzberg MJ, et al. *In vivo* evaluation of Fontan pathway flow dynamics by multidimensional phase-velocity magnetic resonance imaging. *Circulation* 1999;98:2873–2882.

Bridges ND. Early and medium-term outcomes after the fenestrated Fontan operation. *Adv Cardiac Surg* 1999;11:221–231.

Cecchin F, Johnsrude CL, Perry JC, et al. Effect of age and surgical technique on symptomatic arrhythmias after the Fontan procedure. *Am J Cardiol* 1995;76:386–391.

Choussat A, et al. Selection criteria for Fontan procedure. In: Anderson RH, Shinebourne EA, eds. *Pediatric cardiology 1977.* Edinburgh, UK: Churchill Livingstone, 1978.

De leval MR, Kilner P, Gewilling M, et al. Total cavopulmonary connection: a logical alternative to atriopulmonary connection for complex Fontan operations. Experimental studies and early clinical experience. *J Thorac Cardiovasc Surg* 1988;96:682–695.

Emmanouilides GC, Riemenschneider TA, Allen HD, et al., eds. *Moss and Adams: heart disease in infants, children, and adolescents,* 5th ed. Baltimore: Williams & Wilkins, 1995.

Garson A Jr, Bricker JT, Fisher DJ, et al. *The science and practices of pediatric cardiology,* 2nd ed. Baltimore: Williams & Wilkins, 1998.

Gentles TL, Mayer JE Jr, Gauvreau K, et al. Fontan operations in five hundred consecutive patients: factors influencing early and late outcome. *J Thorac Cardiovasc Surg* 1997; 114:376–391.

Kirklin JW, Barratt-Boyes BG. *Cardiac surgery,* 2nd ed. New York: Churchill Livingstone, 1993.

Mahle WT, Wernovsky G, Bridges ND, et al. Impact of early ventricular unloading on exercise performance in preadolescents with single ventricle Fontan physiology. *J Am Coll Cardiol* 1999;34:1637–1643.

Mertens L, Hagler DJ, Sauer U, et al. Protein-losing enteropathy after the Fontan operation: an international multicenter study. PLE study group. *J Thorac Cardiovasc Surg* 1988;115: 1063–1073.

Petrossian E, Reddy VM, McElhinney DB, et al. Early results of the extracardiac conduit Fontan operation. *J Thorac Cardiovasc Surg* 1999;117: 688–696.

Shekerdemian LS, Bush A, Shore DF, et al. Cardiopulmonary interactions after Fontan operations: augmentation of cardiac output using negative pressure ventilation. *Circulation* 1997;96:3934–3942.

Van Praagh R, Plett JA, Van Praagh S. Single ventricle: pathology, embroyology, terminology, and classification. *Hertz* 1979;4:113–150.

Authors: Allan Hordof and Welton M. Gersony

Sinus of Valsalva Aneurysm

Basics

DESCRIPTION

A sinus of Valsalva aneurysm is a congenital or acquired diverticulum of the coronary sinus that, when ruptured, creates a fistula between the aorta and another chamber, typically the right ventricle.

- Right coronary sinus most commonly affected
- Noncoronary sinus is affected in 5%–15% of cases. The left coronary sinus is rarely affected.

EPIDEMIOLOGY

- 3.5% of patients with congenital heart disease that require surgery
- Age 20–40 years
- Males affected more often than females (3:1)

ETIOLOGY

- Lack of continuity between aortic media and annulus fibrosis
- May be more common in Asia than in the western world

CAUSES

- Congenital: lack of fusion of media of aorta with annulus fibrosis of aortic valve
  - —May be associated with connective tissue diseases (e.g., Marfan's syndrome, Ehlers-Danlos syndrome) or other congenital heart diseases (e.g., common supracristal ventricular septal defect with right sinus aneurysm, atrial septal defect, aortic coarctation)
- Acquired: syphilis, rheumatoid heart disease, atherosclerosis, trauma, endocarditis

RISK FACTORS

- Congenital heart disease
- Male gender

PREGNANCY

N/A

ASSOCIATED CONDITIONS

Associated conditions are present in 50%–70% of cases.

- Congenital heart disease
  - —Ventricular septal defect
  - —Atrial septal defect
  - —Coarctation of aorta
- Connective tissue disease
  - —Marfan's syndrome
  - —Ehlers-Danlos syndrome
- Acquired diseases
  - —Aortic valve incompetence
  - —Endocarditis
  - —Rheumatoid heart disease
  - —Syphilitic aortitis

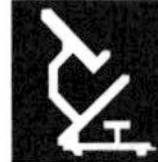

Diagnosis

DIFFERENTIAL DIAGNOSIS

Rupture can present as abrupt onset of dyspnea, weakness, and fatigue. Other cardiovascular disorders can present similarly.

- Congestive heart failure
- Aortic regurgitation
- Aortic dissection

SIGNS AND SYMPTOMS

- Asymptomatic prior to rupture
- Pain with rupture
- Congestive heart failure symptoms (e.g., dyspnea, orthopnea, edema, weakness, fatigue)
- Fistula signs (e.g., bounding pulses; increased pulse pressure; loud continuous murmur, accentuated in diastole, heard best along lower left sternal border; parasternal thrill, hyperdynamic apex)

LABORATORY PROCEDURES

- Blood cultures if endocarditis is suspected

IMAGING STUDIES

- Chest x-ray
  - —Cardiomegaly
  - —Pulmonary edema with acute rupture
- Ultrafast CT scan
  - —Visualizes the aneurysm itself
- Transthoracic echocardiography
  - —2-D echocardiography demonstrates aneurysm in multiple views.
  - —Doppler studies demonstrate flow between the aortic sinus and the chamber into which the fistula empties. In the majority of cases, the fistula is located between the right coronary cusp and right ventricle. It may also be located between the noncoronary cusp and the right atrium.
  - —Contrast echocardiography may demonstrate fistula.
- Transesophageal echocardiography
  - —Enhances visualization of fistula
  - —Aids in planning surgical approach, management
- Cardiac catheterization
  - —Aortography may demonstrate aneurysm or fistula.
  - —Sampling of oxygen saturations reveals step up at level of communication.

SPECIAL TESTS

- ECG
  - —Normal (approximately 20%)
  - —Sinus tachycardia with rupture
  - —Conduction disturbances (including bundle branch blocks)
  - —Ventricular hypertrophy (left and/or right)

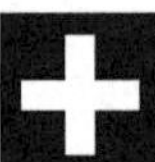

Treatment

GENERAL MEASURES

Acute rupture is an emergency requiring admission to the intensive care unit. Diagnostic procedures are indicated to define the exact location of the aneurysm, as well as associated conditions. Immediate surgical consultation is also indicated because most ruptured sinus of Valsalva aneurysms require surgical intervention.

- Adequate oxygenation
- Afterload reduction with medical therapies listed below
- Diuresis if pulmonary congestion present
- Antibiotics for endocarditis if present

SURGICAL MEASURES

- Cardiac surgery treatment of choice for ruptured aneurysm

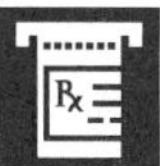

Medications

DRUG(S) OF CHOICE

Angiotensin-converting enzyme (ACE) inhibitors are the standard of care for congestive heart failure that may result from a ruptured sinus of Valsalva aneurysm.

Contraindications

- ACE inhibitors: known allergy, progressive renal failure, renal artery stenosis, hypotension
- Diuretics: hypotension

Precautions

- ACE inhibitors: may cause cough, cause or aggravate renal failure with renal artery stenosis, increase serum potassium levels
- Diuretics: loop diuretics may cause nephrotoxicity, ototoxicity; may deplete potassium, magnesium levels, predisposing to arrhythmias

ALTERNATIVE DRUGS

- Nitrates plus hydralazine
- Sodium nitroprusside

ADMISSION/DISCHARGE CRITERIA

- Chronic sinus of Valsalva aneurysm does not require hospital admission.
- Acute rupture of a sinus of Valsalva aneurysm requires admission to an intensive care unit.

Follow-up

PATIENT MONITORING

Optimal follow-up for nonruptured sinus of Valsalva aneurysms has not been studied. In the absence of clinical data, annual or semiannual physical examination and echocardiography are advisable.

Possible Complications

- Acute rupture
- Pulmonary edema with respiratory failure
- Circulatory collapse with shock
- Endocarditis
- Aortic valve incompetence

EXPECTED COURSE AND PROGNOSIS

- Ruptured sinus of Valsalva aneurysm carries a grave prognosis unless surgically repaired.
- Repaired aneurysms carry an 85% ± 7.4% long-term survival rate.

PATIENT EDUCATION

Activity

- Activity should be limited to bed rest for ruptured aneurysm.
- Activity as tolerated for nonruptured or repaired aneurysm

Diet

Diet may be regular unless on a special diet or NPO for another disorder.

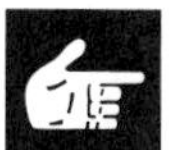

Miscellaneous

ICD-9-CM

441.9 Aortic aneurysms

BIBLIOGRAPHY

Abe T, Komatsu S. Surgical repair and long-term results in ruptured sinus of Valsalva aneurysm. *Ann Thorac Surg* 1988;46:520–525.

Botefeu J-M, Moret PR, Hahn C, et al. Aneurysms of the sinus of Valsalva: report of seven cases and review of the literature. *Am J Med* 1978;65:18–24.

Cheitlin MD, Alpert JS, Armstrong WF, et al. ACC/AHA guidelines for the clinical application of echocardiography. *Circulation* 1997;95:1686–1744.

Chiang CW, Lin FC, Fang B-R, et al. Doppler and two-dimensional echocardiographic features of sinus of Valsalva aneurysm. *Am Heart J* 1988; 116:1283–1288.

Feigenbaum H. Diseases of the aorta. In: Feigenbaum H, ed. *Echocardiography,* 5th ed. Baltimore: Williams & Wilkins, 1994: 646–647.

Friedman WF. Congenital heart disease in infancy and childhood. In: Braunwald E, ed. *Heart disease: a textbook of cardiovascular medicine,* 5th ed. Philadelphia: WB Saunders, 1997:910–911.

Lewis BS, Agathangelou NE. Echocardiographic diagnosis of unruptured sinus of Valsalva aneurysm. *Am Heart J* 1984;107:1025–1027.

Mayer E-D, Ruffman K, Saggau W, et al. Ruptured aneurysms of the sinus of Valsalva. *Ann Thorac Surg* 1986;42:81–85.

McKenny PA, Shemin RJ, Wiegers SE. Role of transesophageal echocardiography in sinus of Valsalva aneurysm. *Am Heart J* 1992;123: 228–229.

Nakamura K, Suzuki S, Satomi G. Detection of ruptured aneurysm of sinus of Valsalva by contrast two dimensional echocardiography. *Br Heart J* 1981;45:219–221.

Authors: Craig M. Brodsky and Nanette K. Wenger

SLE and the Heart

Basics

DESCRIPTION

Systemic lupus erythematosus (SLE) is an autoimmune disease with a wide array of cardiac manifestations, including pericarditis, myocarditis, valvular heart disease, coronary artery disease (CAD), conduction system disease, antiphospholipid antibody syndrome, and hypertension.

Pericardium

- Pericarditis most common cardiovascular manifestation of SLE
- Pericarditis may occur at any time during active disease, and may be persistent or recurrent.
- Tamponade is a rare complication but may be the presenting feature.
- Constrictive pericarditis noted but unusual

Myocardium

- The existence of lupus-related cardiomyopathy remains controversial.
- Clinically evident heart failure is infrequent.

Valvular Heart Disease

- Libman-Sacks lesion: a small verrucous vegetation adherent to the endocardium

Coronary Artery Disease

- Atherosclerotic, thrombotic, embolic or inflammatory (arteritis)
- Typically, medium-sized arteries are affected.
- Accelerated atherosclerosis on corticosteroid therapy
- Severe coronary disease is often associated with pericardial and valvular disease.

Conduction System Disease

- Small vessel vasculitis may injure nodal or other conducting tissue.
- Infiltration of sinus or atrioventricular nodes by fibrous or granulation tissue
- Degrees of heart block and bundle branch block have been described, but complete heart block is rare.
- Atrial fibrillation and flutter may be associated with pericarditis.

Antiphospholipid Antibody Syndrome

- Valvular disease most common manifestation
- Valvular involvement may correlate with anticardiolipin levels and SLE duration.
- Anticardiolipin antibody levels associated with myocardial infarction and graft occlusion
- Intraatrial and ventricular thrombi are rare manifestations.

Hypertension

- Associated with renal disease and corticosteroid therapy

EPIDEMIOLOGY

The prevalence of SLE is 1/2,000 individuals. Autopsy series report a prevalence of cardiovascular involvement that averages nearly 70%. Estimates of clinically apparent disease range from 23% to 60% with an average of 29%. The prevalence of cardiac disease diagnosed by echocardiography is reported to be as high as that in autopsy series.

Predominant Sex

- Females affected more often than males (5:1)

Predominant Age

- 15–40 years

Predominant Race

- African Americans and Hispanics affected more often than whites

Pericardium

- Clinically apparent in 20%–30% of larger series, and up to 39% of echocardiographic studies
- Pericardial effusions occur in up to 42% by echocardiography.

Myocardium

Most clinical studies suggest about 8% affected.

Valvular Heart Disease

- Valvular thickening most common abnormality [50% on transesophageal echocardiography (TEE)], with equal frequency on mitral and aortic valves
- Vegetations in 43% and located on the basal, middle, or tip of leaflets and predominantly on the atrial side of the mitral valve or on the vessel side of the aortic valve
- Libman-Sacks lesions in 60% prior to use of steroids, 35% at autopsy once steroid use common
- Importantly, valvular lesions have been reported to resolve, change, or develop new abnormalities.

Coronary Artery Disease

- The frequency of clinically recognizable CAD is reported to be between 6.1% and 8.9% in adults.
- Thallium scans in asymptomatic individuals with SLE have reported perfusion defects in up to 39%.
- The frequency of coronary atherosclerosis in autopsy series is as high as 45%.

Antiphospholipid Antibody Syndrome

Incidence of antiphospholipid antibodies is up to 50%.

ETIOLOGY

SLE is a disease of unknown etiology in which tissues are damaged by pathogenic autoantibodies and immune complexes. These abnormal immune responses probably depend on interactions between susceptibility genes and environment.

RISK FACTORS

- Genetic predisposition, female gender, flares (ultraviolet B light, alfalfa sprouts)

PREGNANCY

- Antiphospholipid antibody syndrome is characterized by recurrent pregnancy loss.
- Association between maternal lupus and congenital heart block in offspring regardless of maternal disease activity

ASSOCIATED CONDITIONS

- Pleuritis has been noted to accompany pericarditis.
- In a single report, association between lupus myocarditis and peripheral myositis
- Cardiomyopathy and pulmonary hypertension associated with antiphospholipid antibody syndrome

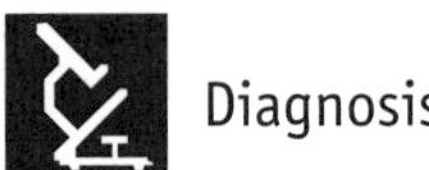

Diagnosis

DIFFERENTIAL DIAGNOSIS

Because SLE has numerous cardiac manifestations, the differential diagnosis includes the potential etiologies for each respective manifestation.

SIGNS AND SYMPTOMS

Almost any symptom or sign that could be attributed to cardiac disease may occur in a patient with SLE, including:

- Inspiratory chest pain, recumbent chest pain relieved by sitting, dyspnea, orthopnea, paroxysmal nocturnal dyspnea, palpitations, angina pectoris, nausea/emesis, diaphoresis, fever, distant heart sounds, elevated jugular venous pressure, pulsus paradoxus, precordial murmur, friction rub, pulmonary rales

LABORATORY PROCEDURES

- Positive antinuclear antibody (ANA) test is not specific for SLE.
- Antibodies to double-stranded DNA (dsDNA) and to Smith are relatively specific for SLE.
- Determining the complete autoantibody profile of each patient helps predict clinical subsets.
- High levels of ANA and anti-dsDNA and low levels of complement usually reflect disease activity.
- CH_{50} levels are the most sensitive measure of complement activation

PATHOLOGIC FINDINGS

Valvular Heart Disease

- Small verrucous vegetation that is adherent to the endocardium
- Ventricular surface of the mitral valve is most commonly affected, but the verrucae can be located on both surfaces of the leaflets of all four valves.
- Rarely, lesions may become large, approaching 10 mm.
- Microscopic: proliferating endothelial cells and myocytes with chronic inflammatory cells
- Granulomatous formation, fibrosis, necrosis, and hematoxylin bodies also present
- Immunoglobulins and complement found on the endoluminal surface of vessels from verrucae

Pericardium

- No pathologic hallmarks of lupus pericarditis
- Histologic: fibrinous exudate, fibrinoid necrosis, and hematoxylin bodies
- Chronic: obliteration of pericardial space with fibrous adhesions
- Pericardial fluid: antinuclear antibodies, LE cells, immune complexes, and a reduced complement level

Myocardium

- No gross lesions
- Role of endomyocardial biopsy unclear but helpful if alternative diagnosis identified
- Histologic: perivascular and interstitial mononuclear cell infiltration, focal fibrinoid necrosis, and infrequent hematoxylin bodies

Coronary Artery Disease

- Arteritis lesions display polymorphonuclear cells in all vascular layers, leading to edema, narrowing, and occasionally obstruction
- Autopsy findings reveal focal or diffuse obstruction of smaller intramural coronary arteries by hyaline deposits and intimal proliferation

IMAGING STUDIES

Echocardiography

- Particularly helpful in diagnosing cardiac manifestations of SLE
- TEE is more sensitive for detecting valvular verrucae

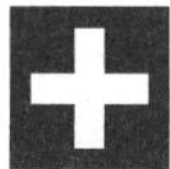

Treatment

GENERAL MEASURES

The treatment of lupus is generally initiated or modified according to its clinical features.

Valvular Heart Disease

- Antibiotic prophylaxis not evidence-based but should be considered
- Infective endocarditis should be ruled out in febrile patients.
- Antiplatelet therapy not evidence-based but suggested to reduce potential cardioembolic complications
- Anticoagulant therapy suggested following hemispheric cerebrovascular accident after vasculitis ruled out
- No consensus on the use of steroids to treat verrucous endocarditis
- Valve replacement has been performed in the mitral and aortic positions but with a high mortality rate (25%).

Pericardial Disease

- Asymptomatic, hemodynamically insignificant effusions are not treated.
- Symptomatic, uncomplicated pericarditis generally responds to nonsteroidal antiinflammatory drugs.
- More severe cases may be treated with corticosteroids.
- Hemodynamically significant effusions treated with percutaneous drainage or pericardial window

Myocardial Disease

- A prolonged 3- to 6-month course of steroid therapy or other immunosuppressants used for myocarditis

Coronary Artery Disease

- Steroid therapy reported to reverse coronary arteritis but steroids should be tapered after stabilization

Follow-up

PATIENT MONITORING

- Serologic tests for disease activity
- Echocardiogram when clinically indicated

EXPECTED COURSE AND PROGNOSIS

- The treatment of SLE and its complications has improved dramatically over the past 30 years.
- However, the morbidity and mortality associated with the cardiovascular complications of SLE are increasing and are reported to be the third most common cause of death in SLE patients.
- Mortality is correlated with serological activity.

PATIENT EDUCATION

Organizations

- Lupus Foundation of America (LFA): www.lupus.org
- National Library of Medicine: http://www.nlm.nih.gov/medlineplus/lupus.html
- Lupus Canada: www.lupuscanada.org
- Clinical Trials Listing Service: www.centerwatch.com

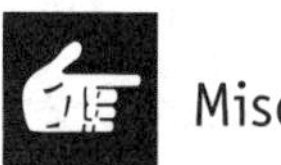

Miscellaneous

ICD-9-CM

Underlying Disease

710.0 Systemic lupus erythematosus
795.79 Antiphospholipid antibody syndrome

Specific Manifestations

424.91 Endocarditis
422.90 Acute myocarditis, unspecified
423.9 Pericardial disease, unspecified
404.90 Hypertension, cardiorenal disease, unspecified

BIBLIOGRAPHY

Doherty NE, Siegel RJ. Cardiovascular manifestations of systemic lupus erythematosus. *Am Heart J* 1985;110:1257–1265.

Ginzler EM. Clinical manifestations of disease activity, its measurement, and associated morbidity in systemic lupus erythematosus. *Curr Opin Rheumatol* 1991;3:780–788.

Mandell BF. Cardiovascular involvement in systemic lupus erythematosus. *Semin Arthritis Rheum* 1987;17:126–141.

Roldan CA, Shively BK, Crawford MH. An echocardiographic study of valvular heart disease associated with systemic lupus erythematosis. *N Engl J Med* 1997;335:1424–1430.

Topol EJ. *Cardiovascular medicine.* Philadelphia: Lippincott Williams & Wilkins, 1998:912–915.

Author: Christopher K. Dyke

Sleep Disturbance and the Heart

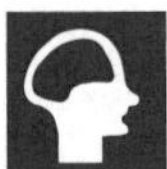

Basics

DESCRIPTION

Obstructive sleep apnea (OSA) is characterized by heavy snoring and oxygen desaturations resulting from anatomic obstruction of the upper airway and periodic apneic episodes. Untreated OSA is associated with an increased risk of myocardial infarction, cardiac arrhythmias, systemic and pulmonary hypertension, and stroke.

ETIOLOGY

Two components of OSA are proposed:

- Obstruction results from prolapse of the soft palate or tongue base during inspiration.
- Apnea results from medullary hyporeactivity to hypercapnia and hypoxia.

Systems Affected

- Cardiovascular, pulmonary, cerebrovascular, and neurologic

Incidence/Prevalence

- Approximately 4% of men and 2% of women over the age of 30 years in the United States

Predominant Age

- Middle age

Predominant Sex

- Male

RISK FACTORS

- Male sex and obesity

ASSOCIATED CONDITIONS

- Systemic hypertension
- Pulmonary hypertension
- Right heart failure
- Cardiac arrhythmias
- Obesity
- Depression

Age-Related Factors

- Pediatric: rare
- Geriatric: incidence declines as weight decreases
- Others: peak incidence in middle age

PREGNANCY

N/A

Diagnosis

DIFFERENTIAL DIAGNOSIS

- Obesity-hypoventilation syndrome (Pickwickian syndrome)
- Tracheal stenosis
- Neuromuscular disorders
- Parenchymal lung disorders

SIGNS AND SYMPTOMS

- Heavy snoring with periodic cessation of breathing
- Daytime hypersomnolence
- Morning headache
- Obesity
- Depression
- Cognitive deficits
- Systemic hypertension
- Pulmonary hypertension
- Nocturnal angina
- Paroxysmal nocturnal dyspnea
- Cardiac arrhythmias, including:
  - —Sinus bradycardia
  - —Sinus arrest
  - —Asystolic episodes
  - —Premature atrial or ventricular contractions
  - —Ventricular tachycardia
- If right heart failure has developed:
  - —Right heart enlargement
  - —Increased pulmonic second sound
  - —Increased jugular venous distention
  - —Tricuspid regurgitation heard at left sternal border
  - —Peripheral edema

LABORATORY PROCEDURES

N/A

Pathologic Findings

- Obesity, right heart enlargement

IMAGING STUDIES

Echocardiography may reveal elevated pulmonary artery pressure and tricuspid valve regurgitation. Right atrial and ventricular dilatation and pulmonic valve regurgitation may be noted in patients with more severe pulmonary hypertension resulting from OSA.

SPECIAL TESTS

N/A

DIAGNOSTIC PROCEDURES

- ECG
  - —Right atrial enlargement (P waves >2.5 mV in lead II)
    - Right ventricular hypertrophy with right axis deviation
    - The polysomnogram sleep study is the standard for diagnosis of OSA. A complete polysomnogram sleep study requires monitoring of electroencephalography, electrooculography, chin electromyography, ECG, airflow, respiratory effort, and oxygen saturation.

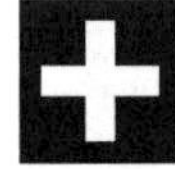

Treatment

GENERAL MEASURES

- Inpatient management may be required for evaluation and treatment of right heart failure in end-stage OSA.
- Inpatient management may be required for evaluation and treatment of right heart failure in end-stage OSA.
- OSA is reversible with administration of continuous positive airway pressure (CPAP).
- CPAP creates a positive pressure in the airway throughout the respiratory cycle, eliminating the obstructive component of OSA.
- Recognition and correction of the side effects associated with CPAP use improves compliance with therapy. Some common problems related to the use of CPAP include:
  - —Claustrophobia
  - —Intolerance to pressure
  - —Discomfort from improper fit of CPAP mask
  - —Weight loss may improve symptoms of OSA in obese patients.

SURGICAL MEASURES

- In patients who fail (or are noncompliant with) CPAP therapy, surgical measures should be considered. Tracheostomy is the only surgical intervention demonstrated to be 100% effective in the treatment of OSA. Other surgical options include:
  - —Uvulopalatopharyngoplasty
  - —Geniohyoid advancement
  - —Laser palatoplasty

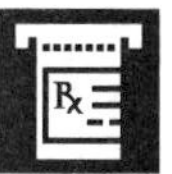

Medications

DRUG(S) OF CHOICE

- Medications have not been demonstrated to significantly improve symptoms of OSA.
- The use of sedatives should be avoided.

ALTERNATIVE DRUGS

N/A

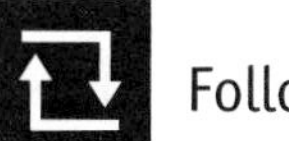

Follow-up

PATIENT MONITORING

- Close outpatient follow-up to evaluate patient compliance with treatment and correction of barriers to compliance

Prevention/Avoidance

Obesity, especially in males, should be avoided.

Possible Complications

- Right heart failure, sudden death

EXPECTED COURSE AND PROGNOSIS

- Successful treatment of OSA may improve the symptoms of right heart failure and pulmonary hypertension, but will not reverse the disease process.
- Early recognition and treatment are critical to prevent development of the irreversible sequelae of OSA.

PATIENT EDUCATION

Educate the patient about the symptoms of OSA.

Activity

Exercise should be encouraged to aid weight loss.

Diet

Calorie restriction and low salt if right heart failure present

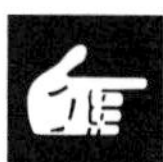

Miscellaneous

ICD-9-CM

780.53

See also: Pulmonary hypertension

BIBLIOGRAPHY

Braunwald E. *Heart disease: a textbook of cardiovascular medicine,* 4th ed. Philadelphia: WB Saunders, 1992.

Coleman J. Complications of snoring, upper airway resistance syndrome, and obstructive sleep apnea syndrome in adults. *Otolaryngol Clin North Am* 1999;32:223–234.

Davidson TM, et al. The sse of ENT-prescribed home sleep studies for patients with suspected obstructive sleep apnea. *Ear Nose Throat J* 1999;78:754–766.

Franklin KA, et al. Sleep apnoea and nocturnal angina. *Lancet* 1995;345:1085–1087.

Piper AJ, Stewart DA. An overview of nasal cpap therapy in the management of obstructive sleep apnea. *Ear Nose Throat J* 1999;78: 776–790.

Young T, et al. The occurrence of sleep-disordered breathing among middle-aged adults. *N Engl J Med* 1993;328:1230–1235.

Author: Timothy C. Bishop

Steal Syndromes

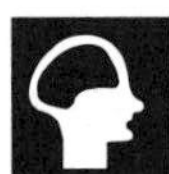

Basics

DESCRIPTION

Steal syndrome is vascular insufficiency secondary to dysfunction of arterial blood flow autoregulation rather than solely due to static flow-limiting occlusions.

Physiology

- Stimulus: increased metabolism
- Response: Arteries dilate to meet higher metabolic demands.
- Normal: Minimal pressure decreases at distal branch points where organs and muscle groups compete for blood flow.
- Abnormal: Inability to vasodilate fully with increased demand
  - —Low "vascular reserve"
- Anatomic stenosis: physical stricture with normal vessel wall, atherosclerosis
- Endothelial dysfunction
- Steal syndrome prerequisites
  - —Abnormal supplying artery
  - —Abnormal branch defaulting to at least one relatively normal arterial branch

Systems Affected

- Cardiovascular
- Cerebrovascular
- Musculoskeletal
- Gastrointestinal

Incidence/Prevalence

- Common
- Vascular diseases of medium-sized branching arteries
  - —Atherosclerosis
  - —Endothelial dysfunction
- Coronary artery steal
- Vertebral artery steal
- Subclavian artery steal

Predominant Age

- Increasing incidence after age 35

Predominant Sex

- More males affected than females

ASSOCIATED CONDITIONS

Atherosclerotic vascular disease

Age-Related Factors

- Pediatric: more associated with congenital vascular anomalies
- Adult: more associated with atherosclerotic vascular disease

RISK FACTORS

- Cigarette smoking
- Hypertension
- Diabetes
- Dyslipidemia
- Male sex
- Family history
- Advanced age

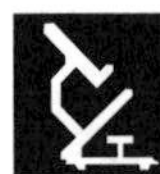

Diagnosis

DIFFERENTIAL DIAGNOSIS

- Fixed obstructive lesions
  - —Normal arterial wall architecture
  - —Atherosclerosis
  - —Kink or bend
- Steal syndrome: unbalanced competition for limited vascular reserve

SIGNS AND SYMPTOMS

- Physical examination
  - —Palpation for unequal pulses
  - —Measurement of unequal blood pressures
  - —Bruits on auscultation
- Myocardium: angina pectoris
- Vertebral arteries: transient neurologic deficits
- Skeletal muscle: claudication
- Intestinal segments
  - —Postprandial abdominal pain
  - —Bowel obstruction

IMAGING STUDIES

- Occlusive plethysmography
- Vascular ultrasonography with Doppler
- Magnetic resonance angiography
- X-ray contrast angiography
- Radionuclide perfusion imaging

SPECIAL TESTS

- Simultaneous pressure tracings via intraarterial catheters

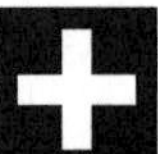

Treatment

GENERAL MEASURES

- Oxygen
- Reduce metabolic demands.
  - —For angina pectoris:
    - Beta-adrenergic blockade
    - Nitroglycerin to decrease preload
  - —For transient cerebrovascular ischemia:
    - Bed rest
    - Lower head of bed.
  - —For claudication
    - Physical exertion should be discontinued.
  - —For gastrointestinal symptoms
    - Nasogastric suctioning
    - NPO status for bowel rest
- Nitroglycerin may overcome endothelial dysfunction.
- Correct anemia if significant.

SURGICAL MEASURES

- Vascular bypass surgery
- Angioplasty

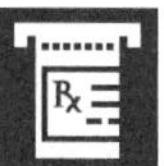

Medications

DRUG(S) OF CHOICE

- Antiplatelets agents such as aspirin
- Lipid-lowering medications such as HMG-CoA reductase inhibitors
- Beta-adrenergic blockers such as metoprolol
- Nitroglycerin to ameliorate spasm caused by endothelial dysfunction
- Calcium channel blockers to prevent subsequent episodes
- Others: aggressive medical treatment of other underlying atherogenic conditions such as hypertension and diabetes

Contraindications

- Preexisting allergy or intolerance

Precautions

Refer to manufacturer's profile for each drug.

Significant Possible Interactions

- Beta-adrenergic blockers combined with nondihydropyridine calcium channel blockers can result in bradyarrhythmias.
- Nitroglycerin should not be administered within 6 hours of Viagra use.

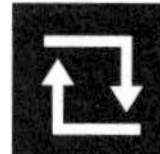

Follow-up

PATIENT MONITORING

- Close regular visits to assess gradually progressive symptoms that may indicate failure of medical therapy

Prevention/Avoidance

- Smoking cessation
- Regular exercise
- Maintain ideal body weight
- Low-fat and low-cholesterol diet
- Surveillance for hypertension, diabetes, and dyslipidemia

Possible Complications

- Acute thrombotic occlusion leading to tissue infarction.

EXPECTED COURSE AND PROGNOSIS

- Progression to fixed occlusive vascular disease with
  - —Tissue infarction
  - —Intractable symptoms
- Medical therapy can potentially slow/halt progression.

PATIENT EDUCATION

- Risk factors for endothelial dysfunction
  - —Cigarette smoking
  - —Dyslipidemia
- Risk factors for progression of atherosclerotic disease

Activity

- Rest as needed.

Diet

- Low fat/cholesterol

INTERNET RESOURCE

- http://www.theheart.org

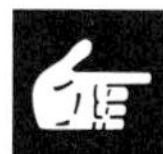

Miscellaneous

ICD-9-CM

413 Angina Pectoris
413.9 Angina, unspecified
435.1 Vertebral artery steal
435.2 Subclavian steal
557.9 Bowel ischemia (transient)

See also: Stable angina pectoris; Claudication; Transient cerebrovascular ischemia; Ischemic bowel

BIBLIOGRAPHY

Alexander RW, Schlant RC, Fuster V, et al. eds. *Hurst's the heart,* 9th ed. New York: McGraw-Hill, 1998.

Harrison DG. Endothelial function and oxidant stress. *Clin Cardiol* 1997;20:11–17.

Harrison DG, Ohara Y. Physiologic consequences of increased vascular oxidant stresses in hypercholesterolemia and atherosclerosis: implications for impaired vasomotion. *Am J Cardiol* 1995;75:75B–81B.

Holmvang G, Fry S, Skopicki HA, et al. Relation between coronary "steal" and contractile function at rest in collateral dependent myocardium of humans with ischemic heart disease. *Circulation* 1999;99:2510–2516.

Ohara Y, Peterson TE, Sayegh HS, et al. Dietary correction of hypercholesterolemia in the rabbit normalizes endothelial superoxide anion production. *Circulation* 1995;92:898–903.

Rosenfield K, Scaainfeld RM, Isner JM. Angioplasty of peripheral blood vessels.

Authors: Andrew B. Chung and Nanette K. Wenger

Sudden Death

Basics

DESCRIPTION

Sudden death is defined as the natural, sudden, unexpected loss of consciousness and death of a person in previously stable condition, with or without known heart disease. It is usually assumed to be a consequence of a ventricular arrhythmia, but bradycardia and noncardiac causes such as pulmonary embolism may be the etiology.

EPIDEMIOLOGY

There are 350,000 sudden, unexpected deaths each year in the United States. Persons of any age may be affected.

ETIOLOGY

- Coronary artery disease is the most common cause, and is not specifically a genetic disease, although there are genetic components.
- There are some clearly inherited disorders of rhythm and conduction such as the long QT syndrome, Brugada syndrome, congenital complete heart block, myotonic dystrophy, Kearn-Sayre syndrome, and, rarely, arrhythmogenic right ventricular dysplasia.
- Cardiomyopathies, both hypertrophic and dilated, are associated with an incidence of sudden, arrhythmic death.

RISK FACTORS

- Same as in coronary artery disease (cigarette use, hyperlipidemia, and hypertension)
- ECG abnormalities, often determined by ambulatory monitoring, including premature ventricular contractions and nonsustained ventricular tachycardia, left ventricular hypertrophy, nonspecific ST-T wave changes, intraventricular conduction delays, increased QT dispersion, T-wave alternans, and decreased heart rate variability
- Decreased functional capacity
- Increased age
- Higher heart rate
- Obesity
- Low left ventricular ejection fraction
- Low vital capacity
- Inducible ventricular tachycardia in high-risk patient (after myocardial infarction, low left ventricular ejection fraction)

ASSOCIATED CONDITIONS

See risk factors above.

PREGNANCY

Pregnancy may precipitate ventricular arrhythmias in long QT syndrome.

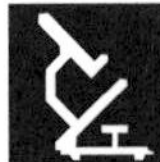

Diagnosis

DIFFERENTIAL DIAGNOSIS

- The cause of sudden, unexpected collapse and death within 1 hour of symptom onset is often elusive.
- Although such events are usually presumed to be cardiac in origin, many other catastrophic events can present with a similar time course, such as pulmonary embolism, aortic rupture, and intracerebral hemorrhage.
- Sometimes postmortem examination can define the cause of sudden death, but even then, the cause cannot always be determined.

SIGNS AND SYMPTOMS

By definition, the unexpectedness makes prodromal symptoms not a necessary component of the syndrome.

- New or worsening chest discomfort, dyspnea, palpitations, or fatigue over weeks or months may be present.
- 40%–50% of all persons who die suddenly have seen a physician in the preceding month because of symptoms not necessarily recognized as being related to the heart.

LABORATORY PROCEDURES

- Cardiac enzymes may identify myocardial infarction.
- If infarction has occurred, the chance for recurrence is low.
- Myocardial infarction as a cause of cardiac arrest would prompt evaluation of coronary anatomy.

IMAGING STUDIES

See Special Tests.

SPECIAL TESTS

- ECG (in the setting of myocardial infarction)
- Cardiac enzymes [creatine kinase (CK), CK with MB fraction, troponin]
- Echocardiogram
- Coronary and left ventricular angiography
- Cardiac MRI (useful in diagnosing arrhythmogenic right ventricular dysplasia)
- Exercise test with perfusion imaging (to assess ischemia)
- Electrophysiologic study
- Many other tests may be appropriate depending on the clinical circumstances. For example, if pulmonary embolus is suspected, ventilation-perfusion imaging, spiral CT scanning, or pulmonary angiography can be considered. If intracranial hemorrhage is suspected, cerebral MRI or CT scanning would be indicated.

PATHOLOGY

- Coronary artery disease usual substrate
- Cardiomyopathy, either hypertrophic or dilated
- Anomalous coronary artery
- Pulmonary embolus
- Cerebral hemorrhage

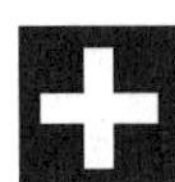

Treatment

GENERAL MEASURES

- Prompt resuscitation
- Management of airway, circulation, and brain

SURGICAL MEASURES

Surgical interventions are dictated by the cause of the cardiac arrest.

- If there is severe coronary artery disease, coronary revascularization is indicated.
- If profound bradycardia is documented, a pacemaker should be implanted.
- If ventricular fibrillation or tachycardia are documented, implantation of an implantable defibrillator should be considered.

ADMISSION/DISCHARGE CRITERIA

- The resuscitation rate in the field is usually <10%.
- If a survivor makes it to the hospital, admission is obviously the only option.
- Even survivors to admission have a high in-hospital mortality rate and often disability if they are discharged alive.

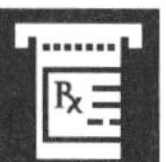

Medications

DRUG(S) OF CHOICE

- Avoid drugs that cause QT prolongation in patients with a history of torsades de pointes ventricular tachycardia and long QT syndrome.
- Amiodarone is indicated if drug treatment strategy is chosen. For cardiac arrest not due to a reversible cause, implantable defibrillators provide a greater chance for long-term survival than does drug therapy.
- Beta-blockers decrease risk of sudden death in patients recovering from myocardial infarction.
- Class IC drugs are contraindicated when coronary artery disease is present. Class IA drugs are also known to cause proarrhythmia.

Follow-up

PATIENT MONITORING

- Assess changes in functional capacity and cardiac symptoms that may be warning of changing ischemic substrate.
- If drug therapy is chosen, assess compliance, drug levels, effect on ECG, and changes in myocardial substrate.
- Device follow-up if implantable defibrillator chosen
- Control of coronary risk factors and prevention of acquired heart disease
- Correct ischemia (surgical or percutaneous revascularization, beta-blockade).
- Improve left ventricular function (angiotensin-converting enzyme inhibitors in coronary artery disease).
- If amiodarone used, follow chest x-ray, thyroid and liver function, and ECG.
- Avoid proarrhythmic drugs.
- Identification of high risk groups by noninvasive (ECG, signal averaged ECG, heart rate variability, baroreflex depression) and invasive (electrophysiologic study) assessment

EXPECTED COURSE AND PROGNOSIS

Outcome depends on the underlying substrate. In the absence of acute myocardial infarction, the chance for recurrent cardiac arrest if sudden death was due to ventricular fibrillation or tachycardia is about 30% at 1 year.

PATIENT EDUCATION

- Genetic testing and counseling, if indicated (e.g., for patients with long QT syndrome or Brugada syndrome)
- Avoidance of drugs that may be proarrhythmic, such as QT-prolonging drugs in patients with long QT syndrome
- Recommendations for diet and activity are specific for the individual patient affected.

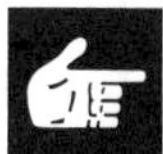

Miscellaneous

SYNONYMS

The following have been used interchangeably but are not synonymous:

- Cardiac arrest (refers to collapse due to ventricular tachycardia or fibrillation)
- Ventricular tachycardia followed by ventricular fibrillation is the usual cause of sudden death.

ICD-9-CM

427.41 Ventricular fibrillation
427.5 Cardiac arrest

See also: Defibrillators, implantable; Premature ventricular contractions; Torsades de pointes ventricular tachycardia; Ventricular fibrillation; Ventricular tachycardia; Brugada syndrome; Long QT syndrome

BIBLIOGRAPHY

Akhtar M, Myerburg RJ, Ruskin JN, eds. *Sudden cardiac death: prevalence, mechanisms, and approaches to diagnosis and management.* Philadelphia: Williams & Wilkins, 1994.

Dunbar SB, Ellenbogen K, Epstein AE, eds. Sudden cardiac death: past, present and future. Armonk, NY: Futura, 1997.

Goldschlager N, Epstein AE, Naccarelli G, et al. Practical guidelines for clinicians who treat patients with amiodarone. *Arch Intern Med* 2000;160:1741–1748.

Poole JE, Bardy GH. Sudden cardiac death. In: Zipes DP, Jalife J, eds. *Cardiac electrophysiology: from cell to bedside. Philadelphia:* WB Saunders, 1995:812–832.

Author: Andrew E. Epstein

Supraventricular Tachycardia

Basics

DESCRIPTION

Supraventricular tachycardia (SVT) is the generic term for paroxysmal, regular supraventricular tachyarrythmias.

- The tachycardia may be due to atrioventricular nodal reentrant tachycardia (AVNRT), AV reentrant tachycardia (AVRT), junctional tachycardia, or atrial tachycardia.
- The term is not generally used for atrial fibrillation or flutter, even if they are paroxysmal, but rather for other usually regular, narrow QRS arrhythmias that occur paroxysmally.

EPIDEMIOLOGY

SVT is common. The prevalence depends on the population studied. SVT is more common in younger groups but can present at any age.

ETIOLOGY

Dual AV nodal pathways, accessory pathway, junctional automaticity, atrial reentry, or automaticity

RISK FACTORS

- None

PREGNANCY

Pregnancy is not contraindicated, but SVTs may be more frequent and precipitated by pregnancy.

ASSOCIATED CONDITIONS

AVNRT and AVRT are usually isolated conditions. Other atrial tachycardias may be associated with structural heart disease.

Diagnosis

DIFFERENTIAL DIAGNOSIS

- AVNRT
- AVRT
- Junctional tachycardia
- Atrial tachycardia
- Atrial flutter with 2:1 AV conduction

SIGNS AND SYMPTOMS

- Palpitations
- Dyspnea
- Dizziness
- Syncope
- Fatigue (sometimes related to drug therapy)
- Chest pain
- Diaphoresis
- Polyuria (usually after tachycardia)

LABORATORY PROCEDURES

- None

IMAGING STUDIES

N/A

SPECIAL TESTS

- ECG: Morphology depends on arrhythmia substrate. See chapters addressing specific SVTs.
- Electrophysiologic study: required if undergoing catheter ablation

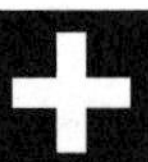

Treatment

GENERAL MEASURES

- Recording of 12-lead ECG extremely important to help with diagnosis
- Due to the problems of long-term drug administration (adverse drug reactions, problem of multiple daily doses/noncompliance, and failure at some time over years of treatment), catheter ablation has emerged as one of the treatments of choice for (recurrent) atrial flutter, atrial tachycardia, AVNRT, and AVRT (Wolff-Parkinson-White syndrome), especially the latter if atrial fibrillation is present.
- The procedure can be performed safely with a low risk of complications; over the long term it improves quality of life compared with drug therapy and is likely cost effective.
- For a single episode, a conservative approach may be adopted, including observation without drug therapy.

SURGICAL MEASURES

Although surgery has been undertaken in the past for SVTs, it has been superseded by catheter ablation. Surgical treatment of SVTs is now primarily of historical interest.

ADMISSION/DISCHARGE CRITERIA

- Patients with SVT usually do not need to be admitted.
- Admission is warranted if SVT is incessant, or if there is a life-threatening associated problem such as atrial fibrillation with rapid conduction over an accessory pathway (shortest preexcited RR interval 250 msec or less).

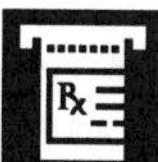

Medications

DRUG(S) OF CHOICE

Treatment depends on arrhythmia substrate. See the chapters addressing specific SVTs.

- Watch for atrial fibrillation if adenosine is used and accessory pathway is present because rapid AV conduction over the accessory pathway can occur and lead to cardiac arrest.
- For patients with structurally normal hearts, "bolus" oral doses of flecainide (300 mg) or propafenone (600 mg) can be used to acutely terminate SVTs on an intermittent basis so that daily drug administration can be avoided.

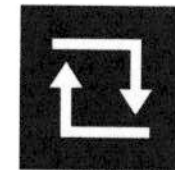

Follow-up

PATIENT MONITORING

- General medical care if on drugs
- If cured by catheter ablation, none required; SVTs are rarely associated with hypotension
- Cardiac arrest can occur if there is rapid conduction over the accessory pathway during atrial fibrillation.

EXPECTED COURSE AND PROGNOSIS

- Excellent

PATIENT EDUCATION

- Relates to treatment options, especially opportunity for cure with catheter ablation
- Vagal maneuvers to terminate arrhythmia

Activity

There are no specific recommendations regarding activity, although SVTs can occasionally be precipitated by exercise and catecholamine increase.

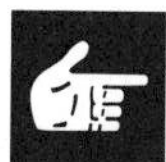

Miscellaneous

SYNONYMS

- Paroxysmal atrial tachycardia (PAT): term now obsolete

ICD-9-CM

427.0 Paroxysmal supraventricular tachycardia

BIBLIOGRAPHY

Ganz LI, Friedman PL. Supraventricular tachycardia. *N Engl J Med* 1995;332:162–173.

Morady F. Radio-frequency ablation as treatment for cardiac arrhythmias. *N Engl J Med* 1999;340:534–544.

Authors: Andrew E. Epstein and John S. Strobel

Syncope, Adult

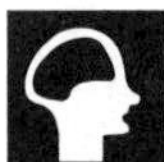

Basics

DESCRIPTION

- Transient loss of consciousness usually accompanied by loss of postural tone
- Precipitated by variety of disorders ranging from benign to fatal

EPIDEMIOLOGY

- 5%–20% of adults experience a syncopal episode by age 75.
- 6% of emergency room visits, 3% of hospital admissions
- Evaluation, treatment for syncope in 1 million people annually
- Incidence increases with age.
- Prognosis worsens with increasing age.
- Most common causes
  - —Neurally mediated (including vasovagal)
  - —Orthostatic
  - —Arrhythmia-related
  - —Seizure

ETIOLOGY

- Any condition leading to decreased cerebral blood flow
- No etiologic diagnosis established in 30%–50% of patients

RISK FACTORS

- Increasing age
- Cardiac disease
- History of neurologic disease
- Peripheral neuropathy

PREGNANCY

- Relatively common, evaluate carefully
- Due to aortocaval compression by enlarged uterus decreasing venous return

ASSOCIATED CONDITIONS

- Cardiac disorders including arrhythmias
- Neurologic disorders
- Chronic illness

Diagnosis

DIFFERENTIAL DIAGNOSIS

- Neurocardiogenic: (vasovagal, situational: cough, micturition, defecation, swallowing)
- Orthostatic
- Cardiac
  - —Arrhythmic: bradyarrhythmia (sinus node disease, heart block, pacemaker malfunction, drug induced), tachyarrhythmia (ventricular, supraventricular), carotid sinus hypersensitivity
  - —Obstructive: aortic stenosis, hypertrophic cardiomyopathy
- Neurologic: seizures
- Vascular: subclavian steal
- Psychiatric: conversion disorder, hyperventilation
- Metabolic: hypoglycemia
- Medications: antidepressants, antihypertensives, analgesics
- Unknown

SIGNS AND SYMPTOMS

History and physical examination identify up to 50% of probable causes.

History

Careful interview of patient, witnesses, medical personnel should be undertaken regarding:

- Situation (description of setting, events leading episode)
- Prodrome (palpitations, dizziness)
- Period of unconsciousness (time course, behavior)
- Residual symptoms (postevent sensations)
- Past medical history
- Medications
- Family history: sudden death, syncope
- Drugs, alcohol

Physical Examination

- Check orthostatic blood pressure: approximately 8% occurrence.
- Check blood pressure in each arm.
- Cardiac examination, including bedside maneuvers (e.g., Valsalva, carotid sinus massage)

LABORATORY PROCEDURES

- Routine laboratory testing not recommended
- Only as specifically suggested by history, physical examination

IMAGING STUDIES

- No routine imaging studies unless suggested by history, physical examination
- Brain imaging (usually with CT scan) if focal neurologic signs noted
- Carotid or transcranial Doppler is indicated if bruits are present or history suggests vertebrobasilar insufficiency. Carotid disease generally does not cause syncope.

SPECIAL TESTS

- ECG: recommended for all patients with syncope
- Echocardiography: useful for suspected organic heart disease
- Exercise testing: consider with exertional syncope, signs of ischemia
- Electroencephalography: performed with history suggesting seizure disorder
- Ambulatory ECG monitoring: history suggesting arrhythmia versus loop event monitoring for recurrent syncope
- Tilt table: if neurocardiogenic syncope suspected
- Electrophysiology: after consultation with cardiology, suspected ventricular arrhythmia

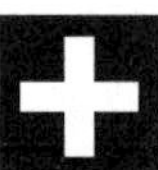

Treatment

GENERAL MEASURES

- Vary, based on etiology of syncope
- Acutely, recumbent position, head down
- Avoid dehydration.
- Volume expansion: increase salt and water intake.
- Avoid precipitating factors and drugs.
- Recognize prodrome.
- Learn adaptive maneuvers.
- Cardiology consultation if further workup indicated; cardiac catheterization, electrophysiology study
- Consider neurology consultation if significant neurologic disease is documented.

SURGICAL MEASURES

The following surgical measures may be considered after electrophysiology consultation and testing:

- Pacemaker
- Implantable defibrillator
- Catheter ablation

ADMISSION/DISCHARGE CRITERIA

- Most patients do not benefit from hospitalization
- Consider hospitalization for elderly patients, suspected arrhythmia
- Consider admission
  - —Severe orthostatic hypotension
  - —Unexplained syncope with injury
  - —New neurologic findings
  - —Concomitant conditions requiring therapy
  - —Structural heart disease
  - —Frequent syncope

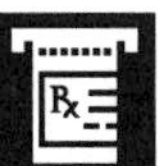

Medications

DRUG(S) OF CHOICE

- Vary with diagnosis
- Empiric drug therapy may increase recurrence.
- For vasovagal syncope
  —Fludrocortisone
  —Beta-blockers
  —Alpha-agonists: midodrine
  —Anticholinergic agents
  —Serotonin reuptake inhibitors
  —Methylxanthines
  —Magnesium
  —Clonidine

Follow-up

PATIENT MONITORING

Follow-up depends on therapy chosen; e.g., pacemakers need regular follow-up with measurement of function and battery life.

EXPECTED COURSE AND PROGNOSIS

- Negative evaluation usually denotes favorable long-term prognosis.
- 45%-50% do not experience recurrence.
- Recurrence over several years associated with good prognosis
- Prognosis worsens with increasing age.
- Mortality risk based on etiology; highest mortality with associated structural heart disease

PATIENT EDUCATION

- Life-style changes to prevent recurrence
- High-salt diet in certain situations: orthostatic, neuropathy
- Restrict driving until cause of syncope is identified and treated.
- Other restrictions based on frequency, etiology (e.g., job restrictions)

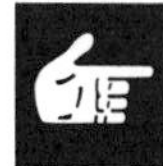

Miscellaneous

ICD-9-CM

780.2

BIBLIOGRAPHY

Boudoulas H, Nelson SD, Schaal FS, et al. Diagnosis and management of syncope. In: Alexander RW, et al., eds. *Hurst's the heart,* 9th ed. New York: McGraw-Hill, 1999:Ch. 35.

Linzer M, Yang E, Estes M, et al. Diagnosing syncope part I. *Ann Intern Med* 1997;126: 989–996.

Linzer M, Yang E, Estes M, et al. Diagnosing syncope part II. *Ann Intern Med* 1997;127: 76–86.

Olahansky B. Evaluating syncope: how to do it efficiently and safely. *J Crit Illness* 1999;14: 423–430.

Authors: Samer Garas and Jonathan Langberg

Syncope, Pediatric

Basics

DESCRIPTION

Syncope is defined as a sudden transient loss of consciousness and postural tone with recovery of sensory perception shortly thereafter (<1 minute).

- Associated physical trauma to the affected patient as a result of the episode is common.
- Consciousness usually returns with assumption of the supine position.
- Episode reflects a transient decrease in cerebral perfusion pressure.
- Rarely life-threatening in children and adolescents

Systems Affected

- Cardiovascular, neurologic, musculoskeletal

Incidence/Prevalence

- Represents 3% of emergency room visits and 6% of hospitalizations for adults in the United States
- Far less frequent in childhood

Predominant Age

- Uncommon in children; increasing frequency through adolescence

Predominant Sex

- Males and females affected equally

ETIOLOGY

- Genetics: variable depending on etiology
- Most common etiology is neurocardiogenic (23%–93% of all childhood syncope)
- Major forms of neurocardiogenic form include vasodepressor, cardioinhibitory, and mixed response.
- Common pathway for all forms of neurocardiogenic syncope is stimulation of the medullary vasodepressor region via the Bezold-Jarrisch reflex.
- Other potential etiologies include bradycardias (sinus bradycardia or atrioventricular block), serious ventricular arrhythmias (e.g., long QT syndrome), supraventricular arrhythmias or congenital lesions associated with reduced antegrade flow such as aortic stenosis, cardiomyopathy, coronary arterial anomalies, severe pulmonary stenosis, and cardiac tumors.

RISK FACTORS

- For neurocardiogenic syncope, prolonged recumbency, physical exhaustion, and pregnancy
- Breath-holding spells in infancy are usually neurocardiogenic in nature.
- For other forms of syncope, presence of Wolff-Parkinson-White (WPW) syndrome on ECG, arrhythmogenic right ventricular (RV) dysplasia, prolongation of the QT interval on ECG or familial history of such, certain forms of congenital heart disease (as noted above and including hypertrophic cardiomyopathy), or serious electrolyte abnormalities

PREGNANCY

- Represents a risk factor for neurocardiogenic syncope in adults

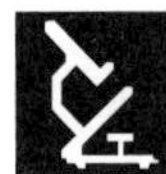

Diagnosis

DIFFERENTIAL DIAGNOSIS

- Neurologic disorders (e.g., seizure disorder, neuropathies, brain arteriovenous malformations), metabolic disorders (e.g., diabetic ketoacidosis), anemia, or ingestions/illicit drug usage

SIGNS AND SYMPTOMS

- History
  —Neurocardiogenic (vasovagal, neurally mediated, common faint)
  —Commonly seen on hot/humid day, on rapidly arising from supine or seated position, in setting of poor nutrition or hydration
  —Standing upright for long periods with venous pooling in lower extremities
  —History of light-headedness with arising from supine position.
  —Positive family history of neurocardiogenic syncope often present.
- Most common signs and symptoms
  —Light-headedness or visual changes are often noted prior to loss of consciousness (neurocardiogenic).
  —When neurocardiogenic in etiology, consciousness returns rapidly with assumption of supine position.
  —When syncope is due to arrhythmic etiology (e.g., LQTS, supraventricular tachycardia, ventricular arrhythmias), often preceded by palpitations or rapid or irregular heart beat; length of syncopal period may be longer than neurocardiogenic
  —For patients with neurocardiogenic syncope, presence of orthostatic changes should be assessed; with this exception, physical examination is often not useful in diagnosis.
  —Patients with congenital heart defects can have multiple findings on auscultation (see chapters on specific heart defects)
  —For patients with syncope due to arrhythmia, ECG/Holter monitoring may offer clues to etiology such as presence of WPW, ventricular or atrial ectopy, or prolongation of the QT interval.

LABORATORY PROCEDURES

- Complete blood count and electrolytes (including magnesium, calcium and glucose); blood and urine for toxicology in cases of potential ingestion or illicit drug use

PATHOLOGIC FINDINGS

For various congenital heart lesions, refer to specific AHA Consult Book chapters. Thinned out, fat-infiltrated RV outflow tract is noted in arrhythmogenic RV dysplasia.

SPECIAL TESTS

- ECG
  —Atrial and ventricular ectopy may be noted
  —Presence of ventricular preexcitation (e.g., WPW) should be assessed
  —Atrioventricular conduction should be reviewed (PR interval)
  —Assessment of precordial voltages and ST-T wave changes in assessing for hypertrophic cardiomyopathy should be made.
  —QTc interval should be measured in all cases.
  —24 hour ambulatory Holter should be screened for ectopy.
  —Home event recording can be useful to detect infrequent arrhythmic events.
- Head-up tilt table test
  —Rarely performed in cases where history and etiology are not clear. Test can be repeated with isoprenaline infusion, although specificity decreases with this addition.
- Electrophysiologic study
  —Performed in patients with syncope and WPW; otherwise, performed primarily in cases where the etiology is unclear and arrhythmia is suspected by history
- Exercise stress study
  —Should be performed in all patients with exercise-induced syncope as well as patients with activity related arrhythmias; often used to assess ventricular ectopy response to high-catechol state in patients with ventricular arrhythmias

IMAGING STUDIES

- Echocardiography
  —Used primarily to rule out congenital heart disease; also useful to assess ventricular function
- Cardiac catheterization
  —May be necessary to diagnose congenital heart disease
  —RV angiography may help in diagnosis of arrhythmogenic right ventricular dysplasia (although not very sensitive)
- Cardiac MRI
  —Demonstrated relatively sensitive for diagnosis of ARVD

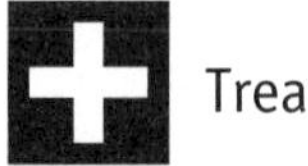

Treatment

GENERAL MEASURES

- For neurocardiogenic syncope, care is most often outpatient. For most other forms, hospitalization for evaluation/observation or intervention may be necessary.

• Self-awareness of symptoms prior to fainting is important to prevention of neurocardiogenic episodes.
  —When symptoms are felt, patients should either sit or assume a supine position.
  —Adequate hydration is the cornerstone of prevention of episodes.
• Rule of thumb is that patients are adequately drinking when the urine is entirely clear (and not concentrated).
• When above measures are carefully followed, they are 95% effective in prevention of further neurocardiogenic syncopal episodes.

SURGICAL MEASURES

• Pacemaker implantation is indicated in cases of bradycardia and may be indicated in rare cases of neurocardiogenic syncope with a predominant cardioinhibitory component.
• Also demonstrated effective in prevention of ventricular arrhythmias in certain forms of LQTS
• Automatic internal cardioverter/defibrillator (AICD) implantation is indicated in patients with documented ventricular arrhythmias unresponsive to or unprotected by medication.
• Stellate gangliectomy has been demonstrated efficacious in certain forms of LQTS in some series.
• Surgery for treatment of associated congenital lesions may be indicated.

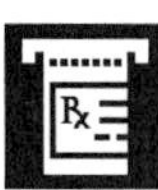

Medications

DRUG(S) OF CHOICE

• Drug therapy is not usually required for neurocardiogenic syncope. For those cases in which it is required, the following are occasionally prescribed:
  —Mineralocorticoid steroid therapy (e.g., fludrocortisone) has been demonstrated useful in certain patients to increase intravascular volume and reduce episodes.
  —Beta blockade had proven efficacious in some patients with this disorder.
  —Methylxanthines have been advocated as treatment for patients with more cardioinhibitory symptomatology.
  —Disopyramide has anticholinergic and negative inotropic effects that have been demonstrated efficacious in certain tilt-table studies.
  —For patients with arrhythmic etiologies, antiarrhythmic therapy (tailored to the individual arrhythmic substrate) is indicated.

Contraindications

For patients with WPW, use of digoxin and verapamil is limited below 1 year of age and absolutely contraindicated above 1 year of age.

Precautions

Refer to manufacturer's profile of each drug.

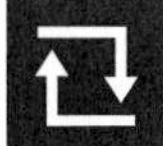

Follow-up

PATIENT MONITORING

Close regular visits for assessment of symptoms and change in such with therapy is indicated.

Prevention/Avoidance

For patients with neurocardiogenic syncope, recognition of signs and symptoms preceding a syncopal episode will often allow prevention of such episodes.

Possible Complications

• Bodily musculoskeletal injury due to falls is common.
• Brain injury due to hypoperfusion of the brain in the setting of prolonged, severe arrhythmias can occur.

EXPECTED COURSE AND PROGNOSIS

• For patients with neurocardiogenic syncope, symptoms usually improve as patients age, with fewer episodes in late adolescence and early adulthood. This may represent self-education at avoidance of activities that induce episodes or recognition of preceding symptoms with subsequent appropriate preventive measures.
• Arrhythmia course is highly variable and is largely related to efficacy of drug or other (e.g., radiofrequency catheter ablation, AICD) therapy.
• Incidence of atrial arrhythmias following Fontan or Mustard/Senning palliation for congenital heart disease increases with time from operation.

PATIENT EDUCATION

• Educate patients with neurocardiogenic syncope to appreciate and note the anticipatory feelings of light-headedness that precede syncopal episodes in order to take appropriate actions (supine position, head between knees, etc.) to avoid syncope.
• For other conditions, understanding the importance of compliance with medical regimen is critical.

Activity

• For patients with aortic outflow obstruction, decreased isometric exercise is indicated.
• Certain LQTS patients may have episodes of torsades des pointes triggered by high catecholamine level activities, and in these patients such activity should be curtailed.

Diet

For patients with neurocardiogenic syncope, high-salt diets with adequate hydration is indicated.

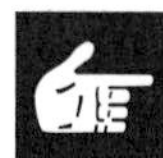

Miscellaneous

SYNONYMS

• For neurocardiogenic syncope, vasovagal, common faint, neurally mediated, and benign syncope

BIBLIOGRAPHY

Fogoros RN, ed. *The evaluation of syncope in electrophysiologic testing,* 2nd ed. Cambridge, MA: Blackwell, 1995.

Kanter RJ. In: Gillette, Garson, eds. *Syncope in clinical pediatric arrhythmias.* Philadelphia: WB Saunders, 1999.

Wiley TM, O'Donoghue S, Platia EV. Neurocardiogenic syncope: evaluation and management. *CVR&R* 1993;October:15–25.

Wolff GS, Young ML, Tamer DF. In: Deal, Wolff, Gelband, eds. *Syncope: diagnosis and management in current concepts in diagnosis and management of arrhythmias in infants and children.* New York: Futura, 1998.

Authors: Robert H. Pass and Welton M. Gersony

Syndrome X

Basics

DESCRIPTION

Syndrome X is characterized by symptoms of angina. Exercise treadmill testing may suggest ischemia and coronary arteries are angiographically normal. Syndrome X excludes patients with chest pain from other cardiac causes including coronary artery spasm, left ventricular hypertrophy, valvular heart disease, systemic hypertension.

Systems Affected

- Cardiovascular

EPIDEMIOLOGY

Incidence/Prevalence

- Up to 30% of patients referred for catheterization

Predominant Age

- Average age 50

Predominant Sex

- 70% of patients women, often premenopausal

ETIOLOGY

Syndrome X most likely represents a spectrum of diseases.

- Myocardial biopsies often normal
- Variable results of laboratory assessment for ischemia, including lactate production
- Proposed mechanisms
  —Abnormal coronary flow reserve from coronary prearteriolar vasodilation with stress causing relative ischemia
  —Abnormal endothelium-mediated vasodilation
  —Altered adenosine metabolism within myocardial cells
  —Minor intramyocardial conduction abnormalities leading to pain from altered myocardial contraction
  —Heightened unusual sympathetic responses to stress
  —Hormonal imbalances, specifically estrogen deficiency promoting vasoconstriction
  —Elevated cardiac pain sensitivity with prominent pain during cardiac manipulation, catheterization, pacing
  —Abnormal central opioid system and lower pain threshold
  —Local release of mediators that cause symptoms with ectopic beats, changes in myocardial blood flow, heart rate fluctuations

PREGNANCY

N/A

ASSOCIATED CONDITIONS

- Underlying psychiatric disorder, especially panic attacks

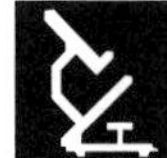

Diagnosis

DIFFERENTIAL DIAGNOSIS

- Coronary atherosclerotic disease
- Hypertensive heart disease
- Coronary artery spasm
- Valvular origin
- Musculoskeletal chest pain
- Gastroesophageal, including esophageal spasm
- Psychiatric, especially panic disorder

SIGNS AND SYMPTOMS

- Chest pain often atypical
  —Prolonged chest pain, often lasting several hours
  —May be exertional, but threshold of onset can vary
  —Rest pain in up to 40%
  —Sublingual nitrates do not bring typical pain relief.
  —Occurs both day and night
- Discomfort often lacks systemic symptoms such as diaphoresis or nausea.
- Lacks ischemia-induced physical findings, including ventricular gallop, mitral regurgitation, precordial heave

LABORATORY PROCEDURES

N/A

IMAGING STUDIES

- Nuclear imaging (positron emission tomography, thallium) abnormal in 20%–30%
- Exercise and dipyridamole imaging shows regional flow differences, wall motion abnormalities, decreases in ejection fraction.
- Decreased response to dipyridamole-induced vasodilation in patients with abnormal imaging
- Diminished coronary flow in normal scans compared with age-matched controls
- Breast attenuation can make nuclear interpretation difficult.

SPECIAL TESTS

- Resting ECG often normal; can show nonspecific ST changes
- Exercise treadmill testing may show ischemic ST segment depression with or without chest pain.
- Continuous ambulatory ECG monitoring may exhibit ST segment depression.
  —ST changes often accompanied by tachycardia
  —Changes typically occur during the day, in contrast to coronary spasm, which shows ST segment elevation typically at night or early morning.
- Exercise and dobutamine stress echocardiography shows variable wall motion abnormalities.
- Left bundle branch blocks (LBBBs) on rest/exercise ECG may exhibit diminished ventricular function during stress testing.

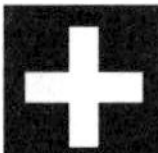

Treatment

GENERAL MEASURES

- Thorough evaluation for causes of chest pain before empirical treatment begun
- Target therapy to cause of problem.
- Chest pain may be disabling, interfering with work.
- Treat traditional coronary risk factors, including hypertension, hyperlipidemia, and diabetes.
- Consider gastroesophageal evaluation in appropriate patients.
- Someday patients with enhanced pain sensation may benefit from spinal cord nerve stimulation.

ADMISSION/DISCHARGE CRITERIA

- Thorough initial evaluation; further workup as outpatient
- Avoid repeated hospitalizations.

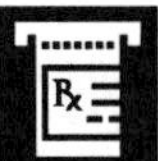

Medications

DRUG(S) OF CHOICE

- Calcium channel blockers, particularly with vasodilating activity (nifedipine, amlodipine, felodipine) are efficacious, possibly due to coronary vasodilation; improve exercise tolerance, symptoms.
- Response to beta-blockers, nitrates often poor; warrant trial
- Angiotensin-converting enzyme inhibitors may be beneficial, reduce angiotensin II effects on coronary vasculature.
- Estrogen therapy may promote vasodilation in postmenopausal women.
- Imipramine may be helpful.
- Avoid narcotics regarding risk of long-term addiction.

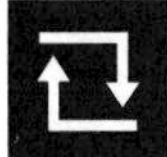

Follow-up

PATIENT MONITORING

- Periodically evaluate therapy effectiveness, life-style modifications.
- Referral to social agencies, support groups

EXPECTED COURSE AND PROGNOSIS

- Long-term outlook favorable, equal to age-matched controls
- Patients with LBBB may represent subgroup with worse prognosis (e.g., worsening left ventricular dysfunction).

PATIENT EDUCATION

- Encourage continuing daily activities as much as possible.
- Avoid known pain precipitants.

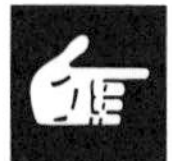

Miscellaneous

ICD-9-CM

786.50 Chest pain NOS

INTERNET RESOURCES

- http//www.nih.gov

BIBLIOGRAPHY

Fedele F, Agati L, Pugliese M, et al. Role of the central endogenous opiate system in patients with syndrome X. *Am Heart J* 1998;136:1003–1009.

Gersh BJ, Braunwald E, Rutherford JD. Chronic coronary artery disease. In: Braunwald E. *Heart disease: a textbook of cardiovascular medicine,* 5th ed. Philadelphia: WB Saunders, 1997: 1343–1344.

Kaski JC, Elliott PM. Angina pectoris and normal coronary arteriograms, clinical presentations and hemodynamic characteristics. *Am J Cardiol* 1995;76:35D–42D.

Ozcelik F, Altun A, Ozbay G. Antianginal and anti-ischemic effects of nisoldipine and ramipril in patients with syndrome X. *Clin Cardiol* 1999;22:361–365.

Schlant RC, Alexander RW. Diagnosis and management of patients with chronic ischemic heart disease. In: Alexander WA, Schlant RC, Fuster V, eds. *Hurst's the heart,* 9th ed. New York: McGraw-Hill, 1998:1295–1297.

Authors: Joseph I. Miller III and Nanette K. Wenger

Syphilitic Heart Disease

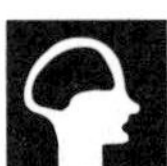

Basics

DESCRIPTION

Syphilitic heart disease results from infection by *Treponema pallidum,* a spirochete, involving the cardiovascular system. Cardiac involvement includes aortitis, coronary ostial stenosis, aortic aneurysm, aortic regurgitation, and gumma infiltration.

• Syphilis acquired by sexual contact, passage through placenta, transmission of saliva, transfusion of blood products, accidental direct inoculation
• Primary infection 14–21 days after inoculation with development of red painless dermal papule called a chancre
• Secondary or disseminated infection 4–10 weeks after initial appearance of primary lesions; involves entire trunk, extremities with papular rash; malaise, fever occur
• Clinical cardiac manifestations of tertiary syphilis develop in approximately 10% of untreated patients after 2–5 years, and may appear decades later.
• Presence of AIDS may accelerate stages.

EPIDEMIOLOGY

• 15–30 years for primary infection (sexually active age group)

ETIOLOGY

Genetics

• Unknown

RISK FACTORS

• Unprotected sexual activity, immunocompromised host

PREGNANCY

• Penicillin in dosage schedules appropriate for stage of syphilis as recommended for nonpregnant patients
• Minimal risk of infection for infant with adequate treatment during pregnancy

Diagnosis

DIFFERENTIAL DIAGNOSIS

• Collagen vascular diseases
• Aortitis from other causes

SIGNS AND SYMPTOMS

Primary

• Chancre
• Inguinal lymphadenopathy
• Condyloma latum

Secondary

• Rash
• Condyloma latum
• Lymphadenopathy
• Hepatitis
• Systemic, including fever, malaise, weight loss
• Neurologic, including headache, meningismus, meningitis, nerve disorders, cerebrovascular accident
• Periostitis
• Uveitis, iritis
• Glomerulonephritis
• Arthritis

Tertiary

• Gummata of skin, subcutaneous tissues, bones, testis, liver
• Neurosyphilis, including tabes dorsalis, paresis, psychosis, dementia, cerebrovascular accidents, meningitis, spinal cord disease
• Cardiac involvement
—Aortic aneurysm: chest pain, hoarseness, cough, dysphagia, pulsation in sternoclavicular joint from enlarging aneurysm; chest pain, hypotension, enlarging cardiac silhouette from ruptured aneurysm
—Aortic insufficiency: diastolic murmur, peripheral "water-hammer" pulses, bisferiens pulse, left ventricular hypertrophy and enlargement, congestive heart failure (dyspnea, orthopnea, lower extremity edema, etc.)
—Coronary ostial stenosis: angina, myocardial infarction, symptoms of ischemic heart disease
—Gumma infiltration: heart block, conduction disorders

Cardiac Manifestations

• Underlying pathologic lesion of cardiovascular syphilis is endarteritis obliterans
• Aortitis from destruction of vasa vasorum of aorta, which results in medial necrosis and destruction of elastic tissue; subsequent aortitis with saccular or fusiform aneurysm formation is most common manifestation
• Predilection to ascending aortic arch, which leads to weakness of aortic valve ring and distortion of valve cusps, resulting in aortic regurgitation
• Involvement of ostia of coronary arteries may lead to ostial stenosis and symptoms of ischemic heart disease; occurs in about 4% of tertiary syphilis.
• Aortic disease may become manifest years after active disease has subsided, probably from continued mechanical stress on already damaged area.
• Gumma, nonspecific granulomatous-like lesions, may involve the myocardium. Involvement at the base of the interventricular septum may result in damage to the conduction system and atrioventricular block.

LABORATORY PROCEDURES

• Nontreponemal (reaginic tests)
—Venereal Disease Research Laboratory (VDRL) test
—Rapid plasma reagin (RPR) test
—Automated reagin test (ART)
• Specific treponemal tests
—Fluorescent antibody absorption (FTA-abs) test
—*T. pallidum* hemagglutination (TPHA and MHA-TP) assay
—Treponemal immobilization (TPI) test
• Dark-field microscopic examination of fluid from chancre

Laboratory Problems

• VDRL test result may remain positive after treatment
• RPR/VDRL may be nonreactive during latent and tertiary phase
• Antibody test results always positive; negative results exclude late syphilis
• Causes of false-positive tests: other infectious diseases (tuberculosis, subacute bacterial endocarditis, leprosy, etc), early HIV, hepatitis, systemic lupus erythematosus, pregnancy, others.

IMAGING STUDIES

• ECG: left ventricular hypertrophy, occasional heart block or conduction disease
• Chest x-ray: cardiac enlargement, ascending aortic enlargement, ascending aortic calcification
• Echocardiogram: aortic insufficiency, aortic dilation with aortic root enlargement, aortic aneurysm, left ventricular hypertrophy, left ventricular enlargement

SPECIAL TESTS

• Cardiac catheterization/angiography: coronary ostial involvement

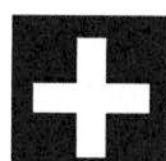

Treatment

GENERAL MEASURES

- Prevention with safe sexual practices
- Patient education
- Early treatment of primary syphilis

SURGICAL MEASURES

- Rare surgical resection of large gumma

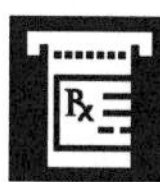

Medications

- Penicillin
  —Intramuscular and oral dosing for primary and secondary syphilis
  —Intravenous dosing for tertiary syphilis
- Doxycycline or tetracycline for penicillin-allergic patients

Precautions

- Jarisch-Herxheimer reaction: systemic reaction occurring 1–2 hours after initial treatment with effective antibiotics
  —Abrupt onset of fever, chills, myalgias, headache, flushing, tachycardia, mild hypotension
  —Usually self-limited, lasts 12–24 hours

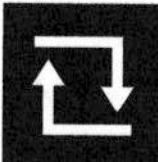

Follow-up

PATIENT MONITORING

- With early or congenital syphilis, repeat nontreponemal tests at 3, 6, and 12 months.
- With secondary syphilis or syphilis of more than 1 year's duration, repeat nontreponemal testing 24 months after treatment.
- Consider retreatment when clinical symptoms progress, nontreponemal test titers are sustained or increase, or polymerase chain reaction test result is positive.

EXPECTED COURSE AND PROGNOSIS

- High likelihood of cure with treatment, especially with earlier stages
- Overall good prognosis with treatment

PATIENT EDUCATION

- Safe sexual practices
- Preventive or epidemiologic treatment to anyone exposed to infectious syphilis in preceding 3 months

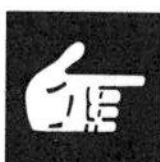

Miscellaneous

ICD-9-CM

865.92

BIBLIOGRAPHY

Alexander RW, Schlant RC, Fuster V. The connective tissue diseases. In: *Hurst's the heart,* 9th ed. New York: McGraw-Hill, 1998:2284–2285.

Alexander RW, Schlant RC, Fuster V. Diagnosis and treatment of diseases of the aorta. In: *Hurst's the heart,* 9th ed. New York: McGraw-Hill, 1998:2461–2466.

Gorbach SL, Bartlett JG, Blacklow NR. *Infectious diseases,* 2d ed. Philadelphia: WB Saunders 1998:2117–2132.

Jackman JD, Radolf JD. Cardiovascular syphilis. *Am J Med* 1989;87:425–433.

Mandell GL, Bennett JE, Dolin R. *Principles and practice of infectious diseases,* 4th ed. New York: Churchill Livingstone, 1995:980–986.

Authors: Mark Steiner and Nanette K. Wenger

Tetralogy of Fallot

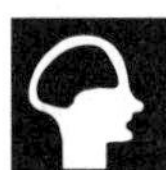

Basics

DESCRIPTION

- The tetrad of tetralogy of Fallot (TOF) includes
  —Ventricular septal defect (VSD)
  —Overriding aorta
  —Infundibular pulmonary stenosis
  —Right ventricular hypertrophy
- The severity of infundibular obstruction ranges from mild stenosis to pulmonary atresia (PA).

EPIDEMIOLOGY

- TOF occurs in about 5%–10% of infants born with congenital heart disease.
- The defect occurs sporadically.
- Found in higher frequency of siblings than would be expected in the general population
- There is no bias to age, race, or sex.

ETIOLOGY

- Unknown; occasionally associated with chromosome 22q deletion

RISK FACTORS

N/A

PREGNANCY

- Women with good surgical results following complete repair should do well with pregnancy.
- Those palliated and remaining cyanotic are at increased risk for maternal and fetal mortality, as well as increased morbidity associated with bacterial endocarditis and cardiovascular deterioration.

ASSOCIATED CONDITIONS

- Although not part of specific hereditary syndromes or chromosomal anomalies, it is commonly found in cardiofacial, VACTERL, and CHARGE syndrome.
- TOF is common in the presence of absent pulmonary valve (PV) syndrome.

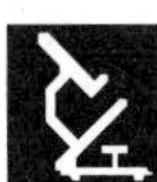

Diagnosis

DIFFERENTIAL DIAGNOSIS

The differential diagnosis of TOF depends on the degree of right ventricular outflow tract (RVOT) obstruction, but includes small VSD, isolated pulmonic stenosis or pulmonary artery (PA) defect or VSD with major aorta pulmonary collateral arteries (MAPCAs).

SIGNS AND SYMPTOMS

- Depends on the degree of RVOT obstruction.
- Acyanotic TOF (left-to-right shunt) is usually asymptomatic with a long systolic murmur along the left sternal border (LSB); these children almost always evolve to cyanotic TOF, usually later in infancy or childhood.
- Shunts may remain balanced, with the patient displaying only minimal cyanosis for decades.
- Cyanotic TOF [right-to-left (R-L) shunt] may have clubbing, dyspnea on exertion and squatting, and a loud and single S2 with a systolic ejection murmur at the upper LSB.
- Hypoxemic spells caused by a decrease in systemic vascular resistance or an increase in infundibular obstruction results in increased R-L shunt with an increase in cyanosis and a decrease in intensity of the RV outflow murmur. This in turn leads to lower pO_2 and elevated pCO_2, causing hyperpnea.
  —Usually in acyanotic TOF
  —Frequently in the morning
  —Usually self limited and responsive to treatment; however, rarely a severe spell may result in syncope, seizures, or death
- TOF/pulmonary atresia, continuous murmurs over both lungs may represent MAPCA flow
- Absent PV syndrome, initial cyanosis when pulmonary vascular resistance high; as PVR decreases the patient may develop heart failure unless the degree of infundibular stenosis is sufficient to limit pulmonary blood flow (PBF)
  —Respiratory distress due to bronchial compression from enlarged aneurysmal pulmonary arteries is a major problem in neonates and infants.

LABORATORY PROCEDURES

In cyanotic patients, a complete blood count identifies polycythemia and iron deficiency anemia.

IMAGING STUDIES

- Chest x-ray
  —Cyanotic TOF: boot-shaped heart caused by an enlarged right ventricle with absence of a radiographic main pulmonary artery segment
  —Decreased pulmonary vascular markings (PVMs)
  —Acyanotic TOF and TOF/pulmonary atresia with MAPCAs, normal to increased PVMs
  —Absent PV, mildly enlarged cardiac silhouette, dilated PAs, hyperinflated lungs
- Echocardiography
  —Aortic override of the ventricular septum, aortic root appears large with fibrous continuity between the mitral and aortic valve
  —Degree of infundibular, main PA and PV stenosis
  —Demonstrate PA continuity, may be discontinuous and connected to the aorta by a patent ductus arteriosus (PDA) or MAPCAs
  —Exclude multiple VSDs
  —Determine arch sidedness, right sided in 25%
  —Absent PV, enlarged right ventricle and main PA with pulmonary insufficiency; absence of PDA demonstrated.
  —Postoperative serial studies, presence of pulmonary insufficiency, residual or progressive right ventricular outflow tract (RVOT) obstruction, and residual VSDs
- Cardiac catheterization
  —RV pressure will equal left ventricular pressure
  —Measure PA pressure, previously shunted patients at risk for pulmonary hypertension
  —Angiography defines various levels of RVOT obstruction, anatomy of PAs, presence of multiple VSDs and coronary anomalies
  —TOF/pulmonary atresia: collaterals originate commonly in the descending thoracic aorta; selective injections are necessary to demonstrate size, distribution, and areas of stenosis in each vessel
  —Pulmonary wedge angiography is sometimes necessary to demonstrate true PAs

SPECIAL TESTS

- ECG
  —Right axis deviation
  —Right ventricular hypertrophy
  —Electrophysiology
  —Evaluate postoperative patients with syncope or suspected arrhythmia
- Interventional catheterization
  —Preoperative balloon dilatation of a stenotic PV may allow for growth of PAs, delaying need for surgical intervention
  —Postoperative use of balloons and stents to relieve native distal areas of pulmonary obstruction or those created at distal anastomotic sites or within conduits
  —Coil embolization of MAPCAs

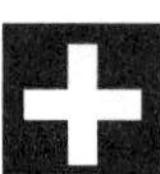

Treatment

GENERAL MEASURES

Medical management involves the effects of hypoxia in individuals with significant RVOT obstruction or hypoxemic spells.

- Resting arterial oxygen saturation in asymptomatic patients may be 70%–90%.
- Adequate oxygen saturations, hemoglobin level 15–17 g/dL, hematocrit 45%–50%
- When hematocrit reaches 65%
  —Changes in clotting status
  —Increased viscosity of blood and R-L shunt increases risk of neurologic events (headaches, seizures, and cerebrovascular accidents).
  —Phlebotomy and exchange transfusion with a plasma substitute may be needed.
- Cyanotic patients are prone to infectious endocarditis and brain abscesses.
  —Headaches in an afebrile patient may represent a brain abscess.

SURGICAL MEASURES

The ultimate goal for patients with TOF and TOF/pulmonary atresia is complete repair.

- TOF
  —Patients with significant resting hypoxia and hypoxemic spells are treated surgically on an urgent basis.
  —Single-stage repair is optimal, but factors may prohibit this: size of patient, small PAs, and coronary anomalies
  —Palliative surgery increases PBF by placing an aorta to pulmonary shunt.
  —Increased PBF may encourage PA growth
  —Complete repair involves patch closing the VSD and relieving RVOT obstruction.
- TOF/pulmonary atresia
  —If true PAs are confluent and of sufficient size and distribution to permit complete repair, establishing continuity between the RV and PA with a conduit and closing the VSD is the procedure of choice.
  —If the PA's are adequate and dual pulmonary blood supply is present, collateral vessels can be ligated at surgery or embolized at cardiac catheterization.
    - In the presence of MAPCAs with small PAs, unifocalization procedures incorporating as many collateral vessels to the true pulmonary arteries are used.
    - Lung totally supplied by unobstructed MAPCAs are at risk for developing pulmonary vascular disease.
    - If true PAs are hypoplastic or maldistributed, staged surgery may be necessary, connecting RV to PAs while leaving the VSD open to increase PBF and increase PA size.
    - Some clinicians advocate early complete repair to allow optimal PA growth rather than the staged approach.
    - Care should be taken to assess PA continuity and intervene appropriately, especially in infants, in whom the PDA provides flow to the left PA. If the PDA closes, the left pulmonary artery stenosis may be lost.
    - Success of surgical repair is directly related to the PA size and distribution.
- TOF with absent PV
  —Patch closing the VSD with a transannular patch
  —PA angioplasty
  —Some clinicians advocate a valued conduit in the pulmonary position to decrease degree of pulmonary insufficiency, but this is not universal.

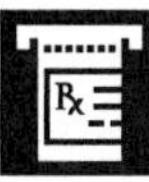

Medications

DRUG(S) OF CHOICE

- Patients with relative anemia (<15 g/dL) are at risk for neurologic events and should receive supplemental iron.
- Treatment of hypoxemic spells include:
  —Place patient in a knee-chest position
  —Oxygen
  —Morphine sulfate 0.1 mg/kg intramuscular (i.v. or s.c.)
  —$NaHCO_3$ 1 mEq/kg
  —Volume, normal saline or albumin 10 mL/kg
  —Propranolol
  —Phenylephrine
  —General anesthesia, but in this situation an emergency shunt should be placed
  —Bacterial endocarditis prophylaxis is needed as recommended by the American Heart Association.

ADMISSION/DISCHARGE CRITERIA

- Patients need admission to a hospital for treatment of medical complications such as polycythemia, neurologic events, bacterial endocarditis, arrhythmia, or congestive heart failure.
- Surgical complications also may warrant hospital admission.
- Discharge is determined by treatment course.

Follow-up

PATIENT MONITORING

- Close regular visits for assessment of progressive cyanosis
- Elective surgery in the latter part of first year
- In TOF/pulmonary atresia with MAPCAs, early cardiac catheterization to define anatomy
- Watch for signs of early congestive heart failure (increased PBF) or increasing cyanosis (decreased PBF) to determine optimal timing of surgery.
- Postoperative, regular follow-up to assess right ventricular function and occurrence of arrhythmia

EXPECTED COURSE AND PROGNOSIS

- Unoperated patients are unlikely to survive into their third decade of life
- A small group survive to adulthood, unoperated or with only a palliative procedure
- Survival to adulthood following excellent repair
- Patients at risk for poor prognosis include:
  —Small PAs such that shunts and relief of outflow obstruction do not improve cyanosis
  —Development of pulmonary vascular disease after a prolonged course with large systemic-pulmonary shunt
  —TOF/pulmonary atresia with no primary PAs
  —Poor RV function
  —Ventricular arrhythmias
- Early postoperative mortality is low.
- Postoperative complications
  —Residual RVOT obstruction, VSD, or both
  —Atrioventricular conduction abnormalities
  —Right bundle branch block
  —Ventricular arrhythmia
  —Pulmonary regurgitation; well tolerated in most patients, but associated with tricuspid regurgitation, RV failure, and arrhythmias in some
  —Risk of sudden death following complete repair is small; when occurring, probably due to sudden arrhythmia
- Routine stress testing and Holter monitoring performed serially following repair
- Absent PV syndrome, prognosis depends on respiratory status in newborns

PATIENT EDUCATION

- Adequate rest and reasonable physical activity
- No dietary restrictions, but those infants with significant heart failure may need increased caloric intake to grow
- Educate parents of the symptoms of hypoxemic spells and what to do they occur.
- There are an estimated 2,140 sites on the Internet about TOF.

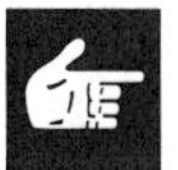

Miscellaneous

ICD-9-CM

745.2 TOF

BIBLIOGRAPHY

Garson A Jr, et al. *The science and practice of pediatric cardiology,* 2nd ed. Baltimore: Williams & Wilkins, 1998.

Park MK. The pediatric cardiology handbook. St. Louis: Mosby Year Book, 1991.

Presbitero P, et al. Pregnancy in cyanotic congenital heart disease: outcome of mother and fetus. *Circulation* 1994:89:2673–2676.

Snider AR, et al. Echocardiography in pediatric heart disease. St. Louis: Mosby Year Book, 1990.

Authors: Jacqueline M. Lamour and Welton M. Gersony

Thrombophlebitis

Basics

DESCRIPTION

Thrombophlebitis is the presence of thrombus within a superficial or deep vein and the associated vessel wall inflammatory response.

- Deep venous thrombosis (DVT) is diagnosed in only 50% of the clinical cases.
- Approximately 45% of femoral and iliac deep vein thrombosis embolize to the lungs (pulmonary embolism; PE).

Systems Affected

- Venous, pulmonary

ETIOLOGY

Genetics

- Hypercoagulable state may be inherited.

Incidence/Prevalence

Approximately 260,000 patients are diagnosed and treated for DVT and PE in the United States each year.

Predominant Age

Incidence increases with age.

Predominant Sex

- None

CAUSES

- Venous stasis
- Vascular injury
- Hypercoagulable state
- Antithrombin deficiency is an autosomal-dominant trait.
- Protein C deficiency is an autosomal-dominant trait.
- Protein S deficiency is an autosomal-dominant trait.
- Factor V Leiden mutation is a genetic polymorphism present in approximately 4%–6% of the population.

RISK FACTORS

As described by Virchow, risk factors include stasis, vascular injury, and a hypercoagulable state.

- Clinical factors
  —Age over 40
  —Prior history of thrombosis
  —Prior major surgery or trauma
  —Immobilization or paralysis
  —Venous stasis
  —Varicose veins
  —Congestive heart failure
  —Myocardial infarction
  —Obesity
  —Oral contraceptive therapy
  —Cerebrovascular accident
  —Cancer
  —Paroxysmal nocturnal hemoglobinemia
  —Antiphospholipid antibody syndrome
  —Inflammatory diseases (e.g., Crohn's disease, systemic lupus erythematosus, thromboangiitis obliterans)
  —Intravascular catheters
  —Disseminated intravascular coagulation
  —Pregnancy (especially the 3rd trimester)
- Heritable factors
  —Antithrombin III (ATIII) deficiency
  —Factor V Leiden mutation
  —Protein S deficiency
  —Protein C deficiency
  —Dysfibrinogenemia
  —Plasminogen disorders
  —Elevation of concentration of Factor VIII
- Age-related factors
  —Pediatric: rare
  —Geriatric: increased incidence and complications

PREGNANCY

Venous thrombosis is increased in pregnancy

- Increased clotting factors
- Increased platelet aggregation
- Decreased fibrinolysis

Diagnosis

DIFFERENTIAL DIAGNOSIS

- Muscle trauma
- Ruptured popliteal cyst
- Lymphedema
- Arterial occlusive disorders

SIGNS AND SYMPTOMS

- History
  —Unilateral leg swelling
  —Warmth
  —Erythema
  —Pain
  —Sudden chest pain or dyspnea if presenting with PE
- Physical findings
  —Leg tenderness
  —Erythema
  —Palpable cord
  —Increased skin turgor
  —Distention of superficial veins
  —Pedal edema
  —Homan's sign (increased pain or resistance with dorsiflexion of foot) is insensitive
  —Chronic stasis dermatitis

LABORATORY PROCEDURES

- D-dimer (low sensitivity and specificity in detecting thrombosis)
- Specific factor levels in heritable causes (e.g., Factor V Leiden, proteins C and S, ATIII)
- Antiphospholipid antibodies
- Lupus anticoagulant

Pathologic Findings

- Venous thrombosis and inflammation

IMAGING STUDIES

- Contrast venography (>90% positive predictive accuracy for deep veins)
- Venous plethysmography (>90% positive predictive accuracy for deep veins)
- Doppler ultrasonography and B-mode ultrasonography (95% positive predictive accuracy for deep veins)
- ^{125}I-fibrinogen scanning (rarely used but better at detecting calf vein thrombosis)
- Impedance plethysmography and duplex ultrasonography are the most commonly used

SPECIAL TESTS

Patients presenting with PE may require additional tests.

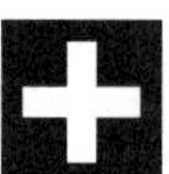

Treatment

GENERAL MEASURES

- Superficial thrombophlebitis or lower extremity DVT can be managed as an outpatient.
- Patients with more proximal DVT or suspected PE should be hospitalized initially.
- Minor symptoms attributable to varicose veins, superficial thrombosis, or calf deep vein thrombosis can be controlled medically as an outpatient with heat, elevation, and nonsteroidal antiinflammatory medications because patients are at no increased risk of PE.
- Documented or suspected DVT requires aggressive management with anticoagulation because there is significant risk of PE (inpatient and outpatient regimens are shown below).
- Documented or suspected PE requires prompt hospitalization and monitoring for possible hemodynamic and respiratory compromise.

SURGICAL MEASURES

N/A

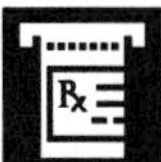

Medications

DRUG(S) OF CHOICE

- Inpatient
  —Unfractionated heparin bolus of 80 U/kg followed by infusion of 18 U/kg adjusted to activated partial thromboplastin time (APTT) of 1.5–2 times control for 5–7 days
  —Simultaneous administration of warfarin dosed to achieve prothrombin time (PT) to 1.3–1.5 times control or INR of 2–3 for 6 months
  —Overlap of heparin and warfarin for 3–4 days: 5,000–10,000 U of heparin given subcutaneously can be given to those where warfarin in contraindicated (adjusted to PTT 1.5–2 times control)
- Outpatient
  —Simultaneous administration of warfarin dosed to achieve PT to 1.3–1.5 times control or INR of 2–3 for 6 months
  —Overlap of heparin and warfarin for 3–4 days
  —Warfarin therapy for 3–6 months
- Treatment of massive DVT
  —Thrombolytic agents can be considered.
  —Streptokinase 250,000 U i.v. loading over 30 minutes followed by 100,00 U/h infusion for 24 hours
  —Urokinase 4,400 U bolus i.v. with 4,400 U/h infusion for 12–24 hours
  —Tissue plasminogen activator i.v. infusion 100 mg over 2 hours
- Recurrent DVT or PE
  —Occurs in 9.5% of patients after 6 months of therapy
  —May require life-long anticoagulation

Contraindications

Active bleeding, recent major surgery, and recent stroke are contraindications for anticoagulation.

Precautions

- Bleeding with anticoagulation (especially thrombolytics)
- Heparin-induced thrombocytopenia (HIT) with platelet count less than 150,000/mm^3 occurs in 5%–10% of patients given unfractionated heparin secondary to heparin-dependent antibodies.

Significant Possible Interactions

Wayfarin can interact with many drugs. See manufacturer's literature.

ALTERNATIVE DRUGS

Low-molecular-weight heparin can be given if warfarin contraindicated and may have a lower incidence of HIT.

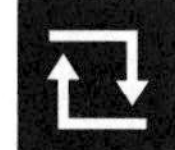

Follow-up

PATIENT MONITORING

- Improvement of presenting symptoms and for recurrence after therapy concluded
- High-risk patients may require repeat imaging to determine response to therapy.

Prevention/Avoidance

- High-risk hospitalized patients should receive DVT/PE prophylaxis, including early postoperative ambulation, pneumatic compression of the lower extremities, or low-dose s.c. heparin 5,000 U every 8 or 12 hours
- Low-molecular-weight heparin (e.g., Enoxaparin TM 30 mg every 12 hours) has been shown to be effective for DVT/PE prophylaxis in surgical patients.

Possible Complications

- Cellulitis
- Chronic stasis dermatitis

EXPECTED COURSE AND PROGNOSIS

- Majority have resolution of symptoms and recannulization of thrombosis
- Recurrence in 9.5% after 6 months of anticoagulation
- Recurrence more likely in patients with ongoing coagulopathy

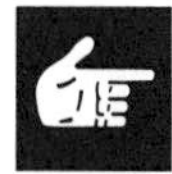

Miscellaneous

ICD-9-CM

451.9 Thrombophlebitis
451.19 Deep vein thrombosis
415.19 Pulmonary embolus

See also: Pulmonary embolus

BIBLIOGRAPHY

Braunwald E. *Heart disease: a textbook of cardiovascular medicine,* 5th ed. Philadelphia: WB Saunders, 1997.

Isselbacher KJ, Braunwald E, Wilson JD, et al. *Harrison's principles of internal medicine,* 13th ed. New York: McGraw-Hill, 1994.

Murphy JG, ed. *Mayo clinic cardiology review.* New York: Futura, 1997.

Topol EJ, ed. *Textbook of cardiovascular medicine.* Philadephia: Lippincott-Raven, 1998.

Author: Robert A. Taylor

Torsades de Pointes Ventricular Tachycardia

Basics

DESCRIPTION

Torsades de pointes (translated from French as "twisting of the pointes") ventricular tachycardia (TdP) is a polymorphic ventricular tachycardia that occurs in the setting of a long QT interval.

- It is recognized by the electrocardiographic appearance of nonuniform but organized rotation, or twisting, of the peaks of the QRS around the central axis of the ECG baseline.
- Although polymorphic, there is a distinct progressive increase and decrease in the amplitude of the QRS within each burst.
- The arrhythmia may occur in the congenital long QT syndrome, as an idiosyncratic response to a variety of drugs, as well as in bradycardia and electrolyte abnormalities, specifically hypokalemia and hypomagnesemia.
- The congenital variety is discussed in the chapter on Long QT Syndrome. The short-term management of the acquired and congenital syndromes have many similarities, but the long-term management and prognosis are different.

EPIDEMIOLOGY

Prevalence depends on population studied, especially on what drugs are used in the population. All age groups can be affected, although presentation of the congenital form occurs more often in the younger age group, and presentation of the acquired form in older patients after drug administration.

ETIOLOGY

Genetic Abnormality/Predisposition

At least six genes have been identified, as discussed in the chapter on the Long QT Syndrome.

- When TdP occurs independently of the congenital form, it is unknown whether there is genetic predisposition that becomes manifest when a precipitating stimulus is present (i.e., drugs listed below, hypokalemia, hypomagnesemia).
- Drugs that prolong repolarization
  - —Hypokalemia
  - —Hypomagnesemia
  - —Hypocalcemia
  - —Bradycardia
  - —Hypothyroidism
- Altered nutritional states (liquid protein diet, anorexia nervosa)
- Neurologic catastrophes, such as subarachnoid hemorrhage, that alter myocardial repolarization.

RISK FACTORS

- Female gender
- Length of QT interval

PREGNANCY

There is not a contraindication to pregnancy. However, arrhythmias are sometimes exacerbated by pregnancy, especially if electrolyte disturbances develop.

ASSOCIATED CONDITIONS

None are known in the congenital form. For the acquired form, patients are usually being treated with a QT-prolonging drug for a specific medical problem.

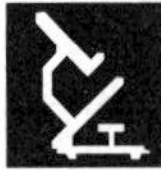

Diagnosis

DIFFERENTIAL DIAGNOSIS

- Recognition of the characteristic pattern in the setting of a prolonged QT interval on the ECG is the foundation of the diagnosis.
- Polymorphic ventricular tachycardia caused by ischemia, or as an idiopathic arrhythmia, Brugada syndrome, central nervous system injury, i.e., disease states that can alter cardiac repolarization, and therefore the QT interval

SIGNS AND SYMPTOMS

- Syncope and presyncope
- Palpitations

LABORATORY PROCEDURES

- None for general use, although genetic screening is done in a research context

IMAGING STUDIES

N/A

SPECIAL TESTS

The ECG is the diagnostic test and shows:

- Polymorphic ventricular tachycardia that varies from beat to beat and appears to rotate around the central axis of the ECG
- Rate variable, usually 160–250 beats/minute
- Long QT interval
- Initiated by long-short coupling interval [e.g., premature ventricular complex (PVC) followed by pause, sinus beat, and late cycle PVC (after peak of T wave)].
- ECG may show T-wave alternans, or variability of T waves before TdP onset.
- Often multiple nonsustained bursts

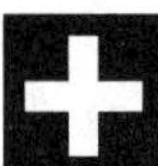

Treatment

GENERAL MEASURES

- See chapter on Long QT Syndrome for management of TdP in that setting.
- For the idiopathic variety, avoidance of and withdrawal of drugs that cause the syndrome is the mainstays of therapy.
- Correction of hypokalemia, hypomagnesemia, and hypocalcemia are essential.
- Pacing can be used to prevent TdP in the acute setting, especially when it occurs in the setting of bradycardia.
- Treat hypothyroidism, if present.

SURGICAL MEASURES

See chapter on Long QT Syndrome for congenital variety.

ADMISSION/DISCHARGE CRITERIA

- Admission is virtually always indicated when this arrhythmia is recorded because it can lead to cardiac arrest.
- Discharge is dictated by resolution of the precipitating cause or management of the congenital long QT syndrome.

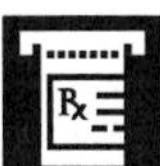

Medications

DRUG(S) OF CHOICE

- Defibrillation if sustained (cardiac arrest)
- Intravenous magnesium (1–2 g acutely)
- Isoproterenol can be used in the acute setting for drug-induced TdP. This is less frequently done today when TdP is acquired because it is frequently ineffective and temporary pacing is so successful.
- Alternatively to isoproterenol, atropine can be used.
- Beta-blockers are the pharmacologic mainstay of therapy in the congenital form (see chapter on Long QT Syndrome).
- Antiarrhythmic drugs, such as lidocaine, bretylium, and phenytoin, yield inconsistent benefit.
- Isolated reports of successful acute suppression with verapamil

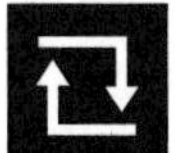

Follow-up

PATIENT MONITORING

See chapter on Long QT Syndrome for follow-up monitoring in the congenital form.

- For acquired TdP, avoidance of precipitating causes is essential.
- If antiarrhythmic treatment is necessary, use drugs that shorten QT (mexiletine, phenytoin). Note that amiodarone can uncommonly cause TdP.
- When in response to precipitating cause, it is idiosyncratic and therefore cannot be predicted.
- Avoid and prevent bradycardia, hypokalemia, hypomagnesemia, hypocalcemia, hypothyroidism, and drugs listed below.

EXPECTED COURSE AND PROGNOSIS

In the acquired form, outcome is excellent if precipitating causes are avoided. See chapter on Long QT Syndrome regarding congenital form.

PATIENT EDUCATION

Contraindications

- Avoid contraindicated drugs, hypokalemia, hypomagnesemia, and hypocalcemia.
- Learn contraindicated drugs.
- See the Appendix for the table on List of QT-Prolonging Drugs.

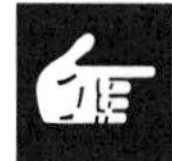

Miscellaneous

SYNONYMS

- Torsades
- Polymorphic ventricular tachycardia with QT prolongation
- Atypical ventricular tachycardia
- Ventricular fibrillo-flutter
- Paroxysmal ventricular fibrillation
- Transient ventricular fibrillation
- Cardiac ballet

ICD-9-CM

427.1 Paroxysmal ventricular tachycardia

BIBLIOGRAPHY

Dessertenne F. La tachycardie ventriculaire à deux foyers opposés variables. *Arch Mal Coeur* 1966;59:263–272.

Haverkamp W, Shenasa M, Borggrefe, et al. Torsades de pointes. In: Zipes DP, Jalife J, eds. *Cardiac electrophysiology: from cell to bedside.* Philadelphia: WB Saunders, 1995:885–899.

Authors: Andrew E. Epstein and John S. Strobel

Trauma, Cardiac

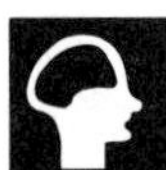

Basics

DESCRIPTION

Cardiac trauma is direct injury to the heart as the result of a violent injury. Injury can be classified as penetrating or nonpenetrating. This discussion will be limited to nonpenetrating injury.

Systems Affected

Cardiovascular

Nonpenetrating injury may involve:

- Contusion of myocardium
- Laceration of any cardiac structure
- Septal perforation
- Pericarditis
- Postpericardiotomy syndrome
- Constrictive pericarditis
- Pericardial laceration
- Hemorrhage with tamponade
- Cardiac herniation
- Rupture of a papillary muscle
- Rupture of chordae tendineae
- Rupture of atrioventricular and semilunar valves
- Coronary artery thrombosis
- Great vessel injury
- Electrical/rhythm disturbances
- Commotio cordis

ETIOLOGY

- Mechanism of injury
  - —Direct force against the chest, either unidirectional or multidirectional
  - —Indirect forces produce increased intravascular hydrostatic pressure and predispose to rupture of fluid-filled cavities.
  - —Deceleration forces, blast forces, and fractures of the ribs or sternum may lead to cardiac trauma.

Incidence/Prevalence

- In persons under the age of 40, violent or traumatic injury accounts for the majority of deaths in the United States.
- Injury is frequently secondary to a motorcycle or automobile accident, work related (e.g., using heavy machinery), or as a result of acts of violence.
- Among these victims, cardiac trauma is one of the leading causes of death.
- Young adult males are the most common sufferers of cardiac trauma because they are most likely to be involved in the acts of violence.

Predominant Age

- Young more affected than elderly

Predominant Sex

- Men affected more than women

ASSOCIATED CONDITIONS

- Trauma to other parts of the body often influence surgical decisions and prognosis.

Age

- Pediatric: unusual
- Geriatric: often fatal

PREGNANCY

- May be injurious to the fetus if cardiac function significantly compromised
- Cardiac surgery often results in fetal loss.

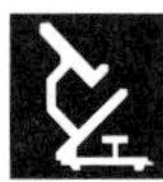

Diagnosis

SIGNS AND SYMPTOMS

- Presentation can range from asymptomatic to cardiogenic shock with rapid progression to death.
- History
  - —Recent blunt trauma to the chest wall, including vehicular impact, either directly or indirectly
  - —Direct blows to the chest wall, direct cardiac compression (e.g., during cardiopulmonary resuscitation, kicks from animals, falls)
  - —The injury pattern in a motor vehicle accident is dependent on the location of the victim in the automobile, the use of seatbelts, and deployment of airbags.
  - —The use of airbags may be associated with rupture of the right atrium.
- Chest pain that is often similar to that of myocardial infarction, frequently precordial, may have a pleuritic component.
- Pain may be difficult to assess secondary to simultaneous musculoskeletal trauma, such as rib fractures
- Congestive heart failure, which may manifest acutely or over several days and can include shortness of breath, dyspnea on exertion, orthopnea, paroxysmal nocturnal dyspnea, restlessness, feeling of uneasiness

PHYSICAL EXAMINATION

- Hypovolemia, which may present as hypotension and tachycardia
- Pericardial involvement: hypotension, oliguria, anuria, distant heart sounds, elevated jugular venous pressure, pulsus paradoxus, pericardial friction rub
- Myocardial contusion: chest wall tenderness, ecchymoses
- Other: holosystolic murmur, which may represent mitral regurgitation or ventricular septal defect, S3, rales
- ECG with non-specific ST-T wave changes or classic findings of pericarditis; ST elevation in coronary thrombosis; pathologic Q waves may represent deep myocardial injury
- Chest x-ray: may show an enlarged cardiac silhouette with pericardial effusion tamponade; evidence of congestive heart failure, pericardial tears with visceral herniation; may reveal air bubbles in the pericardium

DIFFERENTIAL DIAGNOSIS

- No relevant material

LABORATORY PROCEDURES

- Serum enzymes: Creatinine kinase (CK) and CK and MB fraction (CK-MB) are elevated in patients with blunt cardiac trauma, but this is often related to skeletal muscle damage.
- Troponin and T/I are more specific cardiac markers and may increase the sensitivity in picking up myocardial damage.
- Serial cardiac enzymes with MB fraction should be routinely drawn in patients admitted to the hospital with cardiac contusion or trauma.

PATHOLOGIC FINDINGS

- Anatomic considerations
  - —Anterior right ventricular wall is most commonly involved, followed by the anterior interventricular septum and anterior apical left ventricle.
  - —May also involve the conduction system, resulting in bundle branch block

SPECIAL TESTS

N/A

IMAGING STUDIES

- Radionuclide imaging: Technetium pyrophosphate scan can label infarcted myocardium and can be useful in the diagnosis of myocardial necrosis.
  - —Not sensitive enough to identify non-transmural and right ventricular damage
  - —Gated biventricular radionuclide scans can be done at the bedside and can accurately assess wall motion.
  - —Thallium with single-photon CT has been used for the diagnosis of myocardial damage but does not adequately assess the right ventricle.
- Echocardiography can identify contused myocardium by the appearance of increased echogenicity, increased end-diastolic thickness, and impaired systolic function.
  - —The most common echocardiographic finding in cardiac contusion is right ventricular wall motion abnormality with some dilatation.
  - —Presence of wall motion abnormality does not signify a worse outcome if the patient has a normal ECG and enzymes.

—If the patient has had thoracic wall trauma, a transesophageal echocardiogram is the modality of choice because it allows for the visualization of the great vessels.

—Echocardiogram can also be useful in identifying pericardial effusions in patients with pericarditis, post-pericardiotomy syndrome and pericardial tamponade.

- Angiography: If the patient has evidence of coronary artery involvement or thrombosis, coronary angiography is the modality of choice.
- It is useful in defining left ventricular function and coronary artery anatomy.

DIAGNOSTIC PROCEDURES

- Pericardiocentesis may be required to treat tamponade.
- Finding a bloody effusion may confirm the diagnosis of traumatic cardiac/great vessel rupture.

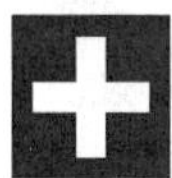

Treatment

GENERAL MEASURES

- Patients with suspected cardiac trauma are usually admitted to a monitored bed.
- Any patient with hemodynamic instability should undergo emergent thoracotomy.
- On arrival, if hemodynamically stable, the patient should give a complete history and undergo a detailed physical examination, ECG, and chest x-ray.
- If no abnormalities are detected, the patient can be observed in the emergency room for 12 hours and then discharged if the observation period is uneventful.
- If the ECG reveals nonspecific ST-T wave changes, the patient should be observed for 24 hours and have serial cardiac enzyme assays.
- Younger patients may be observed on telemetry, with older, more high-risk patients requiring ICU level care.
- If ECG reveals specific abnormalities, the patient should undergo transesophageal echocardiography or TTE.
- Depending on the findings, they should be monitored or have an urgent thoracotomy.
- If the chest x-ray is abnormal, an echocardiogram should be performed.
- If the patient requires other emergent surgery requiring general anesthesia, preoperative cardiac assessment including echocardiography should be performed.
- Intraoperative hemodynamic monitoring is prudent. Patients with marked cardiac risk or known coronary/cardiac disease should be monitored closely.

SURGICAL MEASURES

- Patients who suffer rupture of the cardiac chamber, interventricular septum, or interatrial septum require emergent surgery.
- Myocardial rupture results in sudden death in most patients.
- Patients with ventricular septal defects occasionally present late with heart failure and a holosystolic murmur.
- A small defect can be treated conservatively with supportive measures and subsequent repair if necessary.
- With myocardial rupture, there are often concurrent pericardial tears.

—Tears most often occur on the left.

—Tears also may involve the diaphragmatic pericardium, anterior pericardium, or left pleuropericardium.

- Any of these sites will predispose the patient to cardiac herniation and strangulation.

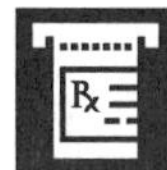

Medications

DRUG(S) OF CHOICE

- Cardiac contusion

—Chest pain is best treated with analgesics; nonsteroidal antiinflammatory drugs (NSAIDs) are not advised because they interfere with myocardial healing and may contribute to increased bleeding.

- Pericardial effusion/postpericardiotomy syndrome

—Pericarditis generally resolves spontaneously.

—Recurrent effusions with associated fever and chest pain are classified as the postpericardiotomy syndrome.

—Usually respond to aspirin or NSAIDs, but steroids are occasionally necessary.

- Treatment with anticoagulants and thrombolytics is generally contraindicated because it can predispose to bleeding and myocardial rupture.

Contraindications

Refer to manufacturer's profile on each drug.

Precautions

Refer to manufacturer's profile on each drug.

Significant Possible Interactions

Refer to manufacturer's profile on each drug.

Follow-up

PATIENT MONITORING

- If the patient is evaluated and discharged, they should have follow-up within a week.
- Those admitted should have follow-up geared to the severity of their injuries.

Possible Complications

Late complications such as arrhythmia, heart failure, aneurysm, valvular regurgitation, late ventricular septum, or free wall rupture have been reported but are rare.

EXPECTED COURSE AND PROGNOSIS

- Young patients who suffer myocardial contusion have an excellent prognosis.
- Although there are similarities between cardiac necrosis caused by trauma and that caused by coronary artery disease, the pathophysiology is quite different.
- Patients with coronary artery disease generally have other comorbidities and are much older. Both of these considerations markedly influence outcome.

PATIENT EDUCATION

- Young patients with minor blunt trauma/myocardial contusion should be treated similarly to those who have suffered a myocardial infarction with a similar amount of myocardium at risk.
- Patients with severe injury requiring surgery should undergo a recovery similar to that of a postoperative coronary bypass patient.
- Cardiac rehabilitation is often useful, especially in the elderly population and those patients with other comorbidities.

Activity

- Bed rest until diagnosis and necessary surgery completed

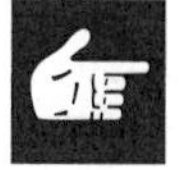

Miscellaneous

ICD-9-CM

861.01 Contusion
861.02 Laceration
861.03 Rupture
860.2 Hemopericardium

BIBLIOGRAPHY

Braunwald E. *Heart disease: a textbook of cardiovascular medicine,* 5th ed. Philadelphia: WB Saunders, 1997.

Dubrow T. Myocardial contusion in the stable patient: what level of care is appropriate? *Surgery* 1989;106:267.

Mattox K. Five thousand seven hundred sixty cardiovascular injuries in 4459 patients: epidemiologic evolution 1958 to 1987. *Ann Surg* 1989;209:698.

Topol E. *Cardiovascular medicine.* Philadelphia: Lippincott-Raven, 1998.

Author: Kathleen M. Allen

Tricuspid Regurgitation

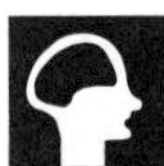

Basics

DESCRIPTION

Tricuspid regurgitation is incompetence of the tricuspid valve resulting in retrograde flow from the right ventricle into the right atrium during systole.

ETIOLOGY

N/A

EPIDEMIOLOGY

Prevalence

- Common

Age

Childhood cases are generally associated with congenital heart disease or pulmonary vascular disease. Most cases are diagnosed in adulthood.

CAUSES

- Secondary tricuspid regurgitation generally results from dilation of the right ventricle and subsequent annular enlargement.
- Common causes of annular dilation with an anatomically normal tricuspid valve include right ventricular failure, left ventricular failure, pulmonic stenosis, primary pulmonary hypertension, right ventricular infarction, Eisenmenger's syndrome, cor pulmonale, and mitral stenosis.
- Primary tricuspid regurgitation with abnormal valvular apparatus is seen in rheumatic disease, infective endocarditis, Ebstein's abnormality, Marfan's syndrome, carcinoid syndrome, and tricuspid valve prolapse.
- Rare causes include cardiac tumors, methysergide treatment, systemic lupus erythematosus, and endomyocardial fibrosis.

RISK FACTORS

Intravenous drug abusers susceptible to *Staphylococcus* endocarditis and tricuspid regurgitation

PREGNANCY

Tricuspid regurgitation generally is well tolerated during pregnancy.

Diagnosis

DIFFERENTIAL DIAGNOSIS

- Mitral regurgitation
- Pulmonic regurgitation

SIGNS AND SYMPTOMS

- Tricuspid regurgitation is well tolerated until pulmonary hypertension develops, at which time cardiac output begins to decline.
- Right-sided heart failure symptoms include edema, ascites, hepatomegaly, splenomegaly, and venous distention.
- Occasionally, throbbing pulsations in the neck and eyes are described. Weight loss, cachexia, cyanosis, jaundice are common. Dyspnea on exertion is frequent, but paroxysmal nocturnal dyspnea is often absent.

LABORATORY PROCEDURES

- The ECG is not specific but may include an incomplete right bundle branch block, right trial enlargement, and a Q wave in V1.
- Atrial fibrillation is common.

SPECIAL TESTS

- Physical examination of the venous pulse shows both a prominent V wave and Y descent, both of which increase with inspiration.
- Occasionally, the right atrium is palpable along the right sternal border.
- The right ventricle is usually hyperdynamic and may have a lift.
- An S3 gallop over the right ventricle may be heard, which is louder with inspiration (Carvello's sign).
- The tricuspid regurgitation murmur is holosystolic, high pitched, and best auscultated in the fourth interspace along the parasternal border.
- The murmur is harsher and longer when tricuspid regurgitation is associated with pulmonary hypertension.
- Dynamic auscultation increases the tricuspid regurgitation under conditions of inspiration, Mueller maneuver (forced inspiration with a closed glottis), liver compression, leg raise, and amyl nitrate inhalation.

PATHOLOGY

- Ebstein's abnormality is associated with downward displacement of the tricuspid valve and anomalous attachment of the leaflets.
- Tricuspid valve tissue is dysplastic, and the apical portion of the right ventricle is atrialized.
- Rheumatic disease results in calcified valve with fusion of the commissures.
- Carcinoid disease is associated with diffuse fibrinous deposits on the valve leaflets.
- Myxomatous degeneration is common with tricuspid valve prolapse.

IMAGING STUDIES

- Chest radiographs often show both right atrial and ventricular enlargement.
- The azygos vein may be dilated if right atrial pressure is elevated.
- Liver congestion often causes right hemidiaphragm elevation.
- Echocardiography usually demonstrates right atrial, right ventricle, and annulus enlargement.
- Right ventricle diastolic overload pattern is common.
- Tricuspid valve prolapse may be noted.
- Doppler echocardiography shows retrograde flow from the ventricle into the atrium as well as systolic flow reversal in the hepatic vein.

DIAGNOSTIC PROCEDURES

- Cardiac catheterization shows elevated end-diastolic pressure.
- The atrial pressure wave form is ventricularized with loss of the Y descent.
- High pulmonary artery pressures are generally associated with secondary tricuspid regurgitation.

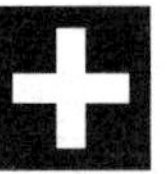

Treatment

GENERAL MEASURES

- Tricuspid regurgitation without pulmonary hypertension is generally well tolerated.
- Symptomatic tricuspid regurgitation with annular dilation is usually treated surgically with tricuspid annuloplasty.
- Rheumatic disease may require commissurotomy if the commissures are fused.
- Endocarditis and Ebstein's abnormality usually require tricuspid valve replacement, although the risk of thrombosis is high in this position because of the low flow rate.
- A large porcine heterograft, without systemic anticoagulation, is preferred.

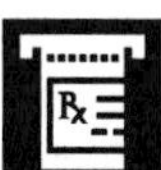

Medications

DRUG(S) OF CHOICE

- Loop diuretics are the drug of choice for edema formation.
- Digoxin can be used for right ventricular failure.
- Peripheral vasodilators are helpful if the tricuspid regurgitation is secondary to left ventricle failure.

Precautions

Low potassium caused by loop diuretic use may potentiate digoxin toxicity.

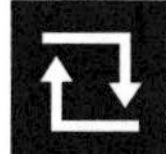

Follow-up

PATIENT MONITORING

Routine echocardiography is not recommended unless there is a change in symptomatology.

Prevention

- Endocarditis prophylaxis

EXPECTED COURSE AND PROGNOSIS

- Generally favorable
- Results of prosthetic tricuspid valve replacement are not as good as annuloplasty, with 30-day morbidity approximately 15% with artificial valve replacement.

PATIENT EDUCATION

Endocarditis prophylaxis is required.

Activity

- No limitations until cardiac output decreases as pulmonary pressures increase.

Diet

- Low sodium diet, especially in the face of edema.

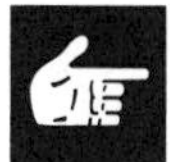

Miscellaneous

ICD-9-CM

424.2

See also: Ebstein's malformation; Rheumatic heart disease

BIBLIOGRAPHY

Alexander RW. *Hurst's the heart.* New York: McGraw-Hill, 1998.

Bonow et al. ACC/AHA guidelines for the management of patients with valvular heart disease. *J Am Coll Cardiol* 1998;32:1486–1588.

Braunwald E, ed. *Heart disease: a textbook of cardiovascular medicine,* 5th ed. Philadelphia: WB Saunders, 1997.

Topol EJ, ed. *Textbook of cardiovascular medicine.* Philadelphia: Lippincott-Raven, 1998.

Authors: Steven Herrmann, Amr El-Shafei, Madhukar Gupta, and Bernard R. Chaitman

Tricuspid Stenosis

Basics

DESCRIPTION

Tricuspid stenosis is a hemodynamic limitation in atrial filling of the right ventricle, resulting in a diastolic pressure gradient between the right atrium and right ventricle.

ETIOLOGY

Genetics

- Almost exclusively rheumatic in origin, with or without associated tricuspid regurgitation.
- Very rare to be only valve associated with rheumatic disease.
- Other causes include infective endocarditis, carcinoid, myxoma/thrombus, Fabry's disease, Whipple's disease, systemic lupus erythematosus, and previous methysergide treatment.

Prevalence

- Found in 15% of autopsy specimens in patients with documented rheumatic heart disease
- More common in females
- Clinically significant tricuspid stenosis occurs in less than 5% of those autopsied with rheumatic disease.
- More commonly seen in India (one-third of autopsied hearts with rheumatic disease) than in the United States or Western Europe.

Age

In the USA, it is most commonly diagnosed between the ages of 20 and 60 years.

PREGNANCY

Anticoagulation with coumadin is contraindicated in pregnancy with mechanical prosthesis.

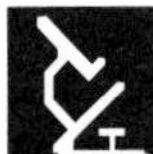

Diagnosis

DIFFERENTIAL DIAGNOSIS

- Congenital tricuspid atresia, right atrial tumors, carcinoid syndrome, endomyocardial fibrosis, tricuspid valve vegetations, extracardiac tumors

SIGNS AND SYMPTOMS

- Low cardiac output results in fatigue and dyspnea with exertion.
- Patients may complain of generalized anorexia.
- Orthopnea and paroxysmal nocturnal dyspnea are rare.
- Passive congestion of the liver and spleen results in abdominal pain.
- Peripheral edema may progress toward anasarca.
- Fluttering in the neck is a result of giant venous *a* waves.
- With severe tricuspid stenosis and mitral valve stenosis, hemoptysis, paroxysmal nocturnal dyspnea, and pulmonary edema (associated with mitral valve stenosis) are usually absent because of decreased right-sided flow across the stenotic tricuspid valve.

LABORATORY PROCEDURES

- Physical examination shows prominent *a* wave in the venous pulsation with decreased Y descent.
- Hepatic pulsation and enlargement along with splenomegaly is common.
- The right atrium may be palpable along the right sternal border with a diastolic thrill that increases with inspiration.
- An opening snap of the tricuspid valve may be appreciated but is usually masked by the mitral valve examination in coexisting mitral valve stenosis.
- The diastolic murmur of tricuspid valve stenosis is best heard along the left parasternal border in the fourth intercostal space and is crescendo-decrescendo in quality.
- Inspiration (Rivero-Carvello sign), right lateral decubitus positioning, leg lift, amyl nitrate, and isotonic exercise increase the auscultatory findings of tricuspid stenosis.
- Pulmonic valve closure is normal.

PATHOLOGIC STUDIES

- Right atrial enlargement with thickened chorda and fibrosis/contracture of the tricuspid valve leaflets and commissural fusion
- Tricuspid valve calcification is rare.
- Mitral valve and aortic valve disease is coexistent in the majority of cases.

IMAGING STUDIES

- Chest radiography shows cardiomegaly with prominence of the right atrial component of the right heart border.
- Pulmonary artery size is normal.
- Pulmonary congestion is usually absent.
- Left atrial enlargement may be noted with coexisting mitral stenosis.

SPECIAL TESTS

- EKG usually shows sinus rhythm with evidence of right atrial enlargement without right ventricular hypertrophy.
- PR segment is often depressed because of abnormal P-wave repolarization.
- Biatrial enlargement is common because of coexisting mitral valve stenosis.
- QRS amplitude may be small in V1 because of the large amount of right atrial tissue between the electrode and the ventricle.
- Transthoracic echocardiogram reveals diastolic doming of the tricuspid leaflets with decreased mobility and thickening of the valve apparatus.
- The tricuspid valve orifice is small. Doppler echocardiography shows increased diastolic velocity with a delayed slope associated with antegrade flow across the tricuspid valve.
- M-mode echocardiography shows reduced E-F slope with increased reflectance of the valve leaflets.

DIAGNOSTIC PROCEDURES

- Cardiac catheterization reveals a diastolic gradient between the tricuspid valve and right ventricle.
- A mean diastolic gradient of 2 mm Hg is sufficient for diagnosis.
- The transvalvular gradient increases as a function of flow during exercise, inspiration, infusion of saline, or administration of atropine.
- Contrast angiography in the right anterior oblique projection may reveal thickening of the valve leaflets and the decreased orifice between the right atrium and ventricle as well as the enlarged right atrium.

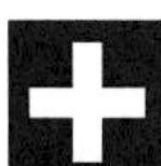

Treatment

GENERAL MEASURES

- Primary therapy for symptomatic tricuspid valve stenosis is tricuspid valve replacement or open valvulotomy.
- Decision for surgery verse valvotomy is often influenced by operative necessity of coexisting valve lesions.
- Candidates for surgery include symptomatic patients with a mean diastolic gradient of 5 mm Hg and/or a valve orifice of less than 2 cm^2.
- Simple finger commissurotomy may result in severe tricuspid regurgitation and is not recommended.
- Porcine prosthesis is recommended over mechanical valves because of the high incidence of thrombosis.
- Tricuspid valve balloon valvuloplasty has been used with favorable results.
- With coexisting tricuspid and mitral stenosis, the tricuspid lesion should not be repaired alone because pulmonary congestion may be unmasked.

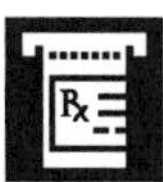

Medications

DRUG(S) OF CHOICE

- Loop diuretics

ALTERNATIVE DRUGS

- Thiazide
- Diuretics
- Digoxin

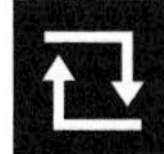

Follow-up

PATIENT MONITORING

- Presence of a diastolic murmur is a class I indication for echocardiography.
- Follow-up echocardiography examinations are based on changes in symptomatology.

Complications

- Valve thrombosis if mechanical valve prosthesis used
- Tricuspid regurgitation if commissurotomy or balloon angioplasty performed

EXPECTED COURSE AND PROGNOSIS

- After valve replacement or repair, outcome is favorable.

PATIENT EDUCATION

Activity

- Should be limited to what is tolerated
- Exercise tolerance is poor with severe tricuspid stenosis.

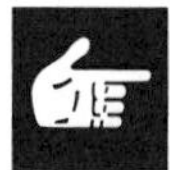

Miscellaneous

ICD-9-CM

424.2

See also: Mitral stenosis; Rheumatic heart disease

BIBLIOGRAPHY

Alexander RW, ed. *Hurst's the heart.* New York: McGraw-Hill, 1998.

Bonow et al. ACC/AHA guidelines for the management of patients with valvular heart disease. *J Am Coll Cardiol* 1998;32:1486–1588.

Braunwald E, ed. *Heart disease: a textbook of cardiovascular medicine,* 5th ed. Philadelphia: WB Saunders, 1997.

Topol EJ, ed. *Textbook of cardiovascular medicine.* Philadelphia: Lippincott-Raven, 1998.

Author: Steven Herrmann

Truncus Arteriosus

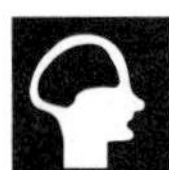

Basics

DESCRIPTION

Truncus arteriosus (TA) is a severe form of congenital heart disease in which a common arterial trunk arises as the sole outlet from both ventricles.

- The common trunk gives rise to the aorta and pulmonary arteries.
- A large ventricular septal defect (VSD) permits unrestricted blood flow from both ventricles to the common trunk.
- TA is classified by the different locations of the origin of the pulmonary arteries from the common trunk.
  —Type I: a common pulmonary artery arises from the left side of the common trunk.
  —Type II. Separate branch pulmonary arteries arise close to each other from the left posterolateral aspect of the common trunk.
  —Type III. Separate branch pulmonary arteries arise from widely separated origins from the common trunk

EPIDEMIOLOGY

- 1%–4% of all cardiac deformities
- Approximately 1/10,000 incidence in the general population

ETIOLOGY

- TA is an early embryonic structure that evolves into the aorta and pulmonary artery.
- There is failure of the TA to septate into the two great vessels.
- Truncal valve does not split into the aortic and pulmonic valves.
- Truncal valve does not migrate inferiorly to meet the left ventricular outflow.
- Crista supraventricularis does not form.
- There is a single, overriding truncus with a single truncal valve and an outlet VSD.

ASSOCIATED CONDITIONS

TA usually occurs as an isolated cardiac malformation but approximately one-third of all cases of TA are associated with DiGeorge's syndrome (the severe form of 22q11 deletion).

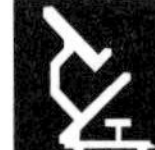

Diagnosis

DIFFERENTIAL DIAGNOSIS

- Isolated large VSD
- Pulmonary atresia with VSD, with secondary source of pulmonary blood flow, such as a patent ductus arteriosus (PDA) or major collateral vessel
- Large PDA
- Aorticopulmonary window

SIGNS AND SYMPTOMS

- In the early newborn period, babies are usually asymptomatic [due to restricted pulmonary flow secondary to high pulmonary vascular resistance (PVR)].
- Babies may present in the newborn nursery with cyanosis or, less likely, with a significant murmur.
- Cyanosis is usually minimal due to complete mixing of saturated and unsaturated blood in the setting of increased pulmonary blood flow.
- If not diagnosed in the newborn nursery, babies usually present in the first few days or weeks of life with signs and symptoms of pulmonary overcirculation and congestive heart failure (CHF), and occasionally with truncal valve insufficiency.
  —Increased respiratory rate
  —Poor feeding with tiring and sweating
  —Poor weight gain
  —Hyperdynamic precordium
  —Systolic murmur and occasional diastolic murmur (pulmonary flow and/or truncal insufficiency)
  —Hepatomegaly
  —Bounding pulses

LABORATORY PROCEDURES

- ECG
  —Usually normal in the first few days of life
  —Biventricular enlargement as PVR decreases and pulmonary overcirculation progresses.

IMAGING STUDIES

- Chest x-ray
  —May be normal in the first few days of life
  —Findings of CHF as PVR decreases; cardiomegaly and increased pulmonary vascular markings
- Echocardiogram
  —Definitive diagnostic study
  —Determines the location of the origins of the pulmonary arteries
  —Pulmonary arteries rarely may be stenotic at their origins
  —Assesses the status of the truncal valve, especially for truncal valve insufficiency
  —Right aortic arch is common.
  —Large, unrestrictive VSD is always present.
- Cardiac catheterization
  —Usually unnecessary unless the diagnosis is in question or the pulmonary artery anatomy is not well defined by echocardiography

SPECIAL TESTS

- Fluorescent *in situ* hybridization for 22q11 deletion

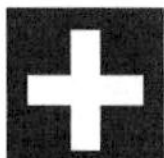

Treatment

GENERAL MEASURES

- If infant presents in the newborn period, surgical intervention is planned within the first few weeks of life.
- When signs and symptoms of CHF develop, treatment with digoxin and furosemide is indicated and usually beneficial.

SURGICAL MEASURES

- Early open heart repair is performed in early infancy.
- Usually in neonate
- Surgery consists of:
  —VSD closure
  —Detaching pulmonary arteries from the arterial trunk
  —Placement of right ventricle (RV) to pulmonary artery (PA) extracardiac conduit (homograft or xenograft) or establishing a direct, nonconduit connection between RV and PA
  —Attaching pulmonary arteries to distal end of the RV–PA connection
- In cases of severe truncal valve insufficiency, if aortic valve replacement is not possible, cardiac transplantation is the only option

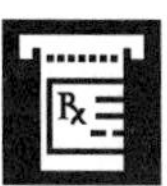

Medications

DRUG(S) OF CHOICE

- Digoxin and furosemide, for treatment of signs and symptoms of CHF

Follow-up

PATIENT MONITORING

- Prior to surgery, monitoring patient for signs and symptoms of CHF, and scheduling surgery prior to deterioration
- In early postoperative period, close follow-up is maintained, including serial physical examinations and appropriate noninvasive laboratory studies.
- In the absence of significant problems, yearly follow-up visits are important, with specific observations for:
  —Progressive abnormalities with the RV–PA connection, such as pulmonary stenosis or insufficiency
  —Truncal valve insufficiency
  —Decreased left and/or right ventricular function
- Surveillance testing usually includes surface ECG, ambulatory ECG, echocardiography, and treadmill exercise testing. Cardiac catheterization is only indicated if hemodynamic data are required for decision making.

EXPECTED COURSE AND PROGNOSIS

- Surgical mortality of complete repair in infancy is approximately 5%.
- If patient does well clinically and ventricular function is excellent in the early post-operative period, long term prognosis is good.
- Reoperations will be required, usually within 10 years, to revise RV–PA conduit.
- Significant truncal valve insufficiency may require aortic valve replacement.

PATIENT EDUCATION

- Routine recreational exercise is usually permitted and encouraged in patients who have had good surgical results.
- Avoid sedentary life-style, significant weight gain.
- Subacute bacterial endocarditis prophylaxis
- Significant symptoms, such as syncope or chest pain, require immediate medical attention.

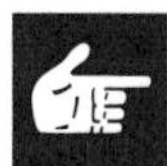

Miscellaneous

ICD-9-CM

745.0

BIBLIOGRAPHY

Anderson RH, et al., eds. *Paediatric cardiology,* 2nd ed. New York: Churchill Livingstone, 2000.

Emmanouilides GC, et al., eds. *Heart disease in infants, children, and adolescents,* 5th ed. Baltimore: Williams & Wilkins, 1995.

Goldmuntz E, et al. Frequency of 22q11 deletions in patients with conotruncal defects. *J Am Coll Cardiol* 1998;32:492–498.

McElhinney DB, et al. Trends in the management of truncal insufficiency. *Ann Thorac Surg* 1998;65:517–524.

Williams JM, et al. Factors associated with outcomes of persistent truncus arteriosus. *J Am Coll Cardiol* 1999;34:545–553.

Authors: Zvi S. Marans and Welton M. Gersony

Turner's Syndrome

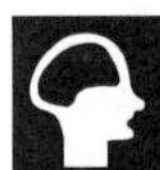

Basics

DESCRIPTION

Turner's syndrome (TS) is the most common chromosomal abnormality in females and is caused by an aneuploidy disorder with only one fully functioning X chromosome. It presents in its classic form with a characteristic phenotype and was first described in 1938 by Dr. Henry Turner.

Systems Affected

Cardiovascular, lymphatic, endocrine, renal, gastrointestinal, otologic, hematologic and neuropsychological

ETIOLOGY

Genetics

Complete absence or partial deletion of X chromosome; chromosome constitution consisting of monosomy X (45,X) karyotype (40%–60% liveborn) or isochromosome (12%–20%) translocation; full penetrance (45,X) or mosaicism (45,X/46,XX or 45,X/46,XY)

Incidence/Prevalence

The overall incidence is 2/4,000 phenotypic females.

Age at Presentation

Fetal to adult

ASSOCIATED CONDITIONS

- Cardiovascular: 22%–35%
  - —Coarctation of the aorta: 5%–15%
  - —Aortic valve disease, stenosis or incompetence: 3%–5%
  - —Bicuspid aortic valve: 15%–35%
  - —Aortic root dilatation with possible dissection or ruptures: 6%
  - —Partial anomalous pulmonary venous return: 3%
  - —Hypoplastic left heart
  - —Idiopathic systemic hypertension
  - —Coronary artery disease: secondary to increased incidence of obesity, systemic hypertension, and gonadal/estrogen deficiency
- Endocrine/reproductive
  - —Gonadal dysfunction, ranging from abnormal menstruation to infertility
  - —Short stature
  - —Osteoporosis
  - —Autoimmune thyroiditis
  - —Carbohydrate intolerance with insulin resistance
- Gastrointestinal
  - —Inflammatory bowel disease
- Renal (50%)
  - —Horseshoe kidney most common
- Otologic
  - —Conductive and sensorineural hearing deficits
- Neuropsychological
  - —Mental retardation (rare)
  - —Developmental problems: speech delay, autism, neuromotor deficits, and learning disabilities

Sex

- Female only

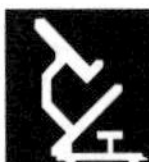

Diagnosis

DIFFERENTIAL DIAGNOSIS

- Other forms of gonadal dysgenesis syndromes such as XY or mixed gonadal dysgenesis, male pseudohermaphrodism, and male TS
- Noonan's syndrome
- The specific diagnosis can be established via both phenotypic differences, such as characteristic associated congenital heart defects, and appropriate chromosomal studies.

Criteria

An abnormal karyotype in at least one tissue characterized by partial or complete absence of the second sex chromosome, usually in association with characteristic phenotypic features.

SIGNS AND SYMPTOMS

The phenotype varies with the age at presentation.

- Fetal
  - —Possible hydrops
  - —Pleural effusion
  - —Cystic hygroma
  - —Typical karyotype on amniocentesis
  - —Brachycephaly or growth retardation
  - —Cardiac and renal abnormalities
  - —Spontaneous abortion
- Infant
  - —Edema of hands and feet
  - —Neck webbing
  - —Wide-spaced nipples
  - —Typical facies: large low-set ears, hypertelorism, epicanthal folds, down-slanting palpebral fissures
  - —Cardiovascular malformations: predominantly coarctation of the aorta or hypoplastic left heart
- Childhood
  - —Short stature
  - —Otherwise few dysmorphic features
  - —Developmental problems
- Adolescence
  - —Delay or absence of puberty: primary or secondary amenorrhea, lack of secondary sexual characteristics
- Adult
  - —Short stature
  - —Obesity
  - —Gonadal dysgenesis: resulting in amenorrhea, infertility, osteoporosis, and premature menopause
  - —Hypertension
  - —Autoimmune thyroiditis
  - —Atherosclerotic coronary artery disease

LABORATORY PROCEDURES

- Chromosome studies of peripheral blood cells (lymphocytes) or other body tissues, including fetal chorion villus or amniocentesis sample revealing either the 45XO karyotype (40%–60% of liveborn Turner's patients) or a mosaic karyotype (30%–40%)
- Endocrine studies such as thyroid function tests, growth hormone, and estrogen levels
- Renal function tests
  - —Urine specific gravity and electrolytes,
  - —Blood urea nitrogen, creatinine, and electrolyte concentrations

IMAGING STUDIES

- Fetal ultrasonography
  - —Subcutaneous edema of nuchal skin folds
  - —Generalized fetal edema
  - —Poly- or oligohydramnios
  - —Brachycephaly
  - —Renal abnormalities
  - —Growth retardation
  - —Cardiac abnormalities
- Transthoracic or fetal echocardiography
  - —Aortic coarctation, aortic valve stenosis or insufficiency, bicuspid aortic valve, or hypoplastic left heart
  - —Anomalous pulmonary venous return
  - —Left ventricular hypertrophy secondary to chronic systemic hypertension
  - —Aortic root dilatation or dissection
- Renal ultrasonography and voiding cystourethrography
  - —Structural renal abnormalities
- Roentgenograms
  - —Chest: enlarged cardiac silhouette secondary to left ventricular hypertrophy or dilatation
  - —Extremity: bone age studies in association with growth hormone therapy for growth retardation

SPECIAL TESTS

- ECG
  - —Left ventricular hypertrophy or dilatation (manifested by increased R-wave voltage in left precordial leads and increased S-wave voltage in right precordial leads) in left heart lesions causing either increased afterload or volume load on the left ventricle
  - —Diminutive left ventricular forces in association with hypoplastic left heart syndrome
  - —May be normal if neither of the above hemodynamics is present
- Audiometry
  - —Sensorineural or conductive hearing losses
- Developmental/psychosocial testing
  - —May reveal varying degrees of cognitive, behavioral, and psychosocial deficits

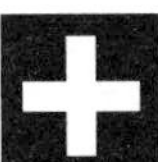

Treatment

GENERAL MEASURES

- Treatment depends on age of diagnosis and/or presentation to medical attention.
  —Prenatal: Parental counseling is advised regarding potentially affected systems, especially cardiac and renal. Timing and mode of delivery should be organized through the efforts of a high-risk perinatal team.
  —Newborn: Patients with fetal hydrops should receive supportive, nutritional, and respiratory care in an experienced center where neonatal, renal, and cardiac care can be provided.
  —Infancy and childhood: early recognition of and intervention for cognitive or developmental delays; identification and management of hearing deficits
  —Adolescence and adulthood
    - Early evaluation and recognition of growth delay
    - Appropriate referral for management of failure to initiate puberty, amenorrhea, absence of secondary sexual characteristics, infertility, or osteoporosis
    - Identification and aggressive management of progressive systemic hypertension
- All individuals with heart lesions associated with an increased risk for endocarditis should receive appropriate prophylaxis prior to dental or invasive procedures.

SURGICAL MEASURES

- Cardiac: repair of left-sided heart lesion
  —End-to-end anastomosis of discrete coarctation of the aorta
  —Norwood, Glenn, and Fontan procedures for hypoplastic left heart syndrome
  —Balloon or surgical valvuloplasty for aortic valve stenosis
  —Aortic valve replacement or Ross procedure for severe aortic valvar stenosis or insufficiency
  —Aortoplasty for severe or progressive aortic dilatation or disruption.
- Orthopedic
  —Leg-lengthening procedures for short stature
- Otologic
  —Placement of hearing-aid devices for sensorineural deficits or myringotomy tubes for conductive hearing loss
- Reproductive
  —Assisted reproduction therapy, such as ovum donation

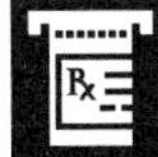

Medications

DRUG(S) OF CHOICE

- Diuretics, digoxin, and/or afterload-reducing medications for appropriate left heart lesions
- Growth hormone therapy beginning as early as 8 years of age for children with growth retardation/short stature
- Hormone/estrogen replacement therapy for delayed puberty, amenorrhea, absence of secondary sexual characteristics, or osteoporosis
- Estrogen replacement therapy for infertility
- Antihypertensive medications for systemic hypertension

Follow-up

PATIENT MONITORING

Routine life-long outpatient visits with attention to systems discussed above, especially cardiovascular, renal, endocrine and otologic. A well-coordinated multidisciplinary approach is required.

PREVENTION/AVOIDANCE

- If cardiac defects present, administer bacterial endocarditis prophylaxis for dental and invasive procedures according to American Heart Association guidelines.
- Aortic disruption or dissection: treat hypertension aggressively in cases of dilation of the aorta.
- Short stature: treat early with growth hormone in collaboration with a pediatric endocrinologist.
- Amenorrhea, infertility, and osteoporosis: Treat with estrogen replacement under obstetric or endocrinologic guidance; artificial fertilization possible.
- Pregnancy: Birth control measures are indicated in TS because, although rare, pregnancy is possible.

POSSIBLE COMPLICATIONS

- Pregnancy
  —Possible in 2% of Turner's cases
  —A large incidence of miscarriages or infants born with malformations (e.g., TS, trisomy 21)
  —38% of pregnancies result in healthy newborns.
- Aortic dissection and rupture: a potentially lethal abnormality usually, but not necessarily associated with a cardiovascular malformation such as bicuspid aortic valve, aortic coarctation, or systemic hypertension

EXPECTED COURSE AND PROGNOSIS

- Overall, the prognosis and outcomes have improved significantly. This is due to early recognition and treatment of associated cardiac malformations, short stature, infertility, systemic hypertension, and osteoporosis.
- Genetic guidance is indicated in pregnant women suspected of carrying a fetus with TS or a woman with TS planning to conceive.

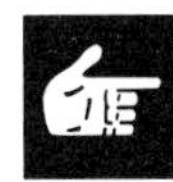

Miscellaneous

SYNONYMS

- XO gonadal dysgenesis
- Gonadal dysplasia
- Ovarian agenesis
- Bonnevie-Ullrich syndrome

BIBLIOGRAPHY

Albertson-Wikland K, Ranke MB. *Turner syndrome in a life span perspective: research and clinical aspects.* Proceedings of the 4th International Symposium on Turner Syndrome, Gothenburg, Sweden, May 18–21, 1995. Amsterdam: Elsevier.

Lin AE, et al. Further delineation of aortic dilation, dissection, and rupture in patients with Turner syndrome. *Pediatrics* 1998;July:102.

Stenberg AE, et al. Otological problems in children with Turner's syndrome. *Hearing Res* 1998;124:85–90.

Tarani L, et al. Pregnancy in patients with Turner's syndrome:; six new cases and review of literature. *Gynecol Endocrinol* 1998;12:83–87.

Telvi L, et al. 45,X/46,XY mosaicism: report of 27 cases. *Pediatrics* 1999;104(part 1):304–308.

Authors: Eric D. Fethke and Welton M. Gersony

Valvular Heart Disease and Surgery

Basics

Aortic Stenosis (AS)

DESCRIPTION

- Severity of aortic stenosis is based on calculated aortic valve area:
  - —Mild AS: >1.5 cm^2
  - —Moderate AS: 1.0–1.5 cm^2
  - —Severe AS: <1.0 cm^2
- Patients with mild aortic stenosis do not need surgical intervention.
- Those with moderate to severe aortic stenosis may need surgical intervention at some stage.

ETIOLOGY

Refer to chapters on Aortic Stenosis.

PREGNANCY

Refer to chapter on Aortic Stenosis, Adult.

Aortic Regurgitation (AR)

DESCRIPTION

Qualitative assessment of severity by cardiac catheterization depends on regurgitation of contrast from aorta to left ventricle (LV) and can be classified as follows:

- Mild (1+): Small amount of contrast enters the LV in diastole, is essentially cleared with one beat, and never fully opacifies the LV.
- Moderate (2+): More contrast enters the LV with each diastole, and faint opacification of entire chamber occurs.
- Moderately severe (3+): LV chamber is well opacified and is equal in density with the ascending aorta.
- Severe (4+): Complete dense opacification of LV chamber with the first beat and appearance that LV is more densely opacified than ascending aorta.

Mitral Stenosis

DESCRIPTION

- Severity of mitral stenosis is based on the calculated mitral valve area.
  - —Mild mitral stenosis >1.5 cm^2
  - —Moderate mitral stenosis: 1.1–1.5 cm^2
  - —Severe mitral stenosis: <1.0 cm^2

Mitral Regurgitation (MR)

DESCRIPTION

Qualitative assessment of severity by cardiac catheterization depends on opacification of left atrium (LA) and can be classified as:

- Mild (1+): never opacifies entire LA and clears with each beat
- Moderate (2+): opacifies LA after several beats, but opacification is less than LV and does not clear with one beat
- Moderately Severe (3+): LA is completely opacified and is equal to LV opacification.
- Severe (4+): opacification of entire LA with one beat, progressively more dense with each beat, and contrast can be seen refluxing into pulmonary vein

Diagnosis

SIGNS AND SYMPTOMS

N/A

LABORATORY PROCEDURES

N/A

IMAGING STUDIES

N/A

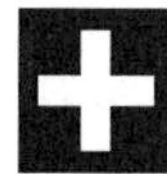

Treatment

Aortic Stenosis (AS)

GENERAL MEASURES

See chapter on Prosthetic Valves.

SURGICAL MEASURES

- Aortic valve replacement (AVR)
- Aortic balloon valvuloplasty

Aortic Valve Replacement

- AVR is definitely indicated in:
  - —Symptomatic patients with severe AS
  - —Patients with severe AS and undergoing coronary artery bypass surgery
  - —Patients with severe AS and undergoing surgery on the aorta or other heart valves
- AVR also may be indicated in patients with moderate AS and undergoing coronary artery bypass surgery or undergoing surgery on the aorta or other heart valves.
- Asymptomatic patients with severe AS and
  - —LV systolic dysfunction
  - —Abnormal response to exercise (e.g., hypotension).
  - —Significant arrhythmias (e.g., ventricular tachycardia)
  - —Marked or excessive LV hypertrophy (≥15 mm)
  - —Valve area <0.6 cm^2

Aortic Balloon Valvuloplasty

- Has an important role in treating adolescents and young adults with AS but a very limited role in older adults
- Immediate hemodynamic results include modest reduction in transvalvular gradient and early symptomatic improvement but at a significant complication rate of about 10%.
- Indications in adults
  - —A bridge to surgery in hemodynamically unstable patients who are at high risk for AVR (cardiogenic shock or moderate/severe heart failure)
  - —Palliation in patients with serious comorbid conditions
  - —Patients who require urgent noncardiac surgery
  - —Patients at extremely high risk for AVR

Aortic Regurgitation (AR)

GENERAL MEASURES

See chapter on Prosthetic Valves.

SURGICAL MEASURES

Aortic Valve Replacement

- AVR is definitely indicated in:
  - —Patients with NYHA functional class III or IV symptoms and preserved LV systolic function, defined as normal ejection fraction at rest (ejection fraction ≥0.50)
  - —Patients with NYHA functional class II symptoms and preserved LV systolic function (ejection fraction >0.50 at rest) but with progressive LV dilatation or declining ejection fraction at rest on serial studies or declining effort tolerance on exercise testing
  - —Patients with Canadian Heart Association functional class II or greater angina with or without coronary artery disease
  - —Asymptomatic or symptomatic patients with mild to moderate LV systolic dysfunction at rest (ejection fraction 0.25–0.49).
  - —Patients undergoing coronary artery bypass surgery or surgery on the aorta or other heart valves
- AVR also may be indicated in:
  - —Patients with NYHA functional class II symptoms and preserved LV systolic function (ejection fraction >0.50 at rest) with stable LV size and systolic function on serial studies and stable exercise tolerance.
  - —Asymptomatic patients with normal LV systolic function (ejection fraction >0.50) but with severe LV dilatation (end-diastolic dimension >75 mm or end-systolic dimension >55 mm) or high left ventricular end-diastolic volume index (≥150 mL/m^2) + PA wedge pressure ≥20 mm Hg

Mitral Stenosis

SURGICAL MEASURES

Percutaneous Mitral Valvotomy

Indications include:

- Symptomatic patients (NYHA functional class II, III, or IV), moderate or severe mitral stenosis (mitral valve area ≤1.5 cm^2), and valve morphology favorable for percutaneous balloon valvotomy

• Asymptomatic patients with moderate to severe mitral stenosis (mitral valve area ≥1.5 cm²) and valve morphology favorable for percutaneous balloon valvotomy who have pulmonary hypertension (pulmonary artery systolic pressure >50 mm Hg at rest or 60 mm Hg with exercise)
• Patients with NYHA functional class III–IV symptoms, moderate or severe mitral stenosis (mitral valve area ≤1.5 cm²), and a nonpliable calcified valve who are at high risk for surgery

Mitral Valve Repair

Indications include:

• Patients with NYHA functional class III–IV symptoms, moderate or severe mitral stenosis (mitral valve area ≤1.5 cm²)
• Patients with NYHA functional class III–IV symptoms, moderate or severe mitral stenosis (mitral valve area ≤1.5 cm²), and valve morphology favorable for repair
• Patients with NYHA functional class III–IV symptoms, moderate or severe mitral stenosis (mitral valve area ≤1.5 cm²), and a nonpliable or calcified valve

Mitral Valve Replacement

Indications include:

• Patients with moderate or severe mitral stenosis (mitral valve area ≤1.5 cm²) and NYHA functional class III–IV symptoms who are not considered candidates for percutaneous balloon valvotomy or mitral valve repair
• Patients with severe mitral stenosis (mitral valve area ≤1 cm²) and severe pulmonary hypertension (pulmonary artery systolic pressure >60–80 mm Hg) with NYHA functional class I–II symptoms who are not considered candidates for percutaneous balloon valvotomy or mitral valve repair

Mitral Regurgitation (MR)

SURGICAL MEASURES

Three different mitral valve operations are currently being used for correction of MR:

• Mitral valve repair
• Mitral valve replacement (MVR) with preservation of part or all the mitral apparatus
• MVR with removal of mitral apparatus

Acute Severe MR

• The patients with acute severe MR are almost always symptomatic.
• These patients need to be assessed by transthoracic or transesophageal echocardiogram for valve morphology.
• If ischemia is not the cause of MR, the patient can have mitral valve repair without the need for cardiac catheterization.

Chronic Severe MR (Nonischemic)

• Surgery is definitely indicated in following patients:
—Acute symptomatic MR in which repair is likely
—Patients with NYHA functional class II, III, or IV symptoms with normal LV systolic function defined as ejection fraction (EF) >0.60 and end-systolic dimension <45 mm.
—Symptomatic or asymptomatic patients with mild LV systolic dysfunction, EF 0.50–0.60, and end-systolic dimension 45–50 mm
—Symptomatic or asymptomatic patients with moderate LV systolic dysfunction, EF 0.30–0.50, and/or end-systolic dimension 50–55 mm
• Surgery also may be indicated in the following patients:
—Asymptomatic patients with preserved LV systolic function and atrial fibrillation
—Asymptomatic patients with preserved LV systolic function and pulmonary hypertension (pulmonary artery systolic pressure >50 mm Hg at rest or >60 mm Hg with exercise).
—Asymptomatic patients with EF 0.50–0.60 and end-systolic dimension <45 mm and asymptomatic patients with EF >0.60 and end-systolic dimension 45–55 mm
—Patients with severe LV systolic dysfunction (EF <0.30 and/or end-systolic dimension >55 mm) in whom chordal preservation is highly likely

Tricuspid Regurgitation (TR)

• Surgical options available for tricuspid regurgitation are:
—Tricuspid valve and chordal reconstruction
—Tricuspid valve annuloplasty
—Tricuspid valve replacement
• Indications
—Annuloplasty for severe long-standing TR and pulmonary hypertension in patients with mitral valve disease requiring mitral valve surgery
—Valve replacement for severe TR secondary to diseased/abnormal tricuspid valve leaflets not amenable to annuloplasty or repair
—Valve replacement or annuloplasty for severe TR with mean pulmonary artery pressure <60 mm Hg when symptomatic; bioprosthesis is preferred over mechanical prosthesis

Tricuspid Stenosis (TS)

Surgical options available for tricuspid stenosis are:

• Tricuspid commissurotomy (closed or open)
• Tricuspid valve replacement

Pulmonary Regurgitation

SURGICAL MEASURES

• Surgical treatment of pulmonary regurgitation is rarely if ever required for intractable right heart failure, usually in patients after multiple surgeries for congenital heart disease.
• Bioprosthesis is preferable because of mechanical valve thrombosis in this position.

Pulmonary Stenosis

SURGICAL MEASURES

• Surgical options available for pulmonic stenosis are either balloon valvuloplasty or valve replacement with or without surgical correction of other abnormalities.
• Balloon valvuloplasty may be indicated in symptomatic patients with pulmonary stenosis and asymptomatic patients with moderate to severe stenosis (peak-to-peak gradient of 50 mm Hg or more).
• Valve replacement is required in patients with dysplastic valve with or without correction of other abnormalities like in patients with Noonan's syndrome.

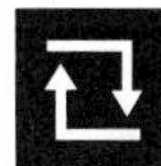

Follow-up

Aortic Stenosis

Complications of AVR

• Significant complications occur at a rate of 2%–3% per year, whereas death due directly to prosthesis occurs at a rate of ~1% per year.
• Risk and complications of anticoagulation for prosthetic metallic heart valve.

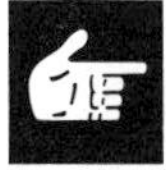

Miscellaneous

BIBLIOGRAPHY

Alexander RW, ed. *Hurst's the heart.* New York: McGraw-Hill, 1998.

Bonow et al. ACC/AHA guidelines for the management of patients with valvular heart disease. *J Am Coll Cardiol* 1998;32:1486–1588.

Braunwald E, ed. *Heart disease: a textbook of cardiovascular medicine,* 5th ed. Philadelphia: WB Saunders, 1997.

Feigenbaum H, ed. *Echocardiography,* 5th ed. Baltimore: Williams & Wilkins, 1993.

Authors: Steve Herrmann and Bernard R. Chaitman

Ventricular Fibrillation

Basics

DESCRIPTION

Ventricular fibrillation (VF) is the rapid, disorganized, and asynchronous contraction of ventricular muscle.

- On the surface ECG, it is characterized by the absence of clearly defined QRS complexes.
- VF represents the final common pathway for death in most patients who experience out-of-hospital cardiac arrest.
- Its rate of recurrence is on the order of 30% in the first year in successfully resuscitated patients.
- Much of the discussion of ventricular tachycardia (VT; see chapter of that name) is relevant to VF.

EPIDEMIOLOGY

Approximately 350,000 sudden, unexpected, arrhythmic cardiac deaths occur each year in the United States.

- The prevalence is variable and depends on the presence or absence of structural heart disease.
- Persons of any age can be affected, but the incidence of VF increases with age because structural heart disease, especially coronary artery disease, is the most common substrate and is more frequently present as we age.
- Although VF is not specifically a genetic disease, there is a genetic component, as in congenital long QT syndrome, Brugada syndrome, and arrhythmogenic right ventricular dysplasia.
- Cardiomyopathies, both hypertrophic and dilated, are associated with VT and VF.

ETIOLOGY

- Coronary artery disease (with or without acute myocardial infarction)
- Myocardial scar from any cause (most commonly coronary artery disease, but also any structural heart disease, and surgical scars)
- Cardiomyopathy (dilated, hypertrophic, arrhythmogenic right ventricular dysplasia)
- Ischemia
- Drug toxicity: includes traditional antiarrhythmic drugs such as class IC agents in coronary artery disease, QT prolonging drugs (torsades de pointes VT)
- Congenital
  - Diseases involving the ventricles (e.g., tetralogy of Fallot)
  - Long QT syndromes
- Valvular heart disease (e.g., aortic stenosis)
- Wolff-Parkinson-White syndrome with rapid ventricular preexcitation during atrial fibrillation
- Myocarditis
- Electrolyte and acid-base abnormalities (hypokalemia, metabolic acidosis)
- Primary electrical disease (idiopathic, Brugada syndrome, nocturnal death in Asians)

RISK FACTORS

- Same as in coronary artery disease (cigarette use, hyperlipidemia, and hypertension)
- Prior myocardial infarction with or without residual ischemia
- Abnormal left ventricular function (i.e., depressed left ventricular ejection fraction, dilated or hypertrophic cardiomyopathy)
- ECG abnormalities
  - ECGs of VF are rarely recorded because efforts are directed at resuscitation during the arrhythmia.
  - Rhythm strips show irregular and disorganized ventricular activity. VF is often preceded by VT.
  - The baseline ECG is often abnormal with nonsustained VT, left ventricular hypertrophy, nonspecific ST-T wave changes, intraventricular conduction delays, increased QT dispersion, T-wave alternans, decreased heart rate variability, and in specific syndromes signature findings (long QT in long QT syndrome, epsilon wave in arrhythmogenic right ventricular dysplasia, incomplete right bundle branch block with ST elevation in leads V1 and V2 in Brugada syndrome).
- Very rarely, VF will spontaneously terminate.
- Increased age
- Glucose intolerance
- Nonsustained ventricular arrhythmias
- Digitalis use
- Inducible VT in a high-risk patient (after myocardial infarction, low left ventricular ejection fraction)

PREGNANCY

- May exacerbate any arrhythmia, and is not uncommon in long QT syndrome

ASSOCIATED CONDITIONS

See list of etiologies and risk factors for VF above.

Diagnosis

DIFFERENTIAL DIAGNOSIS

ECG/monitor shows rapid and disorganized ventricular electrical activity. There is very little that can be confused with VF, other than artifact (e.g., when ECG leads have become dislodged from their positions).

SIGNS AND SYMPTOMS

- Cardiac arrest
- Syncope, sometimes with seizure activity

IMAGING STUDIES

- Echocardiogram (to evaluate cardiomyopathy, localized wall motion abnormalities such as in coronary artery disease)
- Coronary and left ventricular angiography
- Cardiac magnetic resonance imaging (useful in diagnosing arrhythmogenic right ventricular dysplasia)
- Exercise test with perfusion imaging (to assess ischemia)

SPECIAL TESTS

- ECG (myocardial infarction)
- Electrophysiologic study
- Pathology: depends on substrate, including coronary artery disease, any cause of myocardial fibrosis (cardiomyopathy, trauma), fibroadipose infiltration of the myocardium (arrhythmogenic right ventricular dysplasia), or none (Brugada syndrome)

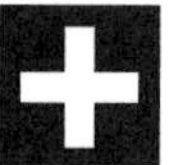

Treatment

GENERAL MEASURES

- Electrical defibrillation is the only definitive, acute treatment.
- Treat underlying heart disease, especially ischemia.
- Treat reversible causes (withdraw toxic drugs, correct electrolyte disturbances).

SURGICAL MEASURES

- VF is not treated by surgery per se.
- Surgery can be used to correct and/or treat reversible causes of VF, such as coronary artery disease and aortic stenosis.
- The Antiarrhythmics Versus Implantable Defibrillators (AVID) Trial showed that survivors of cardiac arrest have a greater survival chance when treated with an implantable cardioverter-defibrillator (ICD) compared with an antiarrhythmic drug.
- In the absence of a reversible cause or reasons to not implant an ICD, one should be offered.

ADMISSION/DISCHARGE CRITERIA

- The resuscitation rate in the field is usually <10%.
- If a survivor reaches the hospital, admission is obviously the only option. Even survivors to admission still have a high in-hospital mortality rate and often disability if they are discharged.

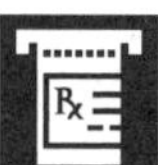

Medications

DRUG(S) OF CHOICE

- Drugs can alter the ease of defibrillation (the defibrillation threshold) by ICDs and the rate of ventricular tachycardia.
- When antiarrhythmic drugs are begun in patients with ICDs, electrophysiologic study should usually be conducted to assess the possibility of adverse drug-device interactions.
- Acutely, external electrical defibrillation is required. In concert with resuscitation efforts, the following drugs are used:
  —Lidocaine
  —Amiodarone
  —Bretylium
  —Rarely procainamide
  —Antidigoxin antibodies if digoxin toxicity suspected
  —Drugs to correct electrolyte abnormalities (e.g., potassium for hypokalemia)
- Chronically (especially, and ideally, in association with ICD in patients with no reversible cause of ventricular fibrillation)
  —Amiodarone
  —Sotalol
- Beta-blockers, to treat ischemia, and as prophylaxis in congenital long QT syndrome
- Class I drugs less effective than class III agents

Follow-up

PATIENT MONITORING

- Patients are followed according to the needs dictated by the cause of their VF.
- Reversible causes of VF must be treated.
- If drug therapy is chosen, assess compliance, drug levels, effect on ECG, and changes in myocardial substrate.
- Device follow-up if ICD chosen

Activity

For VF related to hypertrophic cardiomyopathy, exercise is restricted. Similarly, patients with aortic stenosis (presumably awaiting valve replacement or repair) should not exercise while awaiting surgery.

EXPECTED COURSE AND PROGNOSIS

Outcome depends on underlying heart disease and comorbid conditions. For patients with VF and a structurally normal heart, prognosis is better than if structural heart disease is present. However, the risk for recurrence persists.

PATIENT EDUCATION

- For patients with genetic syndromes, inform regarding need for screening of family members.
- For patients with long QT syndrome, educate regarding drugs to avoid, and for those with the congenital form avoidance of precipitating causes of torsades de pointes VT.
- With regard to specific therapies such as the ICD and drugs with potential organ toxicity (e.g., amiodarone), specialized information must be made available.

Diet

Choose diet appropriate for underlying heart disease (low cholesterol if coronary artery disease, low sodium if congestive heart failure, calorie restricted if diabetic).

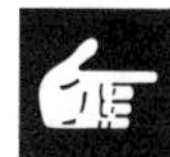

Miscellaneous

SYNONYMS

- Cardiac arrest (refers to collapse due to VT or fibrillation)
- Sudden death (VT followed by VF is usual cause of sudden, unexpected death)

ICD-9-CM

427.41 Ventricular fibrillation

See also: Implantable defibrillators; Premature ventricular contractions; Torsades de pointes ventricular tachycardia; Ventricular tachycardia; Brugada syndrome; Long QT syndrome; Sudden death

BIBLIOGRAPHY

The AVID Investigators (prepared by the AVID Executive Committee: Zipes DP, Wyse DG, Friedman PL, et al.). A comparison of antiarrhythmic drug therapy with implantable defibrillators in patients resuscitated from near-fatal sustained ventricular arrhythmias. *N Engl J Med* 1997;337:1576.

Belhassen B, Viskin S. Idiopathic ventricular tachycardia and fibrillation. *J Cardiovasc Electrophysiol* 1993;4:356.

Echt DS, Liebson PR, Mitchell LB, et al. Mortality and morbidity in patients receiving encainide, flecainide, or placebo: The Cardiac Arrhythmia Suppression Trial. *N Engl J Med* 1991;324:781.

Emergency Cardiac Care Committee and Subcommittees, American Heart Association. Guidelines for cardiopulmonary resuscitation and emergency cardiac care. *JAMA* 1992;268:2171.

Gillum RF. Sudden coronary death in the United States 1980–1985. *Circulation* 1989;79:756.

Klein GJ, Bashore TM, Sellers TD, et al. Ventricular fibrillation in the Wolff-Parkinson-White syndrome. *N Engl J Med* 1979;301:1080.

Maron BJ, Fananapazir L. Sudden cardiac death in hypertrophic cardiomyopathy. *Circulation* 1992;85(suppl I):57.

Viskin S, Belhassen B. Idiopathic ventricular fibrillation. *Am Heart J* 1990;120:661.

Author: Andrew E. Epstein

Ventricular Septal Defect

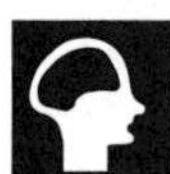

Basics

DESCRIPTION

A ventricular septal defect (VSD) is an anatomic defect that allows intracardiac shunting of blood. VSDs may occur at various positions in the ventricular septum:

- Posterior: inlet distal to the tricuspid valve (endocardial cushion type), may exist as an isolated anomaly or as part of an atrioventricular canal.
- Subaortic (membranous)
- Subpulmonary (supracristal): associated with aortic valve prolapse.
- Muscular: mid or apical; may be multiple

Systems Affected

- Cardiovascular, pulmonary

ETIOLOGY

Genetics

90% of VSDs are "multifactorial" in etiology and not associated with specific chromosomal anomalies. 8% have chromosomal anomalies (trisomy 13,18,21 etc.). 2% may be attributable to environmental causes.

Incidence/Prevalence

- Ventricular septal defect is the most common congenital heart defect, excluding bicuspid aortic valve without obstruction.
- Incidence is 1.5–3.5/1,000 term births and 4.5–7/1,000 premature infants.
- Overall prevalence in children is 1.4/1,000 live births.
- The smaller prevalence in children largely represents spontaneous closure, occurring commonly in the first year of life, but also as late as adult life.

Predominant Sex

- 56% female, 44% male

CAUSES

- Congenital (most common)
- Traumatic
- Ischemic

RISK FACTORS

- Family history of congenital heart disease
- Associated with chromosomal anomalies
- Exposure to teratogens during gestation

ASSOCIATED CONDITIONS

- Failure to thrive
- Congestive heart failure (CHF)
- Pulmonary hypertension
- Pulmonary vascular obstructive disease

Age-Related Factors

- Pediatric: careful evaluation for possible pulmonary hypertension prior to 2 years of life.

PREGNANCY

- Pulmonary hypertension poorly tolerated
- 2%–3% risk of congenital heart disease in offspring

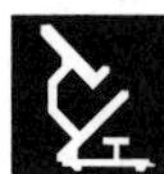

Diagnosis

DIFFERENTIAL DIAGNOSIS

The differential diagnosis of a pansystolic murmur along the left lower sternal border includes atrioventricular valve insufficiency and subaortic stenosis, as well as VSD.

- The infant with CHF and a large left-to-right shunt may have communications between the left and right heart/great arteries other than VSD (atrioventricular canal defect, double-outlet right ventricle (RV), patent ductus arteriosus, single ventricle anatomy without pulmonary stenosis, aortopulmonary window, truncus arteriosus).
- CHF due to severe mitral insufficiency also can be confused with VSD. In addition, other cardiac lesions frequently coexist with VSD.

SIGNS AND SYMPTOMS

- Small restrictive VSD
  - —Asymptomatic
  - —Pansystolic murmur along left lower sternal border
  - —Systolic thrill (occasionally)
- Large unrestrictive VSD with significant shunting (>2:1 Qp/Qs) and hyperkinetic pulmonary hypertension
  - —Loud pansystolic murmur along the left sternal border
  - —Systolic thrill (often)
  - —Diastolic rumble at apex (increased diastolic blood flow across mitral valve)
  - —CHF beginning about 4–8 weeks of age with:
    - Tachypnea
    - Tachycardia
    - Hepatomegaly
    - Rales
    - Fatigue with feeding
    - Poor weight gain
    - Diaphoresis

History

- Murmur
- CHF during infancy (large defects)
- CHF may diminish
  - —With decreasing VSD size
  - —With increasing pulmonary vascular resistance
  - —With development of RV outflow obstruction
- Spontaneous closure may occur, usually in small (but occasionally in large) VSDs. Closure occurs by:
  - —Membranous aneurysm formation
  - —Fibrous proliferation
  - —Muscle bundle hypertrophy with formation of a double-chambered RV
  - —Prolapse of aortic valve leaflet into defect
- Pulmonary vascular obstruction may evolve in older unrepaired patients.
  - —Loud P2
  - —Cardiac murmur less prominent as L-R shunt decreases
  - —Cyanosis as shunt reverses (see chapter on Eisenmenger's syndrome).

PATHOLOGIC FINDINGS

- Anatomic locations
  - —Subaortic, perimembranous
  - —Subpulmonic, outlet
  - —Endocardial cushion, inlet
  - —Muscular (mid-septal, apical, multiple)
- Physiologic findings
  - —Volume overload
  - —Pulmonary congestion
  - —Altered pulmonary compliance
  - —Hyperkinetic pulmonary hypertension
  - —Pulmonary vascular obstructive disease
  - —Late right heart dilatation and hypertrophy
  - —Aortic regurgitation in 5% of patients (40% in Asians)
  - —Infundibular stenosis in up to 7% (evolving tetralogy physiology)

SPECIAL TESTS

- ECG
  - —Small shunts: ECG usually normal.
    - Large shunts: Left atrial enlargement and left ventricular hypertrophy evident; prominent Q waves in the inferior and left lateral leads. In infants, mid-precordial leads may show biventricular enlargement (Katz-Wachtel sign).
    - Pulmonary vascular disease: Right ventricular hypertrophy (RVH) will dominate.

IMAGING STUDIES

Chest X-ray

- Isolated small VSD: normal heart size and vascularity
- Moderate defects with normal pulmonary arterial pressures but high flow: increased vascular markings and varying degrees of cardiomegaly
- Large defects with significant left-to-right shunting: increased pulmonary vascular markings, cardiomegaly, prominent pulmonary artery segments, splaying of the right and left bronchi, and left atrial enlargement
- Large defects with pulmonary vascular disease: RVH with upturned apex and prominent proximal pulmonary artery segments in the absence of increased vascular markings in the periphery. Heart size often appears to be normal.

Echocardiography

Sector Scan

- Number, location of VSDs
- Chamber enlargement or hypertrophy
- Associated lesions

Doppler

- Pulse wave blood flow evaluation
  —VSD demonstrated
  —Valves evaluated
  —Aorta and pulmonary artery anatomy demonstrated
- Continuous wave Doppler evaluation
  —Transseptal gradient determines whether VSD is restrictive
  —Tricuspid regurgitant gradient estimates RV pressure
- Color flow Doppler
  —Shunt location documented
  —Qualitative estimate of shunt

Cardiac Catheterization

- Not routinely indicated in uncomplicated VSD.
- Useful if the VSD is not clearly "restrictive" or has complex associated lesions
- Important data measured or calculated include:
  —Shunt quantitation
  —Pulmonary artery pressure
  —Pulmonary wedge pressure
  —Left ventricular end-diastolic pressure
  —Pulmonary and systemic resistances
- Angiography
  —Documents locations of septal defect(s)
  —Qualitative evaluation of shunt
  —Determination of left and right ventricular function
  —Identification of associated defects

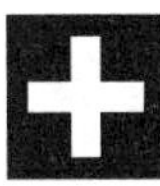

Treatment

GENERAL MEASURES

- Outpatient other than for surgery or management of complications
- Antibiotic prophylaxis
- Small VSDs: High incidence of spontaneous closure, no risk for CHF or pulmonary hypertension. Reassurance should be provided. Although occasional reevaluation may be indicated, in general these patients should not require close follow-up.
- Large VSDs: Close follow-up of infants with large defects is necessary. The clinical course may diverge widely.
- Development of progressive CHF which responds to medical therapy, allowing time for spontaneous closure or subsequent surgical closure prior to 18–24 months of life
  —Development of progressive CHF which does not respond to medical therapy; early surgical closure is required
  —Defects close or become hemodynamically insignificant.
  —Unoperated patients with unrestrictive VSDs may develop increased pulmonary vascular resistance and decreased shunting.
  —RV infundibular hypertrophy may develop, decreasing left-to-right shunting with eventual development of tetralogy physiology.
  —RV muscle bundles may hypertrophy and partially or fully close the VSD, creating a high-pressure subchamber (double-chamber RV).

SURGICAL MEASURES

- Surgical closure is indicated in infants with CHF refractory to medical therapy.
- Older infants with large defects and significant shunts, stable on medical management, still require surgical closure if their defect does not become restrictive. Such patients not repaired by 2 years of life are at significant risk to develop pulmonary vascular disease.
- Timing of surgical closure prior to the end of the second year of life is strongly recommended.
- In contrast, an asymptomatic patient with normal pulmonary arterial pressures rarely will require surgical closure.
- Patients with significant shunts, but normal pulmonary arterial pressures may require closure if failure to thrive, recurrent pulmonary infections, or bronchial compression due to atrial or pulmonary artery dilatation become an issue.

Activity

- Small VSD: unrestricted activity
- Large repaired VSD, no pulmonary vascular disease: If without significant residua (shunt, pulmonary hypertension, myocardial dysfunction), may participate in all activities within 6 months of repair
- Large VSD, repaired, significant arrhythmias: Follow recommendations for specific arrhythmia.

Diet

Adequate calories (139–150 calories/kg/day) should be provided.

PATIENT EDUCATION

- Subacute bacterial endocarditis prophylaxis
- Reassurance with small VSDs
- Emphasize close follow-up of large defects in infancy.
- Anticipate surgical repair of large defects.

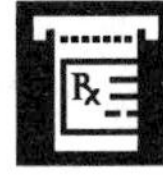

Medications

DRUG(S) OF CHOICE

- Digoxin as an oral cardiotonic agent
- Lasix combined with aldactone for diuretic management of CHF
- Angiotensin-converting enzyme inhibitors may be used for afterload reduction.
- Antibiotic prophylaxis

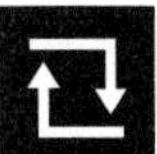

Follow-up

PATIENT MONITORING

- Small defects: close follow-up unnecessary; no restriction of activities
- Large defects: close follow-up for assessment of developing CHF and/or pulmonary hypertension over the first year of life; follow-up after closure; regular activity
- Pulmonary vascular disease: See chapter on Eisenmenger's Syndrome.

Prevention/Avoidance

- Antibiotic prophylaxis (see above)
- Avoid known teratogens during pregnancy.
- Fetal echocardiography for patients with fetus at increased risk for CHD

Possible Complications

- CHF and pulmonary edema
- Pulmonary hypertension and pulmonary vascular disease
- Endocarditis

EXPECTED COURSE AND PROGNOSIS

- Small defects have a benign prognosis. Many will close spontaneously.
- Large defects diagnosed in the first year of life and requiring surgical closure will be repaired prior to 2 years of life. The expected operative mortality should be less than 3%. Long-term prognosis for a "normal life" is excellent.
- Large defects unrepaired or repaired late with pulmonary vascular disease will have a guarded prognosis.

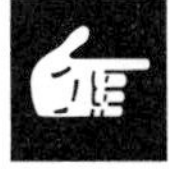

Miscellaneous

ICD-9-CM

745.4 Ventricular septal defect

BIBLIOGRAPHY

Dajani et al. AHA medical/scientific statement: prevention of bacterial endocarditis. *Circulation* 1997:96:358–366.

Elliot LP. *Cardiac imaging in infants, children and adults.* Philadelphia: JB Lippincott, 1991.

Emmanouilides et al., eds. *Heart disease in infants, children and adolescents,* 5th ed. Baltimore: Williams & Wilkins, 1995.

Silverman NH. *Pediatric echocardiography.* Baltimore: Williams & Wilkins, 1992.

Task Force 6. Arrhythmias. *J Am Coll Cardiol* 1994;24:845–899.

Weidman et al. Second natural history study of congenital heart defects. *Circulation* 1993: 87(suppl I) 1–120.

Authors: Donald Leichter and Welton M. Gersony

Ventricular Tachycardia

Basics

DESCRIPTION

Ventricular tachycardia (VT) is wide QRS tachycardia originating in the ventricles due to reentry, triggered activity, or automaticity.

EPIDEMIOLOGY

- Coronary artery disease is the most common cause, and is not specifically a genetic disease, although there is a genetic component.
- Prevalence is variable and depends on presence or absence of structural heart disease.
- All ages can be affected, but VT is more common in older individuals because coronary artery disease is more common.
- Cardiomyopathies, both hypertrophic and dilated, are associated with nonsustained and sustained VT.
- Some clear genetic syndromes, such as long QT syndrome, Brugada syndrome, and arrhythmogenic right ventricular dysplasia, are associated with VT.

ETIOLOGY

- Myocardial scar from any cause
- Drug toxicity [digoxin (bidirectional VT) or QT-prolonging drugs (torsades de pointes VT)]
- Electrolyte abnormalities (hypokalemia)
- Ischemia
- Bundle branch reentry
- Congenital heart disease, especially postoperatively where there has been a ventriculotomy (as in tetralogy of Fallot)
- In structurally normal hearts two VTs can occur:
  - —Right ventricular outflow tract VT
  - —Idiopathic left VT

RISK FACTORS

- Same as in coronary artery disease (cigarette use, hyperlipidemia, and hypertension)
- ECG abnormalities, often determined by ambulatory monitoring, including:
  - —Premature ventricular contractions and nonsustained ventricular tachycardia, left ventricular hypertrophy, nonspecific ST-T wave changes, intraventricular conduction delays, increased QT dispersion, T-wave alternans, and decreased heart rate variability
- Low left ventricular ejection fraction
- Increased age
- Inducible VT in high-risk patient (after myocardial infarction, low left ventricular ejection fraction)

PREGNANCY

Pregnancy may precipitate ventricular arrhythmias in long QT syndrome.

ASSOCIATED CONDITIONS

See Etiology and Risk Factors above.

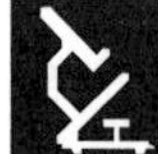

Diagnosis

DIFFERENTIAL DIAGNOSIS

- Supraventricular tachycardia with aberrancy
- Preexcited tachycardia [antidromic reentrant tachycardia, or preexcitation as an innocent bystander such as during atrial flutter with atrioventricular (AV) conduction over a Mahaim accessory pathway]

SIGNS AND SYMPTOMS

Signs and symptoms depend on rate and duration of VT, and extent of underlying heart disease, if any.

- None
- Syncope
- Cardiac arrest
- Dyspnea
- Palpitations
- Chest discomfort/angina

LABORATORY PROCEDURES

- None except to assess electrolytes and drug levels where appropriate

IMAGING STUDIES

- Echocardiogram (to evaluate cardiomyopathy, localized wall motion abnormalities such as in coronary artery disease, arrhythmogenic right ventricular dysplasia)
- Coronary and left ventricular angiography
- Cardiac magnetic resonance imaging (especially useful in diagnosing arrhythmogenic right ventricular dysplasia)
- Exercise test with perfusion imaging to assess ischemia

SPECIAL TESTS

ECG

ECG is the cornerstone of the diagnosis. When a 12-lead ECG is available, the criteria listed below can be used not only to diagnose VT (to distinguish it from supraventricular tachycardia), but also to help guide therapy when ablation is considered.

- General: AV dissociation, extremely wide QRS (>160 msec), QRS axis −90 to 180 degrees, and fusion (capture) beats all favor VT over supraventricular tachycardia with aberrancy.
- Morphology may be uniform (monomorphic) or variable (polymorphic)
- If left bundle branch block morphology, VT suggested if:
  - —In V1 or V2, R wave is >30 msec
  - —In V1 or V2, there is a notch on the downstroke of the QRS
  - —In V1 or V2, the interval from the onset of the QRS to the nadir of the S or Q wave is ≥60 msec
  - —In V6 there is a Q wave
- If right bundle branch block morphology, VT suggested if:
  - —In V1, QRS is monophasic or biphasic, especially if R is greater in amplitude than R′
  - —In V6, R to S ratio is <1 by either amplitude or area under the QRS complex
- Also useful to document if prior or new myocardial infarction present
- Electrophysiologic study

Pathology

Pathology depends on substrate, including coronary artery disease, any cause of myocardial fibrosis (cardiomyopathy, trauma), fibroadipose infiltration of the myocardium (arrhythmogenic right ventricular dysplasia), inflammatory disease (myocarditis, sarcoidosis), or none (right ventricular outflow tract tachycardia, ideopathic left VT, Brugada syndrome).

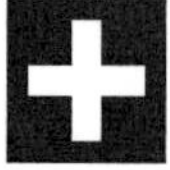

Treatment

GENERAL MEASURES

- Treat underlying heart disease, especially ischemia and left ventricular dysfunction.
- Treat reversible causes (withdraw toxic drugs, correct electrolyte disturbances).
- Be sure to synchronize if performing electrical cardioversion.

SURGICAL MEASURES

Curative therapy is possible with ablation or surgery.

- Catheter ablation is especially useful and efficacious for right ventricular outflow tract and idiopathic left VTs.
- Sometimes VT in the setting of coronary artery disease is amenable to catheter ablation, but ablation is often combined with drug or implantable cardioverter-defibrillator (ICD) therapy.
- In the past, endocardial resection was often used to treat VTs arising from myocardial infarction scars, and is still used today in highly selected patients (presence of surgical coronary artery disease and an anterior aneurysm).
- Because of the mortality and morbidity associated with this operation, ICDs have been used in recent years as an alternative. This approach is further supported by The Antiarrhythmics Versus Implantable Defibrillators (AVID) Trial, which showed superior survival in patients with hemodynamically unstable VTs when treated with ICDs compared with antiarrhythmic drugs.
- In the absence of a reversible cause or reasons to not implant an ICD, one is usually offered (see chapter on ICDs).
- Finally, surgery is used to correct and/or treat reversible causes of VF, such as coronary artery disease and aortic stenosis.

ADMISSION/DISCHARGE CRITERIA

Admission criteria are variable and depend on hemodynamics during VT and the underlying substrate.

- VT from the right ventricular outflow tract and idiopathic left ventricular tachycardias occur in patients with otherwise normal hearts. Hemodynamics are usually preserved, and death due to these VTs does not occur. These patients can be managed in part on an outpatient basis.
- Admission is warranted for radiofrequency ablation of these VTs or the initiation of drug therapy.
- On the other hand, VT in patients with coronary artery disease warrants admission because VT can degenerate to cardiac arrest (ventricular fibrillation).

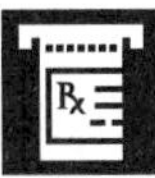

Medications

DRUG(S) OF CHOICE

Acute

- Lidocaine is easy to administer and has few hemodynamic effects.
- Procainamide (but may cause hypotension)
- Amiodarone is very effective.
- Bretylium
- Antidigoxin antibodies if digoxin toxic
- Drugs to correct electrolyte abnormalities (e.g., potassium for hypokalemia)
- For most VTs, intravenous calcium channel blockers remove compensatory peripheral vasoconstriction and lead to (life-threatening) hypotension.

Chronic

- Amiodarone
- Sotalol
- Class IC drugs (flecainide, propafenone) contraindicated if structural heart disease

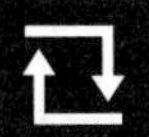

Follow-up

PATIENT MONITORING

- If drug therapy chosen, follow to assess compliance, drug levels, effect on ECG, and changes in myocardial substrate.
- Device follow-up ICD chosen
- Drugs can alter the rate of ventricular tachycardias and the ease of defibrillation (defibrillation threshold) such that when antiarrhythmic drugs are begun in patients with ICDs, electrophysiologic study should be done to assess adverse drug–device interactions.

EXPECTED COURSE AND PROGNOSIS

Outcome depends on underlying heart disease and comorbid conditions. For patients with VT and a structurally normal heart, prognosis is excellent (right ventricular outflow tract and idiopathic left ventricular tachycardias).

PATIENT EDUCATION

Counseling depends in part on the VT substrate.

- For those with genetic syndromes, genetic screening of family members should be discussed.
- Patients with torsades de pointes VT need to be educated about which drugs to avoid, and for those with congenital long QT syndrome avoidance of precipitating causes of VT (startle reflexes).

Exercise

If VT is exercise related, exercise should be restricted.

Diet

Choose diet appropriate for underlying heart disease (low cholesterol if coronary artery disease, low sodium if congestive heart failure, calorie restricted if diabetic).

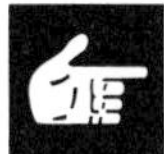

Miscellaneous

SYNONYMS

The following have been used interchangeably but are not synonymous:

- Cardiac arrest (refers to collapse due to ventricular tachycardia or fibrillation)
- VT followed by ventricular fibrillation are the usual causes of sudden death.

ICD-9-CM

427.1 Paroxysmal ventricular tachycardia

See also: Implantable defibrillators; Premature ventricular contractions; Torsades de pointes ventricular tachycardia; Ventricular fibrillation; Brugada syndrome; Long QT syndrome; Sudden death

BIBLIOGRAPHY

The AVID Investigators (prepared by the AVID Executive Committee: Zipes DP, Wyse DG, Friedman PL, et al.). A comparison of antiarrhythmic drug therapy with implantable defibrillators in patients resuscitated from near-fatal sustained ventricular arrhythmias. *N Engl J Med* 1997; 337:1576.

Callans DJ, Schwartzman D, Gottlieb CD, et al. Insights into the electrophysiology of ventricular tachycardia gained by the catheter ablation experience: "Learning while burning." *J Cardiovasc Electrophysiol* 1994;5:877–894.

Kindwall KE, Brown J, Josephson ME. Electrocardiographic criteria for ventricular tachycardia in wide complex left bundle branch block morphology tachycardias. *Am J Cardiol* 1988;61: 1279–1283.

Strickberger SA, Man KC, Daoud EG, et al. A prospective evaluation of catheter ablation of ventricular tachycardia as adjuvant therapy in patients with coronary artery disease and an implantable cardioverter-defibrillator. *Circulation* 1997;96:1525–1531.

Wellens HJJ. The electrocardiogram 80 years after Einthoven. *J Am Coll Cardiol* 1986;7: 484–491.

Author: Andrew E. Epstein

Wolff-Parkinson-White Syndrome

Basics

DESCRIPTION

Wolff-Parkinson-White (WPW) syndrome is defined by the combination of preexcitation on the ECG (delta wave) and supraventricular tachycardia (either atrial fibrillation or reentrant tachycardia using the accessory pathway as part of the circuit). In the purest sense, simple preexcitation without arrhythmias is not the "syndrome."

EPIDEMIOLOGY

Supraventricular tachycardia and WPW syndrome can occur at any age. Conversely, accessory pathway conduction may disappear with aging.

- The prevalence of ECG preexcitation has been reported to range from 0.1 to 3 per 1,000 population.
- The intermittent nature of preexcitation may have led to underestimation of the true prevalence of the disease.
- Accessory pathway–mediated tachycardia accounts for about 30%–40% of paroxysmal supraventricular tachycardias seen in practice.
- WPW syndrome is more frequent in males.

ETIOLOGY

- WPW syndrome results from a developmental abnormality of the atrioventricular (AV) groove.
- During normal cardiogenesis, direct continuity between the atrial and ventricular myocardium is lost by growth of the annulus fibrosis.
- Defects in the annulus leave muscular connection(s) called accessory pathways or Kent bundles between the atrial and ventricular myocardium.
- By bypassing the AV node, these pathways can lead to preexcitation of the ventricles because atrial impulses are not delayed in the AV node.
- Accessory pathways are most often described in electrical terms, with the ECG showing the characteristic delta wave, or they are identified at the electrophysiologic study. The pathways may have "all or none" conduction properties, or have decremental conduction properties, as does the AV node. They may conduct only from the atria to the ventricles (called anterograde or antegrade conduction), only from the ventricles to the atria (called retrograde conduction), or in both directions.
- The majority of patients with WPW syndrome do not have a familial/genetic disorder. However, there have been case reports of autosomal dominant inheritance without associated cardiac disorders.
- Right-sided accessory pathways are associated with Ebstein's anomaly of the tricuspid valve.
- Other conditions that have been associated with WPW syndrome are hypertrophic cardiomyopathy, mitral valve prolapse, and a variety of congenital heart diseases.

RISK FACTORS

- None

PREGNANCY

Pregnancy is not contraindicated, but supraventricular tachycardias may be more frequent and precipitated by pregnancy.

Diagnosis

DIFFERENTIAL DIAGNOSIS

- AV nodal reentrant tachycardia
- Atrial tachycardia
- Atrial flutter with 2:1 AV conduction
- Junctional tachycardia
- ECGs may mask or mimic myocardial infarction, bundle branch block, ventricular hypertrophy, accelerated idioventricular rhythm, ventricular bigeminy, and electrical alternans (the latter two diagnoses when accessory pathway conduction is intermittent).

SIGNS AND SYMPTOMS

- Palpitations
- Dyspnea
- Dizziness
- Syncope
- Fatigue (sometimes related to drug therapy)
- Chest pain
- Diaphoresis
- Polyuria (usually following tachycardia)

LABORATORY PROCEDURES

N/A

IMAGING STUDIES

N/A

SPECIAL TESTS

ECG is the cornerstone of diagnosis:

- The ECG may be normal (if AV nodal conduction is faster that accessory pathway conduction to the ventricles) or abnormal, with varying degrees of preexcitation (depending how much of the ventricles are activated via the accessory pathway and how much via the normal AV node–His-Purkinje system).
- The cardinal ECG features in sinus rhythm are (a) a short PR interval (≤120 msec), (b) a QRS duration of ≤120 msec with a slurred upstroke called a delta wave, and (c) secondary ST-T wave changes.
- In tachycardia, there may be:
  —A narrow, regular QRS rhythm (orthodromic AV reentrant tachycardia) in which AV conduction is via the AV node. P waves may be buried in the QRS complex and not identifiable, or after the end of the QRS in the ST segment or T wave. In these tachycardias, ventriculoatrial conduction is via the accessory pathway.
  —A wide, regular QRS rhythm due to either orthodromic AV reentry with rate-related bundle branch block aberrancy, or antidromic AV reentrant tachycardia, in which AV conduction is via the accessory pathway, and ventriculoatrial conduction is via the AV node
  —An irregular QRS rhythm due to atrial fibrillation. The QRS may be narrow, or wide as a consequence of either rate-related aberrancy or preexcitation of the ventricles via the accessory pathway.
- Electrophysiologic study, required if undergoing catheter ablation

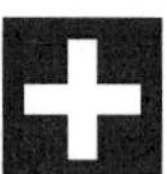

Treatment

GENERAL MEASURES

- 12-lead ECG extremely important to secure the diagnosis
- Digoxin: not desirable drug because if atrial fibrillation occurs, there may be rapid conduction over the accessory pathway and induction of ventricular fibrillation
- Cardioversion is indicated for acute management if atrial fibrillation occurs with rapid conduction over the accessory pathway, or if there is hemodynamic compromise. Cardiac arrest may occur during atrial fibrillation if there is rapid conduction to the ventricles via the accessory pathway.
- Due to the problems of long-term drug administration (adverse drug reactions, problem of multiple daily doses/noncompliance, and failure at some time over years of treatment), catheter ablation has emerged as a (if not the) treatment of choice for recurrent AV reentrant tachycardia.
  —The procedure can be performed safely with a low risk for complications and a high degree of efficacy.
  —Long-term, ablation is likely cost-effective and improves quality of life compared with drug therapy, especially class IA and IC agents.
  —Virtually all deaths attributed to accessory pathway conduction have occurred in patients with prior arrhythmia symptoms, and not as a first event.
  —Thus, electrophysiologic study may be performed to determine the anterograde refractory period of the accessory pathway (or pathways) and the risk of rapid AV conduction during atrial fibrillation before chronic drug treatment is prescribed.

SURGICAL MEASURES

Surgery has been performed in the past. This has been superseded by catheter ablation for cure.

ADMISSION/DISCHARGE CRITERIA

Admission is usually not required.

- Admission is warranted if supraventricular tachycardia is incessant, or if there is a life-threatening associated problem such as atrial fibrillation with rapid conduction over an accessory pathway (shortest preexcited RR interval 250 msec or less, equivalent to a heart rate of 240 beats/min or more).
- Radiofrequency catheter ablation of accessory pathways can be undertaken on a same-day admission schedule.

Medications

DRUG(S) OF CHOICE

Acute Management

To interrupt the reentry circuit:

- Valsalva, and vagal maneuvers
- Adenosine (intravenous), but watch for atrial fibrillation because it may lead to rapid conduction over the accessory pathway and precipitate ventricular fibrillation.
- Although not approved for this indication, ibutilide is effective in blocking conduction in accessory pathways and may have a special place in the treatment strategy of patients with the WPW syndrome and atrial fibrillation.
- Intravenous procainamide may be used acutely because it decreases conduction over the accessory pathway and is safe if anterograde accessory pathway conduction is present in atrial fibrillation. However, intravenous procainamide may cause hypotension.

Chronic Management

- See comments below regarding catheter ablation.
- Drugs that shorten accessory pathway refractoriness and facilitate rapid ventricular rates during atrial fibrillation are contraindicated in patients with anterograde conduction over the accessory pathway because in atrial fibrillation conduction over the accessory pathway may be so rapid that ventricular fibrillation is precipitated.
  —In such patients, class I or class III drugs may be used alone or in combination with an AV nodal blocking agent.
  —Otherwise, a calcium channel blocker such as verapamil, or a beta-blocker can be used. The class IC antiarrhythmic drugs flecainide and propafenone and the class III antiarrhythmic drug sotalol are effective and well tolerated.
- Amiodarone, a class III antiarrhythmic drug, is potentially effective but its use limited by adverse drug reactions.
- Class IA drugs (quinidine, procainamide, and disopyramide) are of limited value due to frequent adverse drug reactions during long-term treatment.

Follow-up

PATIENT MONITORING

General medical care if on drugs. If cured by catheter ablation, none. Recurrence can be prevented by either drug therapy or cure by catheter-based radiofrequency ablation.

EXPECTED COURSE AND PROGNOSIS

If accessory pathways are ablated and the heart is structurally normal, prognosis is normal. The prognosis is also excellent if accessory pathway has a long anterograde refractory period and cannot preexcite the ventricles rapidly during atrial fibrillation.

PATIENT EDUCATION

There are no specific dietary recommendations. Similarly, there are no specific activity recommendations, although arrhythmias can occasionally be precipitated by exercise and catecholamine increase. Otherwise, counseling relates to treatment options, especially opportunity for cure with catheter ablation. Vagal maneuvers to terminate arrhythmia can be taught.

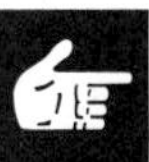

Miscellaneous

SYNONYMS

- Paroxysmal atrial tachycardia (PAT): term now obsolete

ICD-9-CM

426.7 Anomalous atrioventricular excitation

See also: AV nodal reentrant tachycardia; Junctional rhythm

BIBLIOGRAPHY

Al-Khatib SM, Pritchett ELC. Clinical features of Wolff-Parkinson-White syndrome. *Am Heart J* 1999;138:403–413.

Ganz LI, Friedman PL. Supraventricular tachycardia. *N Engl J Med* 1995;332:162–173.

Kay GN, Plumb VJ. Selective slow pathway ablation (posterior approach) for treatment for atrioventricular nodal reentrant tachycardia. In: *Radiofrequency catheter ablation of cardiac arrhythmias: basic concepts and clinical applications.* Armonk, NY: Futura, 1994:171–203.

Jackman WM, Wang X, Friday KJ, et al. Catheter ablation of accessory atrioventricular pathways (Wolff-Parkinson-White Syndrome) by radiofrequency current. *N Engl J Med* 1991:324:1605–1611.

Miles WM, Klein LS, Rardon DP, et al. Atrioventricular reentry variants: mechanisms, clinical features, and management. In: Zipes DP, Jalife J, eds. *Cardiac electrophysiology: from cell to bedside,* 2nd ed. Philadelphia: WB Saunders, 1995:638–655.

Authors: Andrew E. Epstein and John S. Strobel

Appendix

Adenosine

BASICS

Description

Adenosine is an endogenous purine derived from high-energy adenosine phosphates (ATP, ADP, and AMP).

- Intracellular adenosine can cross the cell membrane and diffuse to the extracellular space, where it may act as an autocoid (i.e., it can exert its effects on adjacent cells).
- Adenosine also can be generated in the extracellular space by the ectonucleotidase metabolism of plasma ATP that is released from vascular cells, thrombocytes, and sympathetic nerves during ischemia.
- In the interstitial space, adenosine has a very short half-life. The cell actively reuptakes adenosine, by either simple or facilitated diffusion via a nucleoside transport system that can be pharmacologically inhibited (e.g., by dipyridamole).

Adenosine Receptors

- The physiologic effects of adenosine are mediated by specific G protein–coupled receptors (also known as purinergic P1 receptors) that belong to the family of the seven transmembrane domain receptors.
- At present, four adenosine receptors have been characterized: A1, A2a, A2b, and A3.
  —The A1 and the A3 receptors both couple to inhibitory Gi/o G proteins (hence causing an inhibition of adenyl cyclase), can activate phospholipase C via G protein subunits, and can activate protein kinase C.
  —The high-affinity A2a and the low-affinity A2b receptors both couple to Gs, but the A2b receptor also can couple to Gq/11 to mobilize calcium.

Adenosine Cardiovascular Effects

- Vascular tone
  —Coronary vasodilation (the A2a receptor mainly at the level of resistance vessels and the A2b receptor at the level of conductance vessels), via both KATP channel and NO-mediated mechanisms
  —Renal vasoconstriction (A1)
  —Peripheral vasodilation (A2)
- Electrophysiology
  —Negative chronotropic effect (sinoatrial node, A1)
  —Negative dromotropic effect [atrioventricular (AV) node, A1]
  —Depression of automaticity (A1)
- Mechanical performance
  —Negative inotropic effect (atrial myocardium, A1)
  —Direct positive inotropic effect (A2a receptor, via cyclic AMP (cAMP)-dependent and -independent effects).
  —Indirect negative inotropic effect, by attenuating the cardiac responsiveness to beta-adrenergic stimulation
  —A2 mediated modulation of A1 receptor activity
- Adrenergic responsivity: A1 receptor stimulation attenuates the responsiveness by reducing the beta-adrenergic-mediated increase in cAMP (A1)
  —Presynaptic nerve endings: Adenosine attenuates the release of norepinephrine caused by adrenergic nerve stimulation (A1).
  —Myocardial metabolism: attenuation of the metabolic effects of beta-adrenergic stimulation
  —Endothelial cells: proliferation (and angiogenesis)

Adenosine as a Retaliatory Metabolite

- Adenosine acts as a negative feedback modulator of beta-adrenoceptor–mediated responses in the heart and as a negative feedback regulator that inhibits norepinephrine release from the sympathetic nerve endings. These effects are already present at physiologic adenosine interstitial concentrations.
- In several pathophysiologic conditions, adenosine concentrations in the intracellular space may increase significantly (e.g., during beta-adrenergic catecholamine stimulation, cardiac ischemia, cardiac hypoxia, increased cardiac workload caused by volume or pressure overload). In these situations, characterized by an unfavorable oxygen supply–demand ratio, adenosine can induce coronary vasodilation, attenuate the metabolic and inotropic response to beta-adrenergic stimulation, and modulate the release of norepinephrine from the sympathetic nerve endings.

Cardioprotection Against the Ischemic/Reperfusion Injury

- During ischemia, the antiadrenergic effect of adenosine reduces the norepinephrine available for stimulating the flow-deprived heart and reduces the metabolic and inotropic effects of beta-adrenergic receptor stimulation. At the same time, adenosine is a potent coronary vasodilator.
- Adenosine can therefore protect against ischemia-induced cell death and against reperfusion injury. Moreover, adenosine attenuates ischemia-induced myocardial stunning and decreases the incidence of arrhythmias.

Ischemic Preconditioning

Adenosine plays an important role in triggering and mediating the cardioprotective effect of ischemic preconditioning, via the activation of A1 and A3 adenosine receptors. By mechanisms yet to be completely elucidated, adenosine release during an ischemic episode interacts with KATP channels to induce a protective effect against subsequent periods of acute ischemia. Adenosine-induced protein kinase C activation may be involved as well.

Cardiovascular Diagnosis

Arrhythmias

- The cardiac electrophysiologic actions of adenosine are mediated by the A1 receptor and are either cAMP independent (at the level of nodal or atrial tissue) or cAMP dependent, that is, mediated by the inhibition of the stimulatory effects of adenylyl cyclase (at the level of atrial and ventricular myocytes).
- Due to these electrophysiologic effects, adenosine can be used in the electrophysiology laboratory as a diagnostic tool:
  - —Adenosine may transiently suppress (but not terminate) automatic atrial tachycardia.
  - —Because adenosine may transiently block AV nodal conduction, it plays an important role in the diagnosis of reentrant arrhythmias in which the AV node is a critical component of the tachycardia circuit.
  - —Adenosine causes transient suppression of adrenergically mediated automatic arrhythmias.
  - —Adenosine is useful to identify ventricular arrhythmias due to triggered activity.
  - —Adenosine may be used to diagnose latent preexcitation, to localize the region of the accessory pathway, and to assess the immediate efficacy of accessory pathway ablation.

Ischemic Heart Disease

- In the setting of coronary atherosclerosis artery disease, adenosine-induced coronary vasodilation may induce acute regional ischemia due to flow maldistribution (coronary steal in the myocardial area perfused by a stenotic artery). This paradoxical effect of coronary vasodilation can be exploited as a diagnostic tool by allowing the evaluation of the consequences of acute inducible ischemia. To this end, endogenous adenosine accumulation induced by dipyridamole infusion is used as a pharmacologic stress test in combination with two-dimensional echocardiography or radionuclide perfusion scans. The former will allow the identification of wall motion abnormalities induced by regional ischemia, whereas the latter will assess the relative flow heterogeneity caused by dipyridamole in the presence of coronary artery disease.
- The short-lasting effect of dipyridamole, which acts by blocking the reuptake of adenosine by the cells, and the availability of the antidote theophylline, which blocks adenosine receptors, make dipyridamole stress testing a safe and effective choice for cardiac imaging in ischemic heart disease.

Possible Role in Cardiovascular Therapy

Arrhythmias

- Adenosine can terminate sinus node reentry, paroxysmal reciprocating atrial tachycardia, nodal reciprocating tachycardia, and effort-related ventricular tachycardia due to triggered activity. Dipyridamole-induced increase in endogenous adenosine may slow or terminate AV nodal reentrant tachycardia and AV reciprocating tachycardia.
- Adenosine receptor blockade by theophylline may be effective in treating bradycardia in patients with sick sinus syndrome, in increasing the ventricular response rate in patients with atrial fibrillation, and in reversing complete heart block in the setting of acute myocardial infarction.
- Adenosine administration may cause atrial flutter and/or fibrillation, AV block, sinus bradycardia, and sinus pauses.

Myocardial Cardioprotection

Adenosine is a potentially beneficial additive to cardioplegic solutions during open heart surgery, and it is used to control blood pressure in the setting of postoperative systemic and pulmonary hypertension. Its possible role in protecting the ischemic myocardium during coronary angioplasty and in acute myocardial infarction is under extensive clinical evaluation.

Author: Stefano Perlini and Gerald P. Aurigemma

Angiogenesis

BASICS

Description

Angiogenesis is the growth and development of supplemental collateral coronary vessels that will result in endogenous bypass arteries surrounding occluded coronary arteries.

Mechanism

- A complex process involving endothelial cell proliferation and migration, formation of new capillaries, attraction of macrophages, stimulation of smooth muscle cell proliferation and migration, formation of new vascular structures, and deposition of new matrix

Target Population

Patients with chronic ischemia and anginal symptoms due to advanced coronary artery disease that is:

- Refractory to antianginal medical therapy
- Not amenable to percutaneous interventions
- Not amenable to conventional coronary artery bypass grafting due to small, diffusely diseased distal target vessels
- Found to have significant areas of viable, but underperfused myocardium
- Not a candidate for cardiac transplantation

TYPICAL CANDIDATE PATIENT PROFILE

- Elderly patient with class III or IV angina, mild to moderate reduction in ejection fraction, and multiple prior revascularization procedures
- Most patients have had prior coronary bypass surgery within past 5–10 years and have occluded most bypass grafts.
- Patients frequently have small, diffusely diseased coronary arteries in association with long-standing diabetes mellitus.
- The estimated annual mortality rate for these patients is 15%/year.

Goals of Therapeutic Myocardial Angiogenesis

- Increase growth of new blood vessels
- Increase oxygen delivery
- Decrease angina
- Increase exercise capacity
- Improve quality of life

RATIONALE

Natural History of Collateral Vessels

Collateral vessels form from preexisting vascular structures in response to acute myocardial infarction or chronic ischemia in order to bypass occluded coronary artery territories. This can improve oxygen supply to ischemic muscle.

- Patients suffering AMI have less myocardial damage if collaterals are more abundant.
- There are intra- and interspecies differences in the collateral response to ischemia; collateral development response in humans is intermediate compared with species such as cats and rabbits.
- These differences in collateral development may relate to different levels of endogenous angiogenic factors that would promote this process.
- The signaling for collateral development is upregulated in situations of ischemia and infarction. For example, fibroblast growth factor receptors will be increased in numbers in ischemic myocardium.
- Endogenous angiogenic stimulants include fibroblast growth factors, vascular endothelial growth factors, platelet-derived growth factors, interleukin-8, and tumor necrosis factor alpha.

ANIMAL STUDIES

- Canine and porcine models of acute coronary occlusion or chronic ischemia have been developed in order to assess the response of the coronary arteries to supplemental exogenous angiogenic factors to stimulate coronary collateral growth.
- The following factors stimulate growth of coronary collateral vessels in these animal models:
  - —Basic and acidic fibroblast growth factor (FGF)
  - —Vascular endothelial growth factor (VEGF)
  - —Transmyocardial laser channels inducing inflammation and angiogenesis

Methods

Increased myocardial levels of angiogenic factors have been demonstrated by a variety of methods for the introduction of growth factors in animal models.

- Intracoronary infusions
- Heparin alginate slow release intramyocardial pellets
- Local perivascular delivery
- Intrapericardial infusion
- Direct myocardial injection
- Direct or transthoracic laser channels
- Treatment with genes, plasmids, or virus expressing the angiogenic protein factors rather than with the protein itself.

TREATMENT RESULTS

- VIVA Trial
  —A randomized, placebo-controlled trial of combined intravenous and intracoronary infusions of VEGF in 180 patients with unstable angina
  —No adverse effects reported
  —Although exercise tolerance and anginal symptoms improved in the VEGF arm, they also improved in the placebo arm, thus making definite conclusions about the efficacy of VEGF coronary infusions difficult.
- FIRST Trial
  —A randomized, placebo controlled trial of a 20-minute intracoronary infusion of basic FGF in 337 patients with symptomatic, severe coronary artery disease
    - Trial completed in 1999 and results to be reported in early 2000
    - Trial is based on earlier phase I open label trial of basic FGF in 66 patients with severe symptomatic coronary artery disease demonstrating safety, maximum tolerated dose, and improvement in symptoms and exercise tolerance
    - Transmyocardial laser trials

  —Two randomized, non-blinded trials of transmyocardial laser revascularization in patients with refractory angina have reported improvement in symptoms and possible improvements in exercise tolerance.
  —The mechanism of benefit is unclear and may include formation of new myocardial blood channels, promotion of angiogenesis, and cardiac sympathetic denervation.
  —Results are controversial due to the possibility that a significant placebo effect may be present in patients undergoing surgical procedures.

Future Issues for Therapeutic Angiogenesis

- Proving efficacy versus the placebo effect
- Optimal route of delivery
- Duration of benefit
- Optimal method of angiogenesis: laser, protein or gene therapy
- Long-term safety concerns
  —Neovascularization of nontargeted tissues
  —Tumorigenesis
  —Potential acceleration of atherosclerosis

Bibliography

Engler DA. Use of vascular endothelial growth factor for therapeutic angiogenesis. *Circulation* 1996;94:1496–1498.

Ware JA, Simons M. Angiogenesis in ischemic heart disease. *Nature Med* 1997;3:158–164.

Henry TD, Rocha-Singh K, Isner JM, et al. Results of intracoronary recombinant human vascular endothelial growth factor (rhVEGF) administration trial. *J Am Coll Cardiol* 1998;31:65A.

Horrigan MC, MacIsaac AI, Nicolini FA, et al. Reduction in myocardial infarct size by basic fibroblast growth factor after temporary coronary occlusion in a canine model. *Circulation* 1996;94:1927–1933.

Charney R, Cohen M. The role of coronary collateral circulation in limiting myocardial ischemia and infarct size. *Am Heart J* 1993;126:937–945.

Losordo DW, Vale PR, Symes JF, et al. Gene therapy for myocardial angiogenesis. *Circulation* 1998;98:2800–2804.

Sellke FW, Laham RJ, Edelman ER, et al. Therapeutic angiogenesis with basic fibroblast growth factor: technique and early results. *Ann Thorac Surg* 1998;65:1540–1544.

Kornowski R, Hong MK, Leon MB. Current perspectives on direct myocardial revascularization. *Am J Cardiol* 1998;81:44E–48E.

Schofield PM, Sharples LD, Caine N, et al. Transmyocardial laser revascularization in patients with refractory angina: a randomised controlled trial. *Lancet* 1999;353:519–524.

Laham RJ, Simons M, Pearlman JD, et al. Biosense catheter direct laser myocardial revascularization improves 30 day angina class, regional wall motion, and perfusion of the treated zone using MRI. *J Am Coll Cardiol* 1998;31:333A.

Laham RJ, Hung D, Simons M. Therapeutic myocardial angiogenesis using percutaneous intrapericardial delivery. *Clin Cardiol* 1999;22:6–9.

Author: Harold L. Dauerman

Cytokines

BASICS

Description

Cytokines are locally acting polypeptide mediators, or autocoids, that act as autocrine (acting on the cell of origin), paracrine (acting on neighboring cells), or juxtacrine (acting on adjacent cells) agents. Beyond exerting a crucial role as mediators of inflammatory and immune responses, cytokines play an important role in the pathogenesis of atherosclerosis and in the cardiac dysfunction that accompanies systemic sepsis, viral myocarditis, cardiac allograft rejection, ischemic–reperfusion injury, and congestive heart failure syndromes.

Cytokines and the Heart

- Under different forms of stress (such as mechanical load, oxidative stress, ischemic–reperfusion, lipopolysaccharide exposure), the heart is able to produce different proinflammatory cytokines, namely tumor necrosis factor-alpha (TNF-α), interleukin-1 (IL-1), interleukin-6 (IL-6), and interferon-γ (IFN-γ), that may play an important role in initiating and integrating short-term homeostatic responses within the heart.
- However, when chronically elevated, these stress-activated cytokines have the potential to induce cardiac dysfunction and to modulate peripheral vascular resistance via nitric oxide–dependent and –independent mechanisms.
- Moreover, stress-activated cytokines have been involved in the induction of programmed cell death (apoptosis) of cardiomyocytes and of endothelial cells.
- However, antiinflammatory cytokines such as IL-10, IL-4, and IL-13, secreted by T-helper lymphocytes and other cells, inhibit the production of proinflammatory cytokines.

TNF-α Receptors

- The widespread biologic effects of TNF-α are modulated by two specific receptors: TNF-R1 and TNF-R2. Both receptors are present in equal proportions in normal myocardium, and have a similar affinity for TNF-α.
- However, the negative inotropic effects of TNF-α are mediated by its interaction with TNF-R1 and not with TNF-R2.
- Compared with the nonfailing myocardium, the expression of myocardial TNF-α receptors is decreased in the failing myocardium, whereas the circulating levels of the soluble forms of TNF-R1 and TNF-R2 (namely the soluble TNF-α receptors) are elevated in patients with moderate to severe heart failure.

Cytokines and Contractile Dysfunction

It has been shown that several inflammatory cytokines (particularly TNF-α and IL-1β) induce reversible contractile dysfunction *in vitro* and *in vivo*.

Cytokines and Heart Failure

- The role of stress-induced cytokines in heart failure relates to the observation that many of the untoward pathophysiologic responses of the failing circulation might be explained by these compounds.
- These small molecules appear to cause left ventricular dysfunction and cardiomyopathy, precipitate pulmonary edema, reduce peripheral organ perfusion, induce ventricular remodeling, activate the fetal gene program and the apoptotic process, modify the expression and function of the enzymes regulating nitric oxide production, and induce cachexia, resulting in further skeletal muscle dysfunction.
- Thus, the elaboration of cytokines, similar to the upregulation of neurohormones, may represent a biochemical mechanism that is responsible for producing symptoms in heart failure patients.

Cytokines and Cardiac Cachexia

• TNF-α levels are elevated in patients with chronic heart failure, particularly in patients with cardiac cachexia, a multifactorial neuroendocrine and immunologic disorder characterized by generalized body wasting.
• It has been shown that cardiac cachexia is predictive of poor survival independently of age, functional class, ejection fraction, and exercise capacity.
• In patients with advanced heart failure, the increased levels of TNF-α may be responsible for the induction of body wasting and cachexia.

CARDIAC FAILURE AND SEPSIS

• The possibility that the sera of patients and experimental animals with systemic sepsis (or other forms of systemic inflammatory response) contained a myocardial depressant factor was suggested more than 25 years ago.
• The systemic inflammatory response syndrome (SIRS) is characterized by hypotension, tachypnea, hypo- or hyperthermia, and leukocytosis, as well as other clinical signs and symptoms, including a depression in myocardial contractile function.
• SIRS is a major determinant of survival in patients with advanced viral or bacterial infection, or following severe trauma or burns complicated by multiple organ failure.
• Although the cause of cardiac contractile dysfunction in this syndrome is still largely unknown, cytokines may contribute to the pathogenesis of heart failure in this syndrome.

Cytokines and Ischemic Heart Disease

• Recent evidence has implicated proinflammatory mediators such as TNF-α in the pathophysiology of ischemia–reperfusion injury.
• Clinically, serum levels of TNF-α are increased after myocardial infarction and after cardiopulmonary bypass.
• Each of these represent clinically relevant instances of cardiac ischemia-reperfusion injury.
• Moreover, cytokines may induce cardiac depression and are important in regulating the reparative process, which is activated following myocardial ischemic damage.
• The intense inflammatory reaction following reperfusion of the infarcted myocardium has been implicated as a factor in extension of injury.

CURRENT PERSPECTIVES

• Clarifying the role and the regulation of cytokine production and cellular signaling is an area of active research.
• This may aid the development of drugs that reduce cytokine-mediated cardiac contractile depression, that modulate myocardial damage following ischemic-reperfusion injury, and that prevent progressive cardiomyocyte loss, particularly by inhibiting cytokine-induced apoptosis.
• More broadly, modulation of "stress-activated" cytokines may represent a new frontier in the management of heart failure

Author: Stefano Perlini and Gerard P. Aurigemma

Diastolic Ventricular Function

BASICS

Clinical Importance of Diastolic Dysfunction

Diastolic mechanisms contribute importantly to many, if not most, of the instances of heart failure seen in the United States in view of the following considerations:

- Hypertension is an underlying risk factor in most patients with congestive heart failure.
- The prevalence of hypertension increases substantially with age.
- Roughly one-third to one-half of patients hospitalized with congestive failure have normal systolic ejection fraction at the time of hospitalization or thereafter.
- The proportion of heart failure patients with normal ejection fraction parallels the age of the study population.

Physiology of Ventricular Diastole

Left ventricular (LV) diastolic filling occurs in two phases: passive filling followed by atrial systole. Normal diastolic filling may be characterized as the ability of the ventricle to fill optimally at normal pressures. This capability is influenced by both the active (energy-requiring) and passive (compliance) properties of the LV.

Underlying Mechanisms

- Filling occurs as the LV relaxes and pressure decays; this filling takes place during isovolumic relaxation (time between the aortic second sound and mitral valve opening) and during the early part of diastole, during which rapid filling takes place.
- The rapid pressure decay in the LV, in association with untwisting and elastic recoil of the LV, promotes a pressure gradient (diastolic suction).
- Because the ventricular myocardium is relaxed and distensible during diastole, pressures are low in what is effectively the common chamber, comprising the LV, left atrium, and pulmonary veins. Therefore, filling in the normal ventricle is associated with a low or normal pulmonary capillary wedge pressure.
- Atrial systole, an active process whereby blood is pumped into the LV, assumes greater importance as aging or myocardial disease render the LV myocardium less distensible (increasing stiffness, decreasing compliance).
- Major influences on the compliance of the LV myocardium include the extent of fibrosis (scar from prior infarction, unrelieved pressure and/or volume overload) and whether hypertrophy is present.
- LV and therefore left atrial, pulmonary vein, and pulmonary capillary pressures are also influenced by LV volume. Because even the normal LV does not have infinite compliance, a much larger than normal LV volume will result in abnormal elevation in LV diastolic pressures.

Left Ventricular Filling/ Clinical Assessment

- In the heart failure patient, bedside clinical assessment may not completely distinguish the heart failure patient with normal systolic function from the patient with systolic dysfunction. In both, individual signs of increased central venous and pulmonary venous volume may be present. Therefore, additional testing is necessary. Echocardiography is generally the test of choice in the assessment of the patient with heart failure and is the most common clinical test ordered to assess LV diastolic function.

Role of Echocardiography

- The presence of a normal ejection fraction greatly increases the likelihood that diastolic dysfunction contributes importantly to the heart failure syndrome.
- Doppler echocardiography is used in everyday practice to assess LV filling and to determine the mechanism of congestive heart failure.
- The Doppler inflow pattern consists of two velocity profiles:
  - —Early (E) wave, which corresponds to passive filling
  - —Late (A) wave which corresponds to atrial systole
  - —In normal subjects the ratio of early to late filling is ≥ 1, because the atrial contraction tends not to be particularly forceful.
  - —With advancing age, the ratio of peak E velocity to peak A velocity approaches 1 in normal individuals at around age 70.

Pathophysiology of Diastolic Dysfunction

- As implied by the above discussion, the two major pathophysiologic problems comprise abnormalities in relaxation and abnormalities in LV compliance.
- Some of the more common underlying abnormalities include:
  - —Myocardial hypertrophy (generally associated with long-standing hypertension)
  - —Interstitial fibrosis
  - —Ischemia contributes directly and indirectly to diastolic dysfunction, the latter acting by decreasing the ability of the myocardium to relax and compromising the normal decay in diastolic pressure. Ischemia also increases LV chamber stiffness and thereby alters the normal pressure volume relationship. Thus, in the ischemic LV, the ability of the heart to fill at normal pressure is compromised.
- Diastolic dysfunction generally comprises one or both pathophysiologic mechanisms:
  - —Abnormalities in myocardial relaxation are generally associated with a diminution in the E wave and a prolongation in the time from peak E to zero velocity (diastasis). There is often an accompanying increase in A velocity as the atrial contraction increases in force. This may correspond to the S4 on physical examination.
  - —Compliance abnormalities generally reflect more advanced disease, reflective of myocardial fibrosis. The Doppler pattern associated with compliance abnormalities includes a decrease in the time from peak E to diastasis (deceleration time <140 msec) and a diminution in the A velocity, reflecting increased atrial afterload. Thus, the E to A ratio may increase and approach that seen in normal, healthy adults. In this regard the deceleration time of the E wave will distinguish a pseudonormal E/A ratio from the LV with severe compliance abnormalities.

TREATMENT

General Measures

- Proper patient management is obviously predicated on making the proper diagnosis. An assessment of systolic function, presence of valvular heart disease, extent of hypertrophy, and LV filling is essential. Echocardiography generally provides these data noninvasively. Regional wall motion abnormalities present on the resting echocardiogram imply that coronary heart disease may be a contributing mechanism.
- Once the diagnosis is established, the following measures are in order:
  - —Manage presenting symptoms: these generally include hypertension and coronary artery disease.
  - —Maintenance of normal sinus rhythm and the avoidance of tachycardia have beneficial results.
  - —Reduce congested state: diuretics, salt restriction, angiotensin-inhibitors (or angiotensin II receptor blockers).
  - —Avoid tachycardia and promote bradycardia; this is usually accomplished with beta-blockers and rate-lowering calcium channel blockers.
- Treat ischemia.

Bibliography

Aurigemma GP, Gottdiener JS, Shemanski L, et al. Predictive value of systolic and diastolic function for incident congestive heart failure in the elderly: the Cardiovascular Health Study. *Circulation* 1998;98(suppl):224.

Bonow RO, Udelson JE. Left ventricular diastolic dysfunction as a cause of congestive heart failure. Mechanisms and management. *Ann Intern Med* 1992;117:502–508.

Gaasch WH. Diagnois and treatment of heart failure based on left ventricular diastolic function. *JAMA* 1994;271:1276–1282.

Levy D, Larson MG, Vasan RS, et al. The progression from hypertension to congestive heart failure. *JAMA* 1996;275:1557–1562.

Rakowski H, Appleton C, Chan KL, et al. Canadian consensus recommendations for the measurement and reporting of diastolic dysfunction by echocardiography: from the Investigators of Consensus on Diastolic Dysfunction by Echocardiography. *J Am Soc Echocardiogr* 1996;9: 736–760.

Vasan RS, Larson MG, Benjamin EJ, et al. Congestive heart failure in subjects with normal versus reduced left ventricular ejection fraction. *J Am Coll Cardiol* 1999;33:1948–1955.

Vasan RS, Levy D. The role of hypertension in the pathogenesis of heart failure. A clinical mechanistic overview. *Arch Intern Med* 1996;156:1789–1796.

Authors: Gerard P. Aurigemma and Helge U. Simon

Endothelin

BASICS

Description

Endothelin-1 is a 21-amino acid peptide released by endothelium, which acts locally (paracrine activity) to produce vasoconstriction.

- In fact, endothelin-1 is the most powerful vasoconstrictor yet discovered.
- Messenger RNA coding for endothelin-1 is induced by shear stress, ischemia, and hypoxia.
- Endothelin-1 has a plasma half-life of 4–7 minutes, and 80% is eliminated during its first passage through the lung.
- Plasma endothelin-1 levels may correlate with the severity of heart failure, may give prognostic information, and may be assayed.

DIAGNOSIS

Cardiovascular Pathology

Elevated endothelin levels appear to be an epiphenomenon of endothelial damage and are observed in the following disorders.

Heart Failure

- Endothelin 1 increases angiotensin I to angiotensin II conversion and aldosterone production.
- Angiotensin itself increases endothelin 1 production.
- Hypertrophy induced by angiotensin II can be prevented by blocking endothelin 1.
- Circulating endothelin 1 may contribute to dyspnea caused by direct bronchoconstriction mediated by endothelin receptors.
- Plasma concentration in heart failure is closely related to disease severity.

Ischemia

- Atherosclerosis is generally associated with endothelial dysfunction, both a reduction in nitric oxide and increased endothelin effects.
- Acute injury: in animal models, high endothelin levels are observed downstream from endothelial injury. Anti-endothelin antibody reduces myocardial injury by 40%–45%.
- Nitric oxide, prostacyclin, and arterial natriuretic peptide inhibit endothelin 1 production.
- Reperfusion injury appears to be related to endothelin release.
- Endothelin appears to play a role in restenosis: neointima formation after balloon angioplasty in rats may be linked to mitogenic properties of endothelin and prevented by blocking of the endothelin receptor.
- The mortality rate 1 year after myocardial infarction (MI) correlates with endothelin 1 levels on day 3 following MI.

Hypertension

- No apparent involvement of endothelin in essential hypertension but has been associated with hypertension in preeclampsia (high endothelin levels)

Pulmonary Hypertension

- High local endothelin 1 concentration are found in primary pulmonary hypertension and asthma.

TREATMENT

- Diagnostic uses appear limited:
  —Overlap in conditions associated with endothelin release and plasma levels may underestimate local ET levels and action.
  —Measurements of serum levels are technically difficult (cross-reactivity with precursor big endothelin and endothelin 2 and 3, adherence of the protein to glassware and plastic).

FOLLOW-UP

Expected Course and Prognosis

- Possible future role of endothelin antagonists in chronic heart failure with high neurohormonal activation, to prevent end-organ damage in hypertension and to prevent renal damage from toxic drugs.

MISCELLANEOUS

Bibliography

Benigni A, Remuzzi G. Endothelin antagonists. *Lancet* 1999;353:133–138.

Homcy CJ. Signaling hypertrophy: how many switches, how many wires. *Circulation* 1998;97:1890–1892.

Schrier RW, Abraham WT. Hormones and hemodynamics in heart failure. *N Engl J Med* 1999;341:577–585.

Authors: Helge U. Simon and Gerard P. Aurigemma

Heart Rate Variability

BASICS

Description

Heart rate variability (HRV) is variability of heart rate on a beat-to-beat basis due to dynamic interactions between ongoing perturbations to the cardiovascular system and the response of control mechanisms, which serve to regulate cardiovascular function.

The perturbations may be exogenous or endogenous (e.g., changes in posture, the mechanical effects of respiratory variation in intrathoracic pressure on the filling and emptying of cardiovascular structures, autoregulatory adjustments in local vascular resistance in different tissue beds that lead to fluctuations in total vascular resistance).

DIAGNOSIS

Signs and Symptoms

HRV can be used as a quantitative tool to investigate autonomic function:

- Independent factor of mortality after myocardial infarction (MI)
- Marked derangement of HRV in patients with severe CHF
- Decreased HRV a predictor of death in patients with congestive heart failure

Clinical Use

- One of the most promising quantitative markers of autonomic activity
- There is a significant relationship between the autonomic nervous system and cardiovascular mortality, including sudden cardiac death.

Special Tests

Time–Domain Techniques

- The most simple and straightforward technique involves the detection of each QRS complex in a continuous ECG recording and the determination of normal-to-normal (NN) intervals or the instantaneous heart rate. Ectopic or nonconducted beats are not included.
- Statistical methods: The simplest variable to calculate is the standard deviation of the NN intervals (SDNN), that is, the square root of variance.
- Geometric methods: The series of NN intervals also can be converted to a geometric pattern and a simple formula is used that judges the variability on the basis of the geometric and/or graphic properties of the resulting pattern.

Frequency–Domain Techniques

- The use of spectral analysis implies that the event series can be represented by a sum of sinusoidal components, of different amplitude, frequency, and phase values, using the Fast Fourier transform algorithm (FFT) or on an autoregressive (AR) methodology. The main spectrum calculated from short-term recordings of 2–5 minutes includes very low frequency (VLF), low-frequency (LF), and high-frequency (HF) components. The distribution of the power and the central frequency of LF and HF vary in relation to changes in autonomic modulations of heart period. When the spectrum is calculated from the entire 24-hour period, the result also includes an ultra low frequency (ULF) component.
- In most cases, the results of the frequency-domain analysis are equivalent to those of the time-domain analysis, which is easier to perform.

Physiologic Correlates of HRV

- The HRV reflects modulations of heart rate related to fluctuations in autonomic activity but not mean levels of autonomic tone.
- The efferent vagal activity is a major contributor to the HF component. The LF component is considered either as a marker of sympathetic modulation or as a parameter that includes both sympathetic and vagal influences.
- There is a circadian pattern, with higher values of LF in the daytime and of HF at night. An increased LF is observed during 90 degree tilt, standing, mental stress, and moderate exercise in healthy subjects, and during moderate hypotension, physical activity, and occlusion of a coronary artery or common carotid arteries in conscious dogs. Conversely, an increase in HF is induced by controlled respiration, cold stimulation of the face, and rotational stimuli.

Changes of HRV Related to Specific Pathologies and Clinical Use of HRV

Myocardial Infarction

- To date, the most practical clinical utility of HRV is its prognostic power after MI, which is independent of other factors established for risk stratification.
- For prediction of all-cause mortality, HRV is similar to that of left ventricular (LV) dysfunction. However, HRV is superior to LV dysfunction in predicting arrhythmic events (sudden cardiac death and ventricular tachycardia).
- The general consensus is that HRV should be assessed from 24-hour recordings approximately 1 week after index infarction. A high-risk group may be selected by the dichotomy limits of SDNN <50 msec or HRV triangular index <15.
- For clinically meaningful ranges of sensitivity, the predictive value of HRV alone is modest and should be combined with other factors.
- HRV is decreased early after acute MI and begins to recover within a few weeks; it is maximally but not fully recovered by 6–12 months after MI. HRV measured late (1 year) after acute MI also predicts further mortality.

Myocardial Dysfunction

Although there is poor correlation between HRV and asymptomatic LV dysfunction, reduced HRV has been observed consistently in patients with congestive heart failure. The circadian pattern also reveals an absence of the usual diurnal variation in day–night HRV.

Cardiac Transplantation

- A very reduced HRV with no definite spectral components was reported in patients with a recent heart transplant.

Diabetic Neuropathy

- A reduction in time–domain parameters of HRV seems not only to carry negative prognostic value but also to precede the clinical expression of diabetic neuropathy.

MEDICATIONS

Drug(s) of Choice

- Flecainide and propafenone but not amiodarone decrease time–domain measures of HRV in patients with chronic ventricular arrhythmia.
- Beta-blockade induces a significant increase in HRV parameters in heart failure.

MISCELLANEOUS

Conclusion

- Measurements of HRV offer a simple, noninvasive, and reliable approach to the clinical assessment of the cardiac autonomic modulation in healthy and diseased hearts.
- So far, the clinical utility of HRV resides mainly in the ability to risk-stratify post-MI patients with respect to outcome events.
- Yet, because of its relatively low predictive accuracy, HRV is a useful adjunct when used in conjunction with other measures.

Bibliography

Appel ML, Berger RD, Saul JP, et al. Beat to beat variability in cardiovascular variables: noise or music? *J Am Coll Cardiol* 1989;14: 1139–1148.

Kleiger RE, Miller JP, Bigger JT, et al. and the Multicenter Post-infarction Research Group. Decreased heart rate variability and its association with increased mortality after acute myocardial infarction. *Am J Cardiol* 1987;59: 256–262.

Nolan J, Batin PD, Andrews R, et al. and the United Kingdom Heart Failure Evaluation and Assessment of Risk Trial. Prospective study of heart rate variability and mortality in chronic heart failure. *Circulation* 1998;98:1510–1516.

Saul PJ, Arai Y, Berger RD, et al. Assessment of autonomic regulation in chronic congestive heart failure by heart rate spectral analysis. *Am J Cardiol* 1988;61:1292–1299.

Task force of the European Society of Cardiology and the North American Society of Pacing and Electrophysiology. Heart rate variability: standards of measurement, physiological interpretation and clinical use. *Circulation* 1996; 93:1043–1065.

Zuanetti G, Latini R, Neilson JMM, et al. and the Antiarrhythmic Drug evaluation Group (ADEG). Heart rate variability in patients with ventricular arrhythmias: effect of antiarrhythmic drugs. *J Am Coll Cardiol* 1991;17:604–612.

Authors: Theofanie Mela

Natriuretic Peptides

BASICS

Description

A variety of neurohormones, including the group of natriuretic peptides (ANP, BNP), help maintain fluid homeostasis in the healthy individual. These hormones oppose the actions of the renin–angiotensin–aldosterone system in response to short-term perturbations in fluid balance.

Atrial Natriuretic Peptide (ANP)

- 28-amino acid peptide hormone released from the atria into the circulation
- Main stimulus for release of ANP is atrial stretch.

ANP Effects

- Natriuresis: dilation of the afferent glomerular arteriole and constriction of the efferent arteriole, resulting in increased filtration pressure. Sodium reabsorption is inhibited in the collecting duct; both mechanisms cause increased natriuresis.
- Opposes angiotensin effects on aldosterone and renin release, vascular tone, vascular mitogenesis and renal sodium absorption, further promoting natriuresis; increases vascular permeability
- Antimitotic effect *in vitro*
- Central nervous system effects: decreased salt appetite, decreased thirst, decreased corticotropin release
- All of above effects result in lowered plasma volume and lowered blood pressure.

Brain Natriuretic Peptide (BNP)

- Discovered in brain homogenate
- Secreted in the ventricles, less in the atria
- Similar natriuretic and central effects compared with ANP
- Kidney: natriuresis nearly as strong as ANP

MISCELLANEOUS

Bibliography

Levin ER, Gardner DG, Samson WK. Natriuretic peptides. *N Engl J Med* 1998;339:321–328.

Schrier RW, Abraham WT. Hormones and hemodynamics in heart failure. *N Engl J Med* 1999;341:577–585.

Authors: Helge U. Simon and Gerard P. Aurigemma

Remodeling

PATHOPHYSIOLOGIC BASIS OF CARDIAC REMODELING

• The term *remodeling* is most commonly used in connection with a progressive change in shape of the left ventricle (LV) in response to alterations in load or ischemic damage. More recently, surgical procedures have been undertaken to favorably affect remodeling in patients with dilated cardiomyopathy.
• The LV has the remarkable ability to remodel in order to compensate for alterations in load. The physiologic principle underlying such remodeling is known as the law of Laplace, which dictates that the force borne per unit myocardium, or LV afterload (wall stress, σ), is directly proportional to pressure, directly proportional to ventricular size, and inversely proportional to wall thickness. Thus:

$$\sigma = P \times r/th$$

where σ is afterload (wall stress), P is systolic pressure, r is LV cavity radius, and th is wall thickness. Moreover, end-systolic stress is the force that limits systolic ejection. Accordingly, high wall stress will be associated with reduced systolic ejection performance, even in instances where the intrinsic contractile function of the LV is normal.

ASSESSMENT OF CARDIAC REMODELING

• Echocardiography provides a noninvasive method to assess cardiac remodeling in all forms of heart disease. Hearts can be characterized by whether hypertrophy is present and by the geometry or shape of the LV. Simple M-mode echocardiographic measurements of LV size and wall thickness in diastole are used to estimate the mass (weight) and to characterize LV shape.
• LV mass is estimated by an anatomically validated formula:

$$\text{LV mass} = 0.8\{1.04\,[(\text{STd} + \text{LVIDd} + \text{PWTd})]^3 - \text{LVIDd}^3]\} + 0.6\text{ g}$$

• LV mass, computed from this formula, should be indexed to some measure of body size, either height or body surface area. Hypertrophy is defined as an LV mass index exceeding the value represented by the mean plus two standard deviations of a normal population. Indexation to height will characterize some obese subjects as having hypertrophy, and some clinicians therefore prefer this method of indexation. It has been repeatedly demonstrated that left ventricular hypertrophy carries an ominous prognosis, even when controlling for age and cardiac risk factors.
• The LV can also be characterized by its ratio of wall thickness to cavity size; this measure, the relative wall thickness (RWT) provides an estimate of LV shape. When the RWT exceeds 0.45 (the value that represents mean plus two standard deviations of a normal population), concentric geometry is said to be present.

$$\text{RWT} = 2 \times \text{PWTd/LVIDd}$$

• Thus any population can be subcategorized as to whether hypertrophy is present or not and whether the geometry is concentric or eccentric (high LV mass index, normal RWT). The term *concentric remodeling* has been used to describe the subpopulation of individuals with normal LV mass index but concentric geometry. Some literature suggests that hypertensives with concentric remodeling have a worse prognosis than those with normal mass and geometry; other work suggests that these individuals have mild impairment of systolic function.

REMODELING IN VALVULAR HEART DISEASE

• Cardiac remodeling is an expected finding in chronic valvular heart disease.
—Aortic regurgitation: Ventricular volume is increased as a result of aortic valve incompetence; systolic pressure is increased due to increased forward stroke volume in the face of normal or diminished peripheral vascular resistance. Chronic severe aortic regurgitation is often associated with eccentric hypertrophy.
—Mitral regurgitation: Ventricular volume is increased as a result of chronic mitral valve incompetence, thus contributing, by the Laplace relationship, to increased afterload. By contrast, in acute severe mitral regurgitation, afterload is reduced. Systolic pressure is usually normal. This valvular lesion is generally associated with eccentric hypertrophy, with a lower RWT than seen in chronic aortic regurgitation.
—Aortic stenosis: The important hemodynamic impairment is severe pressure overload, occasioned by the marked increase in intracavitary systolic pressure. In the fully adapted LV, increased wall thickness permits normalization of afterload; LV cavity size is normal to slightly diminished. Severe aortic stenosis would be expected to be associated with concentric hypertrophy.
• Without compensatory ventricular remodeling, afterload "excess" in these three settings would be associated with a diminution in systolic function. However, in chronic valvular regurgitation, the ventricle remodels by series replication of sarcomeres to better bear the increased force associated with a larger circumference. These changes permit ejection of larger volumes of blood and maintenance of normal ejection fraction despite increased heart size and systolic pressure.

REMODELING IN HYPERTENSIVE DISEASE

• These same principles of cardiac remodeling also apply to patients with long-standing hypertension, although ventricular systolic pressures are not expected to be as high as those encountered in severe valvular aortic stenosis. Increases in wall thickness, which often accompany hypertension, normalize wall stress and can keep ejection fraction in the normal range. Ganau and co-workers analyzed a group of untreated middle-aged hypertensive patients and characterized these individuals into one of four categories:
—Normal (roughly 52% of the population)
—Eccentric hypertrophy (28%)
—Concentric hypertrophy (8%)
—Concentric remodeling (12%)

• A review of other studies in the literature suggests that the proportion of hypertensive patients with hypertrophy is roughly 20%, although the prevalence varies considerably depending on race, age, and the prevalence of obesity. Patients with concentric hypertrophy appear to have a worse prognosis than those with eccentric hypertrophy; those with concentric remodeling, in one study, fared less well than patients with normal mass index and geometry.

REMODELING IN ISCHEMIC HEART DISEASE

In many, if not the majority, of patients dying of acute myocardial infarction, pathologic evidence of infarct expansion is found. Following the initial infarction, LV remodeling may be observed. The process comprises myocyte necrosis and subsequent elongation of the infarct zone (infarct expansion). In time, due to altered load on the noninfarcted LV, dilation and dysfunction may ensue. Factors that predispose to infarct expansion and subsequent remodeling include size of the infarction, Q-wave infarction, anterior/apical location, and persistent infarct-related artery occlusion. The pioneering series of studies by Pfeffer and Pfeffer, culminating in the Survival and Ventricular Enlargement (SAVE) study, demonstrated that remodeling could be attenuated by use of angiotensin-converting enzyme inhibitors.

SURGICAL REMODELING OF THE LEFT VENTRICLE

The rationale underlying LV volume reduction surgery is the aforementioned Laplace relationship, which predicts a decrease in end-systolic stress (and an increase in systolic function) with reduction in cardiac size. Batista has reported favorable impact of such surgery (partial left ventriculectomy) on symptom status in patients with class IV patients with low ejection fractions (<20%). It stands to reason that mitral valve repair in patients with severe mitral regurgitation, to the extent that heart size is reduced by removal of the regurgitant leak, might achieve some of the same benefits.

Bibliography

Aurigemma GP, Gaasch WH, Villegas B, et al. Noninvasive evaluation of left ventricular volume, mass, and systolic function. *Curr Probl Cardiol* 1995;20:6:361–440.

Bach DS, Bolling SF. Improvement following correction of secondary mitral regurgitation in end stage cardiomyopathy with mitral annuloplasty. *Am J Cardiol* 1996;78:966–971.

Batista RJ, Santos JL, Takeshita N, et al. Partial left ventriculectomy on left ventricular function in end stage heart disease. *J Cardiol Surg* 1996;11:96–102.

Casale PN, Devereux RB, Milner M, et al. Valve of echocardiographic measurement of LV mass in predicting cardiovascular morbid events in hypertensive men. *Ann Intern Med* 1986; 105:173–178.

Devereux R, Reichek N. Echocardiographic determination of left ventricular mass in man. Anatomic validation of the method. *Circulation* 1977;55:613–618.

Ganau A, Devereux R, Roman M, et al. Patterns of LV hypertrophy and geometric remodeling in essential hypertension. *J Am Coll Cardiol* 1992;19:1550–1560.

Goldfine H, Aurigemma GP, Zile MR, et al. Left ventricular length-force-shortening relations before and after surgical correction of chronic mitral regurgitation. *J Am Coll Cardiol* 1998; 31:180–185.

Hutchins GM, Bulkley BH. Infarct expansion versus extension: two different complications of acute myocardial infarction. *Am J Cardiol* 1978;41:1127–1133.

Levy D, Garrison RJ, Savage D, et al. Prognostic implications of echocardiographically determined left ventricular mass in the Framingham heart study. *N Engl J Med* 1990;322:1561–1566.

McKay RG, Pfeffer MA, Pasternak RC, et al. Left ventricular remodeling after myocardial infarction: a corollary to infarct expansion. *Circulation* 1986;74:693–696.

Pfeffer JM, Pfeffer MA, Fletcher PJ, et al. Progressive ventricular remodeling in rat with myocardial infarction. *Am J Physiol* 1991;260: H1406.

Pfeffer MA, Braunwald E. Ventricular remodeling after myocardial infarction: experimental observations and clinical implications. *Circulation* 1990;81:1161–1170.

Pfeffer MA, Braunwald E, Moye LA, et al. Effect of captopril on mortality and morbidity in patients with left ventricular dysfunction after myocardial infarction: results of the survival and ventricular enlargement trial. *N Engl J Med* 1992;27:669–677.

Ross J Jr. Afterload mismatch in aortic and mitral valve disease. *J Am Coll Cardiol* 1985;5: 811–826.

Sadler D, Aurigemma GP, Williams DW, et al. Systolic function in hypertensive men with concentric remodeling. *Hypertension* 1997;30: 777–781.

Author: Gerard P. Aurigemma

Silent Myocardial Ischemia

Silent ischemia may be defined as the presence of objectively documented myocardial ischemia, occurring without associated angina or an angina equivalent. One of the first studies to establish the importance of silent myocardial ischemia was published by the Framingham Heart Study investigators, who demonstrated that roughly one-third of patients found to have a new myocardial infarction during routine ECG had no antecedent symptoms. Understandably, the incidence of myocardial silent ischemia not associated with myocardial infarction is likely to be much less. However, a precise incidence of silent ischemia in asymptomatic patients is not known. However, there have been some smaller studies that permit an estimate of the incidence of silent ischemia. Such studies have suggested that 25%–45% of patients with documented myocardial ischemia have evidence of myocardial ischemia during daily activities, most of these episodes asymptomatic. Interestingly, most episodes of silent ischemia occur with minimal or no physical exertion.

Possible mechanisms that might explain silent ischemia include the following:

- defective angina warning system
- presence of a higher pain threshold
- shorter duration of ischemic episodes

It is difficult to generalize about the mechanism of silent ischemia in an individual patient. Most have underlying atherosclerotic coronary artery disease but coronary artery vasospasm appears to also play a part in the pathogenesis. Whether decreases in coronary supply versus increases in coronary flow demand are the primary inciting stimulus for silent ischemia has not been completely established, and it is likely that the contribution varies from patient to patient. This is supported by the fact that both beta-adrenergic blockers (which primarily act by lowering heart rate and blood pressure but do not improve myocardial perfusion) and non-rate-lowering calcium channel blockers (which likely act primarily by improving myocardial perfusion) have both been shown to reduce the number of silent ischemia episodes.

Bibliography

Deedwania PC, Carbajal EV. Silent myocardial ischemia—a clinical perspective. *Arch Intern Med* 1991;151:2373.

Author: Gerard P. Aurigemma

Appendix Tables

Appendix Tables

Risk Stratification in Hypertensive Patients

BLOOD PRESSURE STAGES (mm Hg)	RISK GROUP A (NO RF; NO TOD AND/OR CCD)	RISK GROUP B (AT LEAST 1 RF, NOT DIABETES, NO TOD OR CCD)	RISK GROUP C (TOD/CCD AND/OR DIABETES)
High-normal 130–139/85–89	Life-style modification	Life-style modification	Drug therapy[a]
Stage 1 140–159/90–99	Life-style modification (up to 12 mo)	Life-style modification (up to 6 mo)	Drug therapy
Stage 2–3 >169/>100	Drug therapy	Drug therapy	Drug therapy

[a]In those with heart failure, renal insufficiency, or diabetes.

TOD, target organ damage; RF, risk factor.

Risk Stratification Scoring System for Patients Undergoing Coronary Bypass Surgery

PREOPERATIVE FACTORS	SCORE
Emergency surgery	6
Serum creatinine 1.6–1.8	1
≥1.9	4
Severe LV dysfunction (LVEF <35%)	3
Reoperation	3
Mitral regurgitation	3
Age 65–74 yr	1
≥75 yr	2
Prior vascular surgery	2
COPD	2
Anemia (Hct <35)	2
Aortic stenosis	1
Weight ≤65 kg	1
Diabetes not diet controlled	1
Cerebrovascular disease	1

LV, left ventricle; LVEF, left ventricular ejection fraction; COPD, chronic obstructive pulmonary disease; Hct, hematocrit.

Adapted from Higgins, et al. Stratification of morbidity and mortality outcome by preoperative risk factors in coronary artery bypass patients. *JAMA* 1992;267:2344–2348; with permission.

Intravenous Drugs for Cardiac Surgical Patients: Pharmacologic Therapy

DRUG	PEAK EFFECT	DURATION	DOSAGE	COMMENTS
Nitroprusside	Immediate	2–5 min	Initiate 0.1–0.25 μg/kg/min, titrate to max dose 8 μg/kg/min	May use during rewarming of hypothermic patient to maintain MAP 80–90; if CI <2.0 L/min, add inotropic drug
Nitroglycerin	Immediate	2–5 min	5–100 μg/min	Primarily venodilator, useful with high filling pressures, myocardial ischemia
Nicardipine	5–60 min	20–40 min	2.5 mg over 5 min; may repeat four times at 10-min intervals; infusion 2–7.5 mg/h	Potent systemic arterial, coronary vasodilator without coronary steal; no negative inotropy, effects on AV conduction
Hydralazine	15–20 min	3–4 h	5–10 mg bolus; may repeat every 15 min up to 40 mg total	Arterial vasodilator may produce reflex tachycardia
Esmolol	2–5 min	8–10 min	1 min loading infusion 0.25–0.5 mg/kg; sustained infusion 50–200 μg/kg/min	Cardioselective, short-acting i.v. beta-blocker, useful in normal CO, rapid sinus rate
Enaliprat	15–30 min	6 h or more	0.625–1.25 mg slowly over 5 min every 6 h	i.v. ACE inhibitor, useful in hemodynamically stable patient with normal or decreased CO
Diltiazem	3–30 min	3 h	20–25 mg bolus; may repeat in 10 min	Arterial vasodilator with mild negative inotropy, potent negative chronotropy
Verapamil	2–3 min	20–40 min	5–10 mg bolus; may repeat in 10 min	Less potent vasodilator with more potent negative inotropy, chronotropy
Labetalol	5–15 min	2–6 h	20 mg bolus over 2 min; then 40–80 mg boluses every 15 min, until effect achieved (to total 300 mg)	Vasodilator, alpha- and beta-blocker, predominent beta-blocking effect in i.v. form

MAP, mean arterial pressure; CI, cardiac index; CO, cardiac output; AV, atrioventricular; ACE, angiotensin-converting enzyme.

Adapted from Morris DC, St. Claire D Jr. Management of patients after cardiac surgery. *Curr Probl Cardiol* 1999;24:161–228; with permission.

Interpretation of Hemodynamic Patterns in Cardiac Patients

	DECREASED PRELOAD		CARDIOGENIC				
ETIOLOGY	HYPOVOLEMIA	VASODILATION	BRADYCARDIA	LV DYSFUNCTION	RV DYSFUNCTION	TAMPONADE	SEPSIS
Hemodynamics							
RA	<8	<8	≤10	≥10	>10	>15	<10
PCW	<15	<15	>15	>20	≤15	>15	<15
CI	<2.0	<2.0	<2.0	<2.0	<2.0	<2.0	≥2.0
SVR	>1,200	<1,000	>1,200	>1,000	>1,000	>1,000	<600
Other			HR <60		PCW >15 if LV failure present	RA=PCW=PAd	Narrow AVO_2 difference
Management	Fluids; transfuse if Hgb <10; inotropic drugs	Vasopressors	Cardiac pacing	Inotropic drugs; vasopressors; vasodilators; mechanical assistance	Supplemental O_2; pulmonary vasodilators; inotropic drugs; mechanical assistance	Reexploration; inotropic drugs; fluids	Fluids; antibiotics; vasopressors; inotropic drugs

LV, left ventricular; RV, right ventricular; RA, right atrial; PCW, pulmonary capillary wedge; CI, cardiac index; SVR, systemic vascular resistance; PAd, pulmonary artery diastolic pressure; AVO_2, arteriovenous oxygen; Hgb, hemoglobin.

Adapted from Antman E. Medical management of the patient undergoing cardiac surgery. In: Braunwald E, ed. *Heart disease: a textbook of cardiovascular medicine,* 5th ed. Philadelphia: WB Saunders, 1997:1726; with permission.

Intravenous Positive Inotropic Agents

MEDICATION	DOSAGE	COMMENTS
Dopamine	2–20 μg/kg/min	Low dose: dopaminergic effect Moderate dose: inotropic effect High dose: vasopressor effect
Dobutamine	2–20 μg/kg/min	Inotropic drug
Epinephrine	1–4 μg/min	Inotropic drug
Amrinone	10–15 μg/min	Inotropic drug
Isoproterenol	0.5–10 μg/min	Inotropic and chronotropic drug
Norepinephrine	2–12 μg/min	Vasopressor and inotropic drug
Phenylephrine	10–500 μg/min	Vasopressor

Adapted from Morris DC, St. Claire D Jr: Management of patients after cardiac surgery. *Curr Probl Cardiol* 1999;24:161–228; with permission.

Diagnosis of Myocardial Infarction in Patients Undergoing Coronary Bypass Surgery

NEW Q-WAVES ON ECG	CK-MB >30 IU/L	NEW RWMA ON ECHO	DIAGNOSIS OF MI	COMMENTS
Yes	Yes	Yes	Definite	
Yes	No	Yes	Definite	CK-MB missed with infrequent sampling
Yes	Yes	No	Probable	New zone of necrosis may not be evident on echo
No	Yes	Yes	Probable	NQMI
Yes	No	No	Possible	New Q's may be false positive
No	Yes	No	Unlikely	Small NQMI cannot be entirely excluded
No	No	Yes	Unlikely	Removal of pericardium may result in new RWMA, especially high anterior septum
No	No	No	No MI	

CK-MB, creatinine kinase–MB fraction; RWMA, regional wall motion abnormality; NQMI, non–Q-wave myocardial infarction; MI, myocardial infarction.

Adapted from Antman E. Medical management of the patient undergoing cardiac surgery. In: Braunwald E, ed. *Heart disease: a textbook of cardiovascular medicine,* 5th ed. Philadelphia: WB Saunders, 1997:1724; with permission.

Appendix Tables

Activity Recommendations in Patients with Congenital Aortic Stenosis

Mild (gradient ≤20 mm Hg)	Low static/moderate dynamic
No LVH, no symptoms	sports (baseball, tennis or volleyball), low dynamic/moderate
Moderate	static activities (diving or
Mild LVH, no symptoms	equestrian activities)
Moderate with symptoms or severe	No competitive, limited recreational sports
Full participation in recreational and competitive sports	

LVH, left ventricular hypertrophy.

Digitalis Drug Interactions

EFFECT ON DIGOXIN CONCENTRATION	*DRUG*	*MECHANISM*
Increase	Quinidine Propafenone Verapamil	Reduces tubular secretion, inhibits digoxin transport, and decreases volume of distribution
	Amiodarone Diltiazem	Decreases renal tubular secretion
	NSAIDs	Decreases renal clearance
	Spironolactone	Decreases renal clearance and can falsely elevate digoxin levels by interacting with certain laboratory tests
	Erthromycin Tetracycline Clarithromycin	Eliminates gut flora
	Atropine Propantheline	Increases absorption
Decrease	Activated charcoal Antacids Cholestyramine Colestipol Sucralfate Sulfasalazine Phenytoin	Decreases absorption secondary to binding of digoxin
	Cisapride Metoclopramide Probantheline	Decreases absorption secondary to increased intestinal motility
	Thyroxine	Increases volume of distribution and renal clearance
	Albuterol	Increases volume of distribution

NSAID, nonsteroidal antiinflammatory drug.

Classification of Severity of Pulmonary Stenosis

RV-PA GRADIENT	*SEVERITY*
<50 mm	Mild
50–79 mm	Moderate
80+ mm	Severe

RV-PA, right ventrical-pulmonary artery.

Drugs that Can Prolong the QT Interval

- Antiarrhythmic drugs
  - Quinidine (Quinidex extentabs, Quinaglute, Cardioquin, Duraquin)
  - Procainamide (Pronestyl, Procan, Procan SR, Procanbid)
  - Disopyramide (Norpace)
  - Sotalol (Betapace)
  - Amiodarone (Cordarone)
  - Ibutilide (Corvert)
  - Dofetilide
  - Flecainide (Tambocor)[a]
  - Mexiletine (Mexitil)[a]
  - Tocainide (Tonocard)[a]
- Calcium blockers for angina
  - Bepridil (Vascor)
  - Mibefradil (Posicor: withdrawn from market)
- Psychiatric drugs
  - Phenothiazines [prochlorperazine (Compazine), thioridazine (Mellaril), chlorpromazine (Thorazine), fluphenazine (Prolixin), trifluoperazine (Stelazine), perphenazine (Etrafon, Trilafon), etc.]
  - Tricyclics [amitriptyline (Elavil), imipramine (Tofranil), maprotiline (Ludiomil), nortriptyline (Pamelor), protriptyline (Vivactil), amoxapine (Asendin),[a] clomipramine (Anafranil),[a] doxepin (Sinequan),[a] etc.]
  - Haloperidol (Haldol)
  - Pimozide (ORAP)
  - Risperidone (Risperdal)
  - Thiothixene (Navane)
- Antibiotics
  - Azithromycin (Zithromax)
  - Chloraquine (Aralen)
  - Erythromycin (Akne-Mycin, E-Mycin, Ery-Tab, EryPeds, PCE Dispertab, and others)
  - Fluconazole (Diflucan)
  - Halofantrine (Halfan)
  - Itraconazole (Sporanox)
  - Ketoconazole (Nizoral)
  - Pentamadine (Pentacarinat, Pentam, NebuPent)
  - Trimethoprim-sulfa (Septra, Bactrim)
- Antihistamines (especially with antifungals, such as ketoconazole)
  - Terfenadine (Seldane)
  - Astemizole (Hismanal)
  - Clemastine (Tavist)[a]
  - Diphenylhydramine (Benadryl)[a]
- Antihyperlipidemics
  - Probucol (Lorelco)
- Toxins
  - Arsenic
  - Organophosphate insecticides
  - Liquid protein diets
- Anesthetics/antiasthmatics
  - Adrenaline/epinephrine
- Miscellaneous (and potentially risky)
  - Amantadine (Symmetrel)
  - Diuretics without potassium, and sometimes magnesium, supplementation, especially indapamide (Lozol)
  - Chloral hydrate
  - Cisapride (Propulsid) with ketoconazole, fluconazole, itraconazole, miconazole, erythromycin, troleandomycin, clarithromycin
  - Cocaine
  - Fludrocortisone (Florinef)
  - Ipecac
  - Tamoxifen (Nolvadex)
  - Terodiline (Mictrol, Micturin)

[a]Unconfirmed or rarely reported cases of torsades de pointes ventricular tachycardia.

Index

Page numbers in boldface indicate major discussion; page numbers in italics denote figures; those followed by "t" denote tables.

Index